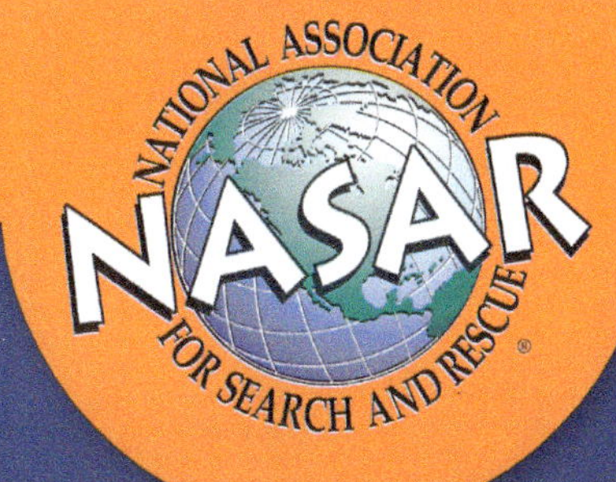

The National Association For Search And Rescue

FUNDAMENTALS OF

SEARCH AND RESCUE

SECOND EDITION

JONES & BARTLETT LEARNING

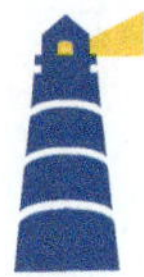

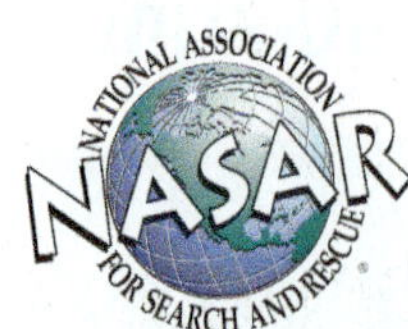

Jones & Bartlett Learning
World Headquarters
5 Wall Street
Burlington, MA 01803
978-443-5000
info@jblearning.com
www.psglearning.com

The National Association For Search And Rescue
P.O. Box 232020
Centreville, VA 20120-2020
703-222-6277
education@nasar.org
www.nasar.org

Jones & Bartlett Learning books and products are available through most bookstores and online booksellers. To contact the Jones & Bartlett Learning Public Safety Group directly, call 800-832-0034, fax 978-443-8000, or visit our website, www.psglearning.com.

Substantial discounts on bulk quantities of Jones & Bartlett Learning publications are available to corporations, professional associations, and other qualified organizations. For details and specific discount information, contact the special sales department at Jones & Bartlett Learning via the above contact information or send an email to specialsales@jblearning.com.

Production Credits
General Manager and Executive Publisher: Kimberly Brophy
VP, Product Development: Christine Emerton
Senior Acquisitions Editor: Tiffany Sliter
Senior Development Editor: Amanda Brandt
Editorial Assistant: Jessica Sturtevant
Editorial Assistant: Ashley Procum
Vendor Manager: Molly Hogue
Director of Marketing Operations: Brian Rooney
VP, Manufacturing and Inventory Control: Therese Connell
Composition and Project Management: S4Carlisle Publishing Services
Cover Design: Kristin E. Parker
Text Design: Scott Moden
Rights & Media Specialist: Robert Boder
Media Development Editor: Troy Liston
Cover Image (Title Page, Part Opener, Chapter Opener): © Courtesy of Michael St. John. Marin County Search and Rescue.
Printing and Binding: LSC Communications
Cover Printing: LSC Communications

Library of Congress Cataloging-in-Publication Data
Names: Cooper, Donald C., editor.
Title: Fundamentals of search and rescue / edited by Donald C. Cooper.
Description: Second edition. | Burlington, Massachusetts : Jones & Bartlett Learning, [2019] | Includes bibliographical references and index.
Identifiers: LCCN 2018012800 | ISBN 9781449642730 (paperback : alk. paper)
Subjects: LCSH: Search and rescue operations.
Classification: LCC TL553.8 .F86 2019 | DDC 363.34/81--dc23 LC record available at https://lccn.loc.gov/2018012800

6048

Printed in the United States of America
25 10 9 8 7

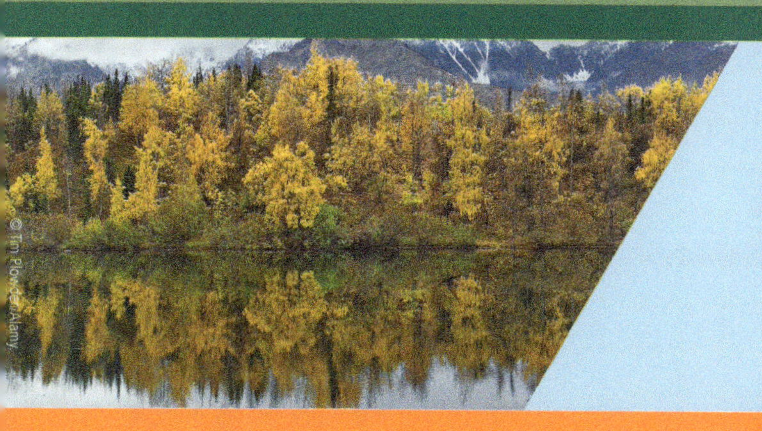

Brief Contents

Contents

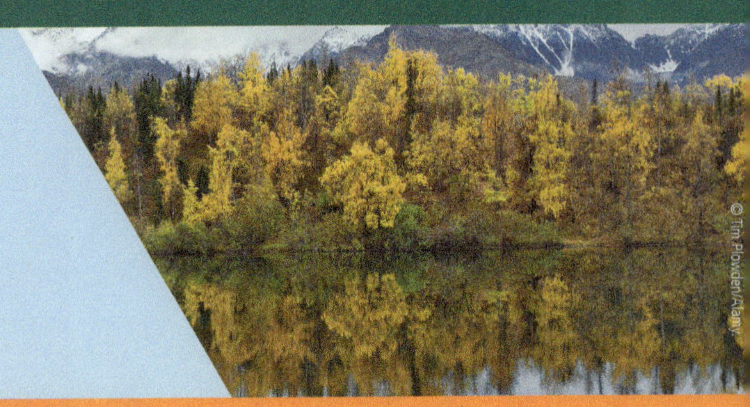

SECTION 3

Search and Rescue Operations

CHAPTER 14

Principles of Search and Related Issues 316

CHAPTER 15

Search Operations 343

CHAPTER 16

Rescue 376

APPENDICES

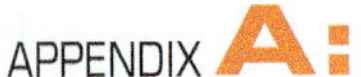

Some of the contents of Chapter 2 were published in *Wilderness Medicine*, Volume 1, D.C. Cooper, PhD and W.R. Smith MD, "Search and Rescue," pp. 687-710, Copyright Elsevier, 2017.

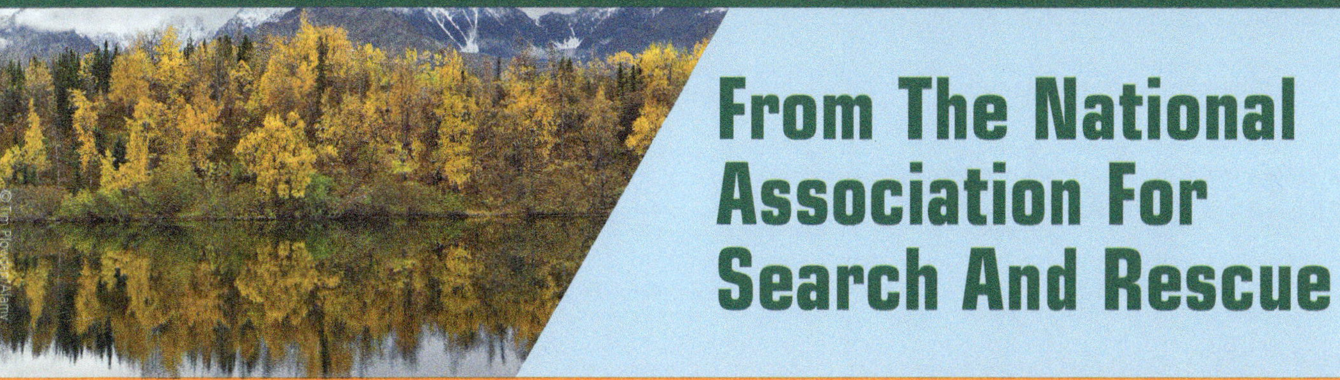

From The National Association For Search And Rescue

Dedication

This book is dedicated to those who commit their lives to the service of others and to those who love and support them.

President's Message

On behalf of The National Association For Search And Rescue (NASAR), I would like to thank all the contributors to the rewrite of the *Fundamentals of Search and Rescue* text. This text has been, and will continue to be, the core of our Search and Rescue (SAR) training program. It is instrumental in providing high-quality education and training to SAR professionals throughout the United States, Canada, and several other countries. I hope that this text assists you in building your career in SAR and serving others in their time of greatest need.

Mike Vorachek
President
The National Association For Search And Rescue

Executive Director's Message

Since 1973, The National Association For Search And Rescue (NASAR) has supported and honored the SAR community through the development of high-quality education and certification materials like this text.

Thank you for answering the call to assist others in need and for being stewards of your community.

Christopher Boyer
Executive Director/COO
The National Association For Search And Rescue

Acknowledgments

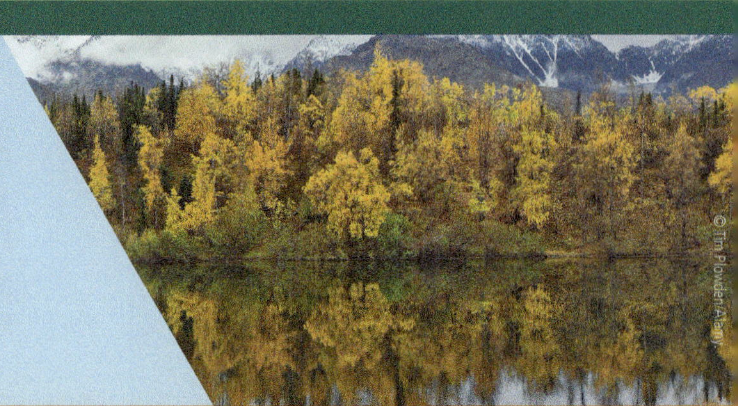
© Tim Plowden/Alamy

Jones & Bartlett Learning and The National Association For Search And Rescue (NASAR) would like to thank the contributors and reviewers of *Fundamentals of Search and Rescue, Second Edition.*

Editor

Donald C. Cooper

Contributors

Chris Boyer
Rob Brewer
David P. Calderone
Donald C. Cooper
Rob Davis
Paul Doherty
Jarod Doke
Bryan Enberg
Joe Flachman
Dallas Lane
Evan Schumann
Craig Spieker
Susan J. Thrasher
Jerry Whaley

Reviewers

Joseph Wayne Bunn
Elvin Burnell
Bryan A. Collett
Kent Courtney
Bryan Courtois
Mike Gorsuch
Shawn Haynes
Michael Hudson
David Johnsen
Jared Kimball
Jeremy Lawson
Antoinette Tharrett
Shannon Pawlowski
Joe Poulin
Ricky Roberts
Keith A. Sharisky
Mark Spangenberg
Neil Van Dyke
Josh Weiner

Contributors to the First Edition

Craig Bannerman
Donald C. Cooper
Frank Fire, Jr.
Steve Foster
John R. Frost
Mike Guzo
Patrick "Rick" LaValla
Jeff Lehman
Winnie Pennington
Timothy Provost
Robert "Skip" Stoffel
Susan J. Thrasher
Edward C. Wolff

The editor and contributors wish to thank the following individuals and groups for their gracious and enlightened review of, and assistance with, this resource:

American Meteorological Society
NASAR Education Committee
Cole Brown III
Roger Bryant
Jacki Golike
Carol Iverson
Georges Kleinbaum
Chris Long
Dave Maynard
Tom Millen
James Newberry
Donald Patch
Larry Pugh
Matthew Scharper
Jim Stumpf
Frank Wysocki

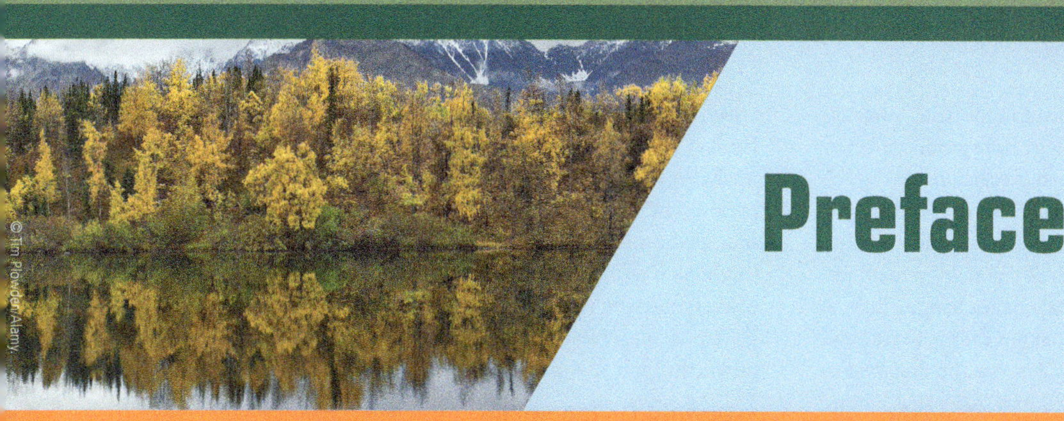

Preface

At the annual conference of The National Association For Search And Rescue (NASAR) in Reno, Nevada, in 1984, a special interest group meeting, chaired by Willis Larson, was held to discuss the potential development of a basic search and rescue (SAR) skills training program that could standardize such skills across the United States. Donald C. Cooper volunteered to coordinate the research and development of the program. Over the following year, research was conducted whereby many experts in the field of SAR were identified and asked to suggest what should be included in such a training program. Their input, combined with research from numerous other sources, was collected and collated to form the initial basis for the first version of this document and its related training program.

The following individuals were involved in the original research: Betty J. Burke, Stan Bush, Donald C. Cooper, Bob Deckwa, Gene Fear, Udo Fischer, John Gallagher, Rick Goodman, Hatch Graham, Paul Green, Dan Hawkins, John F. Hays, Bob Hill, Steve Hudson, Ernie Jesch, A.S.G. "Tony" Jones, Willis Larson, Patrick "Rick" LaValla, M.J. McCartor, Lois Clark McCoy, Greg McDonald, Michael R. McEwan, Mark Pennington, Bill Pierce, G. Wesley Reynolds, George Rice, Jim Segerstrom, Robert "Skip" Stoffel, Adam Ustik, Tom Vines, J.W. "Bill" Wade, and Jon Wartes.

In 1985, the first prototype basic SAR program (later named FUNSAR for Fundamental Search and Rescue Skills Program) was taught at Cuyahoga Community College in Parma, Ohio. Soon thereafter, Western Piedmont Community College in western North Carolina, in cooperation with Burke County Emergency Management, sponsored the second program to train SAR personnel using the prototype developed.

Many programs were taught over the subsequent few years across the United States. Modifications were made to the program, and revisions in the course content made this SAR skills program the most widely accepted standard available at the time. The following gracious individuals and members of the SAR community helped revise and improve the program that ultimately made this textbook possible: Duane Alire, Warren Bowman, MD, Roger Bryant, Burke County Emergency Management, Cuyahoga Valley National Park, Ralph DeCunzo, Charles Erwin, Vikki Fenton, Steve Foster, Lloyd Gallagher, Peter Goth, MD, Jeff Harbour, John F. Hays, J. Hunter Holloway, David H. Hoover, Peter Howells, E. Frank Kirk, Steve Larakis, Norman Lawson, Jr., John McComas, Randy McKinney, Al Musgrove, David Rodgers, Terry Shaeffer, J.W. Shiner, Albert "Ab" Taylor, William V. Vargas, Kirk Waggoner, Nick Waters, and Tim Woods.

NASAR was interested in publishing the materials collected for use in the program but did not have the resources to do it at the time. So, Rick LaValla and Skip Stoffel offered to use their corporate identity (ERI, Inc.) to publish the material as a book, and the first edition was published in 1989. In the first two years of its use, the following people made valuable contributions to the improvement of the contents: Paul Anderson, Michael Cooper, Roger Bryant, Peggy Fisher, Steve Foster, Dan Hawkins, Mark King, Bill Ramsey, MD, David Rodgers, John Stroup, Ab Taylor, and Tom Vines.

Since that early version of the book, certain individuals have offered support and help that far exceed the normal "call of duty." This support sometimes included editing, ideas, and suggestions for modifications. Most often, however, it involved moral support, simple kindness, logistical offerings, and a listening ear. To these individuals, special thanks are due on behalf of anyone who may ever benefit from the contents of this publication. It is individuals and groups such as these that truly make involvement in SAR satisfying: Paul Anderson, Burke County Emergency Management, Roger Bryant, Julie Cooper, Steve Foster, Dan Hawkins, Bob Hill, Peter Howells, A.S.G. "Tony" Jones, Logan County Public Rescue, Willis Larson, Norman Lawson, Jr., Sally Santeford, David Schrader, Rick Tate, Ab & Lillian Taylor, Bill Wade, Nick Waters, and West Virginia SAR Network.

In 2002, NASAR entered into an agreement with Jones and Bartlett Publishers and acquired the rights to the book that was previously published elsewhere. After hundreds of hours of work by dozens of individuals, the book evolved once again in 2005. The individuals and groups that participated in the research, development, and improvement of this material were numerous, and we thank you all for your help in expanding and evolving the material, and for conveying this information to those who need it. You are all the reason for our energy, enthusiasm, and continuing participation in this important field.

Much has happened in the years since the first edition. Technology has advanced significantly. We can now search with flying cameras that return images in real time, "see" through the Earth to search underground, navigate with magnificent accuracy, track searchers in the field in real time on a computer screen, receive extraordinary information from mobile phones carried by nearly everyone in society, acquire video and photographic images in almost any environment and situation, and communicate more clearly than ever before from almost anywhere in the world. Additional research in the field of search and rescue (SAR) has allowed us to confirm some of what we thought we knew, refute some long-standing notions, and identify new opportunities for improvements in the field. Advances in chemistry and manufacturing technology have produced better textiles, clothing, and rescue software than ever before.

Our systems and equipment have been tested in epic disasters, and we have learned a great deal from our successes and mistakes. However, with all the rapidly evolving SAR technology, methods, and research, some notable fundamentals have changed little, if at all. These are the very elements that remain central to safe and effective land-based search and rescue. We must be prepared to operate in the environment in which SAR may take place, and we must be able to survive should even the most significant challenges arise. We must be able to manage when technology fails and be familiar enough with an alternative method to continue to operate safely. We must be willing to work hard in difficult settings for long periods of time in the simple hope of assisting someone in distress. Indeed, the most important elements of SAR—the ones about which this book is written—have changed very little. It is the sincere hope of everyone who participated in the revision of this book that the generous, honorable, and noble people who feel drawn to serve others through SAR might somehow benefit from this work.

—Donald C. Cooper, Ed.

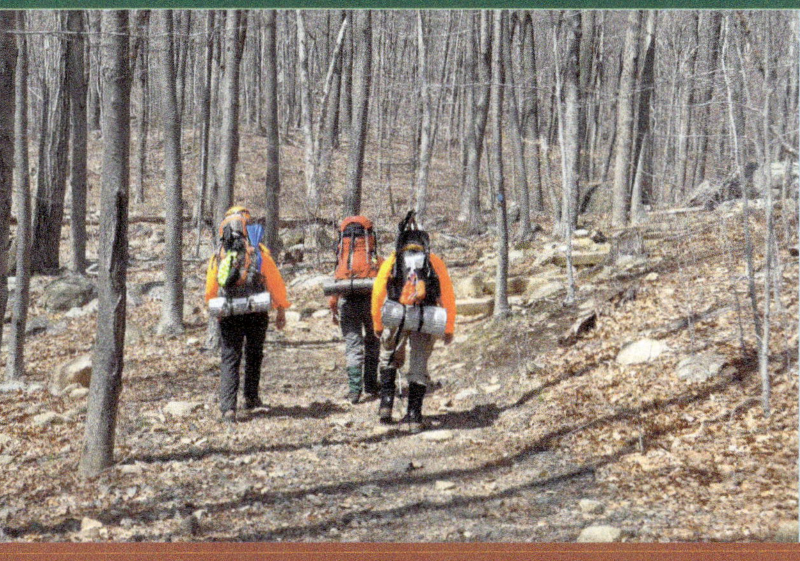

SECTION 1

Search and Rescue Overview

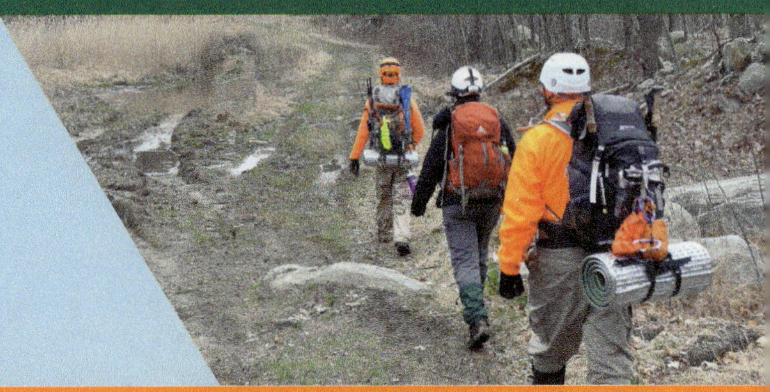

CHAPTER 1

Overview of Land Search and Rescue

OBJECTIVES

Upon completion of this chapter and the related course activities, the student will be able to meet the following objectives:

- Provide a contemporary definition of the terms *search* and *rescue*.
- List the three basic categories of search and rescue (SAR) skills training.
- Describe generally at least one course offering of the U.S. National Search and Rescue School.
- List at least two organizations involved in developing standards and one organization involved in developing regulations.
- Describe at least two significant characteristics of each of the following U.S.-based organizations that provide opportunities for individuals to become involved in SAR:
  - The National Association For Search And Rescue (NASAR)
  - Mountain Rescue Association (MRA)
  - Civil Air Patrol (CAP)
  - U.S. Coast Guard Auxiliary
  - USA Freedom Corps
  - Citizen Corps
  - Community Emergency Response Teams (CERT)
- Identify two international SAR organizations and describe their general role in search and rescue

A Brief History of Search and Rescue

One of the core human beliefs shared across many cultures is the desire to live a long, happy, and healthy life. Thus, applying education, equipment, and technology to help people delay death continues to be a significant goal for many contemporary societies. It is not surprising then that rescue—the act of saving another's life—has become an honorable, respected, and heroic vocation.

Searches and rescues have been carried out around the world for centuries, but it has only been recently that we have referred to these acts collectively as "search and rescue" or "SAR." Ever since humans began traveling into unknown terrain, they have encountered difficulties and required assistance. During these difficulties, others with the appropriate equipment, skills, and knowledge were often compelled, for one reason or another, to help. In the mountains, the locals, often very knowledgeable about the territory and well equipped to deal with it, were called upon to assist when the less skilled and equipped found themselves in distress. In the deserts, oceans, jungles, and other environments around the globe, the same incidents often happened: those who possessed the proper equipment, skills, and knowledge were frequently called upon to search for, and rescue, others in distress.

As technology improved, human populations became more reliant on it and less reliant on the skills that had previously allowed them to survive without technology. As populations expanded into previously isolated areas, the need to assist people in distress became increasingly necessary. In the early part of the 20th century, several countries found it necessary to develop a specific capability to find and recover wartime marine and aircraft crews. This interest, and wartime funding, began what many consider to be the birth of organized government-supported SAR. During this era, the considerable wartime resources of the U.S. government were brought to bear on the problems of finding such things as downed aircraft, missing vessels, unexploded ordnance, and enemy locations, and of rescuing, retrieving, or destroying that which was sought. This attention and funding, as well as improved technology in general, produced the basis for much of organized SAR as it is known today.

Contemporary SAR systems provide the response for overdue, lost, injured, or stranded people in many environments. One type of environment that is often associated with SAR is the wilderness. However, it is important to note that in SAR, wilderness can take on several meanings. For instance, most consider **wilderness** to be a region that is generally uninhabited and devoid of any synthetic (humanmade) amenities. While this certainly describes natural areas such as large parks and rural areas, it also describes many regions, even urban, that have been devastated by a disaster such as an earthquake or a hurricane. This also makes it easy to see why SAR is an extremely important part of nearly every disaster, fire service, law enforcement, emergency medical service (EMS), and military incident. Because most of the world's population resides in urban areas, and because disasters are common, emergency responders, including SAR personnel, are often just as likely to encounter an urban wilderness as they are a natural one (**FIGURE 1-1**).

Types of search and rescue incidents vary nationally and internationally, as do the responders. Programs, equipment, and personnel differ geographically in accordance with local needs and available resources. SAR often involves a great many volunteers and entails a multitude of skills. Consider the following examples of vastly different threats, hazards, and environments requiring widely diverse sets of SAR knowledge and skills:

- St. Tammany deputies search for a Mississippi hunter who was reported missing in the Pearl River Wildlife Management Area.
- Rescue workers search for eight people missing from the TransAsia Airways plane that crashed into a river in Taiwan.
- A young boy with autism disappears on the way home from school and is found playing in a local park by searchers.
- Either straight line winds or a tornado causes multiple occupied buildings to collapse in Central Oklahoma.
- Mount St. Helens in Washington State erupts in 1980.
- Terrorists attack the World Trade Centers and the Pentagon in 2001.
- Multiple Atlantic hurricanes strike the southeastern United States in 2005 (Wilma, Katrina, and Rita) and 2017 (Harvey and Irma) and devastate the Caribbean (Maria).
- A 75-year-old woman with dementia walks away from her care facility and is found, with medical issues, in a local creek bed.
- A girl is kidnapped at age 11 and is found alive years later, living with her abductors in California.
- Two climbers in Yosemite are trapped mid-climb by unexpected winter weather and are rescued by YOSAR.

Management of these SAR operations can range from directing the actions of a few responders in a small community to managing an effort involving thousands of responders in a large regional disaster. Often, large situations involve several geopolitical subdivisions (e.g., cities, counties, states, provinces, countries) and coordination of air, ground, and/or marine resources. Local governments and other agencies that participate in SAR must coordinate diverse, all-hazard responders. Many organizations that collectively support multiagency SAR responses operate under their own specific statutory authority according to relevant law and SAR doctrine.

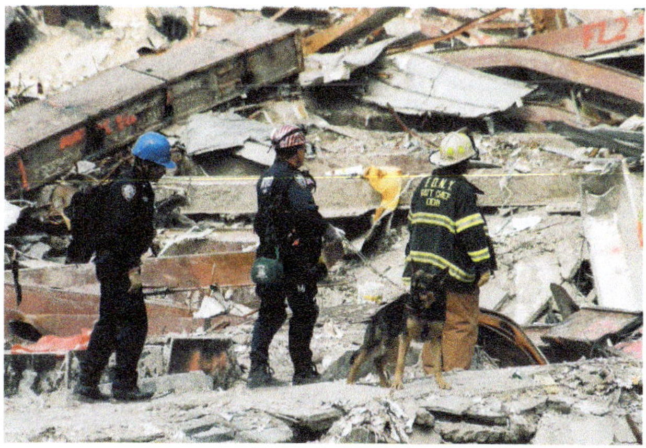

FIGURE 1-1 Wilderness SAR personnel are often just as likely to encounter an urban wilderness as they are a natural one.
Courtesy of Bri Rodriguez/FEMA.

SEARCH AND RESCUE TIP

Wilderness is an uninhabited region devoid of any synthetic amenities.

Time is almost always a factor in SAR operations, which tends to focus efforts on a quick conclusion. The general idea is to find or rescue the missing, lost, or injured subject so that suffering is minimized and before he or she succumbs to the effects of the environment, injuries, or a specific hazard.

Because search and rescue programs, equipment, and personnel vary widely around the world, SAR has many definitions and meanings. The first explicit definition of the term *search and rescue* in the context we use today was likely contained in the proceedings of the Provisional International Civil Aviation Organization (PICAO), circa 1946. In an article in the 1946 *Air Sea Rescue Bulletin* entitled, "Evolution of SAR: An Editorial," the (unknown) author noted that PICAO adopted the term *search and rescue* and recommended that it be defined as, "The act of finding and returning to safety the survivors from an emergency incident." Setnicka (1980) defined SAR as, "...any operation aimed at helping someone in trouble, someone who cannot solve his or her problem alone...." The same author uttered the classic line that SAR was essentially, "a *transportation* problem—of rescuers to the victim and the victim to safety." More contemporary references, such as *The International Aeronautical and Maritime Search and Rescue* (IAMSAR) *Manual* (2016), have found it useful to define "search" and "rescue" separately: **search** is an operation using available personnel and facilities to locate persons in distress, and **rescue** is an operation to retrieve persons in distress, provide for their initial medical or other needs, and deliver them to a place of safety.

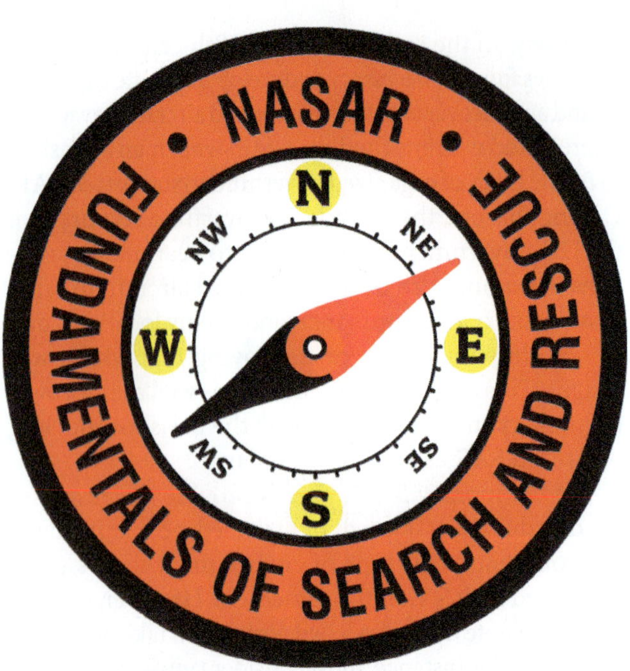

FIGURE 1-2 Fundamental search and rescue skills are a diverse collection of topics that cover many areas.
Courtesy of NASAR.

Foundational Concepts in SAR

Beyond what is taught in NASAR's "Introduction to SAR" course, three concepts are important to grasp before discussing how one gets involved in search and rescue: the SAR training categories, the SAR "tool" acquisition process, and SAR standards and regulations.

SAR Training Categories

Fundamental search and rescue skills are a diverse collection of topics that cover many areas (**FIGURE 1-2**). For the discussion in this text, these skills have been divided into three basic categories for organizational purposes. Those categories are:

- Search
- Rescue
- Survival/support

All the skills and knowledge contained in this text can be grouped into one or more of these categories:

- Search training continues one's education in searching only.
  - Specialties include land search, water search, air search, the application of search theory, search planning, and search dogs—and can be quite technical.
- Rescue training includes diverse specialties that differ in terrain and equipment.
  - Specialties are based in the environments in which they are required, including mountain, wilderness, ice, water, and urban rescue, as well as many others.
  - Equipment differs greatly among rescue types and can be quite complex.
- Survival/support training is an area of study that includes many skills that are also included in search and rescue but are skills that may be required independent of both.
  - Such skills include wilderness survival, signaling, navigation, improvisation, fitness, and communication (**FIGURE 1-3**).

U.S. National Search and Rescue School

The U.S. National Search and Rescue School is operated jointly by the U.S. Air Force (USAF) and the U.S. Coast

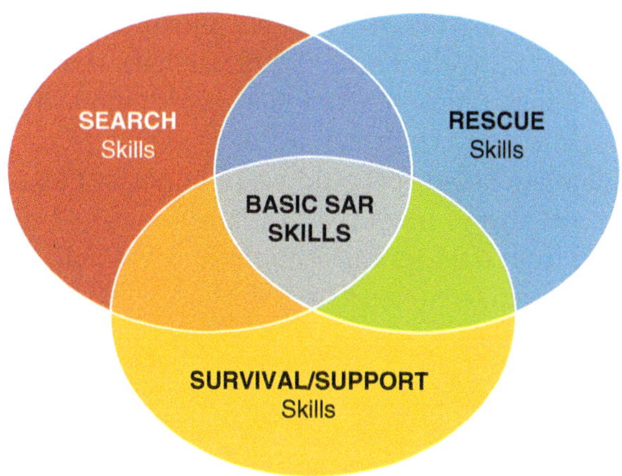

FIGURE 1-3 Basic SAR skills (the fundamentals) are an intersection of search, rescue, and survival/support skills.

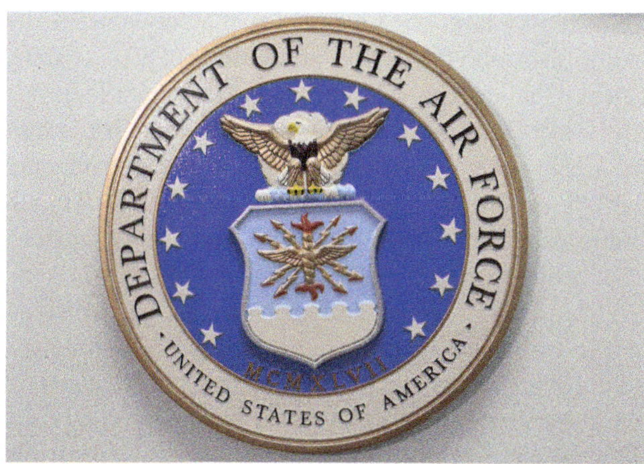

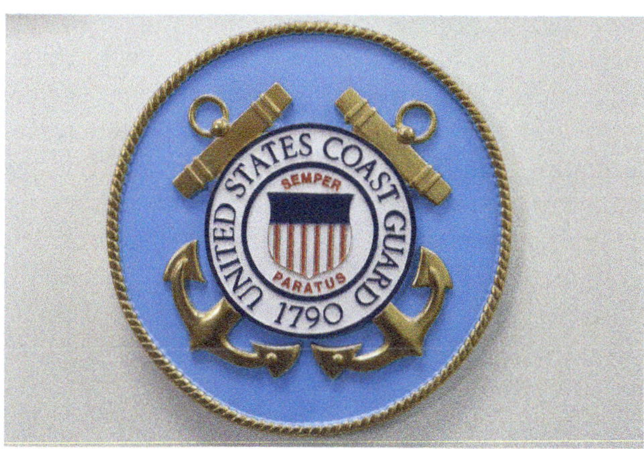

FIGURE 1-4 The U.S. National Search and Rescue School is operated jointly by the U.S. Air Force (USAF) and the U.S. Coast Guard (USCG) at the U.S. Coast Guard Training Center in Yorktown, Virginia.

Guard (USCG) at the U.S. Coast Guard Training Center in Yorktown, Virginia (**FIGURE 1-4**). Each service offers instruction from its own expertise. The school's mission is to provide standardization and professionalism within the SAR community. The joint USCG/USAF teaching staff provides training in oceanic, coastal, and inland search planning procedures to SAR professionals from all U.S. military branches, various U.S. government agencies, volunteer SAR organizations, as well as members of the international SAR community. The inland search and rescue element of the school offers two courses: the Inland SAR Planning Course (ISPC) and the Basic Inland SAR Course (BISC).

The five-day Inland SAR Planning Course is advertised as a graduate-level course designed to teach advanced search and rescue theory and its application to land and air searches for missing persons and aircraft. The focus in this course is on wilderness, not urban, searches. The course consists of classroom lessons and practical, tabletop exercises and does not include field training. Emphasis is on the planning necessary for effective area-type searching during an extended search, and the course does not teach search tactics or technical procedures. The course is directed toward federal, state, and local SAR leaders in emergency services and law enforcement, as well as Civil Air Patrol (CAP) and international and volunteer SAR organizations. The course is meant for those few individuals who are responsible for the planning and overall conduct of inland search missions. The general searcher or search team leader, while arguably the most important part of the SAR team, would likely not find this course useful. Classes are held at various locations around the United States approximately 10 to 12 times per year.

The two-day Basic Inland SAR Course is designed to teach basic federal SAR architecture, resources, and mission coordination with an introduction to search theory. The course is designed as an entry-level SAR management course for federal, state, and local responders (U.S. Coast Guard, 2018b).

Tools for SAR

Search and rescue is an extremely diverse field that involves both art and science. Determining what will and what will not work is often based on the educated opinions of those involved, and these opinions may vary greatly. What works in one situation may not work in others. Because of this, SAR is difficult to learn based on one source or the teachings of one instructor. It is important in SAR, therefore, to gain knowledge from many sources, tempering everything with practicality and experience.

SAR education is a "tool" acquisition process. Specific knowledge and skills are tools to the rescuer, as hammer and nails are to the carpenter. A specific skill (tool) may be used, but situations will occasionally require tools beyond the contents of one's existing tool chest. In SAR, the tools are collected from appropriate sources—through formal education and experience—and then used where necessary to meet an objective. Some tools work better than others in certain situations, but all may be of value at one time or another (**FIGURE 1-5**).

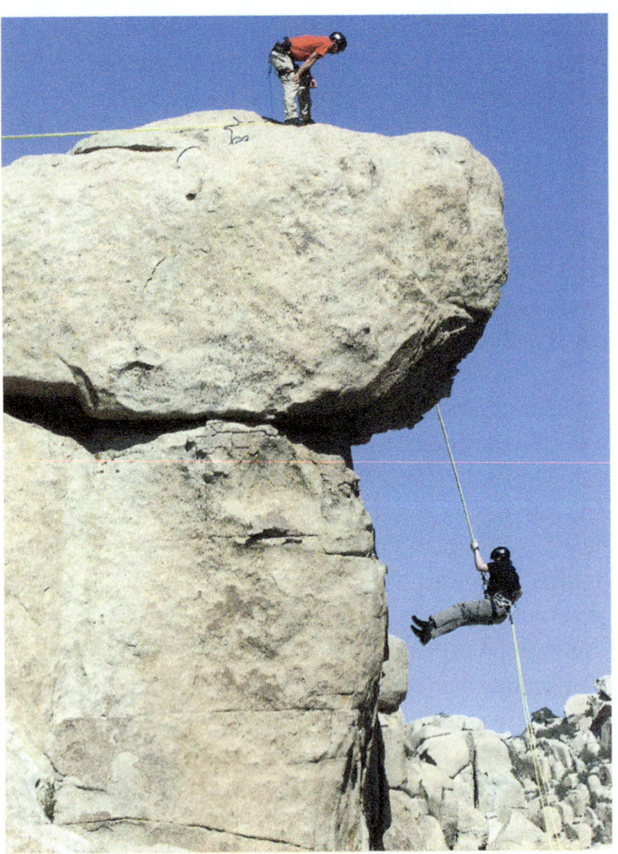

FIGURE 1-5 SAR education is a "tool" acquisition process.
Courtesy of Gerald Nino/U.S. Customs & Border Protection.

Every student or practitioner of SAR should acquire as many "tools" as possible. The more tools you have, the better the chances that you will have what it takes to perform safely and effectively. Specialization may be necessary, but not to the exclusion of a broad base of knowledge and skill. As in most pursuits, a single tool should not be expected to work perfectly for every job. Users vary, and so do the ways in which the tools can be applied to attain a goal; what works for one may not work for another. These tools may eventually serve as the only foundation on which to build a system that is expected to save a life. As such, they must be well chosen and skillfully applied.

Avoid anyone who claims to teach the only truth in SAR. Few things are more dangerous in SAR than an individual who lacks an open mind and thinks that he or she possesses knowledge of the only true way. There are as many ways to perform any search or rescue operation as there are opinions on which is best. Every search and/or rescue operation can be improved. Learning how such improvements can be made is the key to advancing beyond basic tool application.

Standards and Regulations

Standards and regulations relevant to various search and rescue disciplines have evolved significantly over the past few years. They generally fall into three categories: training (individual and organizational), operations (individual and organizational), and manufacturers (equipment and clothing).

Standards and regulations are important because they are always intended to improve safety, usually evolve from tragic events, and may involve penalties if not followed (some may have the force of law).

Regulations (i.e., rules or codes) are compulsory and usually written by government agencies with specific responsibilities for the subject matter. Failure to comply with or adhere to regulations could result in fines or other penalties. A regulation sometimes references a standard, which has the effect of incorporating the standard into the regulation. However, a standard is generally not compulsory unless it is referenced in a regulation or otherwise required by law. The Occupational Safety and Health Administration (OSHA) is an example of a U.S. federal agency that develops and promulgates regulations, and the Ohio Division of State Fire Marshal is an example of a U.S. state agency that develops and promulgates regulations, which are also referred to as "rules" or "administrative law." All U.S. states have multiple agencies that promulgate rules and regulations.

Standards are typically written by committees, often comprising volunteers, working under the aegis of a standard writing organization. "Consensus standards" are distributed to, and then agreed upon, by groups of interested parties prior to publication. The specific process varies among standard writing organizations but is usually well described in their educational literature and on their websites. Each of the standard writing organizations has procedures for initiating standards, fairly developing and revising standards, allowing for public comments, addressing public comments, and publishing the standards. The National Fire Protection Association (NFPA), ASTM International, and the American Society of Safety Engineers (ASSE) are examples of standard writing organizations.

The American National Standards Institute (ANSI) is a nonprofit organization with a mission to enhance the global competitiveness of U.S. businesses by ". . .promoting and facilitating voluntary consensus standards and conformity assessment systems. . ." (ANSI, 2018, para 3). ANSI oversees creation, promulgation, and use of standards and accredits other organizations that develop consensus standards, such as the NFPA and ASTM International.

The European Committee for Standardization (CEN; i.e., Comité Européen de Normalisation) is a nonprofit standards organization that provides, ". . .a platform for the development of European Standards and other technical documents in relation to various kinds of

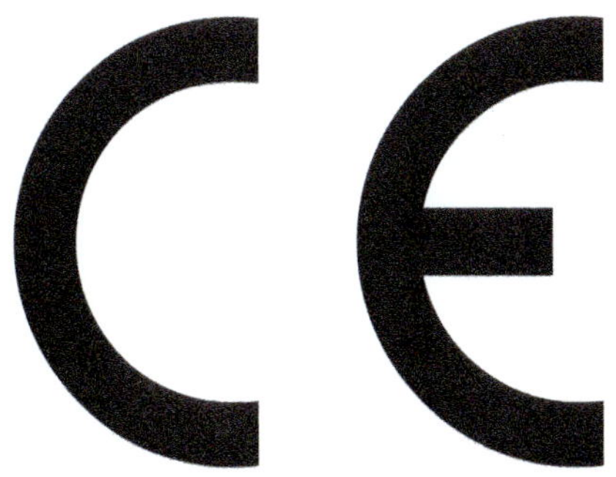

FIGURE 1-6 The familiar CE marking of the European Committee for Standardization (CEN).

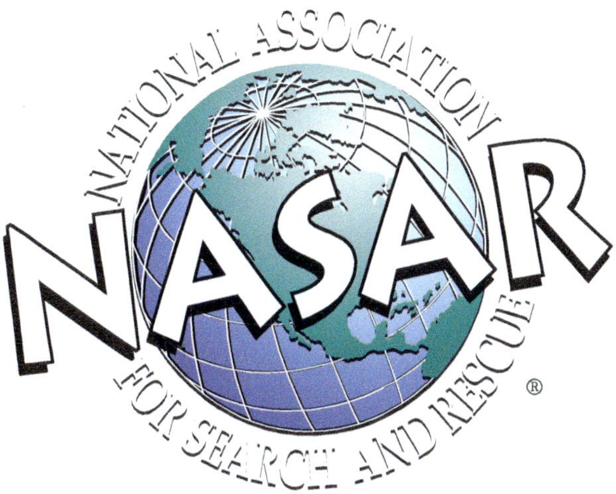

FIGURE 1-7 Seal of The National Association For Search And Rescue (NASAR).

products, materials, services and processes" (European Committee for Standardization [CEN], 2018, para 3). CEN writes standards for a wide variety of fields, including health and safety and personal protective equipment, which can affect the search and rescue field. These standards may also be relevant to SAR personnel because European recreational climbing equipment may bear the familiar CE marking (**FIGURE 1-6**). The CEN collaborates with the International Climbing and Mountaineering Federation (UIAA; i.e., Union Internationale des Associations d'Alpinisme) to harmonize each organization's standards, but the two standards may still be slightly different.

Getting Involved in SAR

There are several organizations through which individuals can get involved in search and rescue in the United States, including NASAR; the MRA; CAP; the U.S. Coast Guard Auxiliary; the USA Freedom Corps; Community Emergency Response Teams (CERT); and other national, state, provincial, and local agencies and organizations.

The National Association For Search And Rescue

Formed in the early 1970s, NASAR is a not-for-profit membership organization of primarily volunteer SAR response professionals (**FIGURE 1-7**). NASAR is the only U.S. national-level SAR education and certification body that focuses on individual SAR responders and local SAR teams. NASAR also acts as an umbrella advocacy organization where people of all SAR specialties can meet, network, and coordinate their wide-ranging skills to establish maximum effectiveness in emergency situations. Since 1972, NASAR has provided its members with educational and certification opportunities; timely publications; and a variety of conferences, workshops, and symposia. NASAR offers formal training opportunities that have grown to include topics ranging from the most rudimentary SAR skills through sophisticated incident management and specialty skills.

In 1991, NASAR developed some of the first national certification criteria for search and rescue personnel. These criteria are referred to as SARTECH III, SARTECH II, and SARTECH I/Crewleader III, and they were developed to evaluate three levels of search responder so that a measurable level of individual and crew capability could be available for incident commanders. The criteria have also been adopted by several states in the United States and by many SAR teams nationwide; the development and acceptance of these criteria continue to grow. NASAR also participates in international standards-making processes such as those of the NFPA and ASTM International. NASAR maintains a specialty bookstore that contains authoritative and often difficult-to-find texts and has established an extensive website.

As an umbrella organization, NASAR has close ties to the widest variety of SAR-related organizations, including all types of public safety agencies. Among the active partner organizations are the MRA, CAP, search dog organizations, numerous local volunteer SAR units, dive rescue units, cave rescue groups, and other related organizations. In the United States, NASAR maintains a close relationship with the National Sheriff's Association (NSA), the Department of Homeland Security (DHS), the Federal Emergency Management Agency (FEMA), the U.S. Air Force Rescue Coordination Center (AFRCC), the National Park Service, the National Forest Service, the U.S. Agency for International Development/Office of Foreign Disaster Assistance (USAID/OFDA), and the U.S. Coast Guard (USCG). NASAR also participates on the National SAR Committee (NSARC). Internationally, NASAR enjoys a close relationship with the Canadian SAR Secretariat and the Royal Canadian Mounted Police (RCMP) and has a growing member presence in countries all over the world (The National Association For Search And Rescue, 2015).

Mountain Rescue Association

In 1927, the MRA started as a group of highly experienced mountaineers that joined forces to conduct mountain rescue services on Mt. Hood, Oregon. While volunteers in terms of pay, they were proficient and professional in their skills. In 1958, the first meeting of the MRA took place at Mt. Hood. Soon thereafter, several national parks, Air Force units, and others joined the MRA, as did teams from Oregon, California, and Colorado. Other states and units from Canada soon followed (MRA, 2018).

In the 1960s, the MRA started to produce rescue training materials, and in 1972, Bill May, and later the Rocky Mountain Rescue Group—an MRA member team—published what was perhaps the first complete text on rescue methods in the United States: *Mountain Search and Rescue Techniques.*

Today, the MRA is a national nonprofit membership association dedicated to saving lives through rescue and mountain safety education. About 100 teams, mostly from the United States, are in the association, which comprises nearly 2,500 individual, professional rescue volunteers. MRA teams perform approximately 5,000 search and rescue operations in the United States each year. The organization holds high standards for maintaining team membership and sponsors highly regarded public education programs, team training, and training publications. The MRA also sponsors numerous programs taught by MRA members and holds renowned semi-annual conferences, one of which (SARCON) is presented in conjunction with NASAR and the Colorado Search and Rescue Board. The MRA also presents the International Technical Rescue Symposium (ITRS), a leading forum for the exchange of state-of-the-art technical rescue research, techniques, and information (Mountain Rescue Association, 2018).

Civil Air Patrol

In 1948, CAP was permanently chartered by the U.S. Congress as the official auxiliary of the U.S. Air Force (**FIGURE 1-8**). This nonprofit organization of volunteers was charged with three primary missions: development of aviation through aerospace education, a cadet youth program, and emergency services. CAP boasts more than 60,000 members, including thousands of cadets between the ages of 12 and 21 years; the world's largest fleet of single-engine, piston aircraft; and access to 1000 emergency service vehicles. It is proud of the fact that nearly 100 lives are saved each year by CAP members.

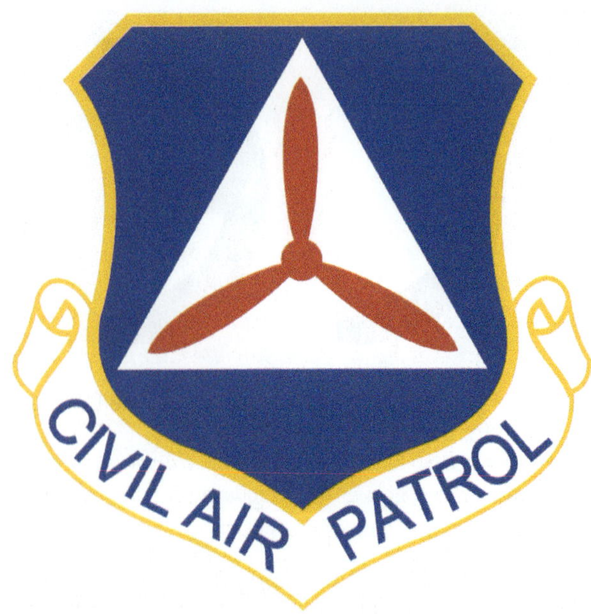

FIGURE 1-8 The seal of the Civil Air Patrol.

Under their emergency services mission, CAP provides SAR mission coordinators, search aircraft, ground teams, personnel on alert status, and an extensive communications network to support emergency response efforts. CAP members provide services to national relief organizations during disasters; transportation of time-sensitive medical materials; and aerial reconnaissance, airborne communications support, and airlift of law enforcement personnel in the national counter-drug effort. When CAP resources are engaged in a SAR mission, they are reimbursed by the U.S. Air Force for communications expenses, fuel and oil, and a share of aircraft maintenance expenses. In addition, CAP members are covered by the Federal Workers' Compensation Act in the event of injury while participating in a SAR mission.

CAP is the AFRCC's prime air resource for the inland area. The AFRCC maintains an alert roster provided by CAP wings in each of the 48 contiguous states and is the central point of contact for CAP participation in SAR missions. The AFRCC also works closely with CAP national headquarters and directly provides input for CAP training in emergency services (Civil Air Patrol, 2018).

U.S. Coast Guard Auxiliary

The USCG Auxiliary is to the USCG what CAP is to the U.S. Air Force (**FIGURE 1-9**). The auxiliary comprises citizens who volunteer time and boats or aircraft to enhance and maintain the safety of boaters. This work is based on the auxiliary's four cornerstones: vessel examination, education, operations, and fellowship. Following passage of the Coast Guard Authorization Act of 1996, the auxiliary assists the Coast Guard, as authorized by the commandant, in performance of any Coast Guard function, duty, role, mission, or operation authorized by law. Today, auxiliarists are civilian volunteers whose activities are directed by policies established by the commandant of the USCG. Although under the authority of the commandant, the auxiliary is internally autonomous, operating on four organizational levels (smallest to largest): flotilla, division, district regions, and national.

When auxiliary resources are engaged under USCG "orders," they are reimbursed by the USCG for communications expenses, fuel and oil, and a share of vessel and aircraft maintenance expenses. In addition, auxiliary members are covered by the federal Workers' Compensation Act in the event of an injury while participating in an authorized mission.

Many members of the auxiliary spend their weekends providing free boating safety courses to the public and free courtesy safety inspections to boaters. However, members also respond to minor SAR incidents, and the local USCG station, group, or district rescue coordination center (RCC) coordinates their activities. Some auxiliarists have become qualified to work in the RCCs or assist regular USCG facilities with regulating and patrolling regattas and other maritime events.

With 30,000 members, the auxiliary saves hundreds of lives each year, in addition to assisting thousands of boaters, performing courtesy marine examinations, teaching public and youth classes, and assisting the USCG in both administrative and operational missions (U.S. Coast Guard, 2018a).

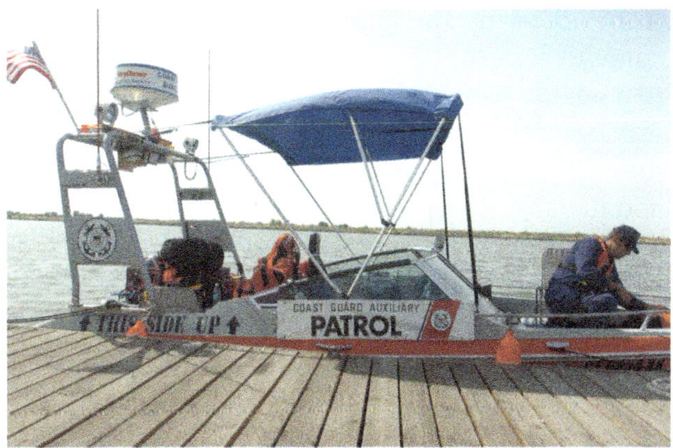

FIGURE 1-9 The U.S. Coast Guard Auxiliary comprises citizens who volunteer time and boats or aircraft to enhance and maintain the safety of boaters.

USA Freedom Corps and the Corporation for National and Community Service

Following the tragic events of September 11, 2001, state and local government officials have increased opportunities for U.S. citizens to become an integral part of protecting their country and supporting local first responders. Officials agree that the formula for ensuring a more secure and safer homeland consists of preparedness, training, and citizen involvement in supporting first responders.

During his 2002 State of the Union address, President George W. Bush called upon every American to get involved in strengthening the country's communities and sharing America's compassion around the world. He called on every American to dedicate at least two years over the course of their lives to the service of others. He included all Americans because everyone can do something, and he created the USA Freedom Corps to help all Americans answer his call.

President Obama expanded this concept into the White House Office of Social Innovation and Civic Participation, which started as a coordinating council housed at the White House and chaired by the president of the United States. The organization worked to strengthen American culture of service and to help find opportunities for every American to start volunteering. This effort eventually expanded to establish the Office of Faith-Based and Neighborhood Partnerships, which incorporated faith-based organizations into the concept and included an advisory council composed of religious and secular leaders and scholars from various backgrounds.

These programs eventually evolved into the Corporation for National and Community Service (CNCS), which today serves more than 50,000 locations across the United States. This federal agency helps millions of Americans improve the lives of their fellow citizens through service as it works to expand and strengthen federal service programs such as the Citizen Corps, AmeriCorps, Social Innovation Fund, Volunteer Generation Fund, and Senior Corps and to raise awareness of and break down barriers to service opportunities with all federal government agencies (Corporation for National & Community Service, 2018).

Citizen Corps

After September 11, 2001, the United States witnessed a wellspring of selflessness and heroism. People in every

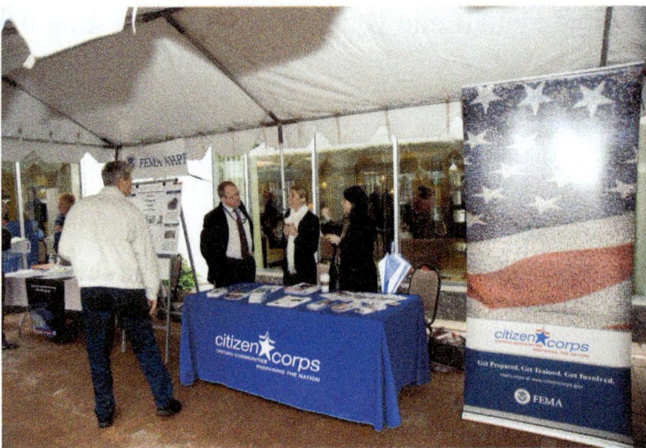

FIGURE 1-10 Citizen Corps was created to help coordinate volunteer activities that make our communities safer, stronger, and better prepared to respond to any emergency situation.
Courtesy of Bill Koplitz/FEMA.

corner of the country asked, "What can I do?" and "How can I help?" Citizen Corps was created to help all Americans answer these questions through public education and outreach, training, and volunteer service (**FIGURE 1-10**).

Citizen Corps, a key component of what was formerly known as the USA Freedom Corps, was created to help answer these questions and coordinate volunteer activities that make American communities safer, stronger, and better prepared to respond to any emergency situation. It provides opportunities for Americans to participate in a range of measures to make their families, their homes, and their communities safer from the threats of crime, terrorism, and disasters of all kinds. Citizen Corps programs build on the successful efforts that are in place in many communities around the country to prevent crime and respond to emergencies. Programs that began through local innovation are the foundation for Citizen Corps and this national approach to citizen participation in community safety.

Citizen Corps is coordinated nationally by FEMA. In this capacity, FEMA works closely with other federal entities, state and local governments, first responders and emergency managers, the volunteer community, and the White House Office of Social Innovation and Civic Participation.

Citizen Corps councils help drive local citizen participation by coordinating Citizen Corps programs, developing community action plans, assessing possible threats, and identifying local resources.

- An expanded Neighborhood Watch Program (NWP) incorporates terrorism awareness and education into its existing crime prevention mission and serves as a way to bring residents together to focus on disaster preparedness and training.
- Volunteers in Police Service (VIPS) provides support for resource-constrained police departments by incorporating civilian volunteers so that law enforcement professionals have more time for frontline duty.
- CERT trains people in neighborhoods, the workplace, and schools in basic disaster response skills—such as fire suppression, urban search and rescue, and medical operations—and helps them take a more active role in emergency preparedness.
- The Medical Reserve Corps (MRC) coordinates volunteer health professionals as well as other citizens with an interest in health issues to provide ongoing support for community public health needs and resources during large-scale emergencies, such as assisting emergency response teams, providing care to victims with less serious injuries, and removing other burdens that inhibit the effectiveness of physicians and nurses.

SEARCH AND RESCUE TIP

The mission of Citizen Corps is to harness the power of every individual through education, training, and volunteer service to make communities safer, stronger, and better prepared to respond to the threats of terrorism, crime, public health issues, and disasters of all kinds (Ready.gov, 2018a).

Community Emergency Response Team

First responders such as fire and EMS personnel arriving at the scene of a major disaster will not be able to meet the demand for their services. Large numbers of victims, communication difficulties, road blockages, and general infrastructure failures will prevent people from accessing the emergency services they have come to expect at a moment's notice through 9-1-1 (**FIGURE 1-11**). Instead of relying on emergency services, citizens will have to depend on each other in these situations to meet their immediate life-saving and life-sustaining needs. Research from large-scale disasters shows that "spontaneous volunteers"—friends, family, and neighbors, or people in the right place at the right time—will save more lives than all trained rescuers combined. During the Mexico City earthquake in September 1985, untrained, impromptu rescuers were credited with saving over 800 lives. Unfortunately, 100 people lost their lives while attempting to save others. It is now thought that the loss of these citizen rescuers could have been prevented through training.

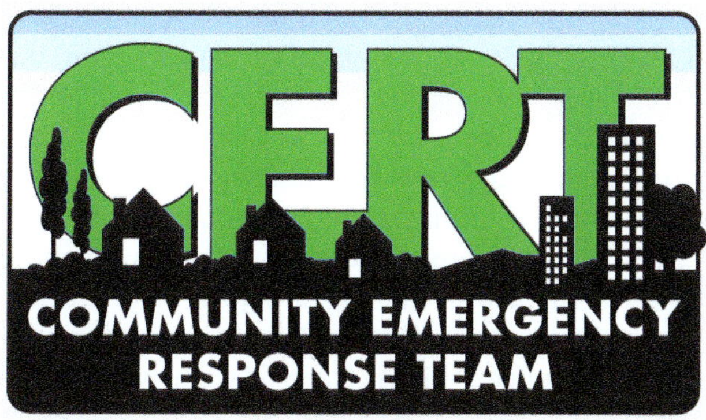

FIGURE 1-11 Community Emergency Response Teams comprise citizens trained to meet immediate life-saving and life-sustaining needs during a major disaster.

Logo is used with permission from FEMA.

If it can be predicted that first responders will not be able to meet immediate needs following a major disaster, and spontaneous volunteering will occur, especially when there is no warning (such as in an earthquake), what can a government do to prepare its citizens better for this eventuality? FEMA makes the following recommendations:

1. Present citizens the facts about what to expect following a major disaster in terms of immediate services.
2. Give the message about their responsibility for mitigation and preparedness.
3. Train them in needed life-saving skills, with emphasis on decision-making skills, rescuer safety, and doing the greatest good for the greatest number of people.
4. Organize teams so that they are an extension of first responder services offering immediate help to victims until professional services arrive.

These are the four elements of a CERT program. The CERT concept was developed and implemented by the Los Angeles City Fire Department (LAFD) in 1985. The Whittier Narrows earthquake in 1987 underscored the area-wide threat of a major disaster in California and confirmed the need for training civilians to meet their own immediate needs. As a result, the LAFD created the Disaster Preparedness Division with the purpose of training citizens, including private and government employees.

The LAFD program furthered the process of citizens understanding their responsibility in preparing for disaster. It also increased their ability to help themselves, their families, and their neighbors safely. These are the reasons FEMA was interested in the program and believed it applicable to all hazards. Today, the Emergency Management Institute (EMI) and the National Fire Academy (NFA) have adopted and expanded the CERT materials to support courses taught nationwide (**FIGURE 1-12**).

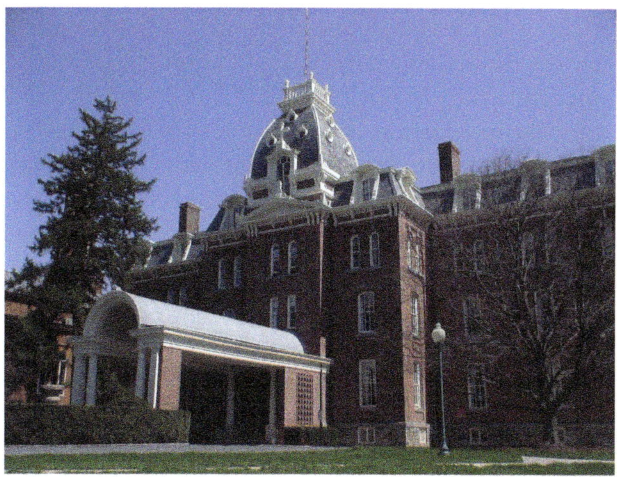

FIGURE 1-12 The National Fire Academy and the Emergency Management Institute, co-located in Emmitsburg, Maryland, train many of today's leaders in disaster and emergency response, operations, and management.

Courtesy of Federal Emergency Management Agency, Mark D. Miller.

The CERT course will benefit any citizen who takes it. This individual will be better prepared to respond to and cope with the aftermath of a disaster. Additionally, if a community wants to supplement its response capability after a disaster, civilians can be recruited and trained as neighborhood, business, and government teams that, in essence, will be auxiliary responders. These groups can provide immediate assistance to victims in their area, organize spontaneous volunteers who have not had the training, and collect disaster intelligence that will assist professional responders with prioritization and allocation of resources following a disaster. Since 1993 when this training was made available nationally by FEMA, hundreds of communities in most U.S. states and Puerto Rico have conducted CERT training (Ready.gov, 2018b).

International Search and Rescue Organizations

The International Commission for Alpine Rescue (ICAR; also known as Internationale Kommission für Alpines Rettungswesen [IKAR] and Commission Internationale du Sauvetage Alpin [CISA]) is a working group of national mountain rescue organizations whose mission is to "provide a platform for mountain rescue and related organizations to disseminate knowledge with the prime goal of improving mountain rescue services and their safety" (Courtesy of ICAR—International Commission for Alpine Rescue [ICAR], 2018). Located in Switzerland,

ICAR is divided into four commissions: terrestrial rescue, air rescue, avalanche rescue, and mountain emergency medicine (i.e., MEDCOM). ICAR is an independent, global organization that promotes international cooperation on mountain rescue services (ICAR, 2018).

The International Climbing and Mountaineering Federation (UIAA), also located in Switzerland, promotes the growth and protection of mountaineering and climbing around the world, mostly through the work of its eight commissions: access, antidoping, ice climbing, medical, mountain protection, mountaineering (including the Training Standards Panel), safety, and youth. Although all commissions do important work, the UIAA Safety Commission may be the most recognizable to climbers because it develops technical safety standards for equipment, which are used by many of the biggest manufacturers of mountaineering equipment around the world. Equipment that has been tested to UIAA standards is permitted to bear the UIAA safety label symbol. The Safety Commission also accredits laboratories that test equipment and offers advice on how to treat their equipment and avoid accidents (International Climbing and Mountaineering Federation [UIAA], 2018).

The International Search and Rescue Advisory Group (INSARAG) is a global network of more than 80 countries and organizations under the United Nations umbrella that deals with urban search and rescue/structural collapse related issues. One goal of the group is to establish minimum international standards for urban search and rescue teams and a methodology for international coordination in earthquake response based on the their own (INSARAG) guidelines endorsed by the 2002 United Nations General Assembly Resolution 57/150 (International Search and Rescue Advisory Group [INSARAG], 2018).

Other Organizations

There is no shortage of opportunities for Americans to help others through volunteering and getting involved with organizations that provide emergency assistance. The American Red Cross, AmeriCorps, and the Corporation for National and Community Service are all examples of organizations that can provide rewarding experiences for those wishing to get involved in emergency service and community support efforts.

Wrap-Up

READY FOR REVIEW

- Searches and rescues have been carried out around the world for centuries, but it has only been relatively recently that we have referred to these acts collectively as "search and rescue" or "SAR."
- Management of SAR operations can range from directing the actions of a few responders in a small community to managing an effort involving thousands of responders in a large regional disaster.
- Beyond what is taught in NASAR's "Introduction to SAR" course, three concepts are important to grasp before getting involved in search and rescue: the SAR training categories, the SAR "tool" acquisition process, and SAR standards and regulations.
- There are a number of organizations through which individuals can get involved in search and rescue in the United States, including NASAR; the MRA; CAP; the USCG Auxiliary; the USA Freedom Corps; CERT, and other national, state, provincial, and local agencies and organizations.

SEARCH AND RESCUE TERMS

Rescue* An operation to retrieve persons in distress, provide for their initial medical or other needs, and deliver them to a place of safety (IMO/ICAO, 2016).

Search* An operation using available personnel and facilities to locate persons in distress (IMO/ICAO, 2016).

Wilderness An uninhabited region devoid of any synthetic amenities.

* Material from the IMO publications IAMSAR Manual Volumes I, II and III (2016 - II960E/IF961E/II962E and 2013 - IH960E/IE961E and IH962E) and/or the IMO website www.imo.org is reproduced with the permission of the International Maritime Organization (IMO), which does not accept responsibility for the correctness of the material as reproduced: in case of doubt, IMO's authentic text shall prevail. Readers should check with their national maritime Administration for any further amendments or latest advice. International Maritime Organization, 4 Albert Embankment, London, SE1 7SR, United Kingdom.

REFERENCES AND SUGGESTED READING

American National Standards Institute. 2018. About ANSI. http://www.ansi.org/about_ansi/overview/overview.aspx.

Civil Air Patrol, U.S. Air Force Auxiliary. 2018. Official web page. http://www.gocivilairpatrol.com.

Corporation for National & Community Service. 2018. Corporation for National & Community Service website. https://www.nationalservice.gov/serve.

European Committee for Standardization. 2018. "Who We Are." https://www.cen.eu/about/Pages/.

"Evolution of SAR: An Editorial." July 1946. *Air Sea Rescue Bulletin*.

International Climbing and Mountaineering Federation. 2018. Official website. http://www.theuiaa.org.

International Commission for Alpine Rescue. 2018. "Our Mission." http://www.alpine-rescue.org/ikar-cisa/documents/2015/ikar20150303001487.pdf.

International Maritime Organization and International Civil Aviation Organization. 2016. *International Aeronautical and Maritime Search and Rescue Manual,* Vol. I. *Organization and Management*, Vol. II. *Mission Co-ordination*, Vol. III. *Mobile Facilities*. London/Montreal: International Maritime Organization and International Civil Aviation Organization.

International Search and Rescue Advisory Group. 2018. Official website. http://www.insarag.org.

May, William Gambrill. 1973. *Mountain Search and Rescue Techniques*, First Edition. Boulder, CO: Rocky Mountain Rescue Group.

Mountain Rescue Association. 2018. Official website. http://www.mra.org.

National Association for Search and Rescue. 2018. Official website. http://www.nasar.org.

Ready.gov. 2018a. Citizen Corps. https://www.ready.gov/citizen-corps.

Ready.gov. 2018b. "Community Emergency Response Team." https://www.ready.gov/community-emergency-response-team.

Setnicka, Tim J. 1980. *Wilderness Search and Rescue*. Kenneth Andrasko, editor. Boston, MA: Appalachian Mountain Club.

U.S. Coast Guard. 2018a. "U.S. Coast Guard Auxiliary." http://www.cgaux.org/.

U.S. Coast Guard. 2018b. "Inland Search and Rescue School." http://www.forcecom.uscg.mil/Our-Organization/FORCECOM-UNITS/TraCen-Yorktown/Training/Maritime-Search-Rescue/Inland-SAR/.

Section Opener: Courtesy of NASAR; Chapter Opener: Courtesy of NASAR; Rescuers carrying victim: Courtesy of NASAR.

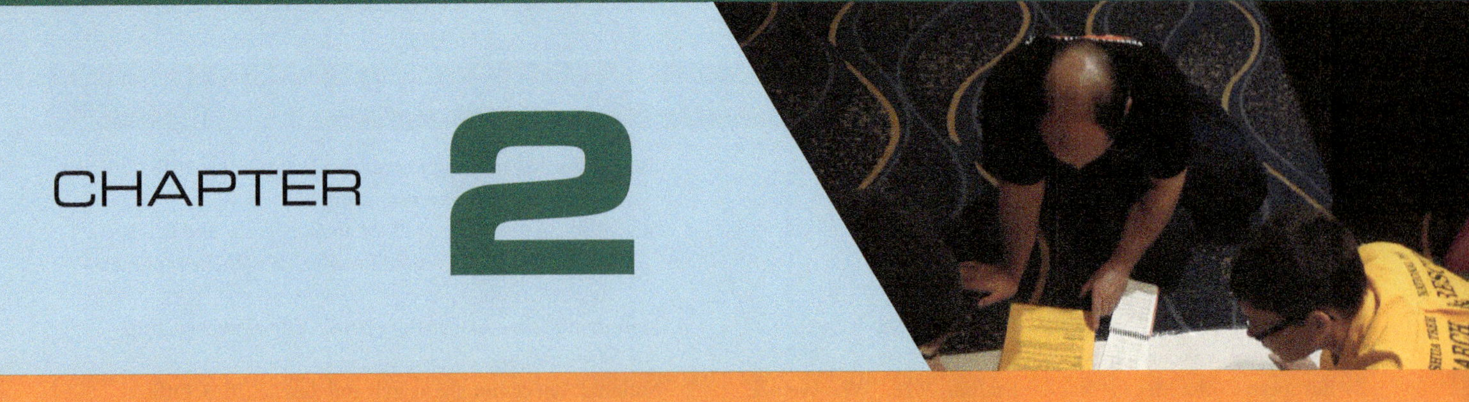

Search and Rescue Systems

OBJECTIVES

Upon completion of this chapter and the related course activities, the student will be able to meet the following objectives:

- List and describe the five international stages of search and rescue (SAR) operations as defined in the *International Aeronautical and Maritime Search and Rescue (IAMSAR) Manual*.
- List and describe the four sequential phases (LAST) of SAR operations.
- Describe the role of the U.S. National SAR Committee and the two documents for which it is responsible.
- Describe the COSPAS-SARSAT system and the roles of the three major types of distress radio beacons within it.
- List the federal SAR coordinators for the United States and describe their respective regions of responsibility.
- Describe the U.S. National SAR Supplement to the *IAMSAR Manual* and the two current U.S. addendums (Land SAR and CISAR).
- Describe the purposes of the National Incident Management System (NIMS) and the National Response Framework (NRF) in the United States.
- Describe at least four typical operations conducted by a FEMA Urban Search and Rescue (US&R) Task Force.
- Define what an Emergency Management Assistance Compact (EMAC) is and summarize how it works.
- Explain how the following miscellaneous tools can be used for SAR:
    - AMBER Alert Program
    - National Center for Missing & Exploited Children

The Global SAR System

Working together, the International Civil Aviation Organization (ICAO) and the International Maritime Organization (IMO) coordinate, on a global basis, member countries' efforts to provide search and rescue (SAR) services. The general goal of ICAO and IMO is to provide an effective, integrated, worldwide system that makes and keeps SAR services available wherever people travel. Pursuant to this goal, these organizations jointly developed the *International Aeronautical and Maritime Search and Rescue (IAMSAR) Manual*. A basic, practical, and humanitarian effect of having such a system is that it eliminates the need for each country to provide SAR services for its own citizens wherever they travel worldwide. Instead, the globe is divided into search and rescue regions (SRRs), each with a **rescue coordination center (RCC)** and associated SAR services, which assist anyone in distress within the SRR without regard to nationality or circumstances (IMO/ICAO, 2016).

International Stages of SAR Operations

The international SAR community has developed an approach to organizing operations not unlike that which has evolved in the land SAR community over the past several decades. This system is documented in the *IAMSAR Manual.* While SAR personnel working in an international maritime environment may find this information useful, the land SAR community in general would do well to seriously consider adopting some or all of these internationally accepted and useful concepts and terms.

The *IAMSAR Manual* describes a series of five stages of a SAR operation through which most SAR events pass: awareness, initial action, planning, operations, and conclusion. The manual suggests that, "These stages should be interpreted with flexibility, as many of the actions described may be performed simultaneously or in a different order to suit specific circumstances" (IMO/ICAO, 2016, Vol. II, p. 1-7)*. The reason the *IAMSAR Manual* does not have a preplanning stage is twofold: First, the five stages of a SAR operation concern what happens in a specific incident. Preplanning can address types of incidents but not specific incidents. Second, the preplanning function is addressed in what are called plans of operations or operations plans (OPLANs). These are standing plans for how to deal with various kinds of situations.

Awareness Stage

A SAR organization cannot respond to an incident until it becomes aware that someone needs assistance. At this stage, information is received that someone (or an aircraft or vessel) is, or will be, in distress. There may not be enough information to initiate action, or action may not be necessary, yet.

Initial Action Stage

When enough information is available, immediate action may be necessary. The first action is always to evaluate the information available, attempt to gain more, and determine the degree of the emergency. The phase of the emergency is used by the SAR authority to describe the level of confidence in the available information and the level of concern it raises about the safety of an aircraft or vessel and the person(s) on board. The *IAMSAR Manual* describes three emergency phases: uncertainty, alert, and distress.

- *Uncertainty phase*—A situation wherein doubt exists as to the safety of an aircraft or vessel and the person(s) on board.
- *Alert phase*—A situation wherein apprehension exists as to the safety of an aircraft or vessel and the person(s) on board.
- *Distress phase*—A situation wherein there is reasonable certainty that a vessel or other craft, including an aircraft or person, is threatened by grave and imminent danger and requires immediate assistance.

An overdue aircraft, as an example, may be late for a wide range of reasons. The phases of the emergency allow those in charge to establish and communicate a summary of the available information that matches its validity, the urgency of action, and the extent of the response required. The *IAMSAR Manual* requires specific initial actions based on the established emergency phase.

Planning Stage

Comprehensive planning of SAR response is crucial, especially when the location of the distress situation is unknown, and the subjects may move. "Proper and accurate planning is critical to SAR mission success; if the wrong area is searched, there is no hope that search personnel will find the survivors, regardless of the quality of their search techniques or the amount of their search effort" (IMO/ICAO, 2016, Vol. II, p. 1-8)*. The *IAMSAR Manual* suggests the use of computers for operational planning, but also includes basic information on manual methods of planning searches.

Operations Stage

The operations stage encompasses all the physical activities involved in finding, providing assistance to, and rescuing people in distress. In short, this is the phase in which the plans are carried out.

Many have also found it useful to think of the operations stage of a SAR event as comprising four sequential phases: locate, access, stabilize, and transport (LAST).

Locate Phase. The first step in addressing any emergency situation is locating the subject or subjects in need of assistance. This may be as simple as asking

* Material from the IMO publications IAMSAR Manual Volumes I, II and III (2016 - II960E/IF961E/II962E and 2013 - IH960E/IE961E and IH962E) and/or the IMO website www.imo.org is reproduced with the permission of the International Maritime Organization (IMO), which does not accept responsibility for the correctness of the material as reproduced: in case of doubt, IMO's authentic text shall prevail. Readers should check with their national maritime Administration for any further amendments or latest advice. International Maritime Organization, 4 Albert Embankment, London, SE1 7SR, United Kingdom.

for an address or as complex as conducting an extended search for a lost person or persons. If the subject is easily found, rescuers can quickly move into the access phase. However, if locating the subject is difficult, this phase may turn into the crux of the SAR problem.

Access Phase. After the subject is located, the search is over. Rescuers must now gain access to the subject to assess and treat injuries, evaluate the situation, and mitigate the problem. Accomplishing these objectives may be as simple as walking up a trail to reach the subject or as complex as reaching a climber on the face of El Capitan in Yosemite National Park. Regardless, planning for this eventuality should be complete and ready to be carried out after the locate phase.

Stabilization Phase. The stabilization phase has three primary components: physical, medical, and emotional. Once rescuers have access to the subject, the scene must be quickly evaluated, or sized up, for immediate physical hazards and threats from the environment. Scene safety is an initial priority in the size-up, and risks to everyone must be weighed against the benefits to be gained. An example of physical stabilization would include an occupied automobile teetering on the edge of a cliff. Before the occupant can be medically assessed, the situation must be stabilized to best protect the rescuers and the patient. Other examples of physical stabilization might include protecting the patient from further injury or removing the hazard.

Once the physical environment is stabilized and free from immediate hazards, medical management and stabilization can begin. This process usually follows accepted procedures, starting with primary and secondary physical examinations and progressing through treatment with basic to advanced life support. The process should treat the identified illness and/or injuries as appropriate, and without exception, the process should include some type of protection from the environment. The goal of medical stabilization is usually to prepare the subject for transportation to a definitive care facility. If medical care is not required, confirming this fact may be all that is necessary at this stage before moving into the transport phase.

Emotional stabilization is necessary because an anxious victim is a hazard to rescuers and to himself or herself. The goal is to best protect both the rescuers and the victim. Simple, calm communication with the patient, slowly describing what happened and what rescuers are doing, is often enough to calm a nervous subject.

Stabilization, like assessment, should continue throughout the transport phase. The overall objective is to prepare the victim for transport to definitive care while maintaining his or her comfort and safety.

Transport Phase. In the fourth phase of SAR operations, the subject is moved to definitive care. For this to occur, the stabilized subject must be packaged so that he or she can be moved safely and efficiently while stabilization and assessment continue. Transportation will range from foot travel, with the subject walking on his or her own, to evacuation by aircraft. If helicopter extraction is going to be used, the injured person must be briefed thoroughly on what to expect. This should include everything from the effects of rotor wash to movement and noise. The appropriate mode of transportation can be determined by weather, type and severity of injuries, overall urgency, terrain, and available resources, among other factors.

Conclusion Stage

The conclusion stage is entered when it is determined that no one is in distress, when the search and/or rescue is concluded, or when nothing was found, and the search is called off. This is the phase in which all SAR resources are notified that the mission is concluded.

International Agreements

International conventions, or written agreements between countries, are often what countries use to establish rules between them. The Convention on International Aviation, the International Convention on Maritime Search and Rescue, and the International Convention for the Safety of Life at Sea (SOLAS) all include rules requiring countries that are a party to them to provide aeronautical and maritime SAR coordination and services for their territories and territorial seas. Coverage of the high seas is apportioned among the member countries by these instruments as well. To carry out its SAR responsibilities, a country usually establishes a national SAR organization, or joins one or more other countries to form a regional SAR organization. In the United States, the national SAR organization is called the National Search and Rescue Committee (NSARC). NSARC is responsible for two documents: the U.S. *National SAR Plan* and the U.S. *National SAR Supplement to the IAMSAR Manual.*

While airborne, virtually all commercial aircraft on international routes are under **positive control** (i.e., followed by radar and in direct communication with air traffic controllers) by air traffic services (ATS) units. ICAO has linked ATS units into a worldwide system. Consequently, SAR agencies are usually notified very quickly when an international commercial flight has an emergency. Commercial aircraft on domestic routes and general aviation aircraft may not be under positive control, which can result in delayed reporting of their emergencies. The international aeronautic distress frequency is 121.5 MHz, and it is monitored by ATS, some commercial airliners, and other aeronautic facilities where needed to ensure immediate reception of distress calls. Emergency locator transmitters (ELTs) are carried in most aircraft and are required in most aircraft flown in the United States (see the section on COSPAS-SARSAT), but none of these technologies or systems necessarily guarantees a quick rescue, especially when vast oceans and wilderness areas are involved. For example, in March 2014, Malaysia Airlines Flight 370, carrying 12 crew and 227 passengers from 15 countries, disappeared while flying from Kuala Lumpur to Beijing. The last voice contact occurred while the aircraft was over the South China Sea, and the aircraft was last plotted by military radar over the Andaman Sea. After a multinational search effort, one believed to be the largest and most expensive in history, there has been no confirmation of any flight debris or crash site as of this writing.

The IAMSAR Manual

To assist countries in meeting their obligations under certain international conventions as well as their own SAR needs, the three-volume *IAMSAR Manual* was developed jointly by ICAO and IMO (**FIGURE 2-1**). In short, the IAMSAR volumes provide guidelines for a common aviation and maritime approach to organizing and providing SAR services while encouraging countries to participate in an integrated, global SAR system (IMO/ICAO, 2016).

Each of the *IAMSAR Manual* volumes is written with specific SAR system duties in mind and can be used as a stand-alone document or in conjunction with the other two volumes as a means to attain a full view of the SAR system. Volume I, *Organization and Management*, discusses the global SAR system concept, establishment and improvement of national and regional SAR systems, and cooperation with neighboring countries to provide effective and economical SAR services. Volume II, *Mission Coordination*, assists personnel who plan and coordinate SAR operations and exercises. Volume III, *Mobile Facilities*, is intended to be carried aboard rescue units, aircraft, and vessels to help with performance of search, rescue, or on-scene coordinator functions and with aspects of SAR that pertain to their own emergencies.

Although no more details of the *IAMSAR Manual* will be offered here, it should be clear that this internationally accepted document has a great deal to offer those interested in all types of SAR, including land SAR. This manual describes concepts and methods that have wide applicability to SAR and makes an outstanding contribution to any serious SAR library. The three-volume *IAMSAR Manual* is available for purchase from ICAO and IMO.

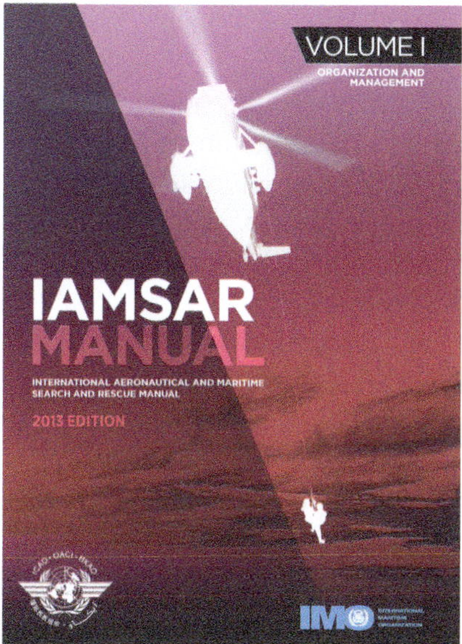

A

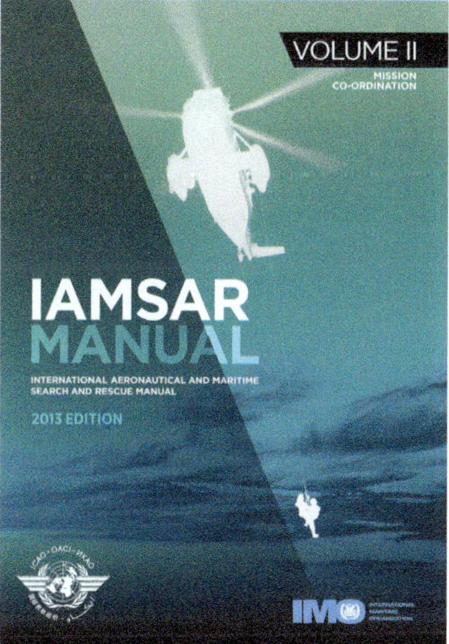

B

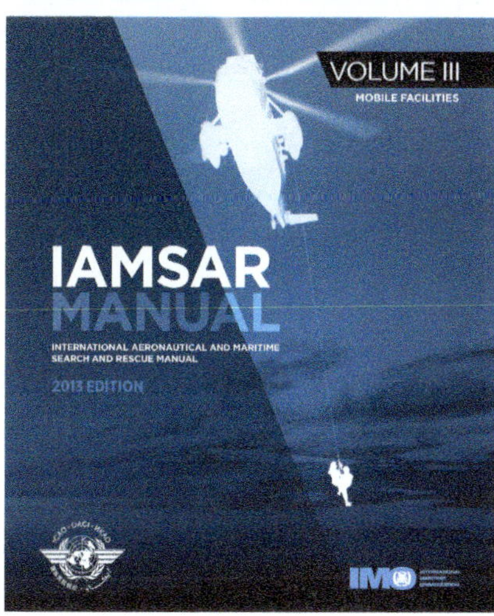

C

FIGURE 2-1 The three volumes of the *International Aeronautical and Maritime Search and Rescue Manual*.

COSPAS-SARSAT

COSPAS-SARSAT is an international humanitarian SAR system that uses satellites to detect and locate emergency beacons carried by ships, aircraft, or individuals. The system consists of a network of satellites, ground stations, mission control centers, and rescue coordination centers.

The SARSAT system was developed in a joint effort by the United States, Canada, and France. In the United States, the National Oceanic and Atmospheric Administration (NOAA) is the lead agency and coordinates national participation in SARSAT and associated international programs. The COSPAS system (*cosmicheskaya sistyema poiska avariynich sudov*; in English, "space system for the search of vessels in distress") was developed by Russia. These four nations banded together in 1979 to form COSPAS-SARSAT, and the system was declared fully operational in 1984. The COSPAS-SARSAT system ceased satellite processing of the original 121.5/243-MHz beacons on February 1, 2009. Second-generation 406-MHz beacons were introduced in 1997 that allow transmission in the 406-MHz message of encoded position data acquired by beacons from global satellite navigation systems such as global positioning systems (GPS), using internal or external navigation receivers. As of this writing, the four original member nations have been joined by many other nations and two regional organizations that operate ground stations and mission control centers that convey alert data to six data distribution regions worldwide (United States, France, Russia, Australia, Japan, and Spain). As of October 2016, the COPAS-SARSAT system had aided in rescuing over 36,000 persons in over 8000 incidents.

When an emergency beacon is activated, the digitally coded signal is sent to a low-Earth-orbit (LEO) satellite and relayed to the nearest available ground receiving station. The ground station, called a local user terminal (LUT), processes the signal and calculates the position from which it originated. This position is transmitted to a mission control center (MCC), where it is joined with identification data and other information on that beacon, if the beacon has been registered with NOAA, which is required by law in the United States. The MCC then transmits an alert message to the appropriate RCC, based primarily on the geographic location of the beacon, which initiates the search and rescue. If the location of the beacon is in another country's SRR, then the alert is transmitted to the appropriate MCC (**FIGURE 2-2**).

COSPAS-SARSAT is in the process of upgrading its system by placing search and rescue repeaters on global navigation satellites (GPS from the United States, Russian Glonass, and European Galileo) orbiting the Earth. These new COSPAS-SARSAT assets are now part

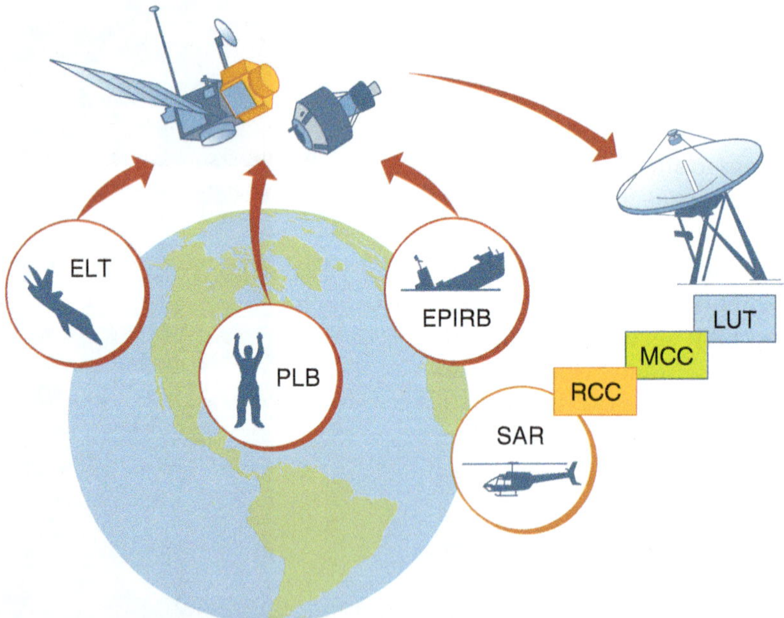

FIGURE 2-2 When a distress radio beacon is activated, the signal is received by a satellite and relayed to the nearest available ground terminal or LUT, which calculates the position from which the signal originated. This position is transmitted to an MCC, where it is joined with identification data and transmitted to the appropriate RCC based on the geographic location of the beacon. The RCC then notifies the appropriate SAR response organization(s).

of a system known as MEOSAR, for Medium-altitude Earth Orbit Search and Rescue system. MEOSAR offers the advantages of the satellite systems used by COSPAS-SARSAT, without many of their limitations, by relaying beacon distress messages and simultaneously calculating the beacon location anywhere on Earth almost instantly as the alert signal is received. The MEOSAR system also allows an optional "return link" transmission back to beacons, which could provide confirmation to the person in distress that their alert message has been received.

Distress Radio Beacons

The most recognizable component of the SARSAT system is the distress radio beacon, also known as a "beacon." There are generally three types of beacons used to transmit distress signals: **emergency position indicating radio beacons (EPIRBs)** designed for maritime use, **emergency locator transmitters (ELTs)** designed for aviation use, and **personal locator beacons (PLBs)** designed for use by individuals and land-based applications. Although the three types of devices are physically different due to the differing environments in which they must operate, they all work on the same principle and in the same way. When turned on (automatically or manually), these devices transmit alert signals on specific frequencies that are intended to be received by COSPAS-SARSAT satellites.

Only a few frequencies are used by these beacons:

- 406 MHz is used in digital beacons and is the only type of beacon currently detected by the COSPAS-SARSAT satellite system.
- 121.5 and 243 MHz are used by many existing analog beacons, but the COSPAS-SARSAT system ceased satellite processing of these signals in 2009. Other devices (such as man-overboard systems and homing transmitters) that operate at 121.5 MHz and do not rely on satellite detection are not affected by the cessation of satellite processing of 121.5 MHz. The 121.5-MHz frequency is still used in aviation for voice communication of an emergency.

SEARCH AND RESCUE TIP

- COSPAS—(in Russian) *Cosmicheskaya Sistyema Poiska Avariynich Sudov* (in English, space system for the search of vessels in distress)
- ELT—Emergency locator transmitter
- EPIRB—Emergency position indicating radio beacon
- PLB—Personal locator beacon
- SARSAT—Search and rescue satellite-aided tracking

Emergency Position Indicating Radio Beacons. EPIRBs are handheld portable radio transmitters for use in maritime applications. They can transmit a signal that will be interpreted as a mayday call. These devices activate when submerged in water but are otherwise operationally equivalent to ELTs.

Emergency Locator Transmitters. ELTs were the first emergency beacons developed, and most aircraft are required to carry them. ELTs were originally intended for use on the 121.5-MHz frequency to alert aircraft flying overhead. Obviously, a major limitation to these is that another aircraft must be within range and listening to 121.5 MHz to receive the signal. One of the reasons the COSPAS-SARSAT system was developed was to provide a better receiving source for these signals. Another reason was to provide location data for each activation (something that overflying aircraft were unable to do).

Different types of ELTs are currently in use. There are thousands of the older-generation 121.5-MHz ELTs in service in the United States. Unfortunately, these have proved to be highly ineffective. They have a 99% false-alert rate, activate properly in only 12% of crashes, and provide no identification data. To fix this problem, 406-MHz ELTs were developed to work specifically with the COSPAS-SARSAT system. These ELTs have unique identifiers and dramatically reduce the false-alert impact on SAR resources, have a higher accident survivability success rate, and decrease the time required to reach accident victims to an average of 6 hours.

Most aircraft operators are now mandated to carry an ELT. Although 121.5/243-MHz ELTs used by some aircraft may still be used, the COSPAS-SARSAT system ceased satellite processing of these beacons in 2009, and alerts from these devices (and from 121.5/243-MHz EPIRBs) are no longer acted on unless detected by an overflying aircraft or ground-based receivers. Therefore, all beacon owners and users must replace their 121.5/243-MHz beacons with 406 MHz beacons as soon as possible and register their beacons with NOAA at www.beaconregistration.noaa.gov.

Personal Locator Beacons. PLBs are portable radio transmitters that operate much the same as EPIRBs or ELTs (**FIGURE 2-3**). These beacons are designed to be carried by an individual person instead of on a boat or in aircraft. Unlike ELTs and some EPIRBs, they can only be activated manually and operate exclusively on 406 MHz in the United States. Like EPIRBs and ELTs, all PLBs also have a built-in, low-power homing beacon that transmits on 121.5 MHz. This allows rescue forces to home in on a beacon once the 406-MHz satellite system has put them within 3.2 to 4.8 kilometers (2 to 3 miles). Some newer PLBs also allow GPS units to be

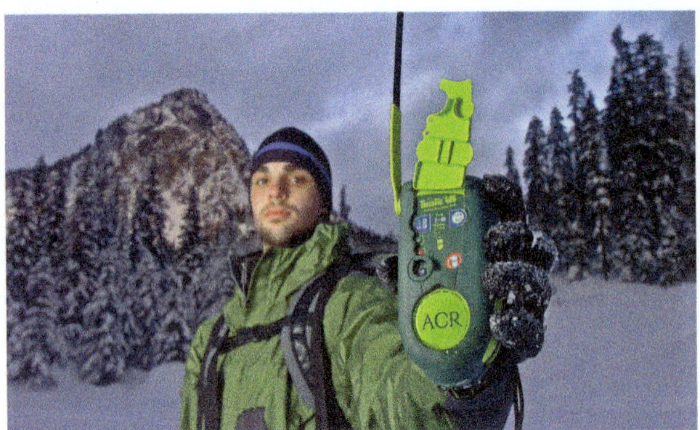

FIGURE 2-3 An example of a personal locator beacon (PLB). Shown is an ACR Electronics Terrafix 406 GPS I/O Personal Locator Beacon (14.5 × 7.7 × 4.4 cm, 340 grams).

integrated into the distress signal. This GPS-encoded position dramatically improves the location accuracy down to within 100 meters.

In the United States, PLBs were in limited use until July 1, 2003, after which they were fully authorized for nationwide use. In 2013, the AFRCC investigated 266 nonmilitary PLB activations that led to 31 missions (SAR operations that require the activation of federal assets) and resulted in five lives saved (USAF, 2015).

NOAA encourages all PLB users to be acutely aware of the responsibility that comes with owning one of these devices. PLBs are a distress-alerting tool and work exceptionally well, but only if registered. PLB users should register their devices at the NOAA website, familiarize themselves with proper testing and operating procedures to prevent false activation, and be careful to avoid their use in nonemergency situations (NOAA, 2015). One misunderstanding of the use of a PLB caused some consternation when the owner thought he was supposed to turn it on when he went out, like an avalanche beacon, and turn it back off when he arrived home. Familiarity with the technology is essential if it is to be helpful when needed.

Satellite Emergency Notification Devices

Distress alerting technology now includes portable emergency notification and locating devices that use commercial satellite systems rather than the COSPAS-SARSAT system. As a category of device, these are generally referred to as satellite emergency notification devices (SEND). These satellite communicators can provide even more accurate geographic location information, texting capabilities, and voice communications through commercial low-Earth orbit satellite networks that have extensive global coverage. Although currently a bit more expensive than a PLB, the cost of these communicators and associated services has decreased in the past few years. These devices allow tracking by remote parties and much more precise geographic location services, which could preclude or replace the need for activation of an emergency beacon like a PLB. Additional features are increasingly being offered, and some newer devices now offer two-way communications via satellite. Delorme offers the inReach™ series of satellite communicators, SPOT™ offers the SPOT Gen3 satellite communicator (**FIGURE 2-4**), and Iridium® offers a number of satellite-based options, including the Iridium GO!®, which is a satellite-based "hot spot" that can allow Internet access and smart phone use almost anywhere on Earth. While this is not an exhaustive list of options, the power of these devices to improve safety for individuals operating in isolated locations is being increasingly recognized.

SAR in the United States

Although most SAR incidents are local issues, a well-tested, comprehensive national search and rescue system exists in the United States to allow for the integration of state, federal, and even international resources into a local event. An awareness of this system and the documents that provide the foundation for it are necessary for a full understanding of where one fits into the bigger picture of SAR in the United States.

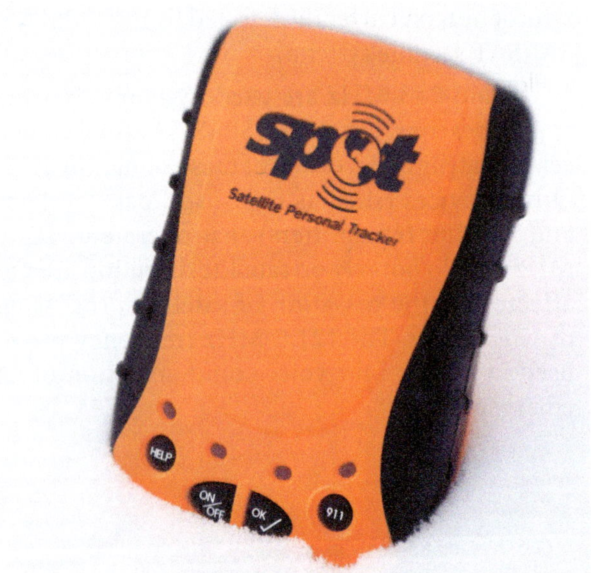

FIGURE 2-4 The SPOT™ Gen3 Satellite GPS Messenger is recommended to be hung on equipment (backpack), in view of the sky, and allows remote tracking of its location, sending custom messages and alerting selected contacts of the need for assistance, of an emergency, or that you are okay (8.5 x 6.5 x 2.5 cm).

The United States National Search and Rescue Plan

The U.S. *National Search and Rescue Plan* (NSP) was developed primarily to provide guidance to signatory federal agencies (agencies who participate in the plan) for coordinating civil SAR services to meet domestic needs and international commitments (**FIGURE 2-5**). The federal government assists with the coordination of certain SAR services, including the coordination of any federal or military resources that may be requested by local or state agencies. Guidance for implementing the NSP is provided in the *IAMSAR Manual*, the *National Search and Rescue Supplement* (NSS, a domestic interagency supplement to the *IAMSAR Manual*), and other relevant directives of the plan participants (NSARC, 2016).

The National SAR Committee (NSARC) is responsible for coordinating and improving federal involvement in civil SAR for the aeronautical, maritime, and land communities within the United States (**FIGURE 2-6**). NSARC is also the federal-level committee formed to sponsor and oversee the U.S. NSP. Member agencies of NSARC are the signatories of the NSP. More information about NSARC may be obtained from the committee's website.

Many U.S. states have chosen to retain established SAR responsibilities within their boundaries for incidents primarily local or intrastate in character. In such cases, agreements have been made between SAR coordinator(s) and relevant state organizations. For land SAR, the federal **search and rescue coordinator** is the U.S. Air Force, which maintains a rescue coordination center (AFRCC) at Tyndall Air Force Base in Panama City, Florida. The relevant state organizations vary from state to state, but agreements exist between each state and the AFRCC.

The *IAMSAR Manual* and the NSP define a **search and rescue region (SRR)** as "an area of defined dimensions, associated with an RCC, within which search and rescue services are provided" (IMO/ICAO, 2016, p. xxiii)**. An RCC is a unit responsible for promoting efficient organization of SAR services and for coordinating the conduct of SAR operations within an SRR. For every SRR, there is one RCC, and the goals are to have no overlaps or gaps between SRRs around the world and to ensure SAR services are available to those in need of them.

In the United States, there are two types of SRRs: maritime and aeronautical. Although only the ocean areas surrounding the United States and its territories fall within the maritime SRRs, both the ocean and land areas of the United States fall within aeronautical SRRs (aircraft can fly over both water and land). The maritime SRRs surrounding the United States include, in the Pacific Ocean, Juneau, Honolulu, Seattle, and Alameda; and in the Atlantic Ocean, Boston, Norfolk, Miami, New Orleans, and San Juan. The oceans surrounding the United States and its territories also fall within aeronautical SRRs whose names and limits coincide with their maritime counterparts. However, with the exception of U.S. islands (Hawaiian, Puerto Rico, etc.) that are contained entirely within maritime SRRs and the Great Lakes (Cleveland Maritime SRR), all U.S. land falls within either the Elmendorf Aeronautical SRR (Alaska) or the Tyndall Air Force Base (Panama City, Florida) Aeronautical SRR (continental United States).

According to the NSP, a SAR coordinator has overall responsibility for, ". . .establishing and providing SAR services, and ensuring that planning for these services is properly coordinated" (NSARC, 2016, p. 2). The SAR coordinators for the United States are as follows:

- The U.S. Air Force for the recognized U.S. aeronautical SRR corresponding to the continental United States other than Alaska.
- The U.S. Pacific Command for the recognized U.S. aeronautical SRR corresponding to Alaska.
- The U.S. Coast Guard (USCG) for all other United States aeronautical and maritime SRRs. This includes the State of Hawaii as well as waters over which the United States has jurisdiction, such as federal navigable waterways of the United States.

Outside these federal SAR coordinators, state and local authorities are responsible for land-based SAR and may designate a person to be "SAR coordinator" within their respective states. State SAR coordinators are important partners of the national SAR coordinators and are critical to providing effective SAR services. In addition, the U.S. Department of the Interior National Park Service (NPS) is responsible for providing emergency services on land and water administered by their agency, and the Federal Emergency Management Agency (FEMA) is responsible for overseeing the national urban search and rescue (US&R) system. All U.S. states have an agreement with the AFRCC that delegates authority for land SAR to the local law enforcement agency, most often the county sheriff, and aeronautical SAR to an appropriate statewide aeronautics or aviation agency.

** Material from the IMO publications IAMSAR Manual Volumes I, II and III (2016 - II960E/IF961E/II962E and 2013 - IH960E/IE961E and IH962E) and/or the IMO website www.imo.org is reproduced with the permission of the International Maritime Organization (IMO), which does not accept responsibility for the correctness of the material as reproduced: in case of doubt, IMO's authentic text shall prevail. Readers should check with their national maritime Administration for any further amendments or latest advice. International Maritime Organization, 4 Albert Embankment, London, SE1 7SR, United Kingdom.

National Search and Rescue Plan of the United States

Policy

1. It is the policy of the signatory Federal departments and agencies to provide a *National Search and Rescue Plan of the United States* (referred to as the "Plan") for coordinating search and rescue (SAR) services to meet domestic needs and international commitments. Implementing guidance for this Plan is provided in the *International Aeronautical and Maritime Search and Rescue (IAMSAR) Manual*, the *National Search and Rescue Supplement (NSS) to the International Aeronautical and Maritime Search and Rescue Manual*, and other relevant directives of the Participants in this Plan.

Purpose

2. This Plan continues, by interagency agreement, the effective use of all available resources in all types of SAR operations to enable the United States to satisfy its humanitarian, national, and international commitments and obligations.

3. The *National Search and Rescue Plan of the United States (2007)* is superseded by this Plan.

Terms and Definitions

4. The following terms and definitions are used in this Plan.[1]

   a. Catastrophic Incident: Any natural or manmade incident, including terrorism, that results in extraordinary levels of mass casualties, damage, or disruption severely affecting the population, infrastructure, environment, economy, national morale, or government functions.

   b. Incident Command System (ICS): a management system designed to enable effective and efficient domestic incident management by integrating a combination of facilities, equipment, personnel, procedures, and communications operating within a common organizational structure. ICS is a subcomponent of the National Incident Management System.

   c. Mass Rescue Operation (MRO): SAR services characterized by the need for immediate response to large numbers of persons in distress, such that the capabilities normally available to SAR authorities are inadequate.

   d. National Incident Management System (NIMS): A systematic, proactive approach to guide departments and agencies at all levels of government, nongovernmental organizations, and the private sector to work together seamlessly and manage incidents

[1] Additional terms and definitions are available in the IAMSAR Manual and the NSS.

FIGURE 2-5 Front page of the U.S. *National Search and Rescue Plan* (NSARC, 2016).
Courtesy of National Search and Rescue Committee.

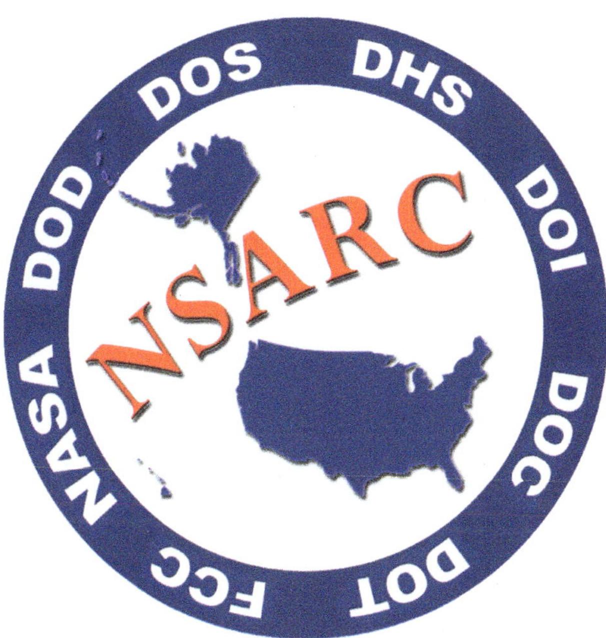

FIGURE 2-6 Emblem of the U.S. National Search and Rescue Committee.
Courtesy of National Search and Rescue Committee.

Because of the unique scale and SAR challenges in Alaska, the USCG is often the lead federal agency for inland SAR incidents in certain areas of the state, including the Alaska Peninsula (south of 58 degrees N), Aleutian Islands, and other coastal islands. The reason for this is simple: In these areas, USCG assets can often respond much more quickly than can those available through the U.S. Alaska Rescue Coordination Center at Ft. Richardson, Alaska, north of Anchorage. For Alaskan inland areas, SAR is carried out by Air National Guard units, the Alaska state troopers, and local borough SAR organizations. Because of the unforgiving environment, all federal, state, and local agencies work together closely in response to SAR missions in Alaska.

SEARCH AND RESCUE TIP

Civilian SAR personnel should be generally familiar with the latest version of the following documents:

- The *National Response Framework*
- The ICAO/IMO *IAMSAR Manual*
- The U.S. *National SAR Plan*
- The *National SAR Supplement to the IAMSAR Manual*
- The *Land SAR Addendum to the National SAR Supplement to the IAMSAR Manual*
- *Catastrophic Incident SAR Addendum to the National SAR Manual*

Participating Federal Agencies

The following U.S. federal agencies are participants in the NSP and members of NSARC (NSARC, 2016):

- Department of Homeland Security (DHS, including the USCG and FEMA)
- Department of Transportation (DOT, including the Federal Aviation Administration [FAA] and the Maritime Administration [MARAD])
- Department of Defense (DOD)
- Department of Commerce (including NOAA, which is the lead federal agency for the COSPAS-SARSAT system)
- Federal Communications Commission (FCC)
- National Aeronautics and Space Administration (NASA)
- Department of the Interior (including the NPS)
- Department of State (DOS)

The National SAR Supplement

NSARC also directs the preparation of the *National SAR Supplement* (NSS) to the *IAMSAR Manual*, which provides guidance to federal agencies concerning implementation of the NSP. The NSS provides specific additional national standards and guidance that build upon the baseline established by the *IAMSAR Manual*. The NSS provides guidance to all federal forces, military and civilian, that support civil SAR operations.

Specifically, the *NSS* is designed to serve as both a training and operational tool for civil SAR operations. SAR planning is both an art and a science, relying greatly on the creativity and experience of the personnel involved. Because of the many variables encountered during SAR operations and the individuality of each SAR case, the guidance provided in the *NSS* must be tempered with sound judgment, having due regard for the individual situation. Very little in the *NSS* is mandatory because it is not intended to relieve SAR personnel of the need for initiative and sound judgment.

Each of the participating agencies of the NSARC (and NSP) may also develop an addendum to the *NSS* for their agency. Such documents could include policies, information, and procedures on civil SAR matters applicable to the agency concerned and consistent with both the *IAMSAR Manual* and *NSS*.

As of this writing, there are currently two addendums to the *NSS*: The Land SAR Addendum and the Catastrophic Incident SAR Addendum.

Land SAR Addendum to the National Search and Rescue Supplement

In 2011, NSARC created the Land SAR Addendum (LSA) to the NSS, which further expands on the implementation of the NSP (**FIGURE 2-7**). In this document, NSARC defines *land SAR* as "the provisioning of civil SAR services for persons in distress or missing within the land areas of the U.S., including persons in distress in aircraft." (NSARC, 2011, p. v) The Land SAR Addendum is intended to provide guidance to federal land SAR

LAND SEARCH AND RESCUE ADDENDUM
to the
National Search and Rescue Supplement
to the
International Aeronautical and Maritime Search and Rescue Manual

Version 1.0

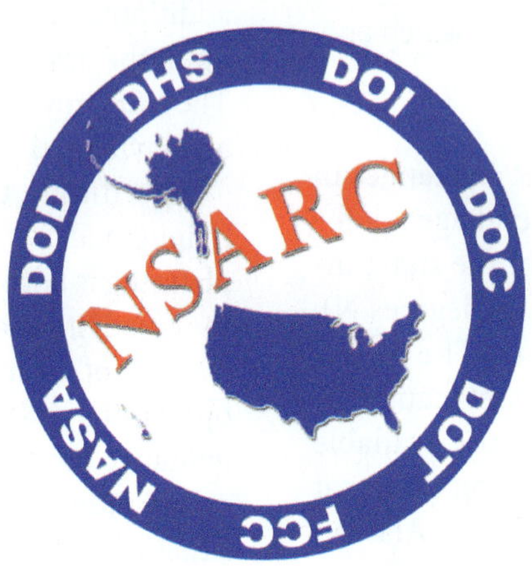

November 2011

Department of Homeland Security
Department of Interior
Department of Commerce
Department of Defense
Department of Transportation
National Aeronautics and Space Administration
Federal Communications Commission
(www.uscg.mil/nsarc)

FIGURE 2-7 Land SAR Addendum to the *National SAR Supplement to the IAMSAR Manual*.
Courtesy of National Search and Rescue Committee.

authorities and offer technical information and best practices for nonfederal SAR training, planning, and operations. The purpose of the document is "...to provide standardized guidance and information concerning land-based SAR operations" (NSARC, 2011, p. xxix).

The Land SAR Addendum emphasizes the importance of standardized search planning theory and describes two general categories of land SAR:

- Aeronautical SAR involving persons in distress in aircraft on or over land areas, particularly in wilderness areas
- Search and rescue of persons missing or in distress

The document describes the U.S. search and rescue system, land SAR resources and capabilities, communications, various types of searches, navigation systems, and search planning, and it is very detailed in its description of the various elements of search theory and their application to land search. In terms of search methodology, it provides a standard, easy-to-follow approach that has evolved from SAR mission experience and advances in search theory. In short, for SAR missions on land in the United States, this document provides the best guidance currently available.

Catastrophic Incident SAR Addendum to the National SAR Supplement

The tragedies of September 11, 2001, Hurricane Katrina in 2005, Hurricane Sandy in 2012, and other calamitous events continue to challenge federal, state, tribal, territorial, and local SAR responders in the planning and execution of large-scale SAR operations. NSARC realized the federal government's response to large-scale **catastrophic incident** SAR (CISAR) needed to improve. As a result, the CISAR Addendum to the NSS was developed to provide guidance for SAR operations during catastrophic incidents and to complement the overarching strategy for a national response to a catastrophic incident provided in the Catastrophic Incident Annex of the NRF (**FIGURE 2-8**). CISAR consists of civil SAR operations carried out as all or part of the response to an emergency or disaster declared by the president, under provisions of the NRF and its emergency support function (ESF) #9, Search and Rescue. This CISAR Addendum does not supersede other federal, state, tribal, or territorial SAR plans.

There are many different federal, state, tribal, territorial, and local SAR response cultures. Each possesses unique capabilities, language, and responsibilities. During a catastrophic incident, NSARC member departments and agencies are required to conduct multiagency SAR operations within a unified command (e.g., a command in which responding agencies and/or jurisdictions with responsibility for the incident share incident management). The CISAR Addendum is intended to (1) provide a concise description of the federal government's civil SAR response to catastrophic incidents; (2) guide federal authorities involved in the response; and (3) inform states, tribes, and territories about what to expect from federal SAR responders.

The primary federal agency responsible for CISAR operations depends on the nature of the SAR operation to be conducted. ESF #9 of the NRF lists FEMA and its urban search and rescue response system as being responsible for US&R; the USCG as being responsible for maritime, coastal, and waterborne SAR; and the U.S. Departments of the Interior (including the NPS) and Defense as being responsible for land SAR during a CISAR event. Regardless of which federal agency takes the lead, the primary agency works closely with the respective federal SAR coordinator in the affected area.

Comprehensive Emergency Management and Disaster Response

No discussion of any type of emergency service, including SAR, would be complete without at least a mention of the idea of comprehensive emergency management. In this concept, *emergency management* is an umbrella system that incorporates all aspects of dealing with emergencies and disasters.

Routine emergencies are daily situations faced by citizens and local emergency services personnel. For example, when fire fighters respond to a call, they are managing an emergency. When an EMS unit responds to a home or arrives at the scene of a traffic accident, the EMS unit is managing an emergency.

Emergency management programs at the local level are responsible for providing overall predisaster planning and other programs such as training and exercises for natural and human-caused disasters that can affect a community. They are the first line of defense in coordinating a large-scale event, such as a hurricane or an earthquake, in any community to ensure an effective response to, and recovery from, such events.

While responsibility for responding to emergencies and disasters begins at the local level, the next higher level of response (county, state, or national) is activated when resources and capabilities are exhausted. At the most basic level, if a homeowner cannot extinguish a fire, the homeowner will call the local fire department. If a local community is overwhelmed and cannot respond to a disaster, it asks the state for assistance. Similarly, when the state's resources are exhausted, it will turn to the federal government for assistance. In the United

CATASTROPHIC INCIDENT
SEARCH AND RESCUE ADDENDUM
to the
National Search and Rescue Supplement
to the
International Aeronautical and Maritime
Search and Rescue Manual

Version 3.0

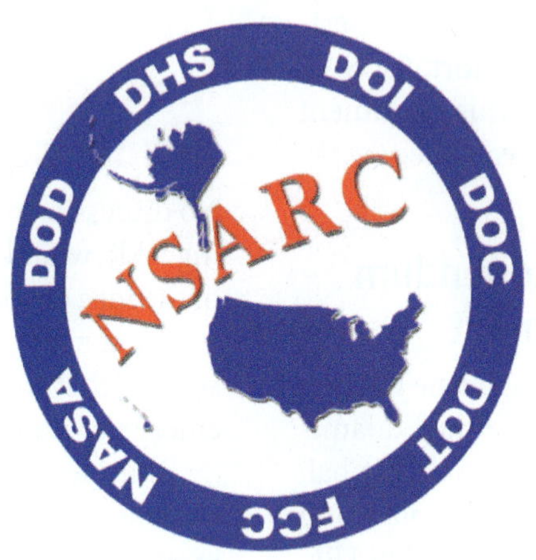

June, 2012

Department of Homeland Security
Department of Interior
Department of Commerce
Department of Defense
Department of Transportation
National Aeronautics and Space Administration
Federal Communications Commission
(www.uscg.mil/nsarc)

FIGURE 2-8 Catastrophic Incident SAR Addendum to the *National SAR Supplement to the IAMSAR Manual.*
Courtesy of National Search and Rescue Committee.

States, this relationship is spelled out in the *Robert T. Stafford Disaster Relief and Emergency Assistance Act*, as amended (Robert T. Stafford Disaster Relief and Emergency Assistance Act, 2013).

The concept used for handling all types of disasters and their consequences is called comprehensive emergency management (CEM). CEM was institutionalized in the United States with the creation of FEMA in 1979. Since that time, many state, local, and tribal governments have accepted CEM and changed the names of their organizations to include the words "emergency management." More importantly, the name change reflects a switch in orientation from preparedness for single hazards or narrowly defined categories of hazards toward an all-hazards approach—attack, natural, and human-made—to potential threats to life and property. The commonalities among all types of human-made and natural disasters suggest strongly that many of the same management strategies will apply to all such emergencies. In a real sense, planning for one means planning for all.

National Incident Management System

The **National Incident Management System (NIMS)**, updated in 2017, provides a systematic, proactive approach to guide departments and agencies at all levels of government, nongovernmental organizations, and the private sector to work together seamlessly during an incident. The idea is that it can be used to manage incidents involving all threats and hazards, regardless of cause, size, location, or complexity, to reduce loss of life and property and harm to the environment. NIMS works hand in hand with the **National Response Framework (NRF)**. NIMS provides the template for the management of incidents, whereas the NRF provides the structure and mechanisms for national-level policy for incident management. NIMS is also the essential foundation to the National Preparedness System and provides the template for the management of incidents and operations in support of all five National Planning Frameworks (prevention, protection, mitigation, response, and disaster recovery). The purpose of NIMS is to provide a common approach for managing incidents. The concepts it contains provide for a flexible but standardized set of incident management practices with emphasis on common principles, a consistent approach to operational structures and supporting mechanisms, and an integrated approach to resource management (DHS, 2017b).

Incidents typically begin and end locally, and they are managed daily at the lowest possible geographical, organizational, and jurisdictional level. There are other instances where success depends on the involvement of multiple jurisdictions, levels of government, functional agencies, and/or emergency responder disciplines. These instances necessitate effective and efficient coordination across this broad spectrum of organizations and activities. By using NIMS, communities are part of a comprehensive national approach that improves the effectiveness of emergency management and response personnel across the full spectrum of potential threats and hazards (including natural hazards, terrorist activities, and other human-caused disasters) regardless of size or complexity (DHS, 2017b).

Three major components make up the systematic approach to incident management: communications and information management, resource management, and command and coordination (DHS, 2017b, pp. 1-2). See Chapter 3, *Incident Management*, for more details on the command and management elements of NIMS.

National Response Framework

The *National Response Framework* (NRF), updated in 2016, is a guide that details how the United States responds to all types of disasters and emergencies, from the smallest local incident to the largest national catastrophe. The NRF describes structures for implementing nationwide response policy and operational coordination for all types of domestic incidents. It establishes a comprehensive, national, all-hazards approach to domestic incident response; identifies the roles and structures that organize national response; and follows these guiding principles:

- Engaged partnerships
- Tiered response
- Scalable, flexible, and adaptable operational capabilities
- Unity of effort through unified command
- Readiness to act

The document describes how communities, states, the federal government, and private sector and nongovernmental partners apply these principles for a coordinated, effective national response. In addition, it describes special circumstances in which the federal government exercises a larger role, including incidents in which federal interests are involved and catastrophic incidents for which a state would require significant support.

The NRF is organized into six parts:

- Roles and responsibilities
- Core capabilities
- Coordinating structures
- Relationships to other mission areas
- Operational planning
- Support resources

The NRF lays the groundwork for a unified national response and is intended to be used by the entire community, not just leaders and emergency responders. The idea is to enable a full range of stakeholders—individuals; families; communities; the private and nonprofit sectors; faith-based organizations; and local, state, tribal, territorial, insular area, and federal governments—to participate in national preparedness activities and to be full partners in incident response. This concept is based on the idea that government resources alone cannot meet all the needs of those affected by a **major disaster**. All elements of the community must be activated, engaged, and integrated to respond to a major or catastrophic incident.

The NRF is built on the same scalable, flexible, and adaptable concepts identified in NIMS and describes specific authorities and best practices for managing incidents that range from small to large and from local to national. The latest version of the NRF is easily located online.

U.S. National Preparedness System

Presidential Policy Directive (PPD) 8 directs the establishment of a national preparedness goal that identified the core capabilities necessary for preparedness and a national preparedness system to guide activities that will provide systematic preparation for national threats, including acts of terrorism, cyberattacks, pandemics, and catastrophic natural disasters. The National Preparedness System outlines an organized process for everyone in the whole community to move forward with their preparedness activities and achieve the National Preparedness Goal. The National Preparedness System has six parts (DHS, 2017):

- *Identifying and assessing risk*. This part involves collecting historical and recent data on existing, potential, and perceived threats and hazards. The results of these risk assessments form the basis for the remaining steps.
- *Estimating capability requirements*. Specific capabilities and activities are determined to best address the identified risks. Some capabilities may already exist, and some may need to be built or improved.
- *Building and sustaining capabilities*. This involves figuring out the best way to use limited resources to build capabilities. The risk assessment can be used to prioritize resources to address the highest probability or highest consequence threats.
- *Planning to deliver capabilities*. Because preparedness efforts involve and affect the whole community, it is important to coordinate plans with other organizations. This includes all parts of the whole community: individuals, businesses, nonprofits, community and faith-based groups, and all levels of government.
- *Validating capabilities*. Are efforts and activities working as intended? Participating in exercises, simulations, or other activities helps identify gaps in the plans and capabilities. It also helps see progress toward meeting preparedness goals.
- *Reviewing and updating*. It is important to regularly review and update all capabilities, resources, and plans. Risks and resources evolve, and so should preparedness efforts.

The **National Preparedness Goal (NPG)** is brief and succinct (DHS, 2015, p. 1):

> A secure and resilient nation with the capabilities required across the whole community to prevent, protect against, mitigate, respond to, and recover from the threats and hazards that pose the greatest risk.

The NPG document describes 41 activities—called *core capabilities*—that address the greatest risk to the United States. Each of these core capabilities is tied to a capability target and organized into five mission areas:

1. *Prevention*. Prevent, avoid, or stop an imminent, threatened, or actual act of terrorism.
2. *Protection*. Protect our citizens, residents, visitors, and assets against the greatest threats and hazards in a manner that allows our interests, aspirations, and way of life to thrive.
3. *Mitigation*. Reduce the loss of life and property by lessening the impact of future disasters.
4. *Response*. Respond quickly to save lives, protect property and the environment, and meet basic human needs in the aftermath of a catastrophic incident.
5. *Recovery*. Recover through a focus on the timely restoration, strengthening, and revitalization of infrastructure, housing, and a sustainable economy, as well as the health, social, cultural, historic, and environmental fabric of communities affected by a catastrophic incident.

The response mission of the NPG includes the capability of "Mass Search and Rescue Operations," which is described as follows (DHS, 2015, p. 16):

> Deliver traditional and atypical search and rescue capabilities, including personnel, services,

animals, and assets to survivors in need, with the goal of saving the greatest number of endangered lives in the shortest time possible.

There are three preliminary targets associated with this capability:

1. Conduct search and rescue operations to locate and rescue persons in distress, based on the requirements of state and local authorities.
2. Initiate community-based search and rescue support operations across a wide, geographically dispersed area.
3. Ensure the synchronized deployment of local, regional, national, and international teams to reinforce ongoing search and rescue efforts and transition to recovery.

The capability targets associated with the core capabilities are not targets for any single jurisdiction or agency; achieving these targets requires a national effort involving whole communities. In fact, each mission area relies on whole communities to ensure success.

For more information on the National Preparedness System, visit the FEMA website.

FEMA Urban Search and Rescue

FEMA serves as the coordinating agency for the NRF's ESF #9, Search and Rescue Annex. As such, FEMA coordinates the efforts of the four primary agencies that have responsibility, "to provide lifesaving assistance to local, state, tribal, territorial, and insular area authorities, including local SAR Coordinators and Mission Coordinators, when there is an actual or anticipated request for Federal SAR assistance" (DHS, 2016b, p. ESF#9-1). As mentioned earlier, the four federal primary agencies responsible for providing SAR support under the NRF are: (1) Department of Homeland Security United States Coast Guard (DHS/USCG), (2) FEMA Urban Search and Rescue (DHS/FEMA), (3) Department of Interior National Park Service (DoI/NPS), and (4) Department of Defense North American Command (DoD/NORTHCOM).

During times of natural or manmade disasters, the USCG is the lead agency for ESF #9 when maritime/coastal/waterborne areas are the primary search area—think hurricanes. When the disaster is urban based, FEMA US&R has the lead—think earthquakes, tornados, or building collapse. The NPS and DoD share joint responsibility for inland SAR support, defined as ". . .operations that require aviation and ground forces to meet mission objectives, other than maritime/coastal/waterborne and structural collapse [S&R] operations. . ." (DHS, 2016b, p. ESF#9-1).

A detailed description of the response capabilities of each of the four ESF #9 primary agencies is beyond this discussion. However, generally, the ESF #9 response elements of the USCG and NPS are assembled from units that perform search and rescue on a day-to-day basis within their assigned areas of operation. The military's response elements are assembled from across the United States and function under doctrine identified in the military's Defense Support of Civil Authorities (DSCA) mission. The 28 task forces of the FEMA National US&R Response System respond under a three-way partnership among the agency that is the sponsoring agency of the task force, the state in which the task force is located, and FEMA.

More information on how the four agencies come together and function in a joint approach to providing search and rescue support is available in the *Catastrophic Incident Search and Rescue Addendum to the National Search and Rescue Supplement* (NSARC, 2009) and the *Response Federal Interagency Operational Plan* (DHS, 2014).

Anatomy of an Urban-Based Search and Rescue Mission

While every disaster assignment is unique, a US&R mission might go something like this:

1. Response always begins at the local level; local rescuers always respond first. If the emergency is great enough, the state can request support from FEMA for federal SAR support or directly from other states through the EMAC (see below).
2. Following the disaster, the local emergency manager requests assistance from the state. If the state chooses to request federal assistance, FEMA coordinates with the four ESF #9 primary agencies to choose the best response element for the requesting state's needs. In an urban environment, this is likely a FEMA US&R task force. FEMA will deploy the requested number of task forces to fill the state's request based on the nearest task forces to the incident location.
3. After the task force arrives at the incident, a reconnaissance (recon) element (consisting of a structural engineer and search, hazmat, and rescue specialists) assesses the assigned area of operation. The engineer and specialists provide direct input to the task force leader (TFL) about structural integrity of the building(s) and the risk of secondary collapses, any identified hazards, the potential to find live victims, and any complications for initiating rescue operations.
4. Following the TFL's authorization, a search for live victims is initiated at the structure. The search

team ventures around and into the collapsed structure attempting to locate trapped victims. A live find canine traverses the structure first. If the canine alerts on a live victim, a second canine is used to confirm the live find. If both canines alert, technical search specialists deploy various methods, including electronic listening devices and search cameras, to pinpoint the victim's location.

5. Once a victim is located, one or two rescue squads (i.e., a squad leader and five rescue specialists) begin the daunting task of breaking and cutting through what may be thousands of pounds of concrete, metal, and wood to reach the victim(s). They also stabilize and support the entry and work areas with wood shoring to prevent further collapse. They may also elect to remove (de-layer) portions of the collapsed structure to access the victim(s).
6. Once an entrapped victim is reached, a medical team, composed of an emergency medicine physician and an emergency medicine/trauma nurse or paramedic with advanced life support training, begins patient care while the final extrication of the victim is completed. Following extrication of the victim from the structure, medical care is continued by the task force's medical staff until the patient is transferred to definitive medical care such as a local hospital or a Health and Human Services (HHS) disaster medical assistance team (DMAT).
7. Throughout the rescue effort, task force hazardous materials specialists (HMS) evaluate the rescue area for the presence of hazardous materials (e.g., chemicals, radiation, biological materials/human waste, or human remains) that may be associated with the structure or disaster. The HMS also monitors the air quality where the rescue and medical personnel are working for presence of sufficient oxygen or a build-up of poisonous or explosive gases. The HMS also completes or supervises the decontamination of rescue and medical team members and any victim(s) removed from the collapse.
8. Should the effort to extricate a victim include the removal of materials overlying the victim, a task force heavy equipment and rigging specialist (HERS) will direct the use of heavy machinery, such as cranes, frontend loaders, and bulldozers, to remove the material. The HERS understands the special dangers of working in a collapsed structure and that removing one piece of collapsed material may cause another to move. The HERS is often assisted by the task force structural engineer.
9. Technical information specialists (TIS) ensure that task force operations are recorded and documented for reporting to higher authorities at the completion of the operational period. The TIS also assists the task force's planning team manager (PTM) to coordinate the task force's future operations with the local authority's incident management team/IC, and to prepare internal task force work documents for the next operational period.
10. Task force operations and support needs are met by a team of logistics specialists (LS) that handle and maintain the more than 29,000 pieces of equipment and 15 vehicles that comprise a FEMA Type I US&R task force. Additionally, the health and welfare needs of the 80 team members of the Type I task force are met by the LS through their maintaining the task force's base of operations (BoO). The task force BoO includes shower and sleeping facilities, toiletries, food, and drinking water. FEMA task forces are required to be self-sufficient for the first 72 hours of operations and then be able to maintain operational tempo for up to 10 days with limited resupply.
11. FEMA task forces are also fully self-sufficient for communications. The task force communication specialist (CS) ensures that all team members can communicate with each other, adjacent FEMA task forces or ESF #9 partner agencies, and the local authority having jurisdiction (AHJ). The CS is responsible for programming and maintaining a cache of DHS portable and mobile radios, two repeater networks, a wireless Internet network, and a robust satellite communications cache.

The FEMA US&R Response System is designed to provide a coordinated response to disasters in the urban environment. Special emphasis is placed on the capability to locate and extricate victims trapped in collapsed structures, primarily of reinforced concrete and steel construction. However, the most common deployment of FEMA US&R task forces is to conduct search and rescue operations over a wide area following disasters that affect a large geographic area; examples include F4 or F5 tornados, hurricanes, and widespread flooding.

The following operations are typical of what FEMA US&R teams conduct:

- Physical and technical search and rescue operations in damaged collapsed structures
- Physical and canine search and rescue operations over wide areas of urban environments
- Emergency medical care to both task force response personnel and entrapped/found victims

- Reconnaissance to assess damage and provide feedback to local, state, and federal officials
- Assessment/shut-off of utilities to buildings
- Hazardous materials surveys/evaluations
- Structural/hazard evaluations of buildings needed for immediate occupancy to support disaster relief operations
- Stabilizing damaged structures, including necessary shoring and cribbing.

Prior to the chemical, biological, radiological, nuclear, and high-yield explosive (CBRNE) upgrade of the FEMA task forces after September 11, 2001, the minimum personnel complement of a FEMA US&R Type I task force was 62 people. With the addition of eight hazardous materials specialists to support the CBRNE mission, the total increased to 70 personnel. In 2004, the system added 10 ground support specialist (GSS) positions (drivers of the various very large vehicles required to deploy a FEMA task force), making the authorized complement 80 personnel for a Type I task force. Then, in 2012, FEMA added a new mission for the task forces: water rescue. FEMA's 80-person Type I task forces now include 14 water rescue specialists (WRS) cross-trained to the technician-level water rescue standards of NFPA 1006, *Standard for Technical Rescue Personnel Professional Qualifications* (NFPA, 2017) (**FIGURE 2-9**). Additionally, in 2012, FEMA allowed task forces that wanted to add canine human remains detection capability to their teams the ability to do so. As of this writing, this is not a requirement of a FEMA task force, and only some of the task forces have elected to build this capability.

Each of the positions within a Type I task force has an even number of personnel filling the position. This ensures the position is filled for both day and night operations.

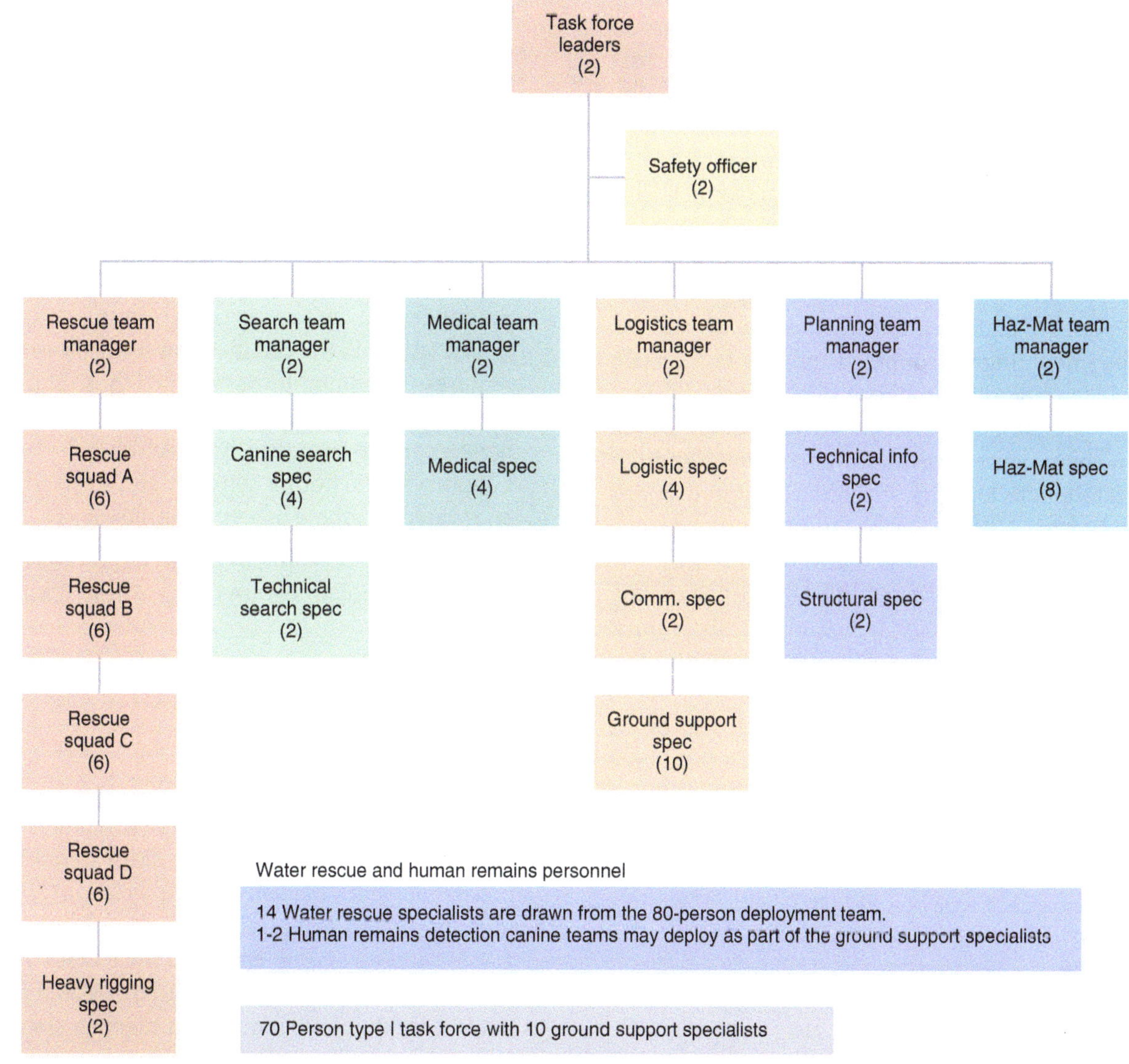

FIGURE 2-9 FEMA Type I Urban SAR task force organization (with WMD upgrade).

To ensure there are always 80 personnel available to deploy at any given time, FEMA requires task forces to maintain three-deep staffing in all deployment positions, or 210 total team members: 70 deployment personnel (excluding ground support specialists) × 3 deep.

Task force personnel are drawn from a combination of local fire and police departments, federal and local governmental agencies, and the private sector (typically physicians, nurses, engineers, and canine handlers)—a true partnership of local, state, federal, and private organizations. Each member of the task force must complete hundreds of hours of general and specialized intensive training and demonstrate the maintenance of their skills on a yearly basis. Specialties in the canine, structural, logistics, and medical positions require 1- to 3-year renewals of their certifications or licenses to remain deployable.

A task force is designed to be self-sufficient for the first 72 hours of operation and to be able to function for up to 10 days before being replaced. Members of the task force divide into two groups and operate in 12-hour shifts on the scene. One group works while the other group rests. All task force members must be sufficiently cross-trained in their skill areas to ensure depth of capability and integrated task force operations. By design, there are two personnel assigned to each identified task force position for the rotation and relief of personnel. This allows for round-the-clock task force operation.

The equipment cache used to support this capability weighs approximately 50,000 pounds, includes more than 29,000 pieces of equipment, is worth about $5 million, and fills (including personnel) a military C-5 or two C-17 (depending on number of vehicles transported) transport aircraft. The equipment cache consists of seven types of equipment: medical, search, rescue, planning/technical support, logistics (including communication's cache), hazmat/CBRNE cache, and the water rescue cache (including boats, motors, and water PPE).

Each task force is designed to be able to be rapidly deployed in an emergency; hence, all members must meet a 4-hour window for mobilization. Depending on the location of the disaster, a task force will respond to the scene either by ground using its own trucks or via a military or civilian aircraft. In general, a task force can be at the scene of a disaster within 12 to 24 hours of activation anywhere in the contiguous United States.

When the task forces are not on a FEMA-requested response, they function as technical rescue teams in their own communities and at the state level as regional or statewide rescue teams.

SEARCH AND RESCUE TIP

Technical rescuers wishing to meet the NFPA 1006 job performance requirements (JPRs) for wilderness search and rescue at the awareness, operations, or technician level should review Chapter 10 of NFPA 1006 (2017). Responders should meet the JPRs in Sections 10.1 for the awareness level, 10.2 for the operations level, and 10.3 for the technician level.

US&R Canine (K-9) Team Evaluation/Certification

Canine teams used as part of a US&R team (dog and handler) must be well trained and certified by FEMA. Some characteristics of this certification include the following:

- Each FEMA US&R canine/handler team must be certified in search and rescue.
- For the handler, certification includes written and verbal tests regarding search and rescue strategies, briefing and debriefing skills, and canine handling skills.
- For the search and rescue canine, certification includes proper command control, agility skills, barking alert skills to notify rescuers of a find, and willingness to overcome innate fears of tunnels and wobbly surfaces under the guidance of the handler.
- There are two levels of certification for the FEMA US&R canine/handler team. Initial certification, Fundamental Skills Ability (FSA), requires the canine to demonstrate obedience and directional ability under the handler's direct supervision and guidance. Advanced certification, Certification Evaluation (CE, the certification for deployability), requires the canine to perform to those standards outside the direct supervision and guidance of the handler and to successfully search and alert on live human scent in both a concrete and a mixed wood and concrete rubble pile environment.
- Canine/handler teams must be re-certified every 3 years to maintain deployability within the FEMA US&R system.

Emergency Management Assistance Compact

EMAC is a national interstate mutual aid agreement that enables states to share resources during a governor-declared emergency or disaster. EMAC is administered by the National Emergency Management Association (NEMA), headquartered in Lexington, Kentucky.

EMAC acts as a complement to the federal disaster response system, providing timely and cost-effective relief to states requesting assistance from member states that understand the needs of jurisdictions that are struggling to preserve life, the economy, and the environment. EMAC can be used either in lieu of federal assistance or in conjunction with federal assistance, thus providing a seamless flow of needed goods and services to an impacted state. EMAC further provides another venue for mitigating resource deficiencies by ensuring maximum use of all available resources within member states' inventories.

Because legislation must be passed by the states involved in the system, once the conditions for aiding a requesting state have been set, the terms constitute a legally binding contractual agreement that makes affected states responsible for reimbursement. The EMAC legislation solves the problems of liability and responsibilities of cost and allows for credentials, licenses, and certifications to be honored across state lines.

How EMAC Works

Requesting and deploying resources is done at the discretion of the impacted (requesting) state, allowing them the ability to pick what they need and for what price. The responding (assisting) state has to offer assistance only if they have the resources and can deploy them. At all times, impacted states retain the choice of seeking resource support from either state or federal, or both, as may be appropriate for their circumstances. Local resources can be deployed under EMAC if the state has adopted intrastate legislation. The EMAC process is outlined below.

1. An EMAC authorized representative confirms the declaration of emergency by the governor.
2. The state assesses needs for resources.
3. The state determines whether it needs an external EMAC A-Team to assist with acquisition of resources or whether it will use its in-state EMAC A-Team and acquire an external A-Team if needed.
4. The state determines the best source for needed resources (EMAC, federal, private sector, etc.).
5. EMAC A-Teams request resources by one or all of the following methodologies:
    a. The team may have direct contact with the state (knows the resource and can go directly to the state that has it—often a recurring mission).
    b. An EMAC resource request is made utilizing the EMAC emergency operations system (EOS) broadcast functionality. States may request broadcast by region (FEMA regions), two regions, or three regions; an individual state; or an individual EMAC-authorized representative or EMAC-designated contact within a state.
    c. Agencies within the states may refer requests and suggested resources to the state emergency management agency for their follow-up.
6. EMAC A-Teams determine cost and availability of resources.
7. The EMAC REQ-A Form is completed by the EMAC-authorized representatives from both the requesting state and the assisting state.
8. Resources are mobilized from the assisting state to the requesting state.
9. Resources check in at state staging areas and deployment locations, and missions are confirmed.
10. Resources complete the mission, relaying any issues back to their home state emergency management agency.
11. Resources are demobilized.
12. Assisting states complete the reimbursement request and, after internal audit, send it to the requesting state.
13. The requesting state reimburses the assisting state.

For more information about EMAC, visit EMAC's or NEMA's website or your state emergency management agency.

Miscellaneous SAR Tools

Three tools are available that can be of great value during a SAR response, and two of them are of particular value when children are the subject of a search: The AMBER Alert Program and The National Center for Missing & Exploited Children.

The AMBER Alert Program™

The AMBER (America's Missing Broadcast Emergency Response) Alert™ program is a voluntary partnership among law enforcement agencies, broadcasters, transportation agencies, and the wireless industry to activate an urgent bulletin in the most serious child abduction cases. The goal of an AMBER Alert is to instantly galvanize the entire community to assist in the search for, and the safe recovery of, the child.

The AMBER Alert program was created in 1996 as a legacy to 9-year-old Amber Hagerman, a little girl who was kidnapped while riding her bicycle and was brutally murdered in Arlington, Texas. The tragedy shocked and outraged the entire community. Residents contacted radio stations in the Dallas area and suggested they broadcast special "alerts" over the airwaves so that they could help prevent such incidents in the future. In response to the community's concern for the safety of local children, the Dallas/Fort Worth Association of Radio Managers teamed up with local law enforcement agencies in northern Texas and developed this innovative early warning system to help find abducted children. Statistics show that when a child is abducted, time is critical.

Once law enforcement determines that a child has been abducted and the abduction meets AMBER Alert criteria, law enforcement issues an AMBER Alert and notifies broadcasters and state transportation officials. AMBER Alerts interrupt regular programming and are broadcast on radio and television and on highway signs. AMBER Alerts can also be issued on lottery tickets, wireless devices such as mobile phones, and over the Internet. Each state program establishes its own AMBER Alert criteria; however, most states' guidelines adhere closely to the U.S Department of Justice guidance on criteria for issuing AMBER Alerts:

- Law enforcement has confirmed that an abduction has occurred.
- The child is in imminent danger of serious bodily injury or death.
- There is sufficient descriptive information of the child, captor, or captor's vehicle to issue an alert.
- The abduction is of a child aged 17 years or younger.
- The child's name and other critical data elements, including the Child Abduction flag, are immediately entered into the FBI's National Crime Information Center (NCIC) system.

If these criteria are met, the alert is issued and distributed by broadcasters, transportation agencies, and through the Emergency Alert System (EAS). They are also sent to the National Center for Missing & Exploited Children, which redistributes the alerts, per a request by the U.S. Department of Justice, to a network of secondary distributors that includes Internet service providers, digital billboards, truckers, and others. The messages are intended as a supplement to the existing EAS, which broadcasts alerts over radio and television. Radio stations interrupt programming to announce the AMBER Alert, and television stations and cable systems run a "crawl" on the screen, along with a picture of the child. Many states now also incorporate electronic highway billboards in their AMBER Alert programs. The billboards, typically used to disseminate traffic information to drivers, now alert the public of abducted children, displaying pertinent information about the child, abductor, or suspected vehicle that drivers might look for on highways.

AMBER Alerts are distributed to cell phones as part of the AMBER Alert program's secondary distribution through the Wireless Emergency Alert (WEA) program, which is also known as the Commercial Mobile Alert System. The WEA program is operated by FEMA. It distributes notifications from authorized federal, state, local, and tribal government agencies that alert customers with capable devices of imminent threats to safety or an emergency situation. The alerts are transmitted simultaneously to all mobile devices within range of the cellular carrier towers in the affected area. The system does not need to know your mobile number, and it does not track your whereabouts; it simply broadcasts the alert, and any mobile devices that can "hear" the alert will display it.

To learn more about the AMBER Alert program, visit the U.S. Department of Justice's AMBER Alert website.

National Center for Missing & Exploited Children®

The National Center for Missing & Exploited Children (NCMEC) works in partnership with the U.S. Department of Justice to help law enforcement find missing children, eliminate child sexual exploitation, and prevent child victimization. NCMEC also assists law enforcement in the prosecution of the criminals who perpetrate these terrible crimes and is authorized by Congress to perform 22 specific tasks described in 42 U.S.C. § 5773.

NCMEC has grown to a team of 350 employees and more than 200 volunteers that make up a high-tech organization with global reach and, most importantly, success. Most NCMEC work is conducted, developed, analyzed, and completed on-site at its headquarters in Alexandria, Virginia, using state-of-the-art technology; highly trained professionals; and committed staff, interns, and volunteers. Two of the many services provided by NCMEC are Team Adam and Project ALERT®.

Team Adam

Named after Adam Walsh, a 6-year-old boy who was abducted and murdered, Team Adam is a resource for law enforcement provided by the NCMEC. Patterned after the National Transportation Safety Board's system for sending trained specialists to the site of serious transportation incidents, Team Adam does the same thing in serious child abduction and child sexual victimization cases. It is an on-site response and support system that provides assistance to local law enforcement agencies and families in serious cases of missing children.

Team Adam comprises a team of specialists who are on call to respond directly to the scene of these incidents. The specialists are chosen based on their expertise and geographic home base to minimize response time and travel costs. Included in the team are retired FBI agents and retired police officers from agencies around the country. NCMEC provides intensive training to ensure that each specialist is prepared to perform the tasks required in a uniform and consistent manner. The specialists work in full coordination with federal, state, and local law enforcement agencies. They advise, assist, and offer NCMEC's extensive resources, including direct access to NCMEC's case management and case analysis systems, lead analysis, and data mining services. If needed, NCMEC also equips the law enforcement agency with computer and communications technology to enable rapid distribution of key information to other agencies and personnel. They are prepared and authorized to provide additional assistance to the investigators, the victim's family, and the media as appropriate.

Team Adam is necessary because time is the enemy in missing child cases. According to a study by the State of Washington's Office of the Attorney General, in 74% of child abduction homicides, the homicides occurred within the first 3 hours after the abduction (Hanfland, Keppel, and Weiss, 1997). Offenders who sexually assault and murder children can do so repeatedly. Rapid capture and prosecution is the best possible remedy. Rapid response is a key factor that correlates directly to the recovery of a child, who is still alive, after being taken by nonfamily abductors.

With 18,000 state and local law enforcement agencies in the United States, some agencies may not be familiar with all available resources. Team Adam helps to ensure a quick and thorough response to these cases, helps to ensure that law enforcement knows of and has access to the best tools and latest technology, and greatly improves the odds of a successful recovery of the victim and prosecution of the assailant.

Project ALERT®

Project ALERT is a team of approximately 170 retired local, state, and federal law enforcement professionals who donate their time and experience to the law enforcement community. Although some members are no longer sworn investigators, they all share their abilities, knowledge, and experience through the Project ALERT program (NCMEC, 2015).

Project ALERT representatives provide technical assistance to law enforcement agencies regarding missing children investigations. They specialize in long-term missing children cases and perform a wide range of functions, including:

- Case review
- Organization and analysis
- Recommendation of investigative strategies
- Follow-up of leads
- Coordination of meetings with law enforcement personnel to discuss additional resources

Project ALERT helps law enforcement access the most current forensic methods to help increase the likelihood of identifying missing children. They integrate NCMEC resources such as age progression, facial reconstruction, poster distribution, DNA protocol, search specialists, and database searches into the investigations. ALERT representatives also collect biometrics and information about missing children and unidentified remains to help supply critical data to the National Missing and Unidentified Persons System, also known as NamUs, and National Crime Information Center databases.

SEARCH AND RESCUE TIP

If My Child Is Missing: Advice from The National Center for Missing & Exploited Children

Act immediately if you believe that your child is missing.

If your child is missing from home, search the house, checking closets, piles of laundry, in and under beds, inside old refrigerators—wherever a child may crawl or hide.

If you still cannot find your child, *immediately call your local law enforcement agency*.

If your child disappears in a store, notify the store manager or security office. Then *immediately call your local law enforcement agency*. Many stores have a Code Adam plan of action—if a child is missing in the store, employees immediately mobilize to look for the missing child. Some stores lock all outside doors until the child is located.

When you call law enforcement, provide your child's name, date of birth, height, weight, and any other unique identifiers such as eyeglasses and braces. Tell them when you noticed that your child was missing and what clothing he or she was wearing. Request that your child's name and identifying information be immediately entered into the National Crime Information Center (NCIC) Missing Person File.

After you have reported your child missing to law enforcement, call the National Center for Missing & Exploited Children on their toll-free telephone number, 1-800-THE-LOST (1-800-843-5678). If your computer is equipped with a microphone and speakers, you may talk to one of the Hotline operators via the Internet.

Unmanned Aircraft Systems

A new area of focus that intersects SAR with the FAA is with unmanned aircraft systems (UAS) or drones. Some local jurisdictions have been using these for SAR on a limited basis for many years, but their increasing use and scrutiny by the FAA and other agencies has brought new attention and concern. UAS can be a very effective SAR tool because they can provide less costly (than a helicopter) aerial assets for a search. Advancement and miniaturization of visual optics, thermal imaging, and forward-looking infrared (FLIR) can be placed on UAS platforms for very effective searching. There is growing concern, however, that as the use of UAS become more prevalent in SAR, personal use, law enforcement, and wildlife management, there is potential for UAS to be used to violate personal liberties or to interfere with general aviation/commercial aircraft.

Current armed conflicts have provided the U.S. military extensive experience in the use of UAS in military controlled airspace. Small, personal UAS platforms in general use have limitations that larger, more durable UAS platforms have overcome. These larger platforms are currently required to operate under an FAA Certificate of Waiver or Authorization (COA) when flying alongside other airspace users (USDOT FAA, 2015b). UAS are evolving from traditional personal remote-controlled vehicles to an effective search tool, but they require appropriate regulation and control. SAR techniques are being tested that use crowdsourcing to help put "more eyes on the ground" through remote viewing of UAS video feeds. In some cases, using UAS may provide a lower risk option than a crewed aircraft, but separation between all aircraft must be maintained at all times.

Wrap-Up

READY FOR REVIEW

- Working together, the International Civil Aviation Organization (ICAO) and the International Maritime Organization (IMO) coordinate, on a global basis, member countries' efforts to provide search and rescue (SAR) services.
- The *IAMSAR Manual* describes a series of five stages of a SAR operation through which most SAR events pass: awareness, initial action, planning, operations, and conclusion.
- The international humanitarian SAR system COSPAS-SARSAT uses a network of satellites, ground stations, mission control centers, and rescue coordination centers to detect and locate emergency beacons carried by ships, aircraft, or individuals.
- The U.S. *National Search and Rescue Plan* (NSP) was developed primarily to provide guidance to signatory federal agencies for coordinating civil SAR services to meet domestic needs and international commitments.
- The National SAR Committee (NSARC) is responsible for coordinating and improving federal involvement in civil SAR for the aeronautical, maritime, and land communities within the United States.
- The National Incident Management System (NIMS) provides a systematic, proactive approach to guide departments and agencies at all levels of government, nongovernmental organizations, and the private sector to work together seamlessly during an incident.
- The three major components to incident management are communications and information management, resource management, and command and coordination.
- The *National Response Framework* (NRF) details how the United States responds to all types of disasters and emergencies, from the smallest local incident to the largest national catastrophe.
- The Emergency Management Assistance Compact (EMAC), a national mutual aid agreement, acts as a complement to the federal disaster response system, providing timely and cost-effective relief to states requesting assistance.
- The AMBER Alert™ Program is a voluntary partnership among law enforcement agencies, broadcasters, transportation agencies, and the wireless industry to activate an urgent bulletin in the most serious child abduction cases.
- The National Center for Missing & Exploited Children (NCMEC) works in partnership with the U.S. Department of Justice to help law enforcement find missing children, eliminate child sexual exploitation, and prevent child victimization.
- A new area of focus that intersects SAR with the FAA is use of unmanned aircraft systems (UAS) or drones. UAS can be a very effective SAR tool because they can provide less costly (than a helicopter) aerial assets for a search.

SEARCH AND RESCUE TERMS

Catastrophic incident Any natural or manmade incident, including terrorism, that results in extraordinary levels of mass casualties, damage, or disruption severely affecting the population, infrastructure, environment, economy, national morale, or government functions (DHS, 2016a, p. 1).

Emergency locator transmitters (ELTs) An emergency radio beacon that usually operates on both 121.5 MHz and 406 MHz; used by most aircraft.

Emergency position indicating radio beacons (EPIRBs) A distress radio beacon for use in maritime applications; used to alert search and rescue services in the event of an emergency. It does this by transmitting a coded message on the 406-MHz distress frequency via satellite and Earth stations to the nearest rescue coordination center. Some EPIRBs also have built-in GPS, which enables the rescue services to more accurately locate the device.

International conventions Written agreements between countries, used to establish rules between them.

Major disaster As defined under the Robert T. Stafford Disaster Relief and Emergency Assistance Act (42 U.S.C. 5122), "any natural catastrophe (including any hurricane, tornado, storm, high water, wind-driven water, tidal wave, tsunami, earthquake, volcanic eruption, landslide, mudslide, snowstorm, or drought), or, regardless of cause, any fire, flood, or explosion, in any part of the United States, which in the determination of the President causes damage of sufficient severity and magnitude to warrant major disaster assistance under this Act to supplement the efforts and available resources of States, tribes, local governments, and disaster relief organizations in alleviating the damage, loss, hardship, or suffering caused thereby" (Robert T. Stafford Disaster Relief and Emergency Assistance Act, 2013).

National Incident Management System (NIMS) "A consistent, flexible, and adjustable national framework within which government and private entities at all levels can work together to manage domestic incidents, regardless of their size, location, or complexity" (DHS, 2008).

National Preparedness Goal U.S. national goal established secondary to Presidential Policy Directive 8 (2011) that identifies the core capabilities necessary for preparedness and a national preparedness system to guide activities that will provide systematic preparation for national threats including acts of terrorism, cyberattacks, pandemics, and catastrophic natural disasters (DHS, 2015). The goal itself is "A secure and resilient nation with the capabilities required across the whole community to prevent, protect against, mitigate, respond to, and recover from the threats and hazards that pose the greatest risk" (DHS, 2015, p. 1).

National Response Framework (NRF) "A guide to how the United States responds to all types of disasters and emergencies. It is built on scalable, flexible, and adaptable concepts identified in the National Incident Management System (NIMS) to align key roles and responsibilities across the Nation. The NRF describes specific authorities and best practices for managing incidents that range from the serious but purely local to large-scale terrorist attacks or catastrophic natural disasters." This framework is always in effect, and elements can be implemented at any time (DHS, 2016a).

Personal locator beacons (PLBs) Portable units that operate much the same as EPIRBs or ELTs. They are designed to be carried by an individual person instead of on a boat or aircraft.

Positive control "The separation of all air traffic within designated airspace by air traffic control" (USDOT FAA, 2015a).

Rescue coordination center (RCC) A unit, recognized by a cognizant international body, responsible for promoting efficient organization of SAR services and for coordinating the conduct of SAR operations within a Search and Rescue Region (SRR) (IMO/ICAO, 2016).

Search and rescue coordinator "As defined in the IAMSAR Manual, one or more persons or agencies within an Administration with overall responsibility for establishing and providing SAR services, and ensuring that planning for those services is properly coordinated" (NSARC, 2016, p. 2).

Search and rescue region (SRR) "An area of defined dimensions, associated with a rescue coordination center (RCC), within which SAR services are provided" (IMO/ICAO, 2016)***.

REFERENCES AND SUGGESTED READING

Federal Aviation Administration, U.S. Department of Transportation. 2017. *Aeronautical Information Manual: Official Guide to Basic Flight Information and ATC Procedures* (AIM). https://www.faa.gov/air_traffic/publications/media/AIM_Basic_dtd_10-12-17.pdf

Federal Emergency Management Agency. 2018. Incident command system resources. https://www.fema.gov/incident-command-system-resources.

Hanfland, Kenneth A., Robert D. Keppel, and Joseph G. Weiss. 1997. *Case management for missing children homicide investigation: Executive summary*. Olympia, Washington: Office of the Attorney General, State of Washington, and U.S. Department of Justice's Office of Juvenile Justice and Delinquency Prevention, May 1997.

International Maritime Organization and International Civil Aviation Organization. 2016. *International Aeronautical and*

*** Material from the IMO publications IAMSAR Manual Volumes I, II and III (2016 - II960E/IF961E/II962E and 2013 - IH960E/IE961E and IH962E) and/or the IMO website www.imo.org is reproduced with the permission of the International Maritime Organization (IMO), which does not accept responsibility for the correctness of the material as reproduced: in case of doubt, IMO's authentic text shall prevail. Readers should check with their national maritime Administration for any further amendments or latest advice. International Maritime Organization, 4 Albert Embankment, London, SE1 7SR, United Kingdom.

Maritime Search and Rescue Manual: Vol. I. Organization and Management, Vol. II. Mission Co-ordination, Vol. III. Mobile Facilities. London/Montreal: The International Maritime Organization (IMO) and the International Civil Aviation Organization (ICAO).

Iridium Communications, Inc. 2015. Website: Iridium GO!®. https://www.iridium.com/products/iridium-go/.

National Center for Missing & Exploited Children. 2015. Website. http://www.missingkids.com/.

National Fire Protection Association. 2017. NFPA 1006: *Standard for Technical Rescue Personnel Professional Qualifications.* Quincy, MA: NFPA.

National Oceanic and Atmospheric Administration. 2015. National Environmental Satellite, Data and Information Service, Search and Rescue Satellite-Aided Tracking (SARSAT). http://www.sarsat.noaa.gov/.

National Search and Rescue Committee. 2018. NSARC website. https://www.dco.uscg.mil/Our-Organization/Assistant-Commandant-for-Response-Policy-CG-5R/Office-of-Incident-Management-Preparedness-CG-5RI/US-Coast-Guard-Office-of-Search-and-Rescue-CG-SAR/NSARC/.

National Search and Rescue Committee. November 2011. *Land SAR Addendum to the National Search and Rescue Supplement to the International Aeronautical and Maritime Search and Rescue Manual*, Version 1.0. https://www.dco.uscg.mil/Portals/9/CG-5R/nsarc/Land_SAR_Addendum/Published_Land%20SAR%20Addendum%20(1118111)%20-%20Bookmark.pdf.

National Search and Rescue Committee. June 2012. Catastrophic incident SAR addendum to the national SAR supplement to the IAMSAR Manual (CISAR), version 3.0, Washington, DC, November 2012. https://www.dco.uscg.mil/Portals/9/CG-5R/nsarc/CISAR%20Addendum%20-%20Version%203-0%20(062112)%20Final.pdf.

National Search and Rescue Committee. 2016. *United States National Search and Rescue Plan.* Washington, DC.: U.S. Superintendent of Documents. https://www.dco.uscg.mil/Portals/9/CG-5R/manuals/National_SAR_Plan_2016.pdf

National Search and Rescue Committee. 2000. *United States National Search and Rescue Supplement to the International Aeronautical and Maritime Search and Rescue Manual.* Washington, DC.: U.S. Superintendent of Documents. https://www.dco.uscg.mil/Portals/9/CG-5R/manuals/Natl_SAR_Supp.pdf

Robert T. Stafford Disaster Relief and Emergency Assistance Act. 2013. 42 U.S.C. 5121, et seq., as amended by the *Disaster Mitigation Act of 2000*, Pub. L. 106-390, 114 Stat. 1552, and the *Sandy Recovery Improvement Act* of 2013, Pub. L. 113-2, 127 Stat. 4 (the Stafford Act).

Setnicka Tim J. 1980. Wilderness search and rescue. Boston, MA: Appalachian Mountain Club.

U.S. Air Force. 2015. 1st Air Force, Air Force Rescue Coordination Center (AFRCC) website. http://www.1af.acc.af.mil/units/afrcc/.

U.S. Coast Guard: U.S. Coast Guard. 2015. U.S. Coast Guard website, *About us.* http://www.uscg.mil/top/about/.

U.S. Coast Guard. 2015. U.S. Coast Guard AMVER website. http://www.amver.com/.

U.S. Department of Homeland Security. 2017a. *National Preparedness System.* Washington, DC.: U.S. Department of Homeland Security. https://www.fema.gov/national-preparedness-system.

U.S. Department of Homeland Security. 2017b. *Response Federal Interagency Operational Plan.* Washington, DC.: U.S. Department of Homeland Security. https://www.fema.gov/media-library/assets/documents/97362.

U.S. Department of Homeland Security. 2016a. *National Response Framework.* Third Edition. Washington, DC.: U.S. Department of Homeland Security. https://www.fema.gov/media-library-data/1466014682982-9bcf8245ba4c60c120aa915abe74e15d/National_Response_Framework3rd.pdf.

U.S. Department of Homeland Security. 2016b. *Emergency Support Function #9 – Search and Rescue Annex [to the National Response Framework].* Washington, DC.: U.S. Department of Homeland Security, June 2016. https://www.fema.gov/media-library-data/1470149567157-f1dc17ef606b8b82629bacf1c358dd55/ESF_9_Search_and_Rescue_Annex_20160705_508.pdf.

U.S. Department of Homeland Security. 2015. *National Preparedness Goal, Second Edition.* Washington, DC.: U.S. Department of Homeland Security. http://www.fema.gov/national-preparedness-goal.

U.S. Department of Homeland Security, U.S. Fire Administration. 2018. *An Overview of Incident Management Teams.* Washington, DC.: U.S. Fire Administration. https://www.usfa.fema.gov/training/imt/imt_overview.html.

U.S. Department of Homeland Security. 2017c. *National Incident Management System* (NIMS), Third Edition. Washington, DC.: U.S. Department of Homeland Security. http://www.fema.gov/media-library-data/1508151197225-ced8c60378c3936adb92c1a3ee6f6564/FINAL_NIMS_2017.pdf.

U.S. Department of Justice Office of Justice Programs. 2018. Amber Alert. http://www.amberalert.gov.

U.S. Department of Transportation, Federal Aviation Administration. 2015a. FAA website: About the FAA. http://www.faa.gov/about/.

U.S. Department of Transportation, Federal Aviation Administration. 2015b. COA: Frequently asked questions. https://www.faa.gov/about/office_org/headquarters_offices/ato/service_units/systemops/aaim/organizations/uas/coa/faq/.

CHAPTER 3

Incident Management

OBJECTIVES

Upon completion of this chapter and the related course activities, the student will be able to meet the following objectives:

- Describe at least eight features and principles of an incident command system (ICS).
- Describe the general duties of the incident commander, the command staff, and the general staff.
- Describe the function of each of the following incident locations and facilities: incident command post, staging area, incident base, camp, helibase, and helispot.
- Describe each of the following: chain of command, unity of command, unified command, and transfer of command.
- Describe at least four resource management processes that are included in the incident command system.
- List and describe at least six elements that are included in a written incident action plan.
- Explain the difference between information and intelligence.

The Incident Command System

Search and rescue (SAR) can take many forms and play an important role in a wide range of **incidents**, such as hurricanes, earthquakes, tornados, floods, fires, and acts of terrorism. SAR skills are also needed to find a lost or missing child or an Alzheimer's patient. Regardless of the nature of the situation, local responders handle most incidents. As the size and complexity of the emergency grows, however, outside assistance is often needed. When this happens, partnerships among local, tribal, state, and federal agencies, as well as nongovernmental and private-sector organizations, become important. To maximize the effectiveness, efficiency, and the margin of safety provided, these partners must respond together in a seamless, coordinated fashion. The **incident command system (ICS)** is the approach to **incident management** used in the United States and many other parts of the world that helps ensure integration and interoperability of response efforts.

SEARCH AND RESCUE TIP

ICS is the system used throughout the United States and many places around the world to manage all of the **functions** of an emergency incident.

ICS is a standardized, on-scene, all-hazard, **all-risk** approach to incident management. ICS allows all responders to adopt an integrated organizational structure that matches the complexities and demands of the incident while respecting agency and jurisdictional authorities. Although ICS promotes standardization, it also allows flexibility. For example, the ICS organizational structure can expand or contract to meet incident needs. ICS also establishes common processes for planning and managing resources, and it allows for the integration of facilities, equipment, personnel, procedures, and communications operating within a common organizational structure.

The ICS was developed following a series of catastrophic fires in California in the 1970s where many died or were injured, and property losses ran into the millions of dollars. The evaluation of the management of these large incidents determined that the worst outcomes were rarely attributed to inadequate resources or improper tactics. Rather, poor outcomes were found to be largely a result of:

- Lack of **situational awareness**
- Lack of accountability (unclear chain of command)
- Poor communications (conflicting codes and terminology)
- Lack of orderly, systematic, and standardized management processes

In the decades since it was first developed, ICS has proven that it works and that it helps ensure the safety of responders, achieve response objectives, and use resources efficiently. Therefore, in the United States, its use is now mandated by the **National Incident Management System (NIMS)** in addition to federal laws such as the Superfund Amendments and Reauthorization Act (SARA) of 1986 (U.S. Environmental Protection Agency, 1986) and the U.S. Department of Labor Occupational Safety and Health Administration (OSHA) Rule 1910.120 (U.S. Department of Labor, 2015), among others.

The ICS is part of the command and management component of NIMS, which, in a larger sense, is intended to provide a consistent framework for incident management at all jurisdictional levels regardless of the cause, size, or complexity of an incident (see the section on NIMS in Chapter 2, *Search and Rescue Systems*). NIMS represents a core set of doctrine, concepts, principles, terminology, and organizational processes that enables effective, efficient, and collaborative incident management. NIMS components—among them, ICS—link together and work in unison to form a comprehensive incident management system. NIMS components include:

- *Preparedness*: Effective incident management begins with a host of preparedness activities well in advance of any potential incident. Preparedness involves an integrated combination of planning, training, exercises, personnel qualification and certification standards, equipment acquisition and certification standards, and publication management processes and activities.
- *Communications and information management*: NIMS identifies the requirement for a standardized framework for communications, information management (collection, analysis, and dissemination), and information sharing at all levels of incident management.
- *Resource management*: NIMS establishes the resource management process to describe, inventory, mobilize, dispatch, track, and recover resources over the life cycle of an incident through defined standardized mechanisms.
- *Command and management*: NIMS standard incident command structures are based on three key organizational systems:
  - The ICS defines the operating characteristics, interactive management components, and structure of incident management and emergency response organizations engaged throughout the life cycle of an incident.
  - **Multiagency coordination systems (MACS)** define the operating characteristics, interactive management components, and organizational structure of supporting incident management entities engaged at the local, regional, state, federal, and tribal levels through mutual aid agreements and other assistance arrangements.
  - Public information refers to processes, procedures, and systems for communicating timely and accurate information to the public and responders during crisis or emergency situations.
- *Ongoing management and maintenance*: This component establishes an activity to provide strategic direction for and oversight of NIMS, supporting both routine review and the continuous refinement of the system and its components over the long term.

SEARCH AND RESCUE TIP

NIMS components include the following:

- Preparedness
- Communications and information management
- Resource management
- Command and management
- Ongoing management

Features and Principles of ICS

ICS incorporates several proven management features and principles that contribute to the overall strength and efficiency of the system. **TABLE 3-1** outlines the 14 key features of ICS with some explanation of each.

Common Terminology

Using the same term to mean the same thing—**common terminology**—is a key feature of ICS. When one

TABLE 3-1 Outline of the Key Features of ICS

Categories	Key Features
Standardization	▪ Common terminology
Command	▪ Establishment, transfer, and termination of command ▪ Chain of command and unity of command ▪ Unified command
Planning and organizational structure	▪ Management by objectives ▪ Modular organization ▪ Incident action planning ▪ Manageable span of control
Facilities and resources	▪ Incident locations and facilities ▪ Comprehensive resource management
Communications/information management	▪ Integrated communications ▪ Information and intelligence management
Professionalism	▪ Accountability • Check-in • Incident action plan • Unity of command • Personal responsibility • Span of control • Resource tracking ▪ Dispatch/deployment of personnel and equipment

definition for any organizational function, incident facility, resource description, and position title is clearly established, accepted, and used by all, communication is significantly enhanced (see Search and Rescue Terms at the end of this chapter). As an example of common terminology, **TABLE 3-2** shows the specific and unique position titles (and support positions) for each supervisory role within ICS. Further, the use of **clear text**—not using radio codes, departmental codes, institution-specific acronyms, or jargon—is also key to effective communications.

Establishment, Transfer, and Termination of Command

The **command** function must be clearly established from the beginning of an incident and must continue until it is passed, transferred, or the incident is stabilized and command is terminated. All incidents, regardless of size or complexity, will have an **incident commander (IC)**. The first-arriving responder establishes himself or herself as the incident commander, then, as necessary, passes command to arriving supervisory personnel. The incident commander is usually the senior supervisor to arrive on the scene, but the person best suited to serve as IC should be the primary consideration for filling this position. The initial IC is also responsible for naming the incident, which is most often related to some feature, such as the name of the city/town, a prominent nearby feature (e.g., mountain, river, valley), or other proximate geographic feature that is unique to the incident.

As an incident grows or becomes more complex, the responsible **jurisdiction** or **agency** may choose to assign another individual as the IC. The process of moving the responsibility for incident command from one individual to another is called *transfer of command*. There are several reasons a transfer of command might take place:

- A more **qualified** incident commander arrives and assumes command.
- A jurisdiction or agency is legally required to take command; for example, the FBI is required to take the lead for investigations of terrorist incidents.
- The incident changes in complexity; for example, an incident starts in a small area but expands into multiple jurisdictions.
- The current IC needs to rest.

TABLE 3-2 ICS Supervisory Position Titles

Organizational Level	Title	Support Position
Incident command	Incident commander	Deputy
Command staff	Officer	Assistant
General staff (section)	Chief	Deputy
Branch	Director	Deputy
Division/group	Supervisor	N/A
Unit	Leader	Manager
Strike team/task force	Leader	Single resource boss

When command is transferred, the process must include a briefing—done face-to-face if possible—that captures and passes on all essential information for continuing safe and effective operations. For more complex transfer of command situations, every aspect of the incident must be documented and included in the transfer of command briefing. The briefing of an oncoming IC should include at least the following:

- Incident history (what happened, what is happening, and what is expected to happen)
- Priorities and objectives
- Current plan and any contingency plans
- Resource assignments
- Resources ordered/needed
- Incident organization (organizational chart)
- Facilities established
- Status of communications
- Any constraints or limitations
- Incident potential
- Introduction to the command staff and general staff members
- Delegation of authority (if applicable)

Once the briefing has taken place, an exact time should be established for the transfer to take place, and the transfer should be communicated to all incident personnel.

Agency policies and incident-specific issues may alter the transfer of command process. In all cases, the information shared should be documented and saved for easy retrieval during and after the incident.

Once the incident is stabilized, the decision is made by the IC to terminate command. The IC should take into consideration all of the following before terminating command:

- Are all personnel accounted for?
- Has safe transportation for all incident personnel been arranged and confirmed?
- Will all bystanders and incident personnel remain safe during termination operations?
- Has the specific responsible party to which the scene will be transferred been selected and notified?
- Has the responsible party to which the scene will be transferred been notified of (a) modifications or damage created during incident operations and (b) all potential or existing hazards?
- Has all damage to and loss of equipment and materials been documented?
- Have all injuries been properly documented?
- Has all documentation been completed and collected (although some may be completed after termination of command)?
- Has a location, date, and time been identified for conducting a post-incident analysis, and has this been communicated to all incident personnel?
- Has the agency administrator (the IC's boss) been notified of the expected termination of command?

Chain of Command and Unity of Command

Chain of command refers to the orderly line of authority that flows down through the ranks of the incident management organization. Chain of command allows **managers** to direct and control the actions of all personnel under their supervision, and it avoids confusion by requiring that orders flow from supervisors. Chain of command does not prevent personnel from directly communicating with each other (informal communications) to ask for or share information that is needed to complete assigned tasks. In fact, this type of informal communication is encouraged.

Unity of command means that every individual in an ICS organization reports to only one ICS supervisor, and this one supervisor serves as the sole source of work assignments. Without adhering to the principles of chain of command and unity of command, multiple conflicting directives are common. Unity of command clears up many of the potential communication problems encountered in managing incidents or events.

Unified Command

In incidents involving multiple jurisdictions, a single jurisdiction with multiagency involvement, or multiple jurisdictions with multiagency involvement, **unified command (UC)** allows agencies with different legal, geographic, and functional authorities and responsibilities to work together effectively without affecting individual agency authority, responsibility, or accountability. (Unified command is discussed in more depth later in this chapter.)

Management by Objectives

ICS is managed by objectives. **Incident objectives** are used to ensure that everyone within the ICS organization has a clear understanding of what needs to be accomplished. **Management by objectives** is an approach borrowed from business that generally includes:

- Establishing overarching priorities and incident objectives
- Subsequently developing assignments, plans, procedures, and protocols
- Directing efforts to attain incident objectives in support of the overarching priorities and defined strategies
- Documenting results to measure performance and facilitate corrective action

Modular Organization

The ICS organizational structure develops in a modular fashion that is based on the size and complexity of the incident, as well as the specifics of the hazard environment created by the incident. As incident complexity increases, the organization expands as functional responsibilities are delegated.

The ICS organizational structure is flexible and scalable. When needed, separate functional elements can be established and subdivided to enhance internal organizational management and external coordination. As the ICS organizational structure expands or contracts, the number of management positions increases or decreases to match organizational needs. Thus, this **modular organization** can readily expand and contract to meet the needs of the incident.

The ICS organization is unique but easy to understand. There is no correlation between the ICS organization and the administrative structure of any single agency or jurisdiction. For example, the highest-ranking official on a police department (police chief) may serve in a subordinate role when deployed under an ICS structure. This is a deliberate feature because confusion over different position titles and organizational structures has been a significant stumbling block to effective incident management in the past.

Incident Action Planning

Every incident, even the smallest, is managed using some form of incident objectives and plans. The plan can be as simple as a list of next actions verbally communicated to others by the IC, or as comprehensive as a detailed, multipage, written document developed by an **incident management team (IMT)**. These **incident action plans (IAPs)**, whether verbal or written, provide a coherent means of communicating the overall incident objectives in a standardized way in the contexts of both operational and support activities. This plan must, at a minimum, specify the incident objectives, state the assignments to be completed (and by whom they will be completed), and cover a specified timeframe, called an **operational period**. Put another way, every IAP must answer at least these basic questions:

- What do we want to do?
- Who is responsible for doing it?
- How do we communicate with each other?
- How do we handle anticipated problems (contingency plans)?
- What is the procedure if someone is injured?

Manageable Span of Control

Span of control is the ICS term used to define the number of individuals or resources that one supervisor can manage safely and effectively during an incident. Properly managing the span of control is key to a successful outcome. In fact, exceeding span of control is a major factor contributing to the breakdown of command. Exceeding span of control compromises situational awareness and the common operating picture, the basis of sound decision-making. Within ICS, the span of control of any individual supervisor should range from three to seven subordinates, and a ratio of one supervisor to five subordinates (1:5) is recommended (**FIGURE 3-1**).

Honoring the concept and principles of span of control improves a supervisor's ability to effectively supervise and communicate with all resources under his or her supervision. Maintaining an effective span of control is critical at incidents where safety and accountability should be top priorities.

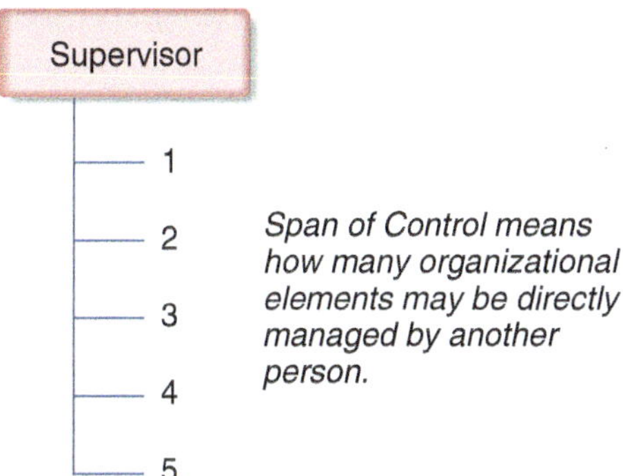

FIGURE 3-1 Important management functions must be delegated to maintain a manageable span of control. Seven is the maximum number of subordinates for each supervisor; five or fewer is preferred.

Incident Locations and Facilities

Various types of operational locations and support facilities are established near an incident to accomplish a variety of purposes. It is important to know and understand the names, functions, and unique purposes of the principal ICS facilities, including incident command posts, staging areas, **mobilization centers**, **coordination centers**, bases, camps, helibases, helispots, and others as required (**TABLE 3-3**). Not all incidents will use all principal ICS facilities. However, an incident command post and a staging area will likely be established on all but the smallest and most routine incidents. Some incidents may require additional facilities beyond standard ICS facilities, such as a triage center or temporary morgue.

Incident Command Post

The location from which the IC (or unified commanders) oversees all incident activities and actions is called the **incident command post (ICP)**. The ICP is where the primary command functions (commanding, planning, logistics, finance, public information, and liaising) are performed. It should be noted that the operations function is not generally performed at the ICP, at least for larger incidents. The operations section chief, who oversees all tactical activity, often establishes a work area much closer to the field of operations. This tactical management post is often referred to as a *forward* or *operational command post.*

A single ICP should be established at all incidents, large or small, and there can be only one ICP for each incident, including multiagency or multijurisdictional incidents operating under a single or a unified command. Space will often be needed at the ICP to allow for various **command staff** and **general staff** (**section** chiefs) functions. Some incidents may be large enough to have an on-site communications center to dispatch **assigned resources**, which is commonly adjacent to the ICP. On a small incident, or early in an expanding incident, the IC may be the only person occupying the ICP. Initially, the ICP may be the vehicle in which the IC arrived. Later, as the command and general staff increase in size, the ICP may be transferred to a larger mobile command vehicle or a structure such as a government building. Regardless of its location, the ICP should be established separate from the primary operational area, when possible, and in a place that can be secured.

TABLE 3-3 Incident Command System Facilities

ICS Facility	Description
Incident command post	The field location at which the primary tactical-level, on-scene incident command functions are performed. This may be co-located with the incident base or other incident facilities and is normally identified by a green rotating or flashing light.
Staging area	Temporary location for available resources. A staging area can be any location in which personnel, supplies, and equipment can be temporarily housed or parked while awaiting operational assignment. The operations section manages staging areas.
Coordination center	A facility used for the coordination of agency or jurisdictional resources in support of one or more incidents. Agency representatives with operational authority gather and provide information, facilitate logistics support and resource tracking, and implement multiagency coordination entity decisions.
Base or incident base	Location at the incident where the primary logistics functions are coordinated and administered. (Incident name or other designator will be added to the term *base*.) The incident command post may be co-located with the base. There is only one base per incident.
Camp	A geographical site, within the general incident area, separate from the incident base, equipped and staffed to provide sleeping, food, water, and sanitary services to incident personnel.
Helibase	The main location for parking, fueling, maintenance, and loading of helicopters operating in support of an incident. It is usually located at or near the incident base.
Helispot	Any designated location where a helicopter can safely take off and land. Some helispots may be used for loading supplies, equipment, or personnel.

Staging Areas

Staging areas are temporary locations where **available resources** are kept while awaiting assignment. Most large incidents have a staging area, and some incidents may have several. All staging areas are managed by a staging area manager who reports to the operations section chief or to the IC if an operations section has not been designated.

There are many reasons for the use of staging areas. They provide locations for immediately available resources to await active assignments and for greater accountability by having available personnel and resources together in one safe location. In addition, staging areas minimize excessive communications of resources calling for assignments and allow the operations section chief or IC to properly plan for resource use and to provide for contingencies.

Resources in a staging area are always in an "available" status, which means they are ready for a specific assignment within three minutes.

Coordination Center

A coordination center is an ICS facility where agency representatives with the authority to make decisions for their respective agencies gather to provide information, facilitate logistics support and resource tracking, and implement the decisions of **multiagency coordination (MAC) entities or groups**. Although a coordination center is not required on most SAR incidents, establishing one can be important when multiple agencies are involved in a large or extended SAR incident and coordination among the agencies involved is needed. Some common examples of coordination centers include:

- *Emergency operations center (EOC)*: This is the physical location at which the coordination of information and resources to support local incident management activities normally takes place. It may also be referred to as *expanded dispatch* and an *emergency command and control center*. EOCs are used in various ways at all levels of government and within the private sector to provide coordination, direction, and control during emergencies such as large, complex, or extended search and rescue operations. Most counties and all states in the United States have an established EOC that is usually managed by the local or state emergency management agency.
- *Joint operations center (JOC)*: In the event of a terrorist incident, the FBI establishes the JOC to coordinate and direct law enforcement and criminal investigation activities related to the incident.
- *Joint field office (JFO)*: This is a temporary federal facility established locally to coordinate operational federal assistance activities to the affected jurisdiction(s) during incidents of national significance. The JFO is a multiagency center that provides a central point of coordination for federal, state, local, tribal, nongovernmental, and private sector organizations with primary responsibility for threat response, incident support, and coordination. Most common in disaster incidents, the JFO accommodates all entities (or their designated representatives) essential to incident management, information sharing, and the delivery of disaster assistance and other support.
- *Joint information center (JIC)*: This is a facility where the public information officer(s) and staff can coordinate and provide information on the incident to the public, media, and other agencies.

Incident Base

The **incident base** is the location at the incident at which primary service and support activities, including logistics section activities, are performed. Few incidents, including SAR, will establish an incident base. However, if and when established, there will be only one incident base for each incident.

Typically, the incident base is the location where unassigned and **out-of-service resources** (personnel and equipment) are located. A base manager manages a base.

Camps

Camps are temporary incident locations, within the general incident area, that are established to provide food, drink, sanitation, and sleeping services for out-of-service personnel. Camps differ from staging areas in that essential support operations are done at camps, and resources at camps are not normally available for immediate assignment. Not all incidents will have camps. In fact, very few search and rescue incidents will ever need to establish one because personnel are commonly demobilized home for rehabilitation.

When established, camps are separate facilities and are not located at the incident base. They may be in place for several days and may be moved depending on incident needs. Very large incidents may have one or more camps located in strategic areas. Camps are used when resources are required to travel long distances from their assignments to the incident base. All ICS functional unit activities performed at the incident base may also be performed at camps. Each camp will have a camp manager assigned.

Helibases and Helispots

An area at which helicopters may be parked, maintained, and fueled is called a **helibase** and is often located at an airport near the incident. It is very difficult, if not

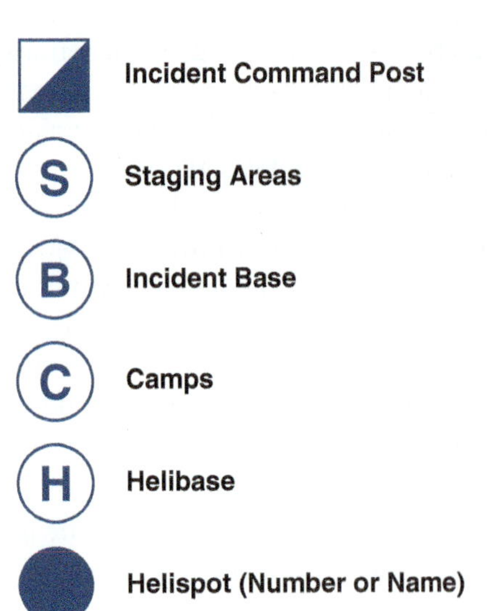

FIGURE 3-2 Map designations for ICS facilities.

Reproduced from FEMA. (2018). Incident Facilities and Map Symbols. Retrieved from https://emilms.fema.gov/IS100b/ICS0102310text.htm

impossible, to construct a helibase outside of an airport because of the many safety and environmental regulations.

Helispots, also referred to as **landing zones (LZs)**, are temporary locations where helicopters can safely land to perform work supporting the incident. Large incidents may have several helispots. Being temporary landing areas, there are often imperfections in the landing environment. Safety must always be a priority when choosing helispot locations and anticipating any potential problems (including the need for fire protection).

Identifying ICS facilities on a map is important, so the map symbols associated with basic incident facilities have been standardized (**FIGURE 3-2**). The development of a wide range of map symbol standards is ongoing. One attempt at this can be found in the Emergency Symbology Reference produced by the Homeland Security Working Group (Federal Geographic Data Committee, 2015).

Comprehensive Resource Management

Resources at an incident must be managed effectively, and maintaining an accurate and up-to-date picture of resource utilization (**resource tracking**) is a critical component of incident management. In ICS, **resources** include personnel and major items of equipment, supplies, and facilities available or potentially available for assignment to incident operations and for which status is maintained. In ICS, **resource management** includes processes for:

- Categorizing, **credentialing**, and identifying resources in advance
- Ordering resources
- Dispatching resources
- Tracking resources
- Recovering resources
- Reimbursement for resources, as appropriate
- **Demobilization** of resources

Resources assigned to an incident will always be in one of these status conditions:

- *En route*: Properly requested and currently responding to an incident
- *Assigned*: Currently tasked with an assignment
- *Available*: Ready for assignment
- *Out-of-service*: Not available for assignment (repairing, servicing, or resting)
- *Demobilized*: Properly released and returning to home agency

Resource Kind and Type

To reduce errors and miscommunications around ordering resources, ICS resources are categorized by kind and type. *Kind* is what the resource is. For example, a dog team, search team, and technical rescuer are **kinds of resources**. **Type** refers to the size, capability, and staffing qualifications of a specific kind of resource. Resource types range from Type 1 (most capable) to Type 4 (least capable). Requesting resources without specifying the proper type and kind often results in the inappropriate utilization of resources (i.e., the personnel are over/under qualified and/or the equipment is not right for the need).

Resource typing is a key component of NIMS. This effort helps all federal, state, tribal, and local jurisdictions locate, request, and track resources to assist neighboring jurisdictions when local capability is overwhelmed.

The **National Integration Center** encourages federal, state, tribal, and local officials to use the NIMS resource typing definitions as they develop or update response asset inventories. All NIMS resource typing definitions and job titles/position qualifications released by FEMA can be found on the Resource Typing Library Tool (RTLT) website, including those that are under review but not yet finalized (U.S. Department of Homeland Security, Federal Emergency Management Agency, 2018).

Unfortunately, not all those who request resources correctly identify the type and kind of resource needed. Thus, resource requests should also include a brief description of the mission/task for which the resource is needed. This is known as *mission tasking*. Including such a description when ordering a resource increases the probability of the resource sent in response to the request matching the need. For example, a request for a Type 1 land search and rescue team might be accompanied by a mission tasking described as "the team is expected to bring its own vehicle that may be required to operate in rough terrain and be able to search in winter conditions in terrain that qualifies as Yosemite Decimal System (YDS) Class 3."

SEARCH AND RESCUE TIP

The Yosemite Decimal System (YDS) is a numeric system for rating the difficulty of climbs. It consists of five general classes, with the fifth "being subdivided with a decimal notation" (Climber.org, 2015, Para 1)*:

Class 1: Trail hiking, bike path, walking on a well-established trail

Class 2: Cross-country (off-trail) travel; hands may be needed for balance; trail may be nonexistent or very uneven

Class 3: Scrambling on rock; requires use of hands for climbing and progress; rope may be used for comfort; do not need to search for handholds

Class 4: Climbing on steep terrain; requires rope belay; serious injury or death may result from a fall, includes any exposed climbing; protection not placed during climb

Class 5: Technical climbing required; placement of protective hardware during climb required; rope belay required; climbing holds not obvious to a novice will be necessary; death very likely with unprotected fall; further subdivided from 5.0 to 5.13.

For more details and information from experienced climbers, visit Climber.org.

*Courtesy of Climber.org

Incidents, like resources, may be categorized into five **incident types** based on complexity. Type 5 incidents are the least complex, and Type 1 are the most complex. Incident typing may be used to make decisions about resource requirements and help determine the need to requisition a formal incident management team (**TABLE 3-4**).

Integrated Communications

The ability to communicate within an ICS organization is essential. Incident communications are facilitated through the development and use of a common communications plan and interoperable communications processes and architectures. A common communications plan is essential for ensuring that responders can communicate with one another during an incident, but this does not mean that all personnel must be able to talk with each other at all times. A good communication plan is one that is designed to allow personnel who must be able to speak with each other the ability to do so through usable and reliable media.

It is best to develop an integrated voice and data communications system (equipment, systems, and protocols) before an incident and to integrate that system into daily operations. This institutionalization of the communication system produces a familiarity with equipment and procedures that improves overall communications during larger, but less frequent, incidents.

An essential part of an effective multiagency incident management system is for all daily communications to be in clear text without the use of jurisdiction-specific terms, codes, and signals. During multiagency responses, such terms will significantly reduce the effectiveness of interagency communications.

SEARCH AND RESCUE TIP

ICS doctrine requires that clear text, not radio codes, be used at all times.

Information and Intelligence Management

In the context of ICS, the distinction between information and intelligence can be subtle but is very important. **Information** is raw or unprocessed data, knowledge, or facts about someone or something gained from somewhere. **Intelligence** is information that has been collected, verified, collated, evaluated, analyzed, and prepared for use in making decisions. The synthesis, analysis, and sharing of information and intelligence is an important component of ICS. The incident management organization must establish a process for gathering, processing, sharing, and managing incident-related information and intelligence that comes from a variety of sources, such as:

- Field observation and damage assessments
- Debriefing response personnel
- Public reports
- Media reports
- Technical specialists (e.g., meteorologists, epidemiologists, search specialists, rescue technicians)
- Event plans
- Emergency operations plans
- Hazard/risk/vulnerability assessments
- Structural plans and vulnerabilities
- National security and classified data
- Threats, including potential violence
- Surveillance of disease outbreak

Without accurate information being transformed into useful intelligence, responders may find it difficult to ensure the safety of responders, prioritize needs, determine incident objectives, and identify the resources needed.

TABLE 3-4 Incident Complexity

Incident Type	Description
Type 5	A Type 5 incident, the smallest and least complex of the five incident types, usually includes one or two single resources (e.g., two search team vehicles) with up to six individual resources (e.g., six searchers). Generally, the IC performs all command and general staff positions, and the incidents are contained within a few hours, at the most, after resources arrive on scene. The IAP is often verbal or limited only to the ICS 201. Examples of a Type 5 incident include a motor vehicle accident, vehicle fire, any injured person (EMS call), or a police traffic stop.
Type 4	A Type 4 incident is larger in size and/or complexity and requires multiple resources—often from different agencies—to work together to manage the incident. Generally, the command and operations sections, and some of the planning section, are activated. Type 4 incidents are usually limited to one operational period, may require a written IAP (at minimum an ICS 201), and may involve expanding dispatch and/or activating the local emergency operations center (EOC).
Type 3	Type 3 incidents are larger still and may involve multiple counties or a region within a state. When capabilities exceed those of the initial attack resources, the appropriate ICS positions should be staffed to match the complexity of the incident. In a Type 3 incident, resources from multiple agencies, counties, and/or region(s) of a state may be required. Most, if not all, of the command and general staff positions are staffed, and division/group supervisors and/or **unit leaders** may be activated. An incident management team may be assigned in a Type 3 incident to manage the significant number of resources. Generally, Type 3 incidents extend into multiple operational periods; may involve a unified command; will require a written IAP for each operational period; and receive support and coordination from local, regional, and/or state emergency operations centers.
Type 2	A Type 2 incident is very large, often complex, and requires regional or national resources to effectively manage. All command and general staff positions, as well as many of the unit- and subordinate-level positions, are filled in a Type 2 incident. The number of personnel in the operations section typically does not exceed 200 per operational period, with the total number of personnel involved in the incident not exceeding 500. A written delegation of authority may be needed, and many different local, regional, state, federal, and private resources will likely be assigned.
Type 1	A Type 1 incident requires national resources and is reserved for only the largest and most complex emergencies or events. This type incident has all the same requirements as a Type 2 incident, but operational personnel often exceed 500 per operational period, and total incident personnel may exceed 1000. With an incident of this size and complexity, the impact on local jurisdiction(s) is high and often requires additional staff for office administrative and support functions. A Type 1 incident may result in a state and/or federally declared disaster; may extend into multiple operational periods lasting days, weeks, or even months; and requires a written IAP for each operational period.

Traditionally, information and intelligence functions are located in the planning section. However, in exceptional situations, the IC may need to assign the information and intelligence functions to other parts of the ICS organization. In any case, information and intelligence must be appropriately analyzed and shared with personnel, designated by the IC, who have proper clearance and a "need-to-know" to ensure they support decision-making.

According to ICS doctrine, the intelligence function may be integrated into an ICS organization in any one of the following ways:

- *Within the command staff by appointing an* **intelligence officer**. This option may be most appropriate in incidents with little need for tactical or classified intelligence, and in which incident-related intelligence is provided by **supporting agency** representatives, through real-time reach-back capabilities. When staffed, the intelligence officer is responsible for managing internal information, intelligence, and operational security requirements supporting incident management activities.
- *As a unit within the planning section.* This option may be most appropriate in an incident with some need

for tactical intelligence, and when no law enforcement entity is a member of the unified command.

- *As a branch within the operations section.* This option may be most appropriate in incidents with a high need for tactical intelligence (particularly classified intelligence), and when law enforcement is a member of the unified command.
- *As a separate general staff section (information and intelligence section).* This option may be most appropriate when an incident is heavily influenced by intelligence factors, or where there is a need to manage and/or analyze a large volume of classified or highly sensitive intelligence or information. This option is particularly relevant to a terrorism incident, for which intelligence plays a crucial role throughout the incident life cycle.

Regardless of how it is organized, the information and intelligence function is also responsible for developing, conducting, and managing information-related security plans and operations as directed by the IC. These can include information security and operational security activities, as well as the complex task of ensuring that sensitive information of all types (e.g., classified information, sensitive law enforcement information, proprietary or personnel information, or export controlled information) is handled in a way that not only safeguards the information, but also ensures that it gets to those who need access to it to effectively and safely conduct their missions. The information and intelligence function also has the responsibility for coordinating information- and operational-security matters with public awareness activities that fall under the responsibility of the public information officer, particularly where such public awareness activities may affect information or operations security.

Formal versus Informal Communications

Some find it useful to define two types of general communications, both of which are essential to the success of an incident: formal and informal communications. Formal communications follow the lines of authority in an ICS organization (i.e., chain of command). The IC communicating the incident objectives for the first operational period to the operations section chief is an example of formal communications. Formal communications must be used when providing/modifying work assignments, requesting/releasing resources, and reporting progress/lack of progress on assigned tasks. It is essential that formal communication be used when one wishes to establish or change standing plans or assignments.

Informal communications involve an exchange of information that does not necessarily follow the chain of command but is nevertheless essential to accomplishing goals and completing assignments. Personnel in an ICS organization are encouraged to share/seek information from any source to fulfill their assigned role or accomplish their assigned task. An example of informal communication would be the **supply unit** leader (logistics section) directly contacting the **resources unit** leader (planning section) to confirm the number of meals that might be needed for the next operational period.

Accountability

Effective accountability—the willingness to assume responsibility and be held accountable for your actions—during incident operations is essential within individual functional areas and at all jurisdictional levels. *Situational awareness*—knowing what is going on around you—is a key component in achieving and maintaining incident accountability. To achieve a helpful level of situational awareness and thus accountability, the following ICS principles must be applied effectively:

- **Check-in**: All responders, regardless of agency affiliation, must report in so that they can be properly tracked and can receive their assignment both in a timely manner and in accordance with the procedures established by the IC.
- *Incident action plan*: The IAP must be relevant to the current operating period, and all personnel and operations must follow the plan.
- *Unity of command*: Individual responders must be assigned to only one supervisor.
- *Span of control*: Supervisors must be assigned to supervise only the number of resources that they can manage efficiently, effectively, and safely.
- *Resource tracking*: All changes of incident status—available, assigned, and out of service—must be immediately reported to supervision and passed on to the resources unit **leader** to maintain proper awareness of incident resource status.

Dispatch/Deployment

Personnel and equipment should respond only when requested or when dispatched by an appropriate authority. Resources not properly requested, coordinated, or controlled by command result in significant accountability and safety issues. Research has consistently determined that self-dispatching and freelancing also create increased safety risks to individuals, other resources, and civilians. In short, self-dispatching and freelancing are unacceptable at the scene of any incident.

After check-in, personnel should locate their incident supervisor and obtain an initial briefing. As a minimum, this briefing should include the following:

- Current assessment of the situation
- Identification of specific job responsibilities
- Identification of coworkers
- Location of work area
- Identification of break areas, as appropriate
- Procedural instructions for obtaining needed resources
- Operational period/work shifts
- Required safety procedures and personal protective equipment (PPE), as appropriate

Incident Commander and Command Staff Functions

Every incident requires that certain management functions be performed. The problem must be identified and assessed and a plan to deal with the identified problems must be developed and implemented with the appropriate resources. There are five major management functions performed at every incident (**FIGURE 3-3**). These five functions are listed below and serve as the foundation upon which the ICS organization develops:

- *Incident command*: Has overall responsibility for the incident and establishes incident priorities, objectives, and strategies
- *Operations*: Directs all operational resources and establishes all tactical assignments that are intended to achieve the incident's objectives
- *Planning*: Supports the incident by collecting and analyzing information, tracking and illustrating situational status, tracking resources, developing contingency plans, maintaining incident-related documents, and leading the preparation and documentation of the IAP
- *Logistics*: Acquires and maintains the resources and services needed to support all incident activities
- *Finance and administration*: Provides accounting, procurement, time recording, and analyses of costs related to the incident

Incident Commander

ICS doctrine requires that the command function be performed, and an IC be assigned, at every incident or **event**, regardless of its size. Further, when subordinate positions are not staffed, such as on smaller incidents or events, the IC must perform the functions until the positions are staffed. For example, during the initial response, or throughout a small SAR incident, the IC may perform all ICS command and general staff functions. He or she may interview the reporting party, request additional resources, plan the search, brief and debrief search teams, deploy resources, maintain an incident log, and write the incident report. In fact, the IC is responsible for all management functions not specifically delegated to another individual.

The IC has overall responsibility for managing the incident. He or she does this by establishing objectives, planning strategies, and implementing tactics. These responsibilities include performing all ICS general staff functions (operations, planning, logistics, and finance/administration) until those functions are delegated to other individuals, known as section chiefs. Further, the IC is responsible for the following command staff functions until they are delegated:

- Ensuring the safety of the responders and public
- Providing information to internal and external stakeholders
- Establishing **liaison** with outside agency representatives

Ensuring the safety of all responders is a primary goal of every IC and may require periodic **personnel accountability reports (PAR)**. In most SAR incidents where no safety officer has been assigned, monitoring safety is an ongoing responsibility of all supervisors, requiring them

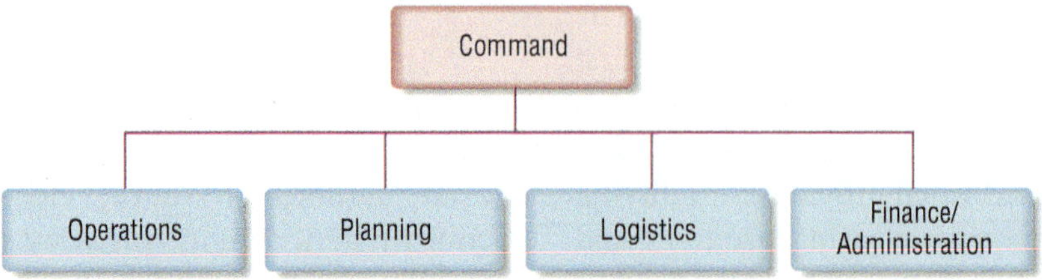

FIGURE 3-3 The five ICS functional sections. These five major functions are performed at every incident.

Data from FEMA. (2018). Introduction to the Incident Command System (ICS 100): Lesson 3: Incident Commander and Command Staff Functions. Retrieved from https://emilms.fema.gov/IS100b/ICS0103summary.htm

to monitor the location and well-being of all operational, administrative, and support personnel. In larger incidents, this task involves the safety officer and his or her assistants monitoring personnel operating on an incident. A PAR can also be useful after a sudden, unexpected situation within the incident, such as a rock fall, avalanche, building collapse, or explosion. A PAR can be requested of all supervisors to immediately account for, confirm, and report on the location and safety of all personnel for which they are responsible. This can be a valuable tool for any SAR leader when the safety of personnel is unknown.

It is critical that command be established from the beginning of an incident, and ICS doctrine requires that the most qualified first-arriving responder assume the role of IC. Not doing so becomes a safety hazard for responders and others. Size-up and decision-making are impossible without a command structure, and it is difficult to expand a disordered organization if the incident escalates.

The IC may appoint one or more deputy ICs. A **deputy**, generally, is a fully qualified individual who, in the absence of a superior, could be delegated the authority to manage or perform a specific task. In the case of a deputy IC, he or she may be asked to assume command, manage a particular aspect of the incident, or perform a specific high-level task.

Because a deputy could act as relief for his or her superior, the deputy must be fully qualified for the position. Deputies differ from **assistants** in that assistants have a particular skill set that supports the superior's position, but deputies must be fully qualified to take over their superior's position. ICS doctrine allows one or more deputies to be assigned only to the IC, members of the general staff (section chiefs), and branch directors. According to ICS doctrine, one or more assistants may be assigned only to command staff positions, but in reality, they are sometimes assigned to help other leadership positions in an ICS organization.

Command Staff

As an incident grows, the need to staff certain positions that answer directly to the IC can arise quickly. These positions are referred to as command staff and consist of the public information **officer**, safety officer, and liaison officer (**FIGURE 3-4**).

The **public information officer** serves as the conduit for information to internal and external stakeholders, including the media and the public. Accurate information is essential, and the public information officer serves as the primary contact for anyone who wants information about the incident and the response to it. The public information officer advises the IC on information dissemination and media relations,

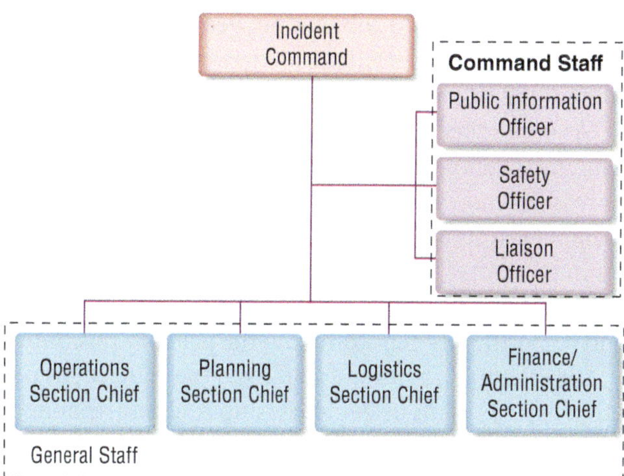

FIGURE 3-4 Functional hierarchy including the command section and command staff.

obtains information from and provides information to the planning section, and obtains information from and provides information to the community and the media. The IC must approve all information released by the public information officer.

The **safety officer**, who monitors conditions and develops measures for assuring the safety of all personnel, is also a member of the command staff. The safety officer works closely with the operations section to ensure safety of field personnel and is responsible for advising the IC on issues regarding incident safety, conducting risk analyses, and implementing safety measures. The safety officer develops the safety plan located in the IAP by working with the ICS 215a Incident Safety Analysis worksheet.

Agencies and jurisdictions that send resources to assist and/or support an incident are characterized as either assisting or cooperating agencies. An **assisting agency** is an agency or organization providing personnel, services, or other resources to the agency with direct responsibility for incident management. A **cooperating agency** is an agency supplying assistance other than direct operational, support functions, or resources to the incident management effort. Do not confuse the two. An assisting agency has direct responsibility for incident response, whereas a cooperating agency is simply offering assistance. An **agency representative** is an individual assigned to an incident from an assisting or cooperating agency. The agency representative must be delegated authority to make decisions on matters affecting that agency's participation at the incident.

Another member of the command staff is the **liaison officer**. This individual assists the IC by serving as a point of contact for agency representatives. The liaison officer also responds to requests from incident personnel for contacts among the assisting and cooperating agencies, monitors incident operations to address any current or potential problems between response agencies, and conducts briefings to answer questions from supporting organizations.

As mentioned earlier, in a large and/or complex incident, members of the command staff may need assistants to help manage their workloads. Each command staff member is responsible for organizing his or her assistants for maximum efficiency. As the title indicates, assistants should have a level of technical capability, qualifications, and responsibility subordinate to the primary positions.

An effective command staff frees the IC to focus on other aspects of his or her leadership role, and although command staff may not be necessary at every incident, every incident requires that at least some command staff functions be performed. The IC should consider staffing command staff positions, especially on complex and/or large incidents.

Unified Command

A single IC may not always be appropriate when multiple jurisdictions or agencies are involved in an incident. In these cases, more than one agency or jurisdiction may have legal responsibility for an incident, which may occur when an incident crosses jurisdictional lines, or when multiple responsible agencies have different legal, geographic, and functional responsibilities at the same incident (**FIGURE 3-5**). Although a single IC may seem easier than two or more, the decision not to use unified command must be weighed against which jurisdictions and/or agencies cannot escape their legal responsibility for an incident or part thereof. When two or more agencies and/or jurisdictions have legal responsibility for an incident, such as when an incident crosses jurisdictional boundaries, establishing a unified command may not only be practical, it may be required.

Searches often involve multiple jurisdictions. When a person is reported missing from a national park, for example, the search area may include the adjoining counties, towns, and/or tribal lands, all of which would have legal jurisdiction within their boundaries. Rather than conducting separate searches within each respective jurisdiction, representatives from each jurisdiction can join together to establish a unified command. This would result in one operational search plan, all information being consolidated and processed through one planning section, and the resources from the various jurisdictions being shared.

To establish a unified command, each agency or organization with legitimate responsibility for an incident, or part of it, provides a senior representative—with the authority to make decisions for the agency/organization represented—to work with other similar individuals. In this way, the unified command collectively acts as a single IC. The multiple individuals within the unified command (i.e., unified commanders or ICs) make joint decisions, speak with one voice, and work together so that none of their respective legal authorities is compromised or neglected. Any differences must be worked out quickly among the unified commanders. With this approach, unity of command is maintained because each responder reports to a single supervisor, and section chiefs (general staff) answer to one individual within the unified command assigned to represent the group (a spokesperson). In a unified command, institutions and responding agencies blend into an integrated, unified team, which results in:

- A shared understanding of restrictions and limitations
- A shared set of priorities
- A single set of incident objectives
- Collaborative strategies and efforts
- Improved internal and external information flow

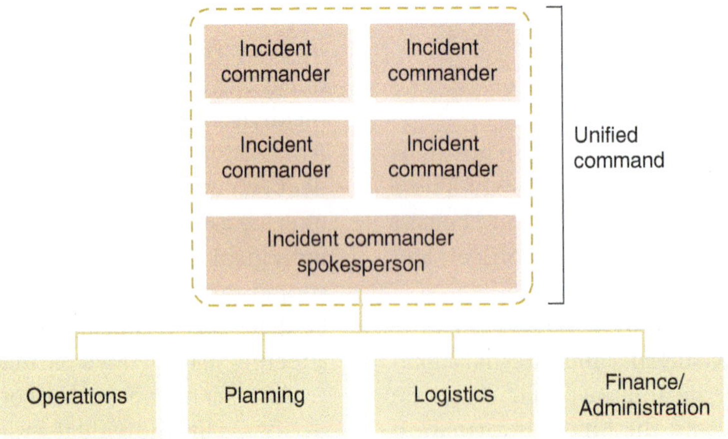

FIGURE 3-5 In unified command, multiple ICs act as one, generate one IAP, and select one operations section chief. Note that one of the ICs may be chosen to serve as spokesperson for the unified command.

- Less duplication of efforts
- Better resource utilization

As a team effort, unified command overcomes much of the inefficiency and duplication of effort that can occur when agencies from different functional and geographic jurisdictions, or agencies at different levels of government, operate without a common system or organizational framework. With a unified command, incident facilities are co-located or shared, rather than duplicated, thus allowing improved efficiency through economies of scale. However, simply placing commanders in the same proximity does not mean there is a unified command. Unified command functions best when the details of how unified command will work are planned, negotiated, and practiced before an incident occurs (pre-planned). This includes planning for how disagreements will be resolved, which is almost always needed.

One key feature of unified command is the development of a single set of incident objectives that are developed in a collaborative, single planning process (similar to the process used in single jurisdiction incidents; see Figure 3-10) that results in a single IAP that addresses all concerns and responsibilities.

Unified command also allows the integration of personnel from multiple agencies and jurisdictions into various functional areas of the ICS organization. Unified commanders jointly select a single operations section chief (usually from the most involved agency), and deputy operation section chiefs can be assigned from other agencies or jurisdictions as warranted. This type of flexibility allows the unified command to distribute expertise throughout the incident leadership to improve overall operations. It is important that the unified commanders concur on the selection of the general staff and that the operations section chief selected has full authority to implement the tactics identified within the IAP.

To take best advantage of a unified command, the ICs within a unified command must work together to establish a coordinated process for single-point ordering of all resources needed. Single-point ordering encourages the most appropriate use of scarce resources, especially to meet high-priority objectives. Unified commanders should also develop agreements on cost sharing—especially for essential services—among those agencies participating in the unified command.

General Staff

As previously mentioned, command (incident or unified) is responsible for all incident management functions, including operations, planning, logistics, and finance/administration. Depending on the incident needs, the IC may delegate some or all of these functions by establishing sections, which may be headed by a **section chief**. If a section chief is assigned, he or she will report directly to the IC. Together, these section chiefs are referred to as the general staff, and each section chief may have one or more deputies (**FIGURE 3-6**).

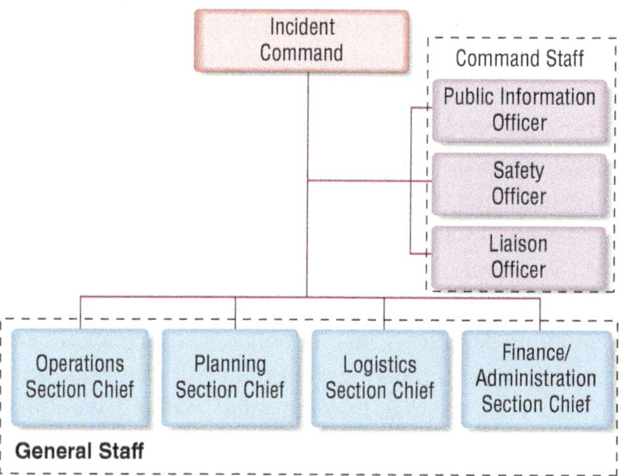

FIGURE 3-6 Organizational chart showing the general staff, which includes each of the section chiefs.

Operations Section

In an expanding incident, the IC first establishes the **operations section** by assigning an operations section chief. The remaining sections are established as needed to support the operations section, which is responsible for all incident tactical operations. The operations section is typically the first section to be staffed. It usually has the most incident resources, and it expands from the bottom up. Practically speaking, the IC should assign an operations section chief early in incidents that are increasing in size or potential. Otherwise, the IC must retain direct responsibility for the operations section, including staging and all tactical assignments, which may quickly exceed span of control requirements and negatively impact operations.

During the initial response to a SAR incident, the IC may personally assign and supervise the first-arriving responders, but as more resources arrive, the IC may quickly become overwhelmed with both command and operations responsibilities. This is when an operations section chief is typically appointed, freeing the IC to focus on command and other general staff functions. As the operations section grows to meet the needs of the incident, divisions, groups, and branches may be added to address span of control issues.

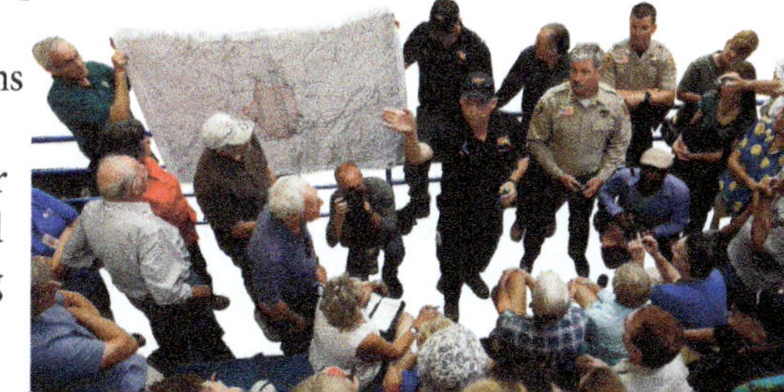

The operations section chief is responsible for developing and implementing

strategy and **tactics** to accomplish the incident objectives for the established operational period. This means that the operations section chief organizes, assigns, and supervises all the tactical or response resources assigned to the incident. Additionally, if a staging area is established, the operations section chief manages it or assigns a staging area manager, who answers directly to the operations section chief.

When an incident involves multiple organizations, assigning deputies from other organizations can increase interagency coordination. For example, for the response to a hazardous materials incident, public works, law enforcement, and hazardous materials responders might work together with one agency taking the lead and representatives from the other organizations serving as deputies.

The ICS organization adheres to a "form follows function" philosophy. The size of the current organization and that of the next operational period is determined through the incident planning process. Because the ICS uses a modular concept, managing span of control is accomplished by organizing resources into teams, divisions, groups, branches, or sections when the supervisor-to-subordinate ratio exceeds seven, or by reorganizing or demobilizing sections, branches, divisions, groups, or teams when the ratio falls below three.

The initial response to most incidents is typically handled by a local 911 dispatcher and emergency responders within a single jurisdiction. Thus, about 95% of all incidents are small and include only an IC (with some command staff support) and a few single resources (**FIGURE 3-7**). A **single resource** is a piece of equipment and its complement of personnel, or a **crew** or team of individuals with an identified work supervisor that can be used on an incident.

On a smaller incident, the operations section may comprise an operations section chief and single resources. A single resource is the smallest deployable element at an incident, but it may not be just one thing or one person. For example, an ambulance with a crew is a single resource. The ambulance cannot be deployed without the crew, and the crew cannot function without the ambulance vehicle, so the ambulance and crew together make up a single resource. SAR resources are organized in the same fashion. A ground search crew may consist of a leader and several members, but the entire crew operates as a single resource.

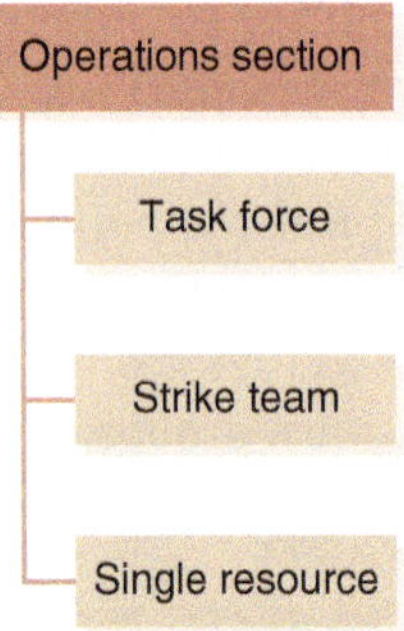

FIGURE 3-7 Task force, strike team, and single resource under the operations section. The IC or the operations section chief may initially work with only a few resources.

Single resources may be combined and organized into teams. Using ICS terminology, the two types of team configurations are:

- **Task forces**: A combination of *mixed resources* with common communications operating under the direct supervision of a leader (e.g., search and rescue task force, which includes both search and rescue resources).
- **Strike teams**: A combination of *similar resources* with common communications operating under the direct supervision of a leader (e.g., four K9 teams are combined to form a K9 strike team).

To maintain span of control, each team should comprise a leader and no more than five to seven members. However, ICS doctrine sometimes allows for a greater number of **individual resources** on a team (e.g., a law enforcement strike team can have 10 law enforcement officers, one of whom is a strike team leader). In search and rescue, search crews and search and rescue task forces are common approaches to resource management.

On a large, complex incident, the operations section may become very large. Using the ICS principle of modular organization, the operations section may add elements to manage span of control. **Groups** are functional collections of resources not necessarily operating in the same geographic region (e.g., search groups, evacuation groups, hazmat groups).

Divisions can also be used to add a level of supervision and are used to divide an incident geographically. The organization chart in **FIGURE 3-8** illustrates how groups and divisions can be used together to maintain span of control within the operations section. The use of divisions would be effective if the incident covered a geographically large or isolated area. For example, a search divided by a river could be broken into two divisions, one on each side of the river. The person leading each group or division is referred to as a **supervisor**.

When necessary, the operations section chief may add **branches** to supervise groups and divisions and further reduce the span of control (**FIGURE 3-9**). Branches can be based on function (e.g., air operations branch) or geography (e.g., west branch). The person in charge of each branch is called a **director**, and a branch director may have one or more deputies. The use of branches is usually reserved only for large incidents but may be used whenever necessary to maintain span of control.

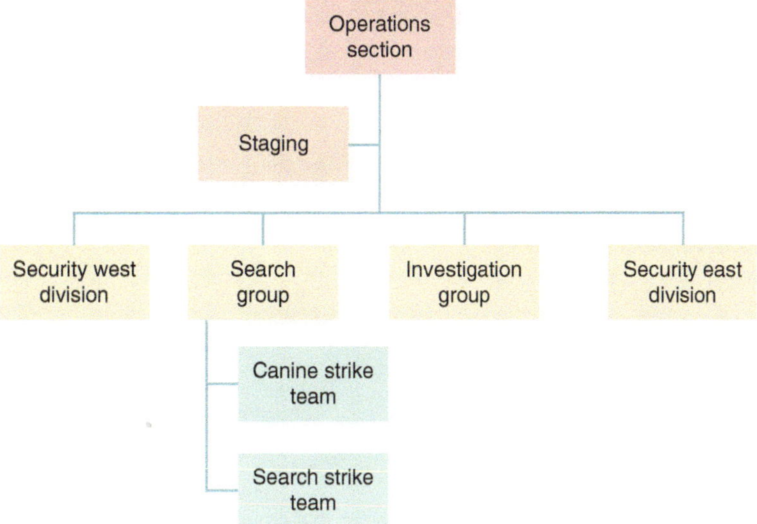

FIGURE 3-8 The operations section showing multiple resources, groups, divisions, and a staging area. Note that the staging area manager reports to the operations section chief, and that divisions and groups are used to maintain span of control.

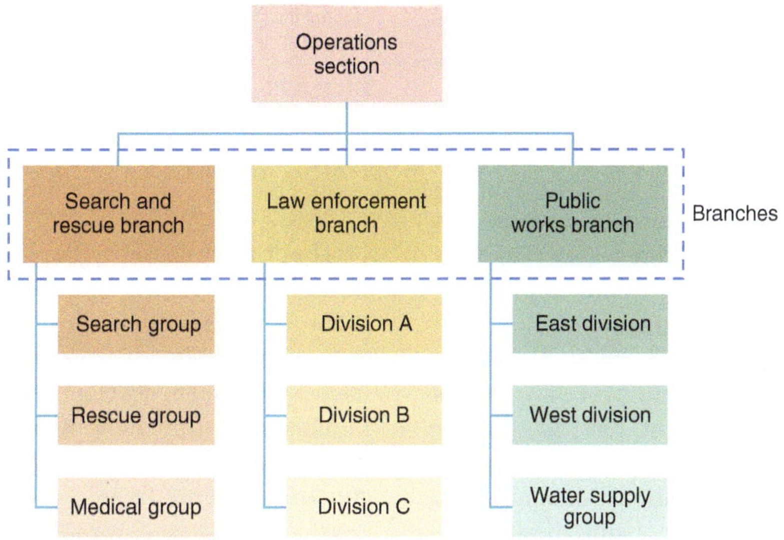

FIGURE 3-9 The operations section with functional branches used to maintain span of control. This approach is usually reserved only for very large and/or complex organizations.

(See Table 3-2 for a summary of unique supervisory position titles and their respective support positions.)

Planning Section

The **planning section** is responsible for the collection, evaluation, and dissemination of operational information related to the incident (**FIGURE 3-10**). It is the responsibility of the planning section to:

- Prepare and disseminate the IAP
- Help promote quality decision-making by providing accurate intelligence
- Maintain information on the current and forecasted situation (situation status)
- Track all incident resources (resource status)
- Provide visual information such as sketches, maps, and floor plans
- Develop appropriate contingency plans

Those involved in the original development of ICS felt there was a need to develop a simple but thorough process for planning that could be used for both smaller, short-term incidents and events, and for longer, more complex incident planning. The planning process may

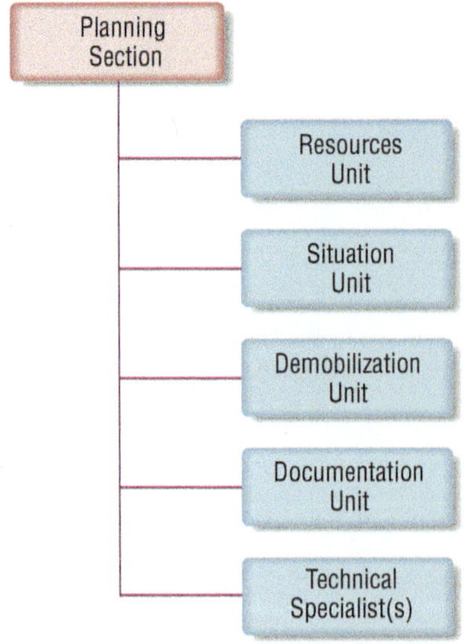

FIGURE 3-10 The functional units of the planning section, which is responsible for the collection, evaluation, and dissemination of operational information related to the incident, and for the preparation and documentation of the IAP. The planning section also maintains information on the current and forecasted situation and on the status of resources assigned to the incident.

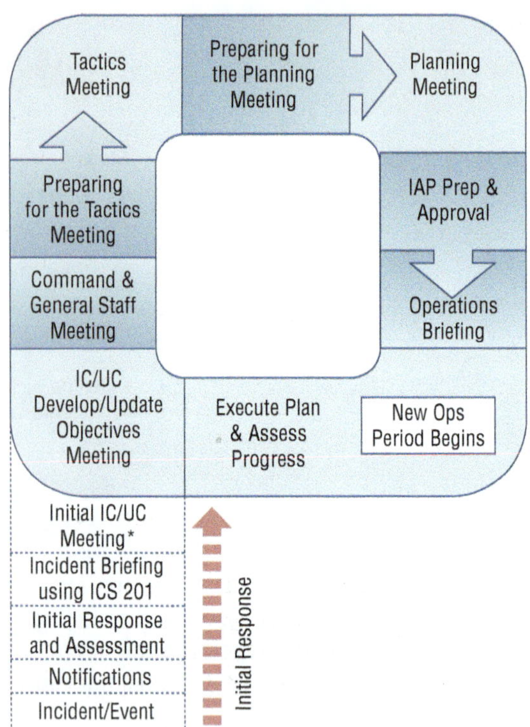

FIGURE 3-11 The Planning "P" is a guide to the ICS planning process and the steps involved in planning within an incident.

begin with the scheduling of a planned event, the identification of a credible threat, or the initial response to an actual or impending event. The process continues with the implementation of the formalized steps and staffing required to develop a written IAP. What was developed to meet this need is the incident planning process, which is depicted by the Planning "P" shown in **FIGURE 3-11**.

The Planning "P" is a guide to the process and steps involved in planning for an incident. The leg of the "P" describes the initial response period: Once the incident/event begins, the steps are notification, initial response and assessment, incident briefing, using the ICS 201 form, and initial incident command (IC)/unified command (UC) meeting. At the top of the leg of the "P" is the beginning of the first operational planning period cycle. In this circular sequence, the steps are:

- IC/UC develops/updates objectives meeting
- Command and general staff meeting
- Preparing for the tactics meeting
- Tactics meeting
- Preparing for the **planning meeting**
- Planning meeting
- IAP prep and approval
- Operations briefing

At this point, a new operational period begins. The next step is to execute the plan and to assess progress, after which the cycle begins again.

The primary phases of the planning process are essentially the same for the IC who develops the initial plan as for the IC and operations section chief revising the initial plan for extended operations, and for the incident management team developing a formal IAP. During the initial stages of incident management, planners must develop a simple plan that can be communicated through concise verbal briefings. Frequently, this plan must be developed very quickly and with incomplete situation information. As the incident management effort evolves over time, additional lead time, staff, information systems, and technologies enable more detailed planning and cataloging of events and lessons learned.

In terms of ICS, planning involves:

- Evaluating the situation
- Developing incident objectives
- Selecting a strategy
- Deciding which resources should be used to achieve the objectives in the safest, most efficient, and most cost-effective manner

The planning, logistics, and finance/administration sections can use **units** to maintain span of control. The planning section includes the **situation unit**, resources unit, **documentation unit**, and **demobilization unit**, as well as **technical specialists** (personnel with special skills that can be used anywhere within the ICS organization and who are activated only when needed).

In a search, the situation unit is important because it can be used to develop maps to display search segments, regions of probability or where the subject is likely to be located, segments that have been searched, and other search progress. In addition, developing this information may require the use of one or more search technical specialists or even a specialized search planning unit, which could be useful in managing the activities necessary to apply the concepts of search theory. Geospatial technical specialists may also be useful in this process by generating any necessary maps and overlaying search data onto them.

The resources unit is also very important in that it tracks the status of all resources assigned to the incident (incident accountability). The operations section chief also tracks the status of all resources assigned to operations (operational accountability). Operational accountability tracks resources with greater detail (exact working location) than incident accountability, which normally tracks incident status (i.e., checked-in/checked-out, available, assigned, and out-of-service).

In large incidents involving many responders, tracking resources may be one of the biggest challenges: knowing exactly when someone arrives (check-in), who is doing what (available, assigned, or out of service), and when someone leaves (check-out). This may also be a significant challenge if many personnel are already operating at an incident when the resources unit is established and staffed. Establishing a secure perimeter and designating adequate check-in locations (staffed by status check-in recorders) is critical in overcoming this sometimes-monumental task.

Logistics Section

The **logistics section** is responsible for providing facilities, services, and material support for the incident (**FIGURE 3-12**). **Logistics** is often critical, especially on more complex incidents. The logistics section chief assists the IC and operations section chief by providing the resources and services required to support incident activities. During an incident, logistics is responsible for ensuring the well-being of responders by providing sufficient food, water, and medical services. Logistics is also responsible for arranging communication equipment, computers, transportation, and anything else needed to support the incident. The logistics section includes the **communications unit**, **medical unit**, and **food unit** (collectively called the **service branch**) and the **supply unit**, **facilities unit**, and **ground support unit** (collectively called the **support branch**). Generally, logistical branches are used only on very large incidents to alleviate span of control issues. Otherwise, each of these units can stand on its own.

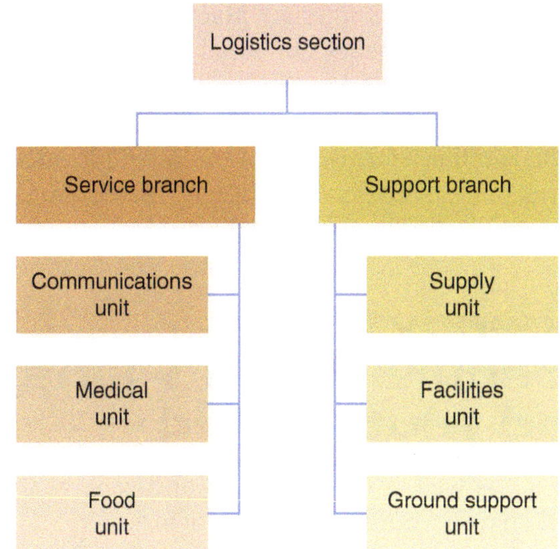

FIGURE 3-12 Branches and units in the logistics section, which are responsible for all of the service and support needs of an incident.

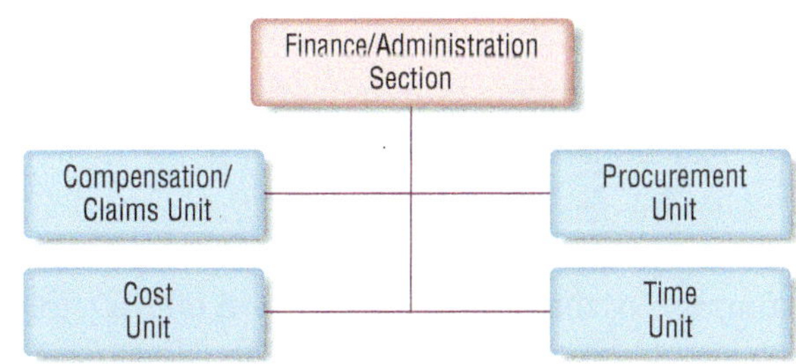

FIGURE 3-13 The organization of the finance/administration section includes four units when fully staffed. This section is responsible for all administrative and financial considerations surrounding an incident.

Finance and Administration Section

Another management function often considered critical by administrators, but typically only established during very large or complex incidents, is finance/administration (**FIGURE 3-13**). The **finance/administration section** is led by a section chief who is responsible for all financial-related aspects of an incident. These include contract negotiation, recording personnel and equipment time, documenting and processing claims for accidents and injuries occurring at the incident, keeping a running tally of the costs associated with the incident (burn rate), and providing cost analysis, as requested. The finance/administration section includes the **time unit**, **procurement unit**, **compensation/claims unit**, and **cost unit**. Rather than establishing a robust finance section, it is common practice for the IC(s) to utilize the home agency's financial resources, policies, and procedures. Good incident documentation—such as unit logs, check-in sheets, resource order forms, situation summary forms, and IAPs—often includes the information needed to address financial issues, especially when recovering costs after the incident.

Agency Preparedness Plans and Mutual Aid

The IC, as well as the command and general staffs, should have a working knowledge of jurisdictional and agency preparedness plans and agreements. Preparedness plans may take many forms, but the most common preparedness plans are:

- Federal, state, or local emergency operations plans (EOPs)
- Standard operating guidelines (SOGs)
- Standard operating procedures (SOPs)
- Jurisdictional or agency policies

EOPs are developed at the federal, state, and local levels to provide a uniform response to all hazards that a community may face. EOPs written after October 2005 should be consistent with NIMS. However, this is not always the case.

Mutual aid is the voluntary provision of resources by agencies or organizations to assist each other when existing resources are inadequate. Mutual aid agreements and assistance agreements are agreements between agencies, organizations, and jurisdictions that provide a mechanism to quickly obtain emergency assistance in the form of personnel, equipment, materials, and other associated services. When combined with NIMS-oriented resource management, mutual aid allows jurisdictions to share resources among mutual aid partners. At a minimum, mutual aid agreements should include the following elements or provisions:

- Definitions of key terms used in the agreement
- Roles and responsibilities of individual parties
- Procedures for requesting and providing assistance
- Procedures, authorities, and rules for payment, reimbursement, and allocation of costs
- Notification procedures
- Protocols for interoperable communications
- Relationships with other agreements among jurisdictions
- Workers' compensation
- Treatment of liability and immunity
- Recognition of qualifications and certifications
- Sharing agreements, as required

Mutual aid agreements and assistance agreements are used at all levels of government:

- Local jurisdictions participate in mutual aid through agreements with neighboring jurisdictions.
- States can participate in mutual aid through the Emergency Management Assistance Compact (EMAC; see Chapter 2).
- Federal agencies offer mutual aid to each other and to states, tribes, and territories under the National Response Framework (NRF; see Chapter 2).

Jurisdictions should be party to agreements with the appropriate agencies and/or organizations from which they expect to receive, or to which they expect to provide, assistance.

In the context of ICS, *authority* is defined as a right or obligation to act on behalf of a department, agency, or jurisdiction. In most jurisdictions, the responsibility for the protection of the citizens rests with the chief elected official (e.g., trustees, mayor, commissioner, etc.). Elected officials have the authority to make decisions, commit resources, obligate funds, and command the resources necessary to protect the population, stop the spread of damage, and protect the environment. In private industry, this same responsibility and authority usually rests with the chief executive officer or business owner.

An IC's authority is derived from existing laws, agency policies and procedures, and/or through a delegation of authority from the **agency administrator** or elected official. A **delegation of authority** is the process of granting authority to another so that he or she may carry out specific functions. It may be issued by the chief elected official, chief executive officer, or agency administrator either in writing or verbally.

Although a delegation of authority does not relieve the granting authority of the ultimate responsibility for the incident, it does allow the IC to assume command where the authority to do so does not otherwise exist. Ideally, this authority will be granted in a written document, but whether it is in writing or verbal, the authorities granted remain with the IC until such time as the incident is terminated, a relief shift IC is appointed, or the IC is relieved of his or her duties for just cause.

A delegation of authority may be needed if the incident is outside the IC's jurisdiction, if the incident scope is complex or beyond existing authorities, or if required by law or procedures. A delegation of authority is not required if the IC is acting within his or her existing authorities. For example, an emergency manager may already have the authority to deploy response resources to a small flash flood, or a fire chief likely has the authority (as part of the job description) to serve as the IC at a structure fire.

Incident Action Plan

Every incident needs a general outline or strategy that covers how the incident response will be conducted. In ICS, this is the IAP. Above all, an IAP should be current, available, and useful to those assigned to work.

At a minimum, the IAP should provide incident objectives, guide operations, establish priorities for action, and describe the number and types of resources required. In shorter, less complex incidents, the IC may develop the IAP by himself or herself and never reduce it to writing; or, for the initial operational period, complete an ICS 201, Incident Briefing Form, which may be the only documentation required. The ICS 201 is a four-page document that contains a scene map/sketch; situation summary; current and planned objective; current and planned actions, strategies and tactics; organization chart; and, resource summary. Using an ICS 201 form also makes it easier to transfer command as the incident grows.

More complex incidents require that the IAP be written so that everyone knows the strategy and tactics being used. Although there may be several incident actions for each operational period (the period of time scheduled for execution of a given set of tactical actions as specified in the IAP), there should be only one IAP at any given time in the incident.

Operational periods can be of various lengths but are usually no longer than 24 hours and no shorter than eight hours. Twelve-hour operational periods are common on many large incidents. The length of an operational period will be based on the needs of the incident and can change over the course of the incident. The planning for an operational period must also be done far enough in advance to ensure that requested resources are available and in place when the operational period begins.

Several forms have been developed to support the ICS planning process. They are each numbered and, although variations exist regarding their layout, the contents of each of the respective forms has been standardized (**TABLE 3-5**).

TABLE 3-5 Incident Command System Forms

ICS Form #	Form Title	Prepared by
201	Incident Briefing (4 pages)	Initial response IC
202*	Incident Objectives	Planning section chief
203*	Organization Assignment List	Resources unit leader
204*	Assignment List	Resources unit leader
205*	Incident Radio Communications Plan	Communications unit leader
205a	Communications List	Communications unit leader
206*	Incident Medical Plan	Medical unit leader
207	Incident Organization Chart	Resources unit leader
208	Safety Message (Site Safety) Plan	Safety officer
209	Incident Status Summary (23 pages)	Situation unit leader
210	Resource Status Change	Resources unit leader
211	Incident Check-in List	Status/check-in recorder
212 (oil)	Resources at Risk	Situation unit leader
213	General Message Form	Anyone

(continues)

TABLE 3-5 Incident Command System Forms (*continued*)

ICS Form #	Form Title	Prepared by
214	Activity Log (2 pages)	All positions
215	Operational Planning Worksheet	Planning and operations Section chiefs
215a	IAP Safety Analysis	Safety officer
216	Radio Requirements Works	Communications unit leader
217	Radio Frequency Assignment	Communications unit leader
218	Support Vehicle/Equipment Inventory	Ground support unit leader
219	Resource Status Card (T-card)	Resources unit
	219-1 Header (gray) 219-2 Crew/Team (green) 219-3 Engine (rose) 219-4 Helicopter (blue) 219-5 Personnel (white)	219-6 Fixed Wing (orange) 219-7 Equipment (yellow) 219-8 Misc. Equip./Task Force (tan) 219-10 Generic (light purple)
220	Air Operations Summary (2 pages)	Operations section chief
221	Demobilization Checkout	Demobilization unit leader
223	Tentative Release List	Supervisors
225	Incident Personnel Performance Rating (2 pages)	Command staff
226	Individual Performance Rating	Supervisors
230	Daily Meeting Schedule	Situation unit leader
230a	Meeting Description	Situation unit leader
259	Resource Order	Supply unit/dispatcher
281	Resource Tracking	Dispatcher/resources unit

* = Required part of incident action plan (IAP)

The essential elements of an IAP are listed in **FIGURE 3-14** along with the ICS forms usually associated with each element. At a minimum, the contents of an IAP should include:

- *Statement of objectives*: Appropriate to the overall incident.
- *Organization*: Describes what parts of the ICS organization will be in place for each operational period
- *Assignments to accomplish the objectives*: These are normally prepared for each division or group and include the strategy, tactics, and resources to be used.
- *Supporting material*: Examples can include a map of the incident, communications plan, medical plan, traffic plan, a blank unit log, etc.

Incident Objectives

As part of the ICS planning process and the IAP, the IC establishes incident objectives, which are statements of guidance and direction necessary for the selection of appropriate strategies and tactics. Incident objectives are based on realistic expectations of what can be accomplished when all allocated resources have been effectively

Item	Complete
*Cover Sheet • Incident name, date, operational period?	
*ICS 202: Incident Objectives • Simple, Measurable, Attainable, Action oriented, Reasonable, Time oriented?	
*ICS 203: Organizational Assignment List • Does 203 match 204?	
*ICS 204: Division Assignment List • Clear, precise, measurable? • Pick up and drop off point/time? • One for each division/group? • Date, time? • Matches communications summary (205)? • Prepared by?	
*ICS 205: Incident Communications Plan • Nets: command, tactical, support? • Match frequencies/talk groups given/coordinated? • Prepared by?	
*ICS 206: Medical Plan • Emergency procedures clear? • Hospitals and ambulance services? • Reviewed by Safety Officer? • Prepared by?	
ICS 220: Air Operations Summary • List of aircraft? • Temporary Flight Restrictions (TFR) in use?	
*Incident Map • Clear, north arrow, scale included, appropriate symbols? • Matches assignments on 204?	
Traffic Plan • Clear, north arrow, scale included, appropriate symbols?	
Approvals on each sheet, signed by appropriate individuals?	
Safety Message • Clear, concise, and applicable to incident?	
Weather Forecast • For operational period and next?	
Logistics and Finance Issues • Anything regarding supplies, facilities, food, ground support, etc.?	
Liaison Officer Issues • Anything for agency representatives and resources?	
Human Resource Message	
Press Release • What is going on with media, media strategy?	
ICS 214: Unit Log (blank)	

* = Mandatory elements

FIGURE 3-14 Checklist: Elements of an Incident Action Plan (IAP).

deployed. Incident objectives must be achievable and measurable, yet flexible enough to allow for strategic and tactical alternatives.

Fully effective incident objectives must be:

- Specific and state what is to be accomplished
- Measurable and include a standard and timeframe
- Attainable and reasonable
- In accordance with the IC's authorities
- Evaluated to determine effectiveness of strategies and tactics

Incident objectives are established by the IC and communicated throughout the entire ICS organization via the incident planning process. The process for the IC establishing and implementing incident objectives involves the following steps:

1. Understand agency policy and direction.
2. Assess the incident situation.
3. Establish incident priorities and objectives.
4. Select appropriate strategy or strategies to achieve objectives.
5. Perform tactical direction.
6. Provide necessary follow-up.

The over-arching priorities for incident objectives are always:

1. Life safety (for both the public and responders)
2. Incident stabilization
3. Property/environmental conservation

Incident priorities and objectives are the first of three parts of a successful incident response. Incident objectives, which are based on established priorities, state what will be accomplished. Then, strategies establish the general plan or direction for accomplishing the incident objectives, and tactics specify how the strategies will be executed.

The IC is responsible for establishing incident objectives and selecting strategies. The operations section is responsible for determining appropriate tactics for each operational period during an incident.

An incident briefing form (ICS 201, see Table 3-5) may be used to record objectives in the initial operational period during the first transfer of command. There should be only one ICS 201 for any incident. A full IAP should be developed after the initial operational period. In subsequent operational periods where a written IAP is used, an ICS 202 form would be used to record objectives.

Common Responsibilities

There are certain responsibilities associated with an incident assignment that are common across all roles within an ICS organization (**FIGURE 3-15**), and meeting these responsibilities can result in a more effective operation:

1. Receive orders to respond from your organization (call out). This should include, at a minimum, a **reporting location** and time, likely length

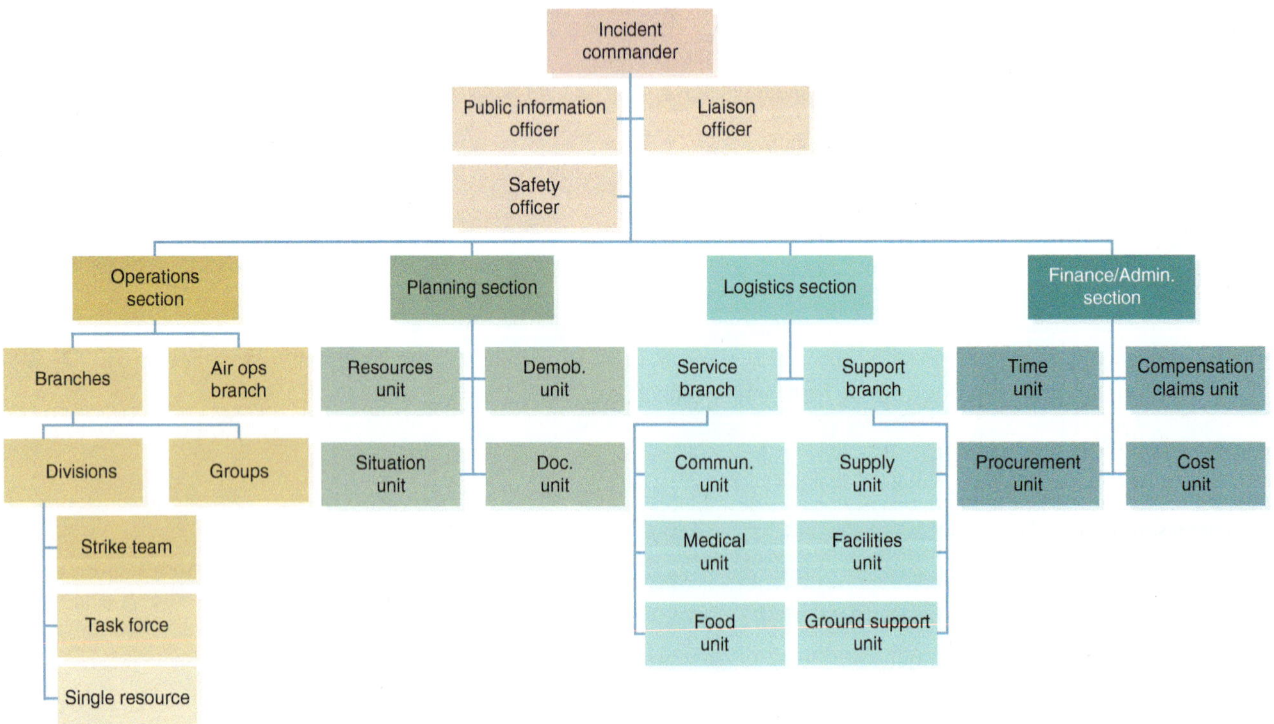

FIGURE 3-15 The ICS organizational model.

Reproduced from FEMA. (2018). ICS for Single Resources and Initial Action Incidents (ICS 200): ICS Organization. Retrieved from https://emilms.fema.gov/IS200b/ICS0102280text.htm

of assignment, brief description of assignment, route information, and a designated communications link if necessary.

2. Begin and maintain an ICS 214 Unit Log.
3. Prepare by bringing any specialized supplies and/or equipment required for your anticipated assignment. Be sure you have adequate personal supplies to last for the expected stay.
4. Check in immediately upon arrival and receive initial instructions.
   - Agency representatives from assisting or cooperating agencies should report to the liaison officer at the ICP after check-in.
5. Use clear text, not radio codes, when speaking on the radio. Refer to incident facilities by the incident name; for example, "Tallmadge Command Post," or "Main Street Staging Area." Refer to personnel by ICS title; for example, "Division C," and not a numeric code or name.
6. Obtain a briefing that you understand from your immediate supervisor.
7. Acquire necessary work materials and locate and set up your work area.
8. Supervisors must maintain accountability for their assigned personnel with regard for exact location(s) and personal safety and welfare at all times, especially when working in or around incident operations.
9. Organize and brief any subordinates assigned to you.
10. Know your assigned radio frequency(s) or talk groups for your area of responsibility and ensure that communication equipment is operating properly.
11. Complete your assignment and report to your supervisor any delays (will finish late), change in status (illness, fatigue, etc.), or obstacles preventing completion of your assignment.
12. Brief your relief at the end of each operational period and, as necessary, at the time you are demobilized from the incident.
13. Complete required forms and reports and submit them to the appropriate person on scene before you leave.
14. Demobilize according to plan.

The safety of all personnel involved in an incident or a planned event is the first duty of ICS leadership. This is the overall responsibility of team leaders, group or division supervisors, branch directors, section chiefs, and all members of the command or unified command staff. Ensuring safe work practices is the top priority within the ICS common leadership responsibilities and is indeed a main reason for the use of ICS. A good operational leader:

- Is proficient at his or her job
- Communicates by giving specific instructions and asking for feedback
- Ensures tasks are understood
- Makes sound and timely decisions
- Supervises the scene of action
- Evaluates the effectiveness of the plan
- Understands and accepts the need to modify plans or instructions
- Ensures safe work practices
- Takes command of assigned resources
- Motivates with a "can do safely" attitude
- Demonstrates initiative by taking action
- Develops subordinates for the future

Wrap-Up

READY FOR REVIEW

- The incident command system (ICS) is the approach to incident management used in the United States and many other parts of the world that helps ensure integration and interoperability of response efforts.
- ICS incorporates several proven management features and principles that contribute to the overall strength and efficiency of the system.
- There are five major management functions performed at every incident: incident command, operations, planning, logistics, and finance/administration.

- Depending on the incident needs, the IC may delegate some or all management functions by establishing sections, which may be headed by a section chief reporting directly to the IC. Together, these section chiefs are referred to as the general staff.
- Preparedness plans may take many forms, but the most common preparedness plans are federal, state, or local emergency operations plans (EOPs); standard operating guidelines (SOGs); standard operating procedures (SOPs); and jurisdictional or agency policies.
- At a minimum, the incident action plan (IAP) should provide incident objectives, guide operations, establish priorities for action, and describe the number and types of resources required.
- The safety of all personnel involved in an incident or a planned event is the first duty of ICS leadership. This is the overall responsibility of team leaders, group or division supervisors, branch directors, section chiefs, and all members of the command or unified command staff.

SEARCH AND RESCUE TERMS

Agency A division of government with a specific function, or a nongovernmental organization (e.g., private contractor, business) that offers a particular kind of assistance. In ICS, agencies are defined as jurisdictional (having statutory responsibility for incident mitigation) or assisting and/or cooperating (providing resources and/or assistance).

Agency administrator A chief executive officer (or designee) of an agency or jurisdiction that has responsibility for the incident.

Agency representative An individual assigned to an incident from an assisting or cooperating agency that has been delegated authority to make decisions on matters affecting that agency's participation at the incident. Agency representatives report to the incident liaison officer.

All-risk Any incident or event, natural or human-caused, that warrants action to protect life, property, environment, public health or safety, and minimizes disruption of government, social, or economic activities.

Assigned resources Resources checked in and assigned work tasks on an incident.

Assistants Subordinates of command staff positions. The title indicates a level of technical capability, qualifications, and responsibility subordinate to the primary positions. Assistants may also be assigned to unit leaders.

Assisting agency An agency or organization providing personnel, services, or other resources to the agency with direct responsibility for incident management.

Available resources Resources assigned to an incident, checked in, and available for a mission assignment, normally located in a staging area.

Branches The organizational level having functional or geographic responsibility for major parts of the operations or logistics functions. The branch level is organizationally between section and division/group in the operations section and between section and units in the logistics section. Branches are identified by Roman numerals or by functional name (e.g., medical, security). A branch is led by a branch director who reports to the operations chief.

Camps Geographical sites, within the general incident area, separate from the incident base, equipped and staffed to provide sleeping, food, water, and sanitary services to incident personnel.

Chain of command The orderly line of authority within the ranks of the incident management organization.

Check-in The process whereby resources first report to an incident. All responders, regardless of agency affiliation, must report in to receive an assignment in accordance with the procedures established by the incident commander. Check-in locations include: incident command post (resources unit), incident base, camps, staging areas, helibases, helispots, and division supervisors (for direct line assignments).

Clear text The use of plain English in radio communications transmissions. No ten codes or agency-specific codes are used when utilizing clear text.

Command The act of directing and/or controlling resources by virtue of explicit legal, agency, or delegated authority. May also refer to the incident commander.

Command staff The staff who report directly to the incident commander, including the public information officer, safety officer, liaison officer, and other positions as required. They may have an assistant or assistants, as needed.

Common terminology Normally used words and phrases—avoiding the use of different words/phrases for the same concepts—to ensure consistency and to allow diverse incident management and support organizations to work together across a wide variety of incident management functions and hazard scenarios.

Communications unit Functional unit in the logistics section responsible for providing communication services at an incident. A communications unit may also be a facility (e.g., a trailer or mobile van) used to provide the major part of an incident communications center.

Compensation/claims unit Functional unit within the finance/administration section responsible for financial concerns resulting from property damage, injuries, or fatalities at the incident.

Cooperating agency An agency supplying assistance other than direct operational or support functions or resources to the incident management effort.

Coordination centers Facilities that are used for the coordination of agency or jurisdictional resources in support of one or more incidents.

Cost unit Functional unit within the finance/administration section responsible for tracking costs, analyzing cost data, making cost estimates, and recommending cost-saving measures.

Credentialing The authentication and verification of the certification and identity of designated incident managers and emergency responders.

Crew See *single resource.*

Delegation of authority A statement provided to the incident commander by the agency executive delegating authority and assigning responsibility. The delegation of authority can include objectives, priorities, expectations, constraints, and other considerations or guidelines as needed. Many agencies require written delegation of authority to be given to incident commanders prior to their assuming command on larger incidents. Also known as *letter of expectation.*

Demobilization The orderly, safe, and efficient return of an incident resource to its original location and status.

Demobilization unit Functional unit within the planning section, responsible for assuring orderly, safe, and efficient demobilization of incident resources.

Deputy A fully qualified individual who, in the absence of a superior, could be delegated the authority to manage a functional operation or perform a specific task. In some cases, a deputy could act as relief for a superior and, therefore, must be fully qualified in the position. Deputies can be assigned to the incident commander, general staff, and branch directors.

Director The ICS title for individuals responsible for supervision of a branch and who answer to the operations chief.

Divisions The organizational level having responsibility for operations within a defined geographic area. A division is located within the ICS organization between the branch and the task force/strike team. (See *group.*) Divisions are identified by alphabetic characters for horizontal applications and, often, by floor numbers when used in buildings. A division is led by a division supervisor.

Documentation unit Functional unit within the planning section responsible for collecting, recording, and safeguarding all documents relevant to the incident.

Event A planned, nonemergency activity. ICS can be used as the management system for a wide range of events, for example, parades, concerts, or sporting events.

Facilities unit Functional unit within the support branch of the logistics section that provides fixed facilities for the incident. These facilities may include the incident base, feeding areas, sleeping areas, sanitary facilities, etc.

Finance/administration section The incident command system section responsible for all administrative and financial considerations surrounding an incident. Includes the time unit, procurement unit, compensation/claims unit, and cost unit.

Food unit Functional unit within the service branch of the logistics section responsible for providing meals for incident personnel.

Functions The five major activities in the incident command system: command, operations, planning, logistics, and finance/administration. A sixth function, intelligence/investigations, may be established, if required, to meet incident management needs. The term *function* is also used when describing the activity involved (e.g., the planning function).

General staff A group of incident management personnel organized according to function and reporting to the incident commander. The general staff normally consists of the operations section chief, planning section chief, logistics section chief, and finance/administration section chief. An intelligence/investigations chief may be established, if required, to meet incident management needs.

Ground support unit Functional unit within the support branch of the logistics section responsible for the fueling, maintaining, and repairing of vehicles, and the transportation of personnel and supplies.

Groups Organizational subdivisions established to divide the incident management structure into functional areas of operation. Groups are composed of resources assembled to perform a special function not necessarily within a single geographic division. (See *Division.*) Groups are located between branches (when activated) and resources in the operations section. A group is led by a group supervisor.

Helibase The main location for parking, fueling, maintenance, and loading of helicopters operating in support of an incident. It is usually located at or near the incident base.

Helispots Any designated locations where a helicopter can safely take off and land. Some helispots may be used for loading of supplies, equipment, or personnel.

Incident action plans (IAPs) Oral or written plans containing general objectives reflecting the overall strategy for managing an incident. It may include the identification of operational resources and assignments. It may also include attachments that provide direction and important information for management of the incident during one or more operational periods.

Incident base Location at the incident where the primary logistics functions are coordinated and administered. (Incident name or other designator will be added to the term *base*.) The incident command post may be co-located with the base. There is only one base per incident.

Incident commander (IC) The individual responsible for all incident activities, including the development of strategies and tactics and the ordering and the release of resources. The IC has overall authority and responsibility for conducting incident operations and is responsible for the management of all incident operations at the incident site.

Incident command post (ICP) The field location at which the primary tactical-level, on-scene incident command functions are performed. The ICP may be co-located with the incident base or other incident facilities and is normally identified by a green rotating or flashing light.

Incident command system (ICS) A standardized on-scene emergency management construct specifically designed to provide for the adoption of an integrated organizational structure that reflects the complexity and demands of single or multiple incidents, without being hindered by jurisdictional boundaries. ICS is the combination of facilities, equipment, personnel, procedures, and communications operating within a common organizational structure, designed to aid in the management of resources during incidents. It is used for all kinds of emergencies and is applicable to small as well as large and complex incidents. ICS is used by various jurisdictions and functional agencies, both public and private, to organize field-level incident management operations.

Incident management The broad spectrum of activities and organizations providing effective and efficient operations, coordination, and support applied at all levels of government, utilizing both governmental and nongovernmental resources to plan for, respond to, and recover from an incident regardless of cause, size, or complexity.

Incident management team (IMT) An incident commander and the appropriate command and general staff personnel assigned to an incident. The level of training and experience of the IMT members, coupled with the identified formal response requirements and responsibilities of the IMT, are factors in determining "type," or level, of IMT.

Incident objectives Statements of guidance and direction necessary for the selection of appropriate strategies and the tactical direction of resources. Incident objectives are based on realistic expectations of what can be accomplished when all allocated resources have been effectively deployed. Incident objectives must be achievable and measurable, yet flexible enough to allow for strategic and tactical alternatives.

Incident types Incidents are categorized by five types based on complexity. Type 5 incidents are the least complex, and Type 1 incidents are the most complex.

Incidents Occurrences or events, natural or human-caused, that require an emergency response to protect life or property. Incidents can, for example, include major disasters, emergencies, terrorist attacks, terrorist threats, wildland and urban fires, floods, hazardous materials spills, nuclear accidents, aircraft accidents, earthquakes, hurricanes, tornadoes, tropical storms, war-related disasters, public health and medical emergencies, and other occurrences requiring an emergency response.

Individual resources One person; in contrast to a "single resource," which describes a piece of equipment and its personnel complement. Individual resources are often called responders or specialists.

Information Data, knowledge, and facts about someone or something gained from somewhere.

Intelligence Information that has been verified, analyzed, collated, evaluated, and prepared for use in making decisions.

Intelligence officer The intelligence officer is responsible for managing internal information, intelligence, and operational security requirements supporting incident management activities. These may include information security and operational security activities, as well as the complex task of ensuring that sensitive information of all types (e.g., classified information, law enforcement sensitive information, proprietary information, or export-controlled information) is handled in a way that not only safeguards the information but also ensures that it gets to those who need access to it to perform their missions effectively and safely.

Jurisdiction A range or sphere of authority. Public agencies have jurisdiction at an incident related to their legal responsibilities and authority. Jurisdictional authority at an incident can be political or geographical (e.g., city, county, tribal, state, or federal boundary lines) or functional (e.g., law enforcement, public health).

Kinds of resources Describe what the resource is (e.g., medic, fire fighter, planning section chief, helicopters, ambulances, combustible gas indicators, bulldozers).

Landing zones (LZs) See *helispots*.

Leader The incident command system title for an individual responsible for a task force, strike team, or functional unit.

Liaison A form of communication for establishing and maintaining mutual understanding and cooperation.

Liaison officer A member of the command staff responsible for coordinating with representatives from cooperating and assisting agencies or organizations. The liaison officer may have assistants.

Logistics The process and procedure for providing resources and other services to support incident management.

Logistics section The section responsible for providing facilities, services, and materials for the incident.

Management by objectives A management approach that involves a five-step process for achieving the incident goal. The management by objectives approach includes the following: establishing overarching incident objectives; developing strategies based on overarching incident objectives; developing and issuing assignments, plans, procedures, and protocols; establishing specific, measurable tactics or tasks for various incident management functional activities and directing efforts to attain them, in support of defined strategies; and documenting results to measure performance and facilitate corrective action.

Managers Individuals within an incident command system organizational unit who are assigned specific managerial responsibilities (e.g., staging area manager or camp manager).

Medical unit Functional unit within the service branch of the logistics section responsible for the development of the medical emergency plan and for providing emergency medical treatment of incident personnel.

Mobilization centers Off-incident locations at which emergency service personnel and equipment are temporarily located pending assignment, release, or reassignment.

Modular organization An organization that can be expanded or contracted as the incident warrants by adding (activating) or removing (demobilizing) organizational elements such as functional sections and units, as needed.

Multiagency coordination (MAC) entities or groups Administrators or executives, or their appointed representatives, working together, who are typically authorized to commit agency resources and funds. A MAC group can provide coordinated decision-making and resource allocation among cooperating agencies and may establish the priorities among incidents, harmonize agency policies, and provide strategic guidance and direction to support incident management activities. MAC groups may also be known as multiagency committees, emergency management committees, or as otherwise defined by the multiagency coordination system.

Multiagency coordination systems (MACS) Systems that provide the architecture to support coordination for incident prioritization, critical resource allocation, communications systems integration, and information coordination. MACS assist agencies and organizations responding to an incident. The elements of a MACS include facilities, equipment, personnel, procedures, and communications. Two of the most commonly used elements are emergency operations centers and MAC groups.

National Incident Management System (NIMS) A set of principles that provides a systematic, proactive approach guiding government agencies at all levels, nongovernmental organizations, and the private sector to work seamlessly to prevent, protect against, respond to, recover from, and mitigate the effects of incidents, regardless of cause, size, location, or complexity, in order to reduce the loss of life or property and harm to the environment.

National Integration Center The U.S. Department of Homeland Security's facility responsible for managing the implementation and administration of the National Incident Management System (NIMS).

Officer The incident command system title for the personnel responsible for the command staff positions of safety, liaison, and public information.

Operational period The time scheduled for executing a given set of operation actions, as specified in the incident action plan. Operational periods can be of various lengths, although usually they last 12 to 24 hours.

Operations section The incident command system section responsible for all tactical incident operations and implementation of the incident action plan. In ICS, the operations section is led by the operations section chief and normally includes subordinate branches, divisions, and/or groups, task forces, strike teams, single resources, and staging areas.

Out-of-service resources Resources assigned to an incident but unable to respond for mechanical, rest, or personnel reasons.

Personnel accountability reports (PAR) Periodic reports verifying the status of responders assigned to an incident.

Planning meeting A meeting held as needed throughout the duration of an incident, to select specific strategies and tactics for incident control operations, and for service and support planning. On larger incidents, the planning meeting is a major element in the development of the incident action plan.

Planning section The incident command system section responsible for the collection, evaluation, and dissemination of operational information related to the incident, and for the preparation and documentation of the incident action plan. This section also maintains information on the current and forecasted situation and on the status of resources assigned to the incident. This section includes the situation, resources, documentation, and demobilization units, as well as technical specialists.

Procurement unit Functional unit within the finance/administration section responsible for financial matters involving vendor contracts.

Public information officer A member of the command staff responsible for interfacing with the public and media or with other agencies with incident-related information requirements.

Qualified A person meeting a recognized level of training, experience, and certification for the assigned position.

Reporting location Location or facility where incoming resources can check in at the incident. (See *check-in*.)

Resource management A system for identifying available resources at all jurisdictional levels to enable timely, efficient, and unimpeded access to resources needed to prepare for, respond to, or recover from an incident. Resource management under the National Incident Management System includes mutual aid agreements and assistance agreements; the use of special federal, state, tribal, and local teams; and resource mobilization protocols.

Resource tracking A standardized, integrated process conducted prior to, during, and after an incident by all emergency management/response personnel and their associated organizations.

Resources Personnel and major items of equipment, supplies, and facilities available or potentially available for assignment to incident operations and for which status is maintained. Resources are described by kind and type and may be used in operational support or supervisory capacities at an incident or at an emergency operations center.

Resources unit Functional unit within the planning section responsible for recording the status of resources committed to the incident. The unit also evaluates resources currently committed to the incident, the impact that additional responding resources will have on the incident, and anticipated resource needs. The resources unit is led by the resources unit leader, who reports to the planning section chief.

Safety officer A member of the command staff responsible for monitoring incident operations and advising the incident commander on all matters relating to operational safety, including the health and safety of emergency responder personnel. The safety officer may have assistants.

Section The organizational level having responsibility for a major functional area of incident management, for example, operations, planning, logistics, finance/administration, and intelligence (if established). The section is organizationally situated between the branch and the incident command and is led by a section chief.

Section chief The incident command system title for individuals responsible for management of functional sections: operations, planning, logistics, finance/administration, and intelligence/investigations (if established as a separate section). A section chief answers to the incident commander.

Service branch A branch within the logistics section responsible for service activities at the incident. Includes the communication, medical, and food units. A branch is led by a branch director who reports to the operations chief.

Single resource A piece of equipment and its personnel complement, or a crew or team of individuals with an identified work supervisor that can be used on an incident.

Situation unit Functional unit within the planning section responsible for the collection, organization, and analysis of incident status information, and for analysis of the situation as it progresses. The situation unit is led by the situation unit leader, who reports to the planning section chief.

Situational awareness The ability to identify, process, and comprehend the critical elements of information about what is happening to the team with regards to the mission. In short, having situational awareness is knowing what is going on around you.

Span of control The number of resources for which a supervisor is responsible, usually expressed as the ratio of supervisors to individuals. (Under NIMS, an appropriate span of control is between 1:3 and 1:7, with optimal being 1:5, or between 1:8 and 1:10 for many large-scale law enforcement operations.)

Staging areas Temporary locations for available resources. A staging area can be any location in which personnel, supplies, and equipment can be temporarily housed or parked while awaiting operational assignment. The operations section manages staging areas.

Strategy The general direction selected to accomplish incident objectives set by the incident commander.

Strike teams Specified combinations of the same kind and type of resources with common communications and a leader.

Supervisor The ICS title for individuals responsible for a division or group.

Supply unit Functional unit within the support branch of the logistics section responsible for ordering equipment and supplies required for incident operations.

Support branch A branch within the logistics section responsible for providing personnel, equipment, and supplies to support incident operations. Includes the supply, facilities, and ground support units. A branch is led by a branch director, who reports to the operations chief.

Supporting agency An agency that provides support and/or resource assistance to another agency. See *assisting agency*.

Tactics The deployment and directing of resources on an incident to accomplish the objectives designated by strategy.

Task forces Combination of single resources assembled for a particular tactical need with common communications and a leader.

Technical specialists Personnel with special skills that can be used anywhere within the ICS organization and who are activated only when needed.

Time unit Functional unit within the finance/administration section responsible for recording time for incident personnel and hired equipment.

Type An incident command system resource classification that refers to capability. Type 1 is generally considered to be more capable than Types 2, 3, or 4, respectively, because of size, power, capacity, or (in the case of incident management teams) experience and qualifications.

Unified command (UC) An incident command system application used when more than one agency has incident jurisdiction or when incidents cross political jurisdictions. Agencies work together through the designated members of the UC, often the senior persons from agencies and/or disciplines participating in the UC, to establish a common set of objectives and strategies and a single incident action plan.

Unit leaders The individuals in charge of managing units within an incident command system (ICS) functional section. The unit can be staffed by many support personnel providing a wide range of services. Some of the support positions are preestablished within ICS (e.g., base/camp manager), but many others will be assigned as technical specialists.

Units The organizational element having functional responsibility for a specific incident planning, logistics, or finance/administration activity.

Unity of command An incident command system principle stating that each individual involved in incident operations will be assigned to only one supervisor.

REFERENCES AND SUGGESTED READING

Climber.org. 2015. *The Yosemite decimal system*. http://climber.org/data/decimal.html.

Federal Bureau of Investigation, Directorate of Intelligence. 2015. *Intelligence defined*. http://www.fbi.gov/about-us/intelligence/defined.

Federal Emergency Management Agency. 2018. *Incident command system resources*. https://www.fema.gov/incident-command-system-resources.

Federal Geographic Data Committee. 2015. Emergency Symbology Reference produced by the Homeland Security Working Group. http://www.fgdc.gov/HSWG/index.html.

U.S. Department of Homeland Security, Emergency Management Institute. 2015. NIMS ICS all-hazards position specific training program official website. Washington, DC.: U.S. Department of Homeland Security. https://training.fema.gov/allhazards/.

U.S. Department of Homeland Security. 2016. *National Response Framework.* Third Edition. Washington, DC.: U.S. Department of Homeland Security. http://www.fema.gov/media-library-data/1466014682982-9bcf8245ba4c60c120aa915abe74e15d/National_Response_Framework3rd.pdf.

U.S. Department of Homeland Security, Federal Emergency Management Agency. 2018. *Resource typing library tool.* Washington, D.C.: U.S. Department of Homeland Security. https://rtlt.preptoolkit.org/.

U.S. Department of Homeland Security, U.S. Fire Administration. 2018. *An overview of incident management teams.* Washington, DC.: U.S. Fire Administration. http://www.usfa.fema.gov/training/imt/imt_overview.html.

U.S. Department of Homeland Security. 2017. National Incident Management System (NIMS), Third Edition. Washington, DC.: U.S. Department of Homeland Security. http://www.fema.gov/media-library-data/1508151197225-ced8c60378c3936adb92c1a3ee6f6564/FINAL_NIMS_2017.pdf.

U.S. Department of Labor, Occupational Safety and Health Administration. 2015. 29 CFR 1910.120, Occupational Safety and Health Standards, Hazardous Materials, Hazardous waste operations and emergency response. https://www.osha.gov.

U.S. Environmental Protection Agency. 1986. Superfund Amendments and Reauthorization Act (SARA) of 1986. http://www.epa.gov/superfund/policy/sara.htm.

CHAPTER 4

Legal Aspects of Search and Rescue

OBJECTIVES

Upon completion of this chapter and the related course activities, the student will be able to meet the following objectives:

- Briefly describe each of the following legal concepts as they apply to search and rescue (SAR):
  - Scope of practice
  - Standard of care
  - Duty to act
  - Engendered reliance
  - Negligence
  - Gross negligence
  - Abandonment
  - Consent
  - Documentation
  - Confidentiality
- Explain how the provisions of the Volunteer Protection Act differ between how they apply to an individual volunteer versus a nonprofit organization.
- Explain the relationship of the Health Insurance Portability and Accountability Act (HIPAA) to the SAR volunteer.
- Describe the three general categories of trespass in the context of SAR.
- List at least three rules that maximize the chances of preserving evidence and maintaining the chain of custody at a SAR scene.
- List at least six suggestions that can minimize liability and legal challenges of the actions of a SAR volunteer.

Do No Harm

A fundamental tenet of emergency care is to do no more harm. Search and rescue (SAR) personnel who act in good faith and according to an appropriate standard of care can usually avoid legal problems, but laws, regulations, and standards vary across the United States and from country to country on all issues related to emergency response, including search and rescue. SAR personnel must be familiar with the various legal aspects of search and rescue (**FIGURE 4-1**).

Situations may also arise that require more than just knowledge of the law. Ethical questions can challenge even the most seasoned SAR professional and must be anticipated.

This chapter is not meant as a substitute for competent legal counsel. Rather, it is meant to guide SAR personnel as they consider legal and ethical issues and serve as an aid to help develop questions to ask legal counsel. Seeking legal counsel is highly recommended for organizations—and individuals—intending to participate in search and rescue operations.

Review of local and state laws cannot be a one-time task. Laws are often revised, and technology, standards, news media, and human interests are constantly changing. SAR organizations and personnel should regularly review the relevant and applicable local and state laws and regulations. They should also seek professional legal advice when questions arise. Some states do not have laws related to SAR, and teams located in those

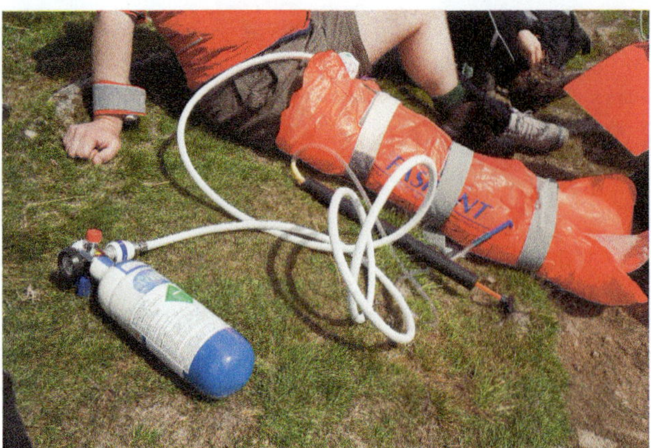

FIGURE 4-1 A fundamental tenet of emergency care is to do no more harm. SAR personnel who act in good faith and according to an appropriate standard of care can usually avoid legal problems.
© Ashley Cooper/Alamy.

states should research their legal position further prior to providing services to the public.

Legal Fundamentals

Some legal issues applicable to the provision of emergency care are so important that they are considered essential knowledge for all SAR personnel. Although a comprehensive overview of legal issues related to SAR cannot be provided here, some of the most important issues related to emergency services personnel will be reviewed in the context of SAR. SAR organizations and personnel have a responsibility to seek competent legal counsel when questions arise.

Scope of Practice

The **scope of practice**, or services a SAR organization can provide, is usually outlined by state law in the United States. Unfortunately, many states do not have SAR-specific laws in place, and other less-specific laws may apply (e.g., legislation regarding volunteers, good Samaritans, and emergency medical services [EMS]). If a SAR organization utilizes the services of medically trained personnel, such as emergency medical technicians (EMTs), the care they render may be guided by a separate scope of practice. There are two important points here to remember: All emergency responders, including SAR personnel, have a responsibility to provide proper and consistent care and services that fall within their authorized scope of practice, and anyone and any team must research their legal position prior to offering SAR services to the public.

Just because an individual is capable of performing certain skills does not mean that those skills are part of the authorized scope of practice. For example, if a team's authorized scope of practice in terms of medical care is only first aid (e.g., stop bleeding, wound care, splinting, cardiopulmonary resuscitation [CPR]), a paramedic on this team may not be able to do any more than is within the authorized scope of practice, even though the individual may be capable of more in terms of treating a patient. Similarly, a search team whose authorized scope of practice includes only wilderness search may exceed its scope of practice if a member—individually qualified or not—chooses to attempt a technical rope rescue while operating as part of the team.

SEARCH AND RESCUE TIP

SAR personnel should completely familiarize themselves with the relevant and applicable local and state laws and regulations before participating in or teaching SAR operations or management. SAR organizations should seek competent legal counsel before developing a response capability.

Standard of Care

All rescue personnel are required by law to act or behave toward others in a certain way regardless of the activity involved. Depending on the situation, one may have a duty to either act or not act. Generally, it is expected that when one's activities have the potential to cause injury or harm, he or she should be concerned about the safety and welfare of others. How one acts or behaves is called a **standard of care**.

Several factors influence the standard of care and, therefore, the appropriateness of one's conduct. Local customs, statutes, ordinances, regulations, and professional and institutional standards all have a bearing on the measure of one's actions.

By definition, standard of care is, "the watchfulness, attention, caution and prudence that a reasonable person in similar circumstances would exercise" (Medical Dictionary for the Health Professions and Nursing, 2012). In other words, it is how a reasonably prudent person with similar training and experience would act under similar circumstances, with similar equipment, and in the same place. Generally, medically trained individuals are expected to conduct themselves the same way as other individuals trained to the same level. For example, an EMT would not be held to the same standard of care as a physician. Similarly, SAR personnel would be held to the same standard of care as other, similarly trained SAR personnel and teams from the same area. Because these standards are often based on locally accepted practices and protocols, a SAR team in Virginia may be held to the same standard as other SAR teams in Virginia but would not likely be held to the same standard as a SAR team from California, even if their training were similar.

In addition, one's conduct will be judged by the current situation (including all the likely confusion), the needs of those who requested assistance, and the specific equipment available. Local customs and practices help define the standard of care required. However, standards of care may also be imposed by statutes, ordinances, regulations, or case law. In many areas, violation of one of these standards is said to cause a type of negligence.

Professional or institutional standards may also come into play in addition to those imposed by law. Organizations and associations involved in SAR can establish standards of care that may be admitted as evidence in determining the appropriateness of one's actions. Any rules and procedures of a specific SAR team, service, or organization with which one is affiliated may also be considered *institutional standards.* The state agency responsible for SAR may have regulations or directives that apply. State or regional SAR teams may have standard practices and procedures that apply. The *National SAR Plan*, the *National SAR Supplement*, the *International Maritime and Aeronautical SAR* (IAMSAR) *Manual*, and similar widely accepted documents may have procedures, policies, and/or guidance that may be relevant to determining the standard of care in any particular SAR situation.

As a minimum, the standard of care is *ordinary care*—the expectation that anyone who offers assistance will exercise reasonable care and act prudently. Anyone who acts prudently, reasonably, and according to the accepted standard minimizes any threat of civil liability.

To maintain this standard of care within the scope of your state's provisions, certification, and licensing requirements, it becomes necessary for all SAR personnel to acquire sufficient training and, during operations, never exceed the level of training received. Creating, updating, following, and training to accepted group training standards also minimizes exposure to liability.

Duty to Act

An individual's responsibility to provide care or services is called **duty to act**. This responsibility may come from law or be secondary to the function being performed.

For example, a bystander is under no obligation to assist a stranger in distress. However, there is likely a duty to act if you are charged with providing SAR services, you are attached to an organization that has a policy that requires you to act, or you are a member of an organization that represents itself to the public as providing SAR services. In these situations, an unpaid volunteer is no different than a paid professional in that once a mission has been accepted, arbitrarily refusing to act is no longer an option.

If you or your organization begins to provide services or treatment, you have a legal duty to continue. If you are out of your jurisdiction and come upon an emergency, you may not have a legal obligation to act, but you have a moral and ethical duty to act because of your special training and expertise.

It is also possible for SAR organizations to enter into agreements with local and/or state government agencies that oblige the organization to respond when called (often called a memorandum of understanding [MOU]). This may constitute a duty to act. The requirements and ramifications of any such agreements must be fully understood by everyone in the organization.

Engendered Reliance

When SAR service users assume that a SAR provider will provide a certain level of service, it is called **engendered reliance**. If the expectations of the users match the capabilities of the providers, there is no problem. But if, for example, the capability of the SAR provider is reduced and the need for, and expectation of, the higher level or specific service remains, a discrepancy arises. If a SAR organization fails to provide the service on which the user has become reliant, the organization may be held liable for the discrepancy. For many reasons, some SAR organizations have advertised a higher level of service based on only one or two individuals' skills and abilities. The advertising of the increased capability may engender reliance on the organization and a level of capability that does not truly exist. This can be a legal problem.

Does your SAR organization advertise a service that it cannot realistically provide? What happens when your organization's ability to provide a service goes away, but the need for the service still exists? Is your organization obligated to find a way to provide SAR service for your area? These are questions to ask of legal counsel when you or your organization seeks to offer services for your response area. One way to help avoid these types of problems is to make sure your group has a clear, concise, and updated mission statement giving the public a realistic expectation of what your group can and cannot do.

Negligence

The outcome of even the best run SAR incident is unpredictable. The subject of a SAR incident may allege that the care rendered, or the rescue performed, was improper, inadequate, or negligent. **Negligence** is the failure to provide the same care someone with similar training and in a similar situation would provide. It is a departure from the accepted standard of care that results in the noticeable harm of another. **Gross negligence** is a form of negligence in which one's failure to exercise reasonable care constitutes an extreme departure from the ordinary standard and, although still unintentional, serves as the worst case of negligence.

In tort law (civil proceedings, in contrast to criminal proceedings), members of society owe a duty to others to act reasonably and in a way that will not hurt another person or another person's property. In the context of SAR, remedy for a private civil wrong is typically sought under a doctrine of negligence. To bring a cause of action under negligence theory, the plaintiff (the party filing the claim) must establish the following four elements:

1. *Duty*: The rescuer (defendant) had a duty to act reasonably within his or her training. To meet this duty, a rescuer must typically adhere to the standard of care established by the rescue profession.
2. *Breach of duty*: The rescuer failed to perform that duty and did not act within the accepted and reasonable standard of care. This breach may occur either through commission or omission of certain acts.
3. *Damages*: The plaintiff must demonstrate damages and that he or she suffered harm to their person, property, or interests.
4. *Cause*: The rescuer's failure was the direct, foreseeable, and proximate cause of the resulting injury. In other words, absent the defendant's conduct, the harm would not have occurred. This is often the most problematic step for plaintiffs.

In all negligence suits, the plaintiff bears the burden of proof in establishing the requisite four elements under a "more probable than not" standard. Said another way, the plaintiff must establish that there was a greater than 50% probability that the defendant's breach of duty caused the harm (Langer and Auerbach, 2017). The heavy burden to prove these four requirements is a strong deterrent against frivolous and unjustified lawsuits.

Abandonment

Generally, in common law countries such as the United States, SAR personnel have no legal duty to provide care for or to rescue endangered strangers, even though a moral obligation may be compelling. However, in countries where the legal system is based in civil law, such as those located in continental Europe, Asia, and South America, a duty to rescue exists (Langer and Auerbach, 2017). "The law presently imposes no liability upon those who stand idly by and fail to rescue a stranger who is in danger" (*Miller v. Arnal Corp.*, 1981). However, when a duty to act is established, one must act or be liable for the consequences.

Abandonment is usually a term applied in the context of medical care where a physician (or other medical caregiver) unilaterally terminates care without adequate notice or the patient's consent (Langer and Auerbach, 2017). However, abandonment might be equally applied to a SAR situation where a rescuer with a duty to act unilaterally terminates rescue activities. In almost all cases, once started, providers have a duty to continue care until an equally competent person assumes responsibility. Not performing this duty can harm the patient and may provide the basis for negligence. Abandonment can result in both civil and criminal actions against SAR personnel and should be taken very seriously.

SEARCH AND RESCUE TIP

Continuing care once initiated is paramount. Once you or your organization begins to provide services or treatment, you may have a legal duty to continue, unless you turn over care to equal or higher-trained personnel.

Consent

Usually, the initiation of care for conscious, mentally competent adults requires permission or consent. If an adult is in control of his or her actions, he or she has the right to refuse care and cannot be treated against his or her will. Furthermore, treating a patient against his or her will may also be grounds for assault and/or battery charges.

SEARCH AND RESCUE TIP

Terms related to consent include the following:

- **Assault**: Unlawfully placing a person in fear of immediate bodily harm without the person's consent.
- **Battery**: Unlawfully touching a person.

Consent can be expressed or implied and may involve the care of a minor or a mentally incompetent person. **Expressed consent** is granted when a person expressly authorizes another—usually verbally—to provide care or transportation. This type of consent must be *informed*. That is, the person granting permission must be made aware of the potential risks, benefits, and alternatives before giving his or her consent. To give expressed consent, a person must be of legal age and be mentally competent to make decisions. This consent may also be limited. For example, a person may grant permission for treatment but not transportation off the mountain or to the hospital.

In a true emergency, when a person is injured or ill and is unable to provide expressed consent, or if a life-threatening situation exists, the law assumes the person would grant permission for treatment and transportation. This is called **implied consent** and applies any time a person is unable to give expressed consent due to either physical or mental impairment. In many situations, the law also allows a spouse or a close relative to give consent for individuals who are unable to give consent for themselves.

In most situations, a parent or legal guardian is required to give consent for the treatment or transportation of a minor. However, depending on the state, a minor may be able to be treated like an adult for the purposes of consenting to medical care if he or she is emancipated, married, or pregnant. Some states also allow minors to give valid consent for medical care depending on their level of maturity and/or age. Implied consent is the same for minors as it is for adults. Regardless, consent should be obtained from a minor's parent or guardian whenever possible.

Incidents involving mentally incompetent adults pose problems like those involving minors because they cannot give informed consent. Therefore, consent should be obtained from someone legally responsible, such as a legal guardian. Because this is often not easy to obtain, many states have protective custody statutes allowing such a person to be taken to a medical facility under the authority of a law enforcement officer. Of course, if a true emergency exists, implied consent can usually be assumed.

Occasionally, forcible restraint may be required of a mentally disturbed individual before emergency care can be rendered. Often, if you believe that an individual will injure himself or herself, or others, state statutes allow you to legally restrain the subject. However, there will always be specific guidelines and procedures to follow to get this accomplished. For example, some states allow only law enforcement officers to restrain people who are a threat to themselves or others. Regardless of the specific state, SAR personnel must be thoroughly informed about local laws, and SAR organizations must have clearly defined protocols describing exactly how to deal with these issues. The thing to remember is that competent adults have the right to expressly refuse assistance, but this refusal should be thoroughly documented.

Documentation

Most legal experts agree that a complete and accurate record of a SAR incident is an important safeguard against legal complications. The absence of such a record, or if such a record is incomplete, may mean that someone would have to testify regarding the events and activities related to the incident from memory alone. In the face of aggressive cross examination, this could be inadequate or embarrassing, and it could raise questions about the appropriateness of other aspects of the incident (**FIGURE 4-2**).

Courts in the United States consider an action or procedure that was not recorded as not being performed. They also consider an incomplete, poorly written, or messy report as evidence of incomplete or unprofessional care. To avoid these potentially dangerous pitfalls, actions and events should be completely, accurately, and neatly documented on appropriate forms. This type of comprehensive documentation can also be used to evaluate how well SAR personnel operated and managed the incident. This can be invaluable when seeking opportunities for improvement.

The requirement to document fully and properly must also extend to training records (both personal and team), equipment usage and maintenance records, and the documentation of any other requirements of SAR teams and personnel. If they are not fully documented, the assumption is that they did not occur. Documentation must be approached with honesty and integrity, documenting only the facts.

The length of time that various records, such as training records, incident records, or equipment maintenance records, must be retained and how they must be disposed of are often addressed in laws or rules called *records retention schedules* that vary from state to state. These schedules provide a description of the various documents and indicate the length of time each must be

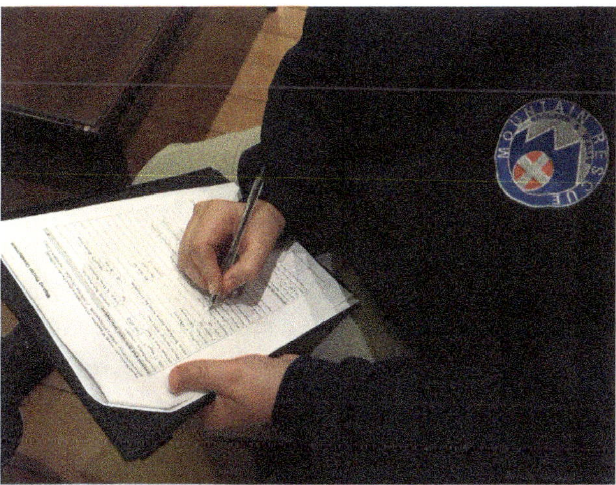

FIGURE 4-2 A complete and accurate record of a SAR incident is an important safeguard against legal complications.
Courtesy of Donald Cooper.

maintained, as well as its ultimate disposition. Retention periods take into consideration local, state, and federal requirements as well as those of professional bodies such as accrediting and licensing agencies that may apply.

With nearly every mobile phone having the capability to take photos and video and record audio, photos and videos have increasingly become a normal part of SAR scene documentation. This has undoubtedly improved these records and is a good thing. However, the device that took a photo may itself become evidence and be confiscated as such, so be warned. If you wish to take a photo, video, or audio recording to help document a SAR scene, do it with a device that you are willing to have confiscated and/or held for an uncertain length of time—such as a disposable camera. This may take some advance planning but is worth the trouble.

Here are some tips on how to record events effectively:

- Use the correct form and write in ink, not pencil.
- Write the incident number or name on every page used.
- Record the complete date and time of each entry.
- Avoid general and vague terms and expressions. Be specific.
- Use standard, accepted abbreviations only.
- Do not use a term if you are unsure of its meaning.
- Document all actions and observations completely.
- Document any changes to situations or conditions already noted.
- Document protective measures used.
- Document activities and procedures only after they are completed, never before.
- When using a pre-printed form, write on every line.
- Sign every entry.
- Fill in omitted items as new entries with the correct time and date. Do not backdate or add to previously written entries.
- Draw a single, thin, horizontal line through errors. Never erase them. Document the date and time of every change.
- Be completely truthful in everything that is written.
- If photos or video are taken, do it with a camera that can itself be put into evidence. You may not have a choice, especially if it is a criminal investigation.
- If photos are used, include in the photo something to show scale, such as a ruler or common object such as a compass, pencil, or coin.

Confidentiality

Communications between rescuers and a patient, especially if medical care has been rendered, are considered confidential and generally should not be disclosed without the expressed permission of the subject (patient). As a minimum, information that must be kept confidential includes the patient's medical history, treatment, and examination findings. However, any information pertaining to a subject's condition and situation and, indeed, all incident-related information should also be kept confidential. Even if the law does not require it, professionalism does.

SAR personnel must also be mindful of what they say during SAR operations. News agencies, interested parties, and family members may ask questions directly of field personnel, and these questions must be referred to the individual(s) tasked with responding to such inquiries by the incident commander. Such inquiries deserve accurate and complete responses, and SAR field personnel are frequently not in the best position to provide the best answers.

The prohibition of communicating unauthorized medical information about a patient also extends to social media. In one case in Florida, a paramedic went to jail for taking selfies with incapacitated patients (nwfdailynews.com, 2018). SAR personnel should be very cautious about discussing the details of, passing information about, or taking photos of subjects of SAR operations, except for official, authorized purposes.

Laws that Affect SAR Personnel

The purpose of some of these laws is to encourage individuals who otherwise do not have a duty to act to assist others without the fear of lawsuits. The actual language of these laws varies greatly from state to state, but many apply to anyone who might aid in an emergency. Other laws protect the patient. Laws that protect the responder do not prevent frivolous lawsuits from being filed, but they do make it more difficult for plaintiffs to prevail when care was rendered in good faith, with consent, and within the scope of the volunteer's training.

Good Samaritan Laws

Good Samaritan laws have been passed in all 50 states in the United States. They are based on the principle that when one person provides reasonable help to another, the helper should not be liable for errors and omissions that are made when the care is provided in good faith. Some requirements of the application of these laws usually include that the care was given in good faith, it was given without compensation, the caregiver did not exceed his or her medical training or license, and the caregiver did not have a preexisting duty to the victim to respond or provide aid. However, these laws do not prevent one from being sued. They just provide an affirmative defense should one get sued for rendering care under the conditions described.

The overriding purpose underlying most Good Samaritan statutes is specifically to ". . .encourage laypersons [and professionals] to help those in need, even when they are under no obligation to do so, by providing immunity from liability claims arising out of an attempt to assist a person in peril" (*Swenson v. Waseca Mut. Ins. Co.*, 2002). In other words, these laws are meant to provide protection to individuals, including SAR personnel, from civil liability for negligent acts or omissions committed while voluntarily providing emergency care.

Laws that grant immunity to official providers of emergency care, such as fire fighters and EMTs, exist, but they vary widely from state to state. In all cases, these types of laws do not protect any care provider from the willful or wanton failure to exercise due care that is characterized by gross negligence.

Since these laws vary from state to state, the applicability of these laws to volunteer SAR personnel and organizations should be investigated thoroughly at the local and state levels.

Volunteer Protection Act of 1997

On June 18, 1997, the Volunteer Protection Act (VPA) was enacted into law by the U.S. Congress (111 Stat. 218). The purpose of the Act is to limit lawsuits against volunteers serving nonprofit public and private organizations and governmental agencies. The VPA was enacted in response to volunteers withdrawing from service to nonprofit organizations because of concerns about liability. By limiting lawsuits against such volunteers, it was thought that the number of volunteers would increase, thus promoting the ability of nonprofit organizations and governmental entities to provide services at a reasonable cost.

Selected Definitions from the Volunteer Protection Act of 1997

According to the VPA (Public Law 105-19, 42 USC 14501, 1997), the term *volunteer* means "an individual performing services for a nonprofit organization or a governmental entity who does not receive:

- Compensation (other than reasonable reimbursement or allowance for expenses actually incurred); or
- Any other thing of value in lieu of compensation, in excess of $500 per year, and such term includes a volunteer serving as a director, officer, trustee, or direct service volunteer."

The term *nonprofit organization* means:

- "Any organization which is described in section 501(c)(3) of the Internal Revenue Code of 1986 and exempt from tax under section 501(a) of such Code and which does not practice any action which constitutes a hate crime referred to in subsection (b)(1) of the first section of the Hate Crime Statistics Act (28 U.S.C. 534 note); or
- Any not-for-profit organization which is organized and conducted for public benefit and operated primarily for charitable, civic, educational, religious, welfare, or health purposes and which does not practice any action which constitutes a hate crime referred to in subsection (b)(1) of the first section of the Hate Crime Statistics Act (28 U.S.C. 534 note)."

It is important to note that although the VPA provides immunity from lawsuits filed against a volunteer for a non-profit organization, it does not provide immunity for the organization itself. Rather, the VPA was intended to protect the individual volunteer from litigation. Common law will hold nonprofit organizations liable for the negligence of its volunteers, even if that volunteer enjoys immunity under the VPA or similar state law. In addition, the immunity is a qualified immunity and protects the volunteer only against claims of negligence and not against claims of gross negligence; willful or criminal misconduct; reckless misconduct; or conscious, flagrant indifference to the rights or safety of the individual harmed by the volunteer (Nonprofit Coordinating Committee of New York, 2015).

To make the most of the protection provided by the VPA, clear direction must be provided to nonprofit volunteers, including defining the scope of each volunteer's authority. For the VPA to apply, four requirements must be met. Volunteers must:

- Be acting within their scope of responsibility in their organization
- Be properly licensed or certified (i.e., authorized)
- Not cause harm by gross negligence or any similarly inappropriate type of misconduct
- Not cause harm by the operation of a motor vehicle, aircraft, or other vehicle for which an operator's license or insurance is required by the state

Although the VPA preempts state statute where "such laws are inconsistent with the act," except where state laws provide better or additional coverage, there are ways that states can preempt or restrict parts or all of this law for their area based on certain criteria. SAR volunteers and organizations that use volunteers must research carefully and know how the law applies to them in their respective states.

Health Insurance Portability and Accountability Act of 1996

The Health Insurance Portability and Accountability Act (HIPAA) of 1996 took effect in the United States in 2003. It was the first-ever set of federal privacy standards to protect patients' medical records and other health information provided to health plans, doctors, hospitals, and other healthcare providers. Developed by the U.S. Department of Health and Human Services (HHS), these standards provide patients with access to their medical records and more control over how their personal health information is used and disclosed. They represent a uniform, federal floor of privacy protections for consumers across the country. State laws providing additional protections to consumers are not affected by this rule.

HIPAA applies only to a *covered entity*, which includes healthcare providers who transmit any health information electronically in connection with transactions for which HHS has adopted standards (45 CFR 160.103). This may include a SAR team that provides medical care to patients. Any SAR team providing medical care often does so under the supervision of a medical advisor (usually a physician) who, in his or her practice, undoubtedly meets the definition of a covered entity. Thus, by extension, SAR teams who provide medical care may be required to meet the privacy requirements of HIPAA. The determination of whether this is required should be done in consultation with a team's medical adviser and legal counsel.

The privacy of protected health information (PHI) is covered by HIPAA and is defined as any information about health status, provision of health care, or payment for health care that can be linked to a specific individual. Thus, the privacy of individually identifiable health information, transmitted or maintained in any form or medium by a covered entity or its business associate, must be maintained according to HIPAA rules. Included in this definition of individually identifiable health information is demographic information and information that relates to an individual's physical or mental health or the provision of or payment for health care. Sources of PHI include patient care reports, dispatch records, incident reports with patient information, billing information, verbal communications between healthcare providers, patient records from nursing homes and hospitals, and physician certification statements. Any of these may be part of a SAR incident/investigation and should be treated as PHI.

A healthcare provider (covered entity) may use and disclose PHI to carry out essential healthcare functions such as treating a patient and consultation between relevant healthcare providers, so discussing the medical condition of your SAR patient with healthcare providers who will take over the care of the patient is explicitly permitted (45 CFR 164.501) under HIPAA.

In January 2013, the HHS Office for Civil Rights announced a final rule that implements several provisions to HIPAA. Designed to strengthen the privacy and security protections for health information and incorporate rules from the Health Information Technology for Economic and Clinical Health (HITECH) Act, the provisions include many changes, including more severe penalties for violation of PHI privacy requirements. The length of time PHI must be protected was also changed from indefinite to 50 years after death.

Covered entities are required to comply with HIPAA and HITECH mandates for protection of PHI and protected health records (PHR). Although SAR personnel and organizations are not specifically mentioned in the law, there is a possibility that the strict requirements of this law could apply to both. It is important that SAR organizations obtain legal counsel regarding how this might affect their group and operations.

Even if your service is not a covered entity, it is still important to have strict policies on confidentiality of patient information and procedures for release of patient care reports. HIPAA has become a standard of care when it comes to patient privacy, so even if you are not covered under the law, your team should institute reasonable safeguards that are similar to the HIPAA privacy rule to ensure that you are following the best practices possible. In short, the Golden Rule of HIPAA is to respect the privacy of patient information as you would your own. A safe way to achieve this is to make sure that anything associated with a specific patient that you hear and/or see is not shared once you leave the scene.

In addition to federal laws, there are many state and local laws that affect SAR personnel and organizations. Laws and protocols are often very different from state to state or even jurisdiction to jurisdiction, and this can present special challenges for SAR responders responding to those areas. In all cases, SAR groups must do their homework and research the laws for their areas of responsibility to know exactly how they will be affected.

Other Legal Considerations

SAR personnel usually have no more right to trespass than anyone else, but an understanding of what constitutes trespassing, how to avoid it, and when it is not an issue is important to staying out of legal trouble.

Because everything discovered at a SAR incident should be treated as if it were evidence of a crime, some understanding of the legal responsibilities of SAR personnel at the scene where evidence or a subject is found is also important.

Trespassing

Trespassing is the act of passing beyond a boundary onto one's property (land) without the owner's permission. Property owners usually convey their interest in preventing trespassing by posting a sign that clearly states, "No Trespassing" (**FIGURE 4-3**). However, many states do not require the use of an actual sign to prohibit trespassing. The simple existence of a fence is sufficient in some states, and a visible swatch of paint placed on a tree or pole at eye level is sufficient in others. In fact, the legal requirements for indicating no trespassing vary widely from state to state and even county to county in the same state. SAR personnel must therefore familiarize themselves with the applicable laws and methods used in their area of operation.

In SAR, a searcher might be trespassing if he or she travels on or across property without proper permission. Generally, SAR personnel have no more right to trespass than anyone else, but there may be some exceptions.

Trespassing falls into three general categories:

1. *Criminal trespass*, where someone willfully enters property that he or she knows has been posted "No Trespassing" or refuses to leave upon being notified to do so by the owner or occupant.
2. *Innocent trespass*, where someone enters the property in such a way that he or she is unaware that the land is posted.
3. *Trespass to save a life*, where someone is able to see a person in distress on the posted property and justify the trespass.

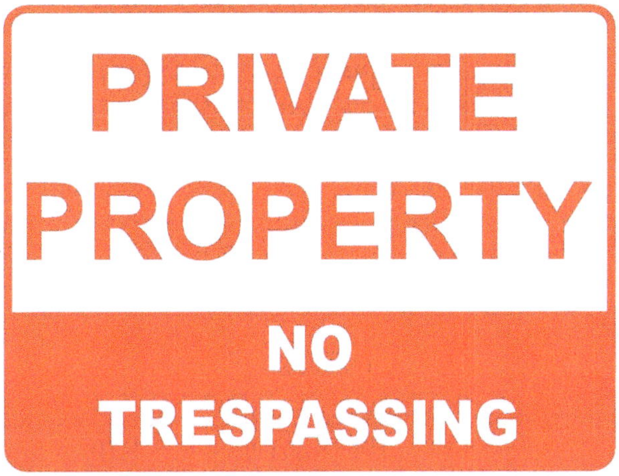

FIGURE 4-3 Property owners often convey their interest in preventing trespassing by posting a "No Trespassing" sign. However, many states do not require the use of an actual sign to prohibit trespassing.
Courtesy of Donald Cooper.

Before traveling onto private property, it is always advisable to obtain permission from the property owner. If permission is denied, entry should not be made, and the refusal must be documented and reported to the incident commander. In most cases, a call by the local law enforcement agency is sufficient to convince a land owner to permit SAR personnel to access the property, but a search warrant may occasionally be necessary.

If a landowner asks searchers to leave, even if the property is not posted, searchers must honor the request. You can minimize problems by including uniformed law enforcement officers on a team that may need to cross posted property.

Incident Site Procedures

Because "what happened?" is a question that will always be asked after an incident, and because a crime could have been committed, everything discovered at a SAR incident should be treated as if it were evidence in a criminal investigation. By following a few simple rules, the chances of preserving evidence and maintaining the chain of custody can be maximized.

Secure the Area

SAR personnel arriving first on the scene have a responsibility to secure the area and prevent others from contaminating or modifying evidence. Toward this end, the area should be cordoned off as best as possible, and access to the immediate area should be controlled. Of course, care must be provided to injured subjects, but beyond this, nothing should be disturbed. In addition, anything that was changed by the treatment of injuries should be noted.

Document the Scene

After securing the scene and controlling access, someone on site should fully document the scene, including anything added, removed, moved, or changed by SAR personnel, even if it was unintentional (**FIGURE 4-4**). This process, however, should not delay summoning the responsible law enforcement agency to the scene (if not already there) to accept responsibility for the scene from SAR personnel. The scene should not be vacated for any purpose after it is secured, or it could affect the acceptability of certain evidence. Once established,

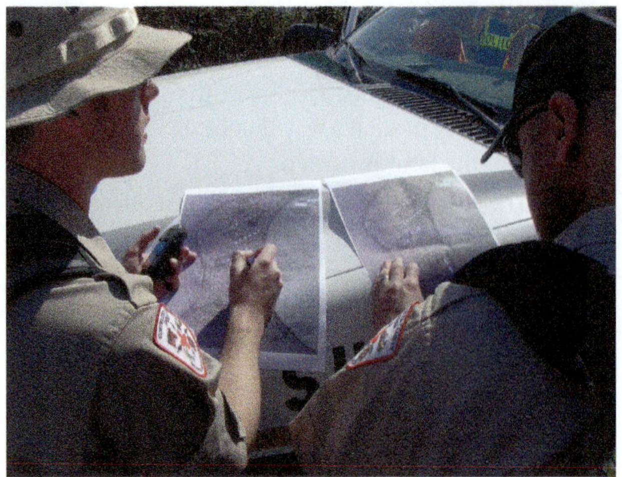

FIGURE 4-4 Fully document the scene, including notations of any changes (intentional or unintentional) made by SAR personnel.
Courtesy of NASAR.

someone should always retain control over the scene to maintain the chain of custody.

Preserve the Scene

Carter (2002) described a useful set of guidelines for preserving the scene at a SAR incident, which is paraphrased below.

- If the subject(s) appears to be dead when first approached, do the minimum possible to confirm death.
- If the subject is hanging, do not cut down.
- If there is a firearm present, use caution; it may be cocked and have a live round in the chamber. Many weapons chamber a new round after firing and are immediately ready to fire again.
- Do not add anything to the scene, such as cigarette butts, candy wrappers, or scrap paper.
- Do not remove anything from the scene, such as a weapon or the subject's wallet.
- Document the scene exactly with notes, sketches, and photographs. Note any additions, deletions, or alterations (your footprints are additions). Photograph from at least four angles. Investigating authorities will confiscate all notes.
- Note the date and the time for all actions and the names and functions of all people present.
- If you are the first on scene, you are responsible for scene security. Do not leave until relieved by a properly identified law enforcement officer. Always get a signed receipt for the scene. It may be necessary to prove later that you were properly relieved.
- Always remember that you may have to testify in court as to what you saw, what you did, and why you did it.

Specific information about handling evidence is in Chapter 14, *Principles of Search and Related Issues.*

General Suggestions

It is impossible to summarize all relevant aspects of the law as it relates to SAR in this text. However, following some simple suggestions can minimize both liability and legal challenges:

- Do not work in constant fear of being sued. Knowing your job and doing it well go a long way toward minimizing liability.
- Always act in good faith and according to an appropriate standard of care. Do what you know you should.
- Seek professional legal advice when specific legal questions arise.
- Provide proper and consistent care at all times. Treat everyone with the same high level of care.
- Become familiar with the standard of care in your area. At a minimum, act prudently, reasonably, and according to the accepted standard.
- Acquire sufficient and appropriate training and, during operations, never exceed the level of training received.
- Keep training up to date.
- Become and stay familiar with any local and state agreements entered into by your organization.
- Do not advertise or suggest a higher level of capability than you or your organization can realistically provide.
- Once started, continue care until properly relieved.
- Become familiar with the various types of consent and receive consent before providing care and/or transportation.
- Maintain and become familiar with the local protocol that describes how to deal with situations that may require forcible restraint.
- Fully and properly document the following: all activities and observations at a SAR incident, all training (both personal and team), and all equipment usage and maintenance.
- Treat all information related to a SAR incident as confidential.
- Become familiar with, and abide by, Good Samaritan laws; the Volunteer Protection Act; HIPAA; and other local, state, and federal laws that affect SAR personnel in your area.
- Become and stay familiar with the procedures used locally in handling evidence at a SAR incident site.

Wrap-Up

READY FOR REVIEW

- Search and rescue (SAR) personnel who act in good faith and according to an appropriate standard of care can usually avoid legal problems.
- Some legal issues applicable to the provision of emergency care are considered essential knowledge for all SAR personnel. SAR organizations and personnel have a responsibility to seek competent legal counsel when questions arise.
- Laws that protect the responder do not prevent frivolous lawsuits from being filed, but they do make it more difficult for plaintiffs to prevail when care was rendered in good faith, with consent, and within the scope of the volunteer's training.
- An understanding of what constitutes trespassing (how to avoid it, and when it is not an issue) and how to treat a scene as evidence is important to staying out of legal trouble.
- Always act in good faith and according to an appropriate standard of care.

SEARCH AND RESCUE TERMS

Abandonment The unilateral termination of care without assuring continuation of care at the same level or higher.

Assault Unlawfully placing a person in fear of immediate bodily harm without the person's consent.

Battery Unlawfully touching a person.

Duty to act An individual's responsibility to provide care or services. This responsibility may come from law or be secondary to the function being performed.

Engendered reliance The assumption by SAR service users that a SAR provider will provide a certain level of service.

Expressed consent Consent granted when a person expressly authorizes another—usually verbally—to provide care or transportation.

Good Samaritan laws Laws that limit liability when one person provides reasonable help to another in good faith.

Gross negligence A form of negligence in which one's failure to exercise reasonable care constitutes an extreme departure from the ordinary standard.

Implied consent Consent granted when a person is injured and unable to provide expressed consent, and the law assumes the person would grant permission for treatment and transportation.

Negligence Deviation from the accepted standard of care resulting in further injury to the patient. Components include a duty to act, breach of that duty, injury/damages inflicted (physical or psychological), and that the actions of the individual rendering care caused the injury/damage.

Scope of practice In health care, the procedures, actions, and processes that a healthcare practitioner is permitted to undertake in keeping with the terms of his or her professional license. In the context of SAR, the services a SAR organization is able to provide.

Standard of care How a reasonably prudent person with similar training and experience would act under similar circumstances, with similar equipment, and in the same place.

Trespassing The act of passing beyond a boundary onto one's property without the owner's permission.

REFERENCES AND SUGGESTED READING

Carter, David. 2002. *Field Team Member Manual*, 4th Ed., edited by White, W., Mark Pennington, and R. Glen. Ruther Glen, VA: Search and Rescue Training Associates, Inc.

Langer, Carolyn S. and Brian S.S. Auerbach. 2017. Medical liability and wilderness emergencies. In *Wilderness Medicine*, 7th Edition, edited by Paul Auerbach, pp. 2253–2261. St. Louis, MO: Elsevier.

Medical Dictionary for the Health Professions and Nursing. 2012. https://medical-dictionary.thefreedictionary.com/standard+of+care.

Miller v. Arnal Corp. 1981. 632 P.2d 990 (Ariz. App. 1981). http://www.leagle.com/decision/1981613129Ariz484_1492/MILLER%20v.%20ARNAL%20CORP.

nwfdailynews.com. 2018. 'Selfie war' paramedic sentenced to 6 months in jail. *Northwest Florida Daily News.* http://www.nwfdailynews.com/news/20170920/selfie-war-paramedic-sentenced-to-6-months-in-jail.

Nonprofit Coordinating Committee of New York. 2015. Volunteer Protection Act of 1997. http://www.npccny.org/info/gti2.htm.

Public Law 105-19, 42 USC 14501. 1997. Volunteer Protection Act of 1997. http://www.gpo.gov/fdsys/pkg/PLAW-105publ19/pdf/PLAW-105publ19.pdf.

Swenson v. Waseca Mut. Ins. Co. 2002. 653 NW2d 794, 797 [Minn Ct App 2002]. https://scholar.google.com/scholar_case?case= 5385032154010252345&hl=en&as_sdt=6,36&as_vis=1.

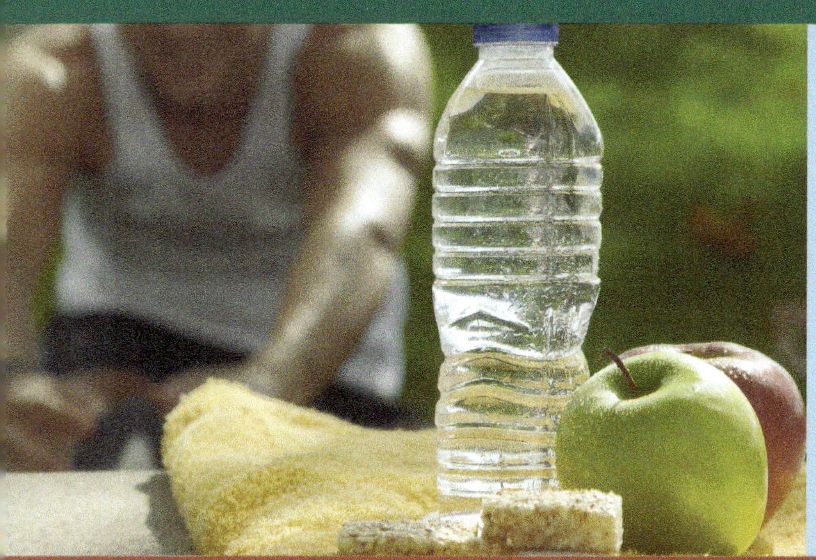

SECTION 2

Support Information, Skills, and Equipment

CHAPTER 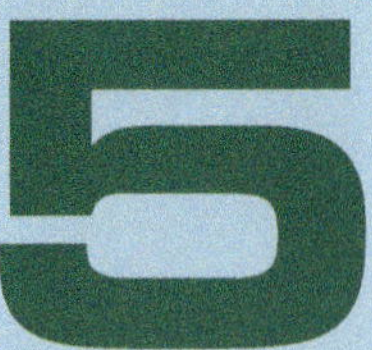

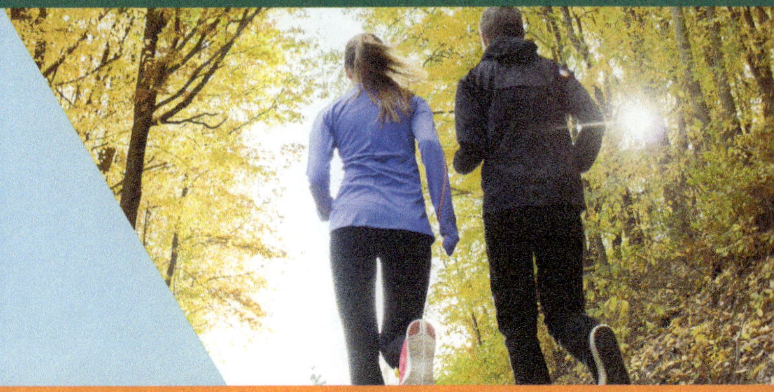

Physiology and Fitness

OBJECTIVES

Upon completion of this chapter and the related course activities, the student will be able to meet the following objectives:

- Describe how activity levels and environmental factors affect the body's caloric requirements.
- Describe the effects on the body of increasing levels of dehydration (water loss).
- Describe the basic water and chemical needs of the human body.
- Describe how, in each of the following processes, the human body loses heat:
  - Conduction
  - Radiation
  - Convection
  - Evaporation
- Discuss the importance of fitness for search and rescue (SAR) personnel.
- List the health conditions for which one should obtain medical clearance before participating in SAR activities.
- Define *physical fitness*.
- List the four basic components of fitness.
- Discuss the importance of weight control as an aspect of fitness.
- Describe the role and importance of knowing one's personal limitations in SAR work.
- Explain how an individual can mentally prepare for SAR work.

Physiology

The foundation for comfortably living and working in the outdoors is an understanding of the human body. This understanding need not be on the level of a physician, but one should have some comprehension of how the body reacts to or is affected by the environment. In short, search and rescue (SAR) personnel must have a working knowledge of human biological survival (the necessities and priorities of life), including a fundamental understanding of issues related to nutrition, hydration, and thermoregulation.

Food and Nutrition

It takes several hours for most foods to become available to the body as energy. The old saying, "You are what you eat," is an accurate statement, but more accurate is the statement, "What you eat today is what you run on tomorrow." To be optimally prepared, SAR personnel must eat a well-balanced diet every day so that they are best prepared for peak performance when they are called.

Because excellent references are readily available on this topic, proper nutrition and diet will not be addressed here in any detail. However, this does not

TABLE 5-1 Estimated Daily Calorie Needs of Athletes by Activity Level

Activity Level	Male Calories per Pound of Weight	Female Calories per Pound of Weight
Light	17	16
Moderate	19	17
Heavy	23	20

Reprinted with permission from Baechle, T.R., & Earle, R.W. (2000). Essentials of Strength and Conditioning, p. 253 (2nd ed.). *The National Strength and Conditioning Association*. Champaign, IL: Human Kinetics.

mean that these subjects are not important to SAR personnel. They are critically important, so much so that they should receive comprehensive examination beyond what is possible here. The U.S. Department of Health publishes dietary guidelines with which all SAR personnel should be familiar. Nutritional planning and discipline are essential if one expects to be able to work today at a SAR incident on the fuel he or she ingested yesterday.

Humans in arctic or cold environments consume more calories than those in warm climates. It has been estimated that this increase could be as great as 2000 extra calories per day. For this reason, long-lasting, high-energy foods become more of a critical factor in cold weather than in other climates. As a point of reference, the basic metabolic rate measured under standard conditions is about 1400 to 1800 calories per day just to maintain the body at its least active waking level, though this varies from individual to individual. **TABLE 5-1** shows estimated caloric needs of individuals by level of activity. Using this table, it can be shown that a 165-pound (75-kilogram) male participating in heavy activity, such as field SAR operations, would require just over 3700 calories per day.

Water and Hydration

Water is essential for proper body function. The human body may be able to survive for as long as a month without food but only a matter of days without water. Approximately two-thirds of one's body weight is water. Two-thirds of this water is inside body cells (intercellular), and the other one-third is in the veins, body cavities, and other spaces. Maintaining adequate fluid balance is vitally important to survival, let alone being able to work under stress. No other nutrient affects athletic or work performance more than water, so consuming an adequate amount of water is vital to being able to perform any sort of activity, including SAR (Jeukendrup and Gleeson, 2010).

Water is so essential that as little as a 1% decrease in body weight from water loss (1.5 pints [720 mL] in a 150-pound [68-kilogram] person) makes us thirsty. Thus, when you first become thirsty, you are already dehydrated. A 2% decrease in body weight from water loss (3 pints [1440 mL] in a 150-pound [68-kilogram] person) impairs exercise performance. At first, when body water levels fall below a certain level, saliva decreases, the throat gets dry, and the urge to drink follows. As the body continues to lose water, the viscosity of the blood increases, blood volume decreases, the ability to dissipate heat decreases, core temperature increases, early fatigue sets in, and muscle cramping may occur. Headache, dizziness, nausea, irritability, and vomiting are also signs and symptoms of dehydration (*signs* can be detected, and *symptoms* are experienced by the patient). A 6% drop in body weight from water loss impairs thinking and judgment, and a 10% drop can be fatal. The time required for such a large fluid loss depends on environmental circumstances and what types of conservation methods are used (Jeukendrup and Gleeson, 2010).

During hard work, the muscles produce an excess of heat, which must be dissipated or the body will overheat. This is why you sweat. For every 600 calories of heat the body generates, you can lose about 1 liter of fluid in the form of sweat. Clothes that do not allow the evaporation of sweat, or a humidity level that does the same, will cause overheating in a hot environment. It is the actual evaporation of moisture from the skin that cools the body, not just the sweating.

Approximately 80% of a person's total daily water intake comes from drinking water and beverages, and the rest comes from food. The general recommendation for daily water intake for women is approximately 2.7 liters (91 ounces)—from all beverages and foods—and men an average of approximately 3.7 liters (125 ounces) daily. An average inactive person might require a bit less than these amounts, and high humidity and physical exertion can easily double these requirements. It is not unusual to require 8 to 10 liters of water per day under extreme conditions (Institute of Medicine, 2005).

In moderate temperatures, people have survived 17 days without water. Conversely, in a hot desert environment, one might last only a few hours, since physical exertion under these conditions can cause the loss of 2 to 3 liters of water per hour to sweat. Beyond normal methods of water loss, vomiting, sickness, excessive urination, and diarrhea can all contribute to rapid dehydration.

Proper re-hydration requires one to drink water slowly until the urine is a pale-yellow color. The color of the urine is a good test for dehydration: deep amber urine (usually in small quantities) signifies dehydration; pale yellow (usually in great quantities) signifies adequate hydration. For activities lasting less than one hour, water is the ideal fluid replacer. For those activities lasting more than 60 to 90 minutes, sports drinks containing carbohydrates or electrolytes may be useful both during and following exercise (Sawka et al., 2007; Puhl and Buskirk, 1998). The taste of commercial sports drinks may also encourage one to drink more, which is important because most people stop drinking fluids before they are adequately re-hydrated. Research shows that people will drink more of a flavored beverage than plain water (Passe, Horn, and Murray, 2000; Wilk and Bar-Or, 1996), so it is recommended that a dry, flavored sports drink mix (Gatorade®, Powerade®, Badger Max®, Propel®, Crystal Light®, Dr. Price's Electrolyte Mix®, etc.) be carried with water. Treated water also can be made more palatable by adding a flavored mix.

It is possible to drink large amounts of water and have little fluid increase due to salt or electrolyte deficiency. Salt deficiency is often underestimated when a person is not acclimated to the heat and sun. Typical hot weather appetite loss adds to possible imbalance. Salt in pill form taken by mouth or directly dissolved in fluid may be recommended for persons perspiring heavily in hot weather. However, salt or salt pills should be taken cautiously and ideally under the direction of a physician. Without adequate water, salt tablets can do more harm than the deficiency they are intended to correct. Salt tablets should never be taken if water is in short supply. In addition, many commercial salt tablets tend to nauseate some people to the point of vomiting, which can worsen dehydration and electrolyte imbalance. Buffered salt tablets seem less troublesome to most people. Some people also have trouble digesting the tablets and pass them straight through their digestive system. The bottom line is that a physician should be involved if salt tablets are considered for use (American College of Sports Medicine, 2014; Greenleaf, 1992).

SEARCH AND RESCUE TIP

Key points in staying hydrated include the following:

- Water is more essential than food, and lack of it will kill you quicker than lack of food.
- It is impossible to physically perform at any reasonable level without the adequate intake of fluids.
- Food should be eaten only when there is enough water to drink. Do not eat if water is scarce.
- For long periods of exercise or when water must be treated, use flavored sports drink mixes to encourage fluid intake.
- Use salt tablets with caution and, ideally, only under the direction of a physician.

Body Temperature Regulation

As warm-blooded creatures (homeotherms), humans possess a thermal regulatory system that maintains the body temperature at about 99°F (37°C), regardless of environmental fluctuations. Since the body constantly produces heat, heat must be transferred to the environment for the body to maintain a constant temperature. Heat balance (thermal equilibrium) is the balance between the rate of heat production and the rate of heat loss.

Balancing Heat Production and Heat Loss

Those interested in maintaining a normal body temperature must do two things: maintain a healthy, well-nourished body (control of heat production) and adjust the clothing system as required (control of heat loss). Nutrition is discussed in the previous section, and clothing systems are addressed in Chapter 7, *Search and Rescue Clothing*.

The body's primary method of regulating its temperature involves finely adjusting the flow of heated blood between its core (brain, heart, and lungs) and periphery (skin, arms, and legs). Generally, blood is pushed to the skin and extremities for cooling and shunted to the core to preserve heat.

The human body is constantly producing heat through metabolism and muscle movement. The body may also absorb heat from its environment. Much of this heat must be dissipated to our clothing and the environment if a constant inner body core temperature is to be maintained. For brief periods, the body can even store a little excess heat in its outer tissues. If heat loss exceeds production, the body will draw on this stored heat. In the end, heat loss must equal heat production and absorption if a thermal equilibrium is to be maintained.

Heat is produced in the body in two ways: as a natural by-product of certain chemical reactions (exothermic metabolism) and as a by-product of muscle movement (work). However, the body can also derive heat through absorption of radiant energy from the sun or other heat source.

An individual's metabolic rate (or **calorie** production) is highly variable and differs from person to person. For the average male, it can range from 70 calories per hour while sleeping to 524 calories per hour during strenuous work (Hedge, 2015).

On a clear day, the unclothed body can absorb as much as 230 calories per hour of the sun's heat energy (Cornell University Ergonomics Web, 2015). In very hot environments, radiated heat gain can cause overheating problems, so the body must be protected from it. In cold environments, layers of clothing and/or shelter can reduce radiated heat loss. The color of clothing can also make a difference. The darker the clothing, the more radiant heat energy is absorbed. The lighter the clothing color, the more radiant heat energy is reflected, so when possible, wear dark-colored clothing in cold environments and light-colored clothing in hot environments.

As the body's core temperature begins to rise, two things happen: blood vessels in and near the surface of the skin dilate (enlarge) to help release the blood's latent heat to the environment, and sweating begins. The subsequent evaporation of perspiration from the skin releases a tremendous amount of heat energy. The hot blood being pumped from the body's core to the skin is also cooled by convection, conduction, and radiation.

The reverse takes place when the body is exposed to a cold environment or its core temperature drops (**FIGURE 5-1**). Blood vessels constrict, and circulation to the surface of the skin and periphery is limited to reduce heat loss. Less blood going to the surface of the skin means less heat lost to the environment. Shivering also begins. In extreme circumstances, circulation may be cut off almost entirely to the most distant appendages (fingers, toes, ears, and nose), thus predisposing them to local cold injuries such as frostbite.

Since the brain is a critical core organ, the head and neck continue to receive full blood flow even under cold stress. Because these areas of the body are very vascular (contain many blood vessels, some quite large), the blood flowing to these areas can release a great deal of heat to the environment if they are not protected. Therefore, it is critically important to cover and protect the head and neck in cold environments.

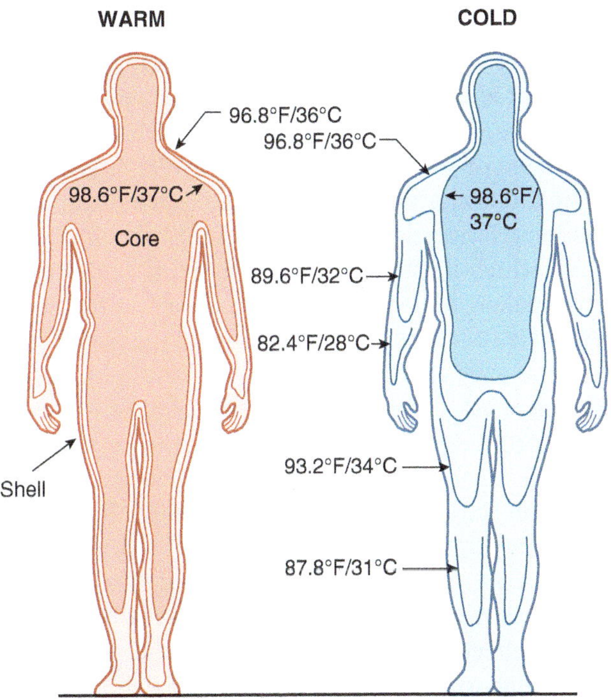

FIGURE 5-1 Reaction of the body to cold (F°/C°).
Courtesy of Donald Cooper.

Muscular activity can increase one's metabolic rate for short periods by as much as 750%. However, different types of muscular activity produce different results. Shivering and isometric exercises (working one muscle group against another without movement) makes heat immediately available to the body without heavy perspiration. Thus, these methods are preferred over running or strenuous activity. In addition, isometrics can be done in a sleeping bag or sitting in a chair. At least 10 minutes of continuous exercise may be needed for the desired effect.

Methods of Heat Transfer

Heat transfer is the movement of heat between the body and the environment. Heat flows from higher temperatures to lower temperatures and flows fastest when the difference between the two is the greatest. There are several methods by which this process occurs, including conduction, radiation, convection, and evaporation. Perspiration and respiration also cause body heat loss but are considered variants of evaporation (**TABLE 5-2**). The effects of various skin and core temperatures on the body are listed in **TABLE 5-3**.

Conduction is heat transfer between objects that are in direct contact, and it normally plays a very small part in total heat loss during everyday activities (Charkoudian et al., 2017). However, this method of heat loss can be a major source of discomfort and cause serious problems in severe climates and hostile environments. For example, sitting or lying directly on snow, ice, the cold ground,

TABLE 5-2 Body Heat Loss Breakdown—At Rest

Percent	Cause
60	Radiation (from nude body in a thermoneutral environment; 69.8°F [21°C])
18	Convection (air close to body absorbs heat)
15	Evaporation (evaporation of water through the outer layer of skin [insensible perspiration] or from the skin surface when it is wetted by sweat or something else
7	Evaporation from lungs (respiration)
3	Excretion of feces and urine (considered evaporation)
3	Conduction (direct contact with skin or clothing)

Note: Percentages are averages and may not sum to 100%.
Data from Cornell University Ergonomics Web. (2015). DEA3500: Ambient environment: Thermal regulation. Retrieved from http://ergo.human.cornell.edu.

TABLE 5-3 Effects of Various Surface (Skin) and Core Temperatures

Skin (Shell) Temperature			Core Temperature		
°C	°F	Condition	°C	°F	Condition
>45	>113	Burns	>42	>108	Fatal
42	108	Pain	41	106	Coma, convulsions
40	104	Uncomfortably hot	39.5	103	Upper acceptable limit, drowsiness
25	77	Uncomfortably cold	37	98.6	Normal
5	41	Numbness	35.5	96	Lower acceptable limit, mental dullness
0	32	Frostbite	34.5	94	Shivering diminishes, extreme mental slowness
<–0.6	<31	Skin freezes	33	91	Coma
			<33	<91	Deep coma, death
			27	81	Heart stops, death

Data from Hedge, A. (2015). Thermal sensation and thermoregulation. Cornell University. Retrieved from www.ergo.human.cornell.edu.

rock, metal, or any good conductor of heat results in continual loss of valuable calories from the body. The only effective way to prevent conductive heat loss is to separate your body from any cold surface or introduce an insulating layer between the two. Moisture imbedded in clothing reduces the amount of trapped air and thus increases conductive heat loss through the material.

A nonconductive or insulating material is one that when heated on one side stays cool on the other. The most efficient insulating material is air, and clothing systems take advantage of this fact by trapping air to enhance insulation. Unfortunately, air that is not trapped circulates and can cause convective heat loss. As free moving air next to the body absorbs heat, it expands and rises. Immediately, new cooler air moves in and replaces this moving warm air. This is natural convection, and it takes place because of both wind and the bellows action of clothing as the wearer moves. Even though air is a poor conductor, it can facilitate the transfer of heat because of its mobility within a clothing system. To properly utilize air's insulation qualities, it must be trapped and prevented from moving.

All objects emit and receive energy through space without an intervening medium. At physiologic (body) temperatures, this is most often via infrared radiation (Schmidt-Nielsen, 1997). *Radiation* during a cold day amounts to about 5% of the total heat loss from a clothed body but 45% or more from a naked body (Charkoudian et al., 2017). Heat lost by radiation is that which escapes from bare skin and usually reaches the outer layer of clothing. The higher the temperature of the radiating surface, the faster heat is lost through this method. The harder one works, the hotter the skin becomes, and the greater the heat that is released by radiation. Therefore, in an emergency situation in the cold, when survival is the issue, one should monitor physical activity because it could be the source of significant heat loss.

Convection is a type of conduction enhanced by the movement of the molecules in a gas or liquid (Charkoudian et al., 2017). To prevent convective heat loss, air movement (wind) around the body must be either eliminated or significantly reduced. Under emergency cold conditions, just getting out of the wind can be a lifesaver. Convection is the reason for the wind chill index, which illustrates how one can feel colder than the actual air temperature when exposed to the wind (**FIGURE 5-2**). Wind chill is based on the rate of heat loss from exposed skin caused by wind and cold. As the wind increases, it draws heat from the body through convection, driving down skin temperature and eventually the core temperature. Therefore, the wind makes the body feel much colder. If the air temperature is 0°F (–18°C) and the wind is blowing at 15 mph (24 kph), the wind chill is –19°F (–28°C). At this wind chill temperature, exposed skin can freeze in minutes. Unlike human flesh, the only effect wind chill has on inanimate objects, such as car radiators and water pipes, is to shorten the amount of time it takes for the object to cool. An inanimate object does not cool below the actual air temperature,

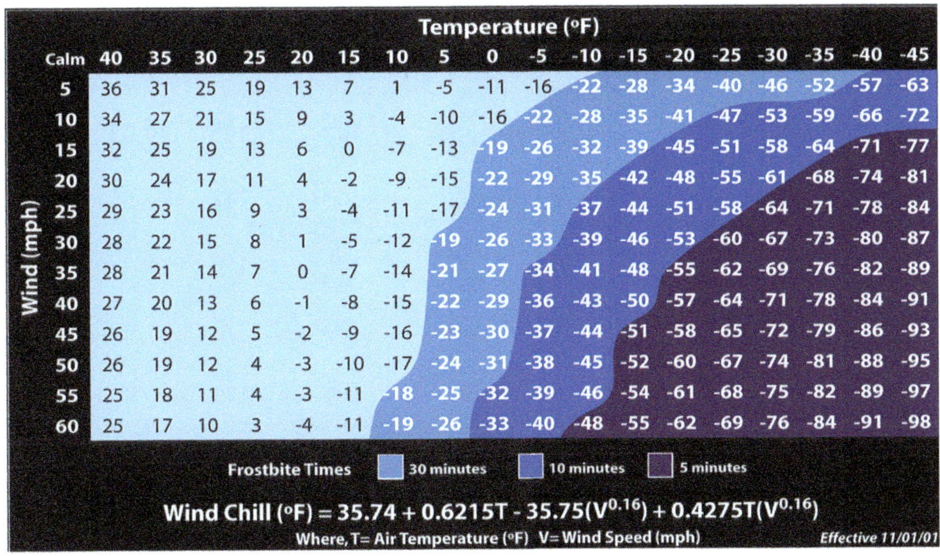

Wind Chill Chart

Wind (mph)	Temperature (°F)																	
Calm	40	35	30	25	20	15	10	5	0	-5	-10	-15	-20	-25	-30	-35	-40	-45
5	36	31	25	19	13	7	1	-5	-11	-16	-22	-28	-34	-40	-46	-52	-57	-63
10	34	27	21	15	9	3	-4	-10	-16	-22	-28	-35	-41	-47	-53	-59	-66	-72
15	32	25	19	13	6	0	-7	-13	-19	-26	-32	-39	-45	-51	-58	-64	-71	-77
20	30	24	17	11	4	-2	-9	-15	-22	-29	-35	-42	-48	-55	-61	-68	-74	-81
25	29	23	16	9	3	-4	-11	-17	-24	-31	-37	-44	-51	-58	-64	-71	-78	-84
30	28	22	15	8	1	-5	-12	-19	-26	-33	-39	-46	-53	-60	-67	-73	-80	-87
35	28	21	14	7	0	-7	-14	-21	-27	-34	-41	-48	-55	-62	-69	-76	-82	-89
40	27	20	13	6	-1	-8	-15	-22	-29	-36	-43	-50	-57	-64	-71	-78	-84	-91
45	26	19	12	5	-2	-9	-16	-23	-30	-37	-44	-51	-58	-65	-72	-79	-86	-93
50	26	19	12	4	-3	-10	-17	-24	-31	-38	-45	-52	-60	-67	-74	-81	-88	-95
55	25	18	11	4	-3	-11	-18	-25	-32	-39	-46	-54	-61	-68	-75	-82	-89	-97
60	25	17	10	3	-4	-11	-19	-26	-33	-40	-48	-55	-62	-69	-76	-84	-91	-98

Frostbite Times: 30 minutes; 10 minutes; 5 minutes

$$\text{Wind Chill (°F)} = 35.74 + 0.6215T - 35.75(V^{0.16}) + 0.4275T(V^{0.16})$$

Where, T= Air Temperature (°F) V= Wind Speed (mph)

Effective 11/01/01

FIGURE 5-2 The wind chill index considers the rate of heat loss from exposed skin caused by wind and cold. To use the chart, find the approximate temperature on the top of the chart. Read down until you are opposite the appropriate wind speed. The number that appears at the intersection of the temperature and wind speed is the wind chill index.

Courtesy of NWS/NOAA.

with or without wind. (More information on wind chill is available on the National Oceanic and Atmospheric Administration (NOAA) website.)

When heat and humidity combine to reduce the amount of evaporation of sweat from the body, outdoor physical activities become dangerous even for those in good shape. Similar to the wind chill index, the heat index is used to measure the amount of discomfort during the summer months when heat and humidity often combine to make it feel hotter than it actually is (**TABLE 5-4**).

Convective heat loss also occurs in water where body heat is lost 25 times faster than in air as the water contacts and moves across the skin (**TABLE 5-5**). Swimming in cold water causes more body heat loss and significantly reduces survival time. The reason: Cold water absorbs more heat than cold air as it moves across the body.

When water changes state—liquid to gas or gas to liquid—a large amount of energy is either given off or absorbed. This is the principle behind perspiration *evaporating* off the skin (water changing from liquid to vapor) to cool the body. In a neutral thermal environment, perspiration is generally not produced, and evaporation accounts for only about 15% of the body's heat loss. Approximately half of this is produced by respiration (breathing) and evaporation through the respiratory tract. The rest is evaporation of water that diffuses passively through the skin (Charkoudian et al., 2017), which is also called insensible perspiration.

The normal skin temperature of a person is about 95°F (35°C). The evaporation of 1 gram of water (0.035 ounces) off the surface of skin at this temperature requires approximately 0.58 **kilocalorie** of energy. Thus, the heat absorbed by the evaporation of 100 cc of water (3.4 fluid ounces), especially if facilitated by fanning, cools the body about 1 degree Celsius (1.8°F) (Schmidt-Nielsen, 1997).

In most environmental circumstances, respiratory heat loss is not considered significant. However, in an extremely cold environment, the respiratory system is converting subzero temperature air to 98.6°F in less than 18 inches of space (the length of the airway and lungs). This requires a substantial investment of calories by the body. With the addition of a simple rebreather (an improvised thickness of clothing, material, or structure that preheats inhaled air, e.g., a scarf, piece of clothing, sock, or tube-shaped hood), one can significantly reduce respiratory heat loss.

Fitness

Research shows that less than 5% of adults participate in 30 minutes of physical activity each day (U.S. Department of Agriculture, 2010), only 1 in 3 adults receives the recommended amount of physical activity each week (U.S. Department of Health and Human Services [USHHS], 2010), and more than 80% of adults do not meet national guidelines for both aerobic and muscle-strengthening activities (USHHS, 2016). In addition, about one-third of

TABLE 5-4 Heat Index

	Apparent Temperature								
Relative Humidity	**Air Temperature (degrees F)**								
	80	**85**	**90**	**95**	**100**	**105**	**110**	**115**	**120**
30	79	83	88	97	102	112	122	135	148
35	79	84	89	99	105	116	128	143	
40	80	84	91	99	109	122	136	151	
45	80	85	93	102	113	128	145		
50	81	87	95	105	118	134	152		
55	81	89	98	110	126	142			
60	82	90	100	114	129	149			
65	83	91	102	119	138				
70	85	93	106	124	144				
75	86	95	109	130					
80	86	97	113	136					
85	87	99	117						
90	88	102	122						
95	89	105							
100	91	108							

The Effects on the Human Body	
≥130°F	Heat/sunstroke highly likely with continued exposure
105–129°F	Sunstroke, heat cramps, or heat exhaustion likely, and heatstroke possible, with prolonged exposure and/or physical activity
90–104°F	Sunstroke, heat cramps, or heat exhaustion possible with prolonged exposure and/or physical activity
80–89°F	Fatigue possible with prolonged exposure and/or physical activity

Reproduced from U.S. Department of Commerce, National Oceanic and Atmospheric Administration [NOAA], National Weather Service [NWS] (2016a).

TABLE 5-5 Cooling Rate of a Body in Water

Water Temperature		Core Body Cooling Rate
°F	°C	°C/Hour
68	20	0.5
59	15	1.5
50	10	2.5
41	5	4.0
32	0	6.0

Note: In cold water, body heat is lost 25 times faster than in cold air due to convective heat loss.

Data from Hedge, A. (2015). Thermal sensation and thermoregulation. Cornell University. Retrieved from http://ergo.human.cornell.edu

U.S. adults (33.8%) are obese, as are approximately 17% of children and adolescents (aged 2–19 years) (Centers for Disease Control and Prevention [CDC], 2011). There are many reasons to believe that these statistics are also relevant to the SAR community.

The importance of **physical fitness** in SAR, or why being fit contributes to field SAR operations, should be obvious. What may need to be stated, though, is that a lack of conditioning and fitness has been repeatedly identified as one of the most common problems faced in the field by SAR personnel. This has undoubtedly resulted in reduced effectiveness and increased safety risk. Administrative (nonfield) personnel, such as search and rescue planners and managers, may also experience mental and physical stress, which can have a negative impact on their health. In short, all SAR personnel should be fit—physically and mentally—to operate at their optimum during a SAR mission, regardless of one's assignment.

It has been said that the best way to prepare for a wilderness venture is to "be in the wilderness on a regular basis" (Schoene, 2017, p. 2183). The same could be said for search and rescue: the best way to prepare for it is to do it. Training for and participating in SAR operations are great ways to stay prepared physically for this demanding work. However, for those who do not do it full time or frequently enough to benefit fully from the repetition, additional conditioning is likely required.

Maintaining a regular program of physical conditioning provides a head start toward coping with stressful emergencies in hostile environments. Not everyone must be a flawless physical specimen, but a reasonable fitness level—especially in terms of aerobic fitness—is necessary for optimal and safe performance, both in the field and in the command post. Running and other serious exercise may not be for everyone. Fortunately, there can be a place in SAR for virtually anyone who wants to participate, as long as every individual recognizes and shares both his or her strengths and limitations.

Because physical fitness has been recognized as such a widespread problem in SAR—much like it has been recognized as a problem in modern society in general—it seems prudent to review some of the very basic issues related to this important topic.

SEARCH AND RESCUE TIP

Worse than being in poor physical condition during a search and rescue mission or survival situation is not realizing that you are unfit.

Making a Commitment

The first important step on the path to physical fitness is to seek information, and the second is to firmly decide that you are going to be physically fit. The information provided here is designed to help you reach that decision and your related goals.

The decision to carry out a physical fitness program to prepare for SAR cannot and should not be taken lightly. It requires a lifelong commitment of time and effort. Exercise must become one of those things that you do without question, like bathing and brushing your teeth. Unless you are convinced of the benefits of fitness and the risks of unfitness, you will not succeed.

Patience is essential. Do not try to do too much too soon, and do not quit before you have a chance to experience the rewards of improved fitness. You cannot regain in a few days or weeks what you have lost in years of sedentary living, but you can get it back if you persevere. The prize is worth the price.

The following sections contain the basic information you need to begin and maintain a personal physical fitness program. These guidelines are intended for the average healthy adult and explain what your goals should be, as well as how often, how long, and how hard you must exercise to achieve them. Information is also provided that will make your workouts easier, safer, and more satisfying. The rest is up to you.

Health Check

If you are under 35 years old and in good health, you probably do not need to see a doctor before beginning an exercise program, but if you are over 35 and have been inactive for several years, you should consult your physician, who may or may not recommend a graded exercise test. Other conditions that indicate a need for medical clearance before proceeding are:

- High blood pressure
- Heart trouble
- Family history of early stroke or heart attack deaths
- Frequent dizzy spells
- Extreme breathlessness after mild exertion
- Arthritis or other bone problems
- Severe muscular, ligament, or tendon problems
- Obesity (body mass index [BMI] of 30 or greater)
- Other known or suspected disease

Vigorous exercise involves minimal health risks for persons in good health or those following a doctor's advice. Far greater risks are presented by habitual inactivity and obesity.

Defining Fitness

Physical fitness is to the human body what fine-tuning is to an engine. It enables us to perform up to our potential. Fitness can be described as a condition that helps us look, feel, and do our best. According to the President's Council on Physical Fitness and Sports, physical fitness is:

> The ability to perform daily tasks vigorously and alertly, with energy left over for enjoying leisure-time activities and meeting emergency demands. It is the ability to endure, to bear up, to withstand stress, to carry on in circumstances where an unfit person could not continue, and is a major basis for good health and well-being (PCFS&N, 2016).

Physical fitness involves the performance of the heart, the lungs, and the muscles of the body, and since what we do with our bodies also affects what we can do with our minds, fitness influences to some degree qualities such as mental alertness and emotional stability.

As you undertake your fitness program, it is important to remember that fitness is an individual quality that varies from person to person. It is influenced by age, sex, heredity, personal habits, exercise, and eating practices. You cannot do anything about the first three factors. However, it is within your power to change and improve the others where needed.

Fitness: The Basics

Physical fitness is most easily understood by examining its four basic components:

- *Cardiorespiratory endurance.* The ability to deliver oxygen and nutrients to tissues and to remove wastes over sustained periods of time. Long runs and swims are among the methods employed in measuring this component.
- *Muscular strength.* The ability of a muscle to exert force for a brief period of time. Upper-body strength, for example, can be measured by various weight-lifting exercises.
- *Muscular endurance.* The ability of a muscle, or a group of muscles, to sustain repeated contractions or to continue applying force against a fixed object. Pushups are often used to test endurance of arm and shoulder muscles.
- *Flexibility.* The ability to move joints and use muscles through their full range of motion. The sit-and-reach test is a good measure of flexibility of the lower back and backs of the upper legs.

SEARCH AND RESCUE TIP

The four basic components of fitness are:

- Cardiovascular endurance
- Muscular strength
- Muscular endurance
- Flexibility

Body composition is often considered a component of fitness. It refers to the makeup of the body in terms of lean mass (muscle, bone, vital tissue, and organs) and fat mass. An optimal ratio of fat to lean mass is an indication of fitness, and the right types of exercises will help you decrease body fat and increase or maintain muscle mass.

Body mass index (BMI) is a useful measure of overall body composition and obesity and is calculated from one's height and weight. BMI is an estimate of body fat and a good gauge of one's risk for diseases that can occur with more body fat. The higher your BMI, the higher your risk for certain diseases such as heart disease, high blood pressure, type 2 diabetes, gallstones, breathing problems, and certain cancers (**FIGURE 5-3**). BMI can be used as a screening tool but is not by itself diagnostic of the health of an individual (CDC, 2016).

BMI[2]	19	20	21	22	23	24	25	26	27	28	29	30	31	32	33	34	35
Height (inches)	Body Weight (pounds)																
58	91	96	100	105	110	115	119	124	129	134	138	143	148	153	158	162	167
59	94	99	104	109	114	119	124	128	133	138	143	148	153	158	163	168	173
60	97	102	107	112	118	123	128	133	138	143	148	153	158	163	168	174	179
61	100	106	111	116	122	127	132	137	143	148	153	158	164	169	174	180	185
62	104	109	115	120	126	131	136	142	147	153	158	164	169	175	180	186	191
63	107	113	118	124	130	135	141	146	152	158	163	169	175	180	186	191	197
64	110	116	122	128	134	140	145	151	157	163	169	174	180	186	192	197	204
65	114	120	126	132	138	144	150	156	162	168	174	180	186	192	198	204	210
66	118	124	130	136	142	148	155	161	167	173	179	186	192	198	204	210	216
67	121	127	134	140	146	153	159	166	172	178	185	191	198	204	211	217	223
68	125	131	138	144	151	158	164	171	177	184	190	197	203	210	216	223	230
69	128	135	142	149	155	162	169	176	182	189	196	203	209	216	223	230	236
70	132	139	146	153	160	167	174	181	188	195	202	209	216	222	229	236	243
71	136	143	150	157	165	172	179	186	193	200	208	215	222	229	236	243	250
72	140	147	154	162	169	177	184	191	199	206	213	221	228	235	242	250	258
73	144	151	159	166	174	182	189	197	204	212	219	227	235	242	250	257	265
74	148	155	163	171	179	186	194	202	210	218	225	233	241	249	256	264	272
75	152	160	168	176	184	192	200	208	216	224	232	240	248	256	264	272	279
76	156	164	172	180	189	197	205	213	221	230	238	246	254	263	271	279	287

Note 1: Although BMI can be used for most men and women, it does have some limits:

- It may overestimate body fat in athletes and others who have a muscular build.
- It may underestimate body fat in older persons and others who have lost muscle.

Note 2: Underweight = BMI < 18.5
Normal = BMI 18.5 – 24.9
Overweight = BMI 25.0 – 29.9
Obese = BMI ≥ 30.0

FIGURE 5-3 Body mass index (BMI), calculated from one's height and weight, is a useful measure of overall body composition and obesity.

Reproduced from National Heart, Lung, and Blood Institute. (2018). Body mass Index Table 1. Retrieved from https://www.nhlbi.nih.gov/health/educational/lose_wt/BMI/bmi_tbl.htm; and Centers for Disease Control and Prevention [CDC]. (2016). Defining adult overweight and obesity. Retrieved from http://www.cdc.gov/obesity/adult/defining.html.

A Workout Schedule

How often, how long, and how hard you exercise, and what types of exercises you do should be determined by what you are trying to accomplish (**FIGURE 5-4**). Your goals, present fitness level, age, health, skills, interests, and convenience are among the factors you should consider. For example, an athlete training for high-level competition would follow a different program than a person whose goals are good health and the ability to meet work and recreational needs.

Any exercise program should include something from each of the four basic fitness components (cardiovascular endurance, muscular strength, muscular endurance, and flexibility). Each workout should begin with a warm-up and end with a cool-down. As a rule, space your workouts throughout the week and avoid consecutive days of hard exercise.

Here are what many sources suggest as the amounts of activity necessary for the average healthy person to maintain a minimum level of overall fitness (PCFS&N, 2016; American Heart Association, 2016). Included are some of the popular exercises for each category.

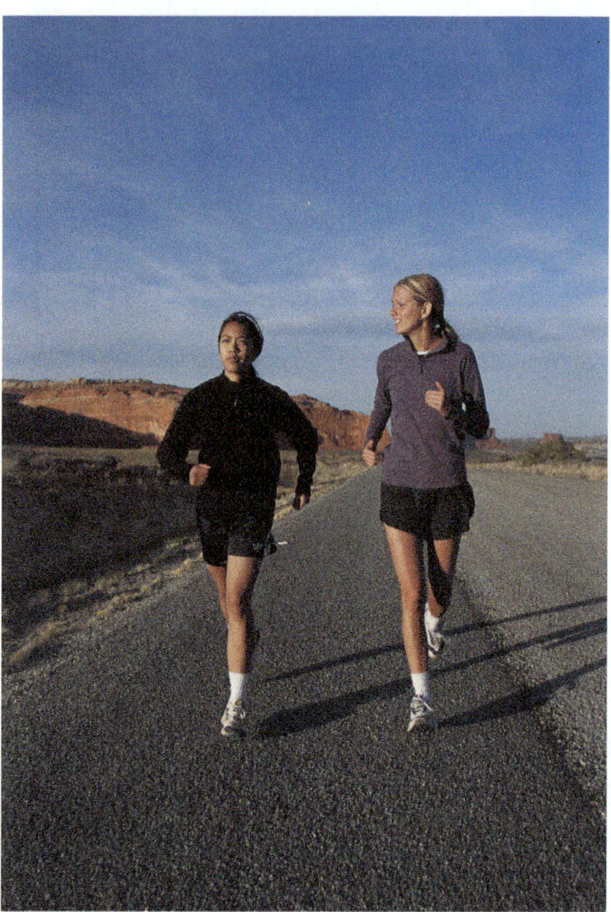

FIGURE 5-4 How often, how long, and how hard you exercise, and what types of exercises you do should be determined by what you are trying to accomplish. Field SAR work is physically demanding and requires a moderate to high level of fitness.

- *Warm-up.* Five to 10 minutes of exercise such as walking, slow jogging, knee lifts, arm circles, or trunk rotations. Low-intensity movements that simulate movements to be used in the activity can also be included in the warm-up.
- *Muscular strength.* The best strengthening activities work all the major muscle groups: legs, hips, back, chest, stomach, shoulders, and arms. These activities may include lifting weights, push-ups, sit-ups, and working with resistance bands. Common household items such as soup cans and bottled water can replace free weights.
- *Muscular endurance.* At least three 30-minute strengthening sessions each week build muscular endurance. Any of the strengthening activities listed above will work.
- *Cardiorespiratory endurance.* Adults between the ages of 18 and 64 should get a minimum of 150 minutes (2.5 hours) per week of moderate-intensity aerobic physical activity. These activities should be done for at least 10 minutes at a time because shorter intervals do not have the same health benefits. Popular aerobic conditioning activities include brisk walking, jogging, ballroom dancing, swimming, cycling, rope jumping, rowing, cross-country skiing, soccer, martial arts, and some continuous action games such as racquetball, handball, and basketball.
- *Flexibility.* Ten to 12 minutes of daily stretching exercises performed slowly, without a bouncing motion. This can be included after a warm-up or during a cool-down.
- *Cool-down.* A minimum of 5 to 10 minutes of slow walking, low-level exercise, combined with stretching.

A Matter of Principle

The keys to selecting the right kinds of exercises for developing and maintaining each of the basic components of fitness are found in the following principles:

- *Specificity.* Pick the right kind of activities to affect each component. Strength training results in specific strength changes. Also, train for the specific activity in which you are interested. For example, optimal hiking performance is best achieved when the muscles involved in walking are trained for the movements required. It does not necessarily follow that a good runner is a good swimmer.

- *Overload.* Work hard enough, at levels that are vigorous and long enough to overload your body above its current level, to bring about improvement.
- *Regularity.* You cannot hoard physical fitness. At least three balanced workouts a week are necessary to maintain a desirable level of fitness.
- *Progression.* Increase the intensity, frequency, and/or duration of activity over periods of time in order to improve.

Some activities can be used to fulfill more than one of your basic exercise requirements. For example, in addition to increasing cardiorespiratory endurance, running builds muscular endurance in the legs, and swimming develops the arm, shoulder, and chest muscles. If you select the proper activities, it is possible to fit parts of your muscular endurance workout into your cardiorespiratory workout and save time.

What Kind of Exercise?

Although any kind of physical movement requires energy (calories), the type of exercise that uses the most energy is **aerobic exercise**. The term *aerobic* is derived from the Greek words meaning "with oxygen" (Dictionary.com, 2016). Jogging, brisk walking, swimming, biking, cross-country skiing, and ballroom dancing are some popular forms of aerobic exercise. Aerobic exercises use the body's large muscle groups in continuous, rhythmic, sustained movement, and require oxygen to produce energy. When oxygen is combined with food, which can come from stored fat, energy is produced to power the body's musculature. The longer you move aerobically, the more energy is needed, and the more calories are used. Regular aerobic exercise improves your cardiorespiratory endurance, which is the ability of your heart, lungs, blood vessels, and associated tissues to use oxygen to produce energy needed for activity. You will build a healthier body while getting rid of excess body fat.

In addition to the aerobic exercise, supplement your program with muscle strengthening and stretching exercises. The stronger your muscles, the longer you will be able to keep going during aerobic activity, and the less chance of injury.

How Much, How Often?

Experts recommend that adults between the ages of 18 and 64 get a minimum of 150 minutes (2.5 hours) per week of moderate-intensity aerobic physical activity, in intervals of not less than 10 minutes each. Of course, if this is too much, you could start with less time each week and gradually build up to the minimum. Then gradually progress until you can work aerobically for 2.5 hours per week. If you need to lose a large amount of weight, you may want to do your aerobic workout five times a week, but only after conferring with your physician.

It is important to exercise at an intensity vigorous enough to cause your heart rate and breathing to increase. How hard you should exercise depends to a certain degree on your age and is determined by measuring your heart rate in beats per minute.

The heart rate you should maintain during exercise is called your **target heart rate**. The American Heart Association (AHA) recommends determining your target heart rate by first determining your maximum heart rate (subtracting your age from 220) and then taking 50–85% of that figure. Beginners should maintain the 50% level; more advanced individuals can work up to the 85% level. This is just a guide, however, and people with any medical limitations should discuss this formula and their target heart rate with their physician (AHA, 2016).

You can and should vary the types of aerobic activities, such as walking one day and riding a bike the next. Make sure you choose an activity that can be done regularly and is enjoyable for you. Do not skip too many days between workouts or health and fitness benefits will be lost. If you must lose a few days, gradually work back into your routine.

Controlling Your Weight

Just about everybody seems to be interested in weight control. Some of us weigh just the right amount; others need to gain a few pounds. Most of us "battle the bulge" at some time in our life. Whatever our goals, we should understand and take advantage of the important role of exercise in keeping our weight under control (AHA, 2016).

Few of today's occupations require vigorous physical activity, and much of our leisure time is spent in sedentary pursuits. Recent estimates indicate that 78 million American adults, and 12.5 million children and adolescents, are considered obese (20% above desirable weight). Also, there has been an increase in body fat levels in children and youth over the past

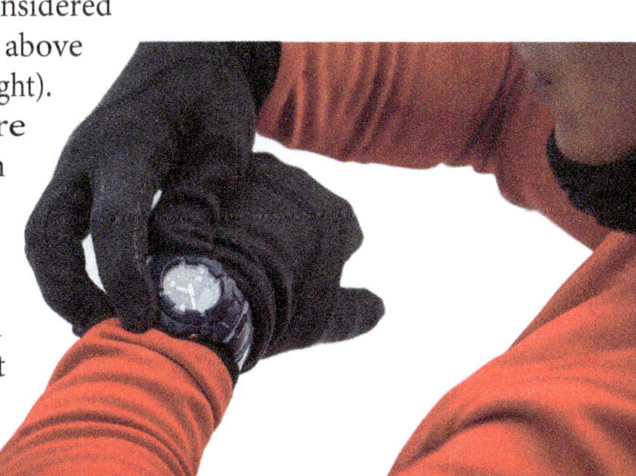

20 years. After infancy and early childhood, the earlier the onset of obesity, the greater the likelihood of remaining obese. Excess body fat has been linked to such health problems as coronary heart disease, high blood pressure, osteoporosis, diabetes, arthritis, and certain forms of cancer. Some evidence now exists showing that obesity has a negative effect on both health and long life (PCFS&N, 2016).

Exercise is associated with the loss of body fat in both obese and normal weight persons. A regular program of exercise is an important component of any plan to help individuals lose, gain, or maintain their weight.

The key to weight control is keeping energy intake (food) and energy output (physical activity) in balance. When you consume only the calories your body needs, your weight usually remains constant. If you take in more calories than your body needs, you put on excess fat. If you expend more energy than you take in, you burn excess fat.

Exercise plays an important role in weight control by increasing energy output, calling on stored calories for extra fuel. Studies show that not only does exercise increase metabolism during a workout, but it causes your metabolism to stay increased for a period of time after exercising, allowing you to burn more calories (AHA, 2016).

How much exercise is needed to make a difference in your weight depends on the amount and type of activity and the amount you eat. Aerobic exercise burns body fat. A medium-sized adult would have to walk more than 30 miles to burn 3,500 calories, the equivalent of 1 pound of fat. Although that may seem like a lot, you don't have to walk the 30 miles all at once. Walking a mile a day for 30 days achieves the same result, providing you don't increase your food intake to negate the effects of walking (Livestrong.com, 2014a).

If you consume 100 calories a day more than your body needs, you will gain approximately 10 pounds in a year. You could take that weight off, or keep it off, by doing 30 minutes of moderate exercise daily. The combination of exercise and diet offers the most flexible and effective approach to weight control.

Muscle tissue weighs more than fat tissue, and exercise develops muscle to a certain degree. Well-muscled individuals, with relatively little body fat, invariably are overweight according to standard weight charts. If you are participating in a regular program of strength training, your muscles will increase in weight, resulting in an overall body weight increase. Body composition is a better indicator of your condition than body weight.

Lack of physical activity causes muscles to become soft, and if food intake is not decreased, added body weight is almost always fat. Once-active people who continue to eat as they always have after settling into sedentary lifestyles tend to suffer from creeping obesity.

Benefits of Exercise in a Weight Control Program

The benefits of exercise are many, from producing physically fit bodies for SAR to providing an outlet for fun and socialization. When added to a weight control program, these benefits take on increased significance.

It has already been noted that proper exercise can help control weight by burning excess body fat. It also has two other body-trimming advantages: (1) exercise builds muscle tissue, and muscle burns calories at a faster rate than body fat; and (2) exercise helps reduce inches, and a firm, lean body looks slimmer even if your weight remains the same.

Remember, fat does not turn into muscle, as is often believed. Fat and muscle are two entirely different substances, and one cannot become the other. However, muscle does use calories at a faster rate than fat, which directly affects your body's metabolic rate or energy requirement. Your **basal metabolic rate (BMR)** is the amount of energy (number of calories) required to sustain the body's functions at rest, and it depends on your age, sex, body size, genes, and body composition (BMI). People with high levels of muscle tend to have higher BMRs and use more calories in the resting stage (Livestrong.com, 2014b; Livestrong.com, 2015).

Some studies have even shown that your metabolic rate stays elevated for some time after vigorous exercise, causing you to burn more calories throughout your day. Additional benefits may be seen in how exercise affects appetite. A lean person in good shape may eat more following increased activity, but the regular exercise burns up the extra calories consumed. On the other hand, vigorous exercise has been reported to suppress appetite. Physical activity can be used as a positive substitute for between-meal snacking.

Better Mental Health

The psychological benefits of exercise are equally important to the weight conscious person. Exercise can decrease stress and relieve tensions that might otherwise lead to overeating. Exercise builds physical fitness, which in turn builds self-confidence, enhanced self-image, and a positive outlook. When you start to feel good about yourself, you are more likely to want to make other positive changes in your lifestyle that help keep your weight under control.

In addition, exercise can be fun, provide recreation, and offer opportunities for companionship. The exhilaration and emotional release of participating in sports or other activities are a boost to mental and physical health. Pent-up anxieties and frustrations seem to disappear when you are concentrating on returning a serve, sinking a putt, or hiking that extra mile.

SEARCH AND RESCUE TIP

Physical and mental fitness are integral to the primary SAR objective of working for the victim.

Tips to Get Started

Hopefully, you are now convinced that you must include exercise in your daily routine. Here are some tips to get you started:

1. Check with your doctor first. If you are carrying around some extra weight, it is wise to get your doctor's "OK" before embarking on an exercise program.
2. Choose activities that you think you will enjoy. Most people will stick to their exercise program if they are having fun, even though they are working hard.
3. Set aside a regular exercise time. Whether this means joining an exercise class or getting up a little earlier every day, make time for this addition to your routine, and do not let anything get in your way. Planning ahead helps you get around interruptions in your workout schedule, such as bad weather and vacations.
4. Set short-term goals. Do not expect to lose 20 pounds in two weeks. It has taken a while for you to gain the weight; it will take time to lose it. Keep a record of your progress and tell your friends and family about your achievements.
5. Vary your exercise program. Change exercises or invite friends to join you to make your workout more enjoyable. There is no best exercise—just the one that works best for you. It will not be easy, especially at the start. However, as you begin to feel better, look better, and enjoy a new zest for life, you will be rewarded many times over for your efforts.

Tips to Keep Going

To continue to manage your weight, and indeed your health, adopt a specific exercise plan, commit it to writing, and share it with others so they can support your efforts. Maintain realistic goals and remind yourself of them often by any convenient means (e.g., post on a wall). Avoid injuries by pacing yourself and including a warm-up and cool-down period as part of every workout. Keep a log of progress and keep it current. Include weight and other measures, such as BMI, on your log to track trends—both improvements and opportunities for improvement. As your fitness improves, adapt (upgrade) your plan accordingly so that improvements continue. Make sure to include family and friends in your plan to help support and accompany you on your journey. Keep others updated on your progress so they can help celebrate your accomplishments, and do not hesitate to celebrate with them for a job well done.

Admitting Limitations

You must make a realistic assessment of your physical abilities without being nostalgic and recalling earlier athletic achievements. Males reach their physiological prime in their late teens and females in their early teens. This does not rule out fitness later in your life, however. If you are to maintain optimum performance, you must not try to do more than you can achieve. Assess your physical limitations realistically and restrict your activities accordingly. There is as much to do for those who are not up to arduous field work as there is for the marathon runner. Do not compare yourself with others; we all set our own limits. Everyone is different.

In general, when you are prepared physically, you will know the limits of that condition. Being prepared is preferred to finding out about your lack of conditioning after a futile and dangerous attempt at working in the field. Remember that when search and rescue personnel become disabled, injured, or ill, focus is drawn away from the victim. Knowing when to stay out of the field is a prime example of when your brain becomes your primary survival tool.

Mental Preparedness

Keeping your body in condition virtually assures your ability to think clearly and concentrate for long periods of time. Both mental and physical conditioning are required for search, rescue, and survival. The time will come when alertness, resourcefulness, and mental toughness will get you through a tight spot. You must be prepared for that eventuality.

In everything you do—work, play, school, relationships, etc.—mental preparedness can be accomplished by following some simple "self" guidelines. The following tips also help in maintaining a proper attitude of safety, in life as well as SAR.

- *Be thorough.* When you begin something, do it well and finish what you start. Perseverance is an essential survival tool. Do not give up.
- *Be confident and willing to learn.* Confidence comes through training and experience. Learn essential skills and practice what you learn. If you do something right or do something wrong, apply what you learned when you are next confronted by a similar situation. Learn something from every experience.
- *Be conscientious.* There is a good chance that no one will be around to watch what you are doing. Your activities must be guided by your own standards. Set them high. Your peace of mind and satisfaction in a job well done may be your greatest, and sometimes only, rewards.
- *Be assertive.* Take advantage of new experiences. Push yourself beyond what you have done in the past without being foolish. Take the lead to get things accomplished. Do not be afraid to take a safer route, recheck your bearings, or change your mind.

Wrap-Up

READY FOR REVIEW

- Search and rescue (SAR) personnel must have a working knowledge of human biological survival (the necessities and priorities of life), including a fundamental understanding of issues related to nutrition, hydration, and thermoregulation.
- To be optimally prepared, SAR personnel must eat a well-balanced diet every day so that they are best prepared for peak performance when they are called.
- No other nutrient affects athletic or work performance more than water, so consuming an adequate amount of water is vital to being able to perform any sort of activity, including SAR.
- Heat balance (thermal equilibrium) is the balance between the rate of heat production and the rate of heat loss.
- All SAR personnel should be fit—physically and mentally—to operate at their optimum during a SAR mission, regardless of one's assignment.
- The first important step on the path to physical fitness is to seek information, and the second is to firmly decide that you are going to be physically fit.
- Physical fitness involves four basic components: cardiorespiratory endurance, muscular strength, muscular endurance, and flexibility.
- How often, how long, and how hard you exercise, and what types of exercises you do should be determined by what you are trying to accomplish.

SEARCH AND RESCUE TERMS

Aerobic exercise Exercise that combines food (often fat) with oxygen to produce energy for the body and that leads to cardiorespiratory endurance.

Basal metabolic rate The amount of energy required to sustain the body's functions at rest.

Calorie The amount of heat required to raise the temperature of 1 gram of water 1 degree Celsius.

Heat transfer The movement of heat between the body and the environment through radiation, conduction, convection, or evaporation.

Kilocalorie One thousand calories, or the amount of heat required to raise the temperature of 1 kilogram of water 1 degree Celsius.

Physical fitness The ability to perform daily tasks vigorously and alertly, with energy left over for enjoying leisure-time activities and meeting emergency demands (PCFS&N, 2016).

Target heart rate The heart rate you should maintain during exercise.

REFERENCES AND SUGGESTED READING

American College of Sports Medicine. 2011. Selecting and effectively using hydration for fitness. http://www.acsm.org/docs/brochures/selecting-and-effectively-using-hydration-for-fitness.pdf.

American Heart Association. 2016. Healthy living. http://www.heart.org/HEARTORG/HealthyLiving/Healthy-Living_UCM_001078_SubHomePage.jsp.

Armsey, Thomas D. and Gary A. Green. 1997. Nutrition supplements: Science vs hype. *The Physician and Sports Medicine*, 25(6), 76–84.

Baechle, Thomas R. and Roger W. Earle. 2000. *Essentials of Strength and Conditioning* (2nd ed.). Champaign, IL: Human Kinetics.

Centers for Disease Control and Prevention. 2016. Defining adult overweight and obesity. http://www.cdc.gov/obesity/adult/defining.html.

Centers for Disease Control and Prevention. 2011. U.S. obesity trends. http://www.cdc.gov/obesity/data/trends.HTML.

Charkoudian, Nisha and Larry Crenshaw. 2017. Thermoregulation, in *Wilderness Medicine*, Seventh Edition. Edited by Paul Auerbach. St. Louis, MO: Elsevier, Inc., pp. 120–134.

Cornell University Ergonomics Web. 2015. DEA3500: Ambient environment: Thermal regulation. http://ergo.human.cornell.edu/studentdownloads/DEA3500notes/Thermal/thregnotes.html.

Dictionary.com. 2016. Website of definitions. www.dictionary.com.

Greenleaf, John E. 1992. Problem: Thirst, drinking behavior, and involuntary dehydration. *Medicine and Science in Sports and Exercise*, 24, no. 6: 645–656.

Hedge, Alan. 2015. Thermal sensation and thermoregulation. Cornell University. http://ergo.human.cornell.edu/studentdownloads/dea3500pdfs/thermreg.pdf.

Institute of Medicine of the National Academies. 2005. *Dietary Reference Intakes for Water, Potassium, Sodium, Chloride, and Sulfate*. Washington, DC: The National Academies Press.

Jeukendrup, Asker, and Michael Gleeson. 2010. *Sports Nutrition: An Introduction to Energy Production and Performance*. 2nd Edition. Champaign, IL: Human Kinetics.

Kenefick, Robert W., Samuel N. Cheuvront, Lisa Leon, and Karen K. O'Brien. 2017. Dehydration and Rehydration. In *Wilderness Medicine*, Seventh Edition, edited by Paul Auerbach, pp. 2031–2043. St. Louis, MO: Elsevier, Inc.

Livestrong.com. 2014a. How to lose 10 pounds a month by walking. http://www.livestrong.com/article/164608-how-to-lose-10-pounds-a-month-by-walking/.

Livestrong.com. 2014b. Is it a myth that muscle burns more calories than fat? http://www.livestrong.com/article/447243-is-it-a-myth-that-muscle-burns-more-calories-than-fat/.

Livestrong.com. 2015. How to lose your BMR to lose weight. http://www.livestrong.com/article/266994-how-to-lose-weight-with-bmr/.

Passe, Dennis, M. Horn, and R. Murray. 2000. Impact of beverage acceptability on fluid intake during exercise. Barrington: IL, Gatorade Sports Science Institute.

President's Council on Fitness, Sports & Nutrition. 2016. Research and reports. http://www.fitness.gov/resource-center/research-and-reports/.

Puhl, S. M., and E. R. Buskirk. 1998. Nutrient beverages for exercise and sport. In *Nutrition in Exercise and Sport*, 3rd ed., edited by Ira Wolinsky and J. F. Hickson. London: CRC Press.

Sawka, M., L. Burke, E. Eichner, M. Bergeron, M. Hargreaves, and R. Maughan. 2007. American College of Sports Medicine position stand. Exercise and fluid replacement. *Medicine and Science in Sports and Exercise*, 39, no. 2, pp. 377–390. http://journals.lww.com/acsm-msse/Fulltext/2007/02000/Exercise_and_Fluid_Replacement.22.aspx.

Schmidt-Nielsen, Knut. 1997. *Animal Physiology: Adaptation and Environment*, Fifth Edition. Cambridge, MA: Cambridge University Press.

Schoene, Robert. B. 2017. Physiology of Exercise, Conditioning, and Performance Training for Wilderness Adventure, in *Wilderness Medicine*, Seventh Edition. Edited by Paul Auerbach. St. Louis, MO: Elsevier, Inc., pp. 2183–2191.

Sterns, Richard H. 2014. Maintenance and replacement fluid therapy in adults. http://www.uptodate.com/home.

U.S. Department of Agriculture. 2010. Dietary guidelines for Americans. http://www.cnpp.usda.gov/dietaryguidelines.htm.

U.S. Department of Commerce, National Oceanic and Atmospheric Administration, National Weather Service. 2016a. NWS heat index. http://www.nws.noaa.gov/om/heat/heat_index.shtml.

U.S. Department of Commerce, National Oceanic and Atmospheric Administration, National Weather Service. 2016b. NWS wind chill chart. http://www.nws.noaa.gov/om/winter/windchill.shtml.

U.S. Department of Health and Human Services. 2010. Healthy people 2010. http://www.cdc.gov/nchs/healthy_people/hp2010.htm.

U.S. Department of Health and Human Services. 2016. Healthy people 2020. http://www.healthypeople.gov/2020/default.aspx.

Wilk, B., and O. Bar-Or. 1996. Effect of drink flavor and NaCl on voluntary drinking and hydration in boys exercising in the heat. *Journal of Applied Physiology,* 80, no. 4. pp. 1112–1117.

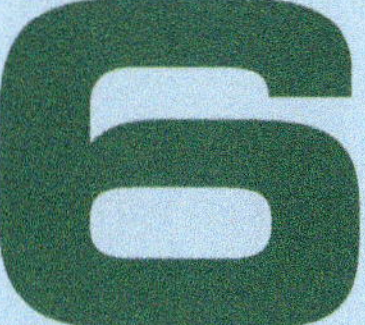

CHAPTER 6

Survival and Improvisation

OBJECTIVES

Upon completion of this chapter and the related course activities, the student will be able to meet the following objectives:

- Explain the significance of positive mental attitude (PMA) for the search and rescue (SAR) professional.
- List and prioritize the necessities of life.
- Describe the three responses to stress according to the general adaptation syndrome (GAS) model.
- List at least five ways to control fear in yourself and others.
- Explain the survival situation plan, STOP (stay/stop, think, observe, plan/proceed).
- List the six steps of the improvisation process.
- Identify at least three important considerations in constructing a shelter.
- Describe at least one method of constructing a fire.
- Describe the four signals recommended for use by SAR professionals.
- List the four minimum recommended water treatment methods for SAR professionals.
- Discuss considerations regarding personal waste disposal.
- Describe at least three methods used for personal cleanliness in the outdoors.

Survival in the Context of Search and Rescue

Traditional definitions of survival imply primitive conditions, living off the land, or battling the elements to live through some precarious predicament in the wilderness. Depending on one's perspective, survival means different things to different people. In terms of SAR, survival is about rescuers being able to take care of themselves, and perhaps one another, in harsh, challenging, or less than optimal circumstances. It is not about being able to snare a rabbit or start a fire with two sticks. It is about being prepared to care for yourself and others in austere circumstances when necessary.

At its core, a survival situation is one in which an individual's very existence is threatened, and some kind of action is necessary to alleviate a threat to life. To survive is to continue existing, to live despite some event or adverse set of circumstances. At its best, survival may be no more than a realization that comfort is not essential to survival. At its worst, survival is simply living a minute longer by any means possible. In SAR, this type of situation might arise when operating in an isolated area and unpredicted severe weather materializes that forces you and your team to shelter in place; or, when a member of your team is severely injured and unable to travel, so you must improvise a shelter and protect them (and you) from the elements until help arrives.

Advancements in communications and other technologies have significantly reduced the time one might need to survive until rescue, usually to a day or two at most. In SAR situations, where the locations to which personnel are deployed is known and SAR planning and resource tracking is taking place, this survival time can be reduced even further, but technologies can fail, and plans can be rendered useless by unpredictable weather, injuries, and other unforeseen circumstances, so one entering an environment in which SAR is required must be prepared to provide or improvise whatever it takes to survive until help arrives or until the situation can be overcome.

To establish an effective, rational response to any survival situation, it is imperative to realize that actions and needs must be prioritized. Preconceived, uninformed ideas about survival can precipitate inappropriate actions when one is stressed, and the results can be fatal. First-hand accounts and interviews of survivors substantiate the fact that the decisions made in the first hours or minutes of an emergency have a great bearing on the ultimate outcome (**FIGURE 6-1**).

It is essential to understand the human body, not as thoroughly as a physician understands it, but how it reacts to or is affected by environmental stress. A working knowledge of how to manage your body properly in an emergency is the key to survival. *Proper body management* is defined as the maintenance and control of your essential (limited) body resources and problem-solving capabilities. If mismanaged, body upsets will result and directly affect one's ability to survive in any environment for any period of time.

The greatest obstacle an individual must overcome is an inappropriate mental attitude. Since so much of survival is dealing with psychological challenge, the brain becomes the individual's most important survival tool.

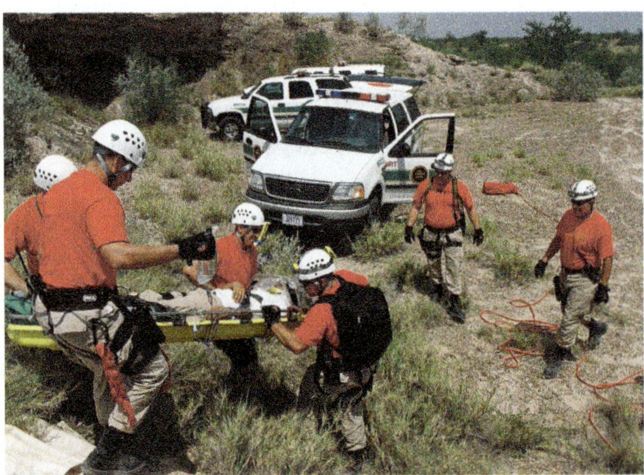

FIGURE 6-1 Decisions made in the first hours or minutes of an emergency have a great bearing on the ultimate outcome of the situation.
Courtesy of James Tourtellotte/U.S. Customs & Border Protection.

Recognizing and acquiring the body's physical needs will always require the capacity for analytical thought that is based in previous experience and training. Thus, the body and mind are inseparable when it comes to survival.

People live, work, and play in a **comfort zone**. Just as people differ in their abilities, comfort zones and their limits also differ from person to person. Since people are creatures of habit, and the technology they have created takes much of the unexpected out of their lives, most rarely venture outside of their comfort zones. Studies of those who perform high-risk and challenging activities show that those who operate on the outskirts of their comfort zones and continually push their limits react better in an emergency. Under repeated stress situations, people learn to make more effective adjustments. However, most people rarely experience an emergency, so their typical response is to display disorganized and shock-like behavior. Rational, coherent thinking that calls upon similar situations from past training and experience will, in most cases, be the most effective method for gaining control of the situation.

Modern technology has accustomed people to light-switch conveniences that eliminate thirst, hunger, cold, heat, and, in most cases, fear. In an unexpected survival situation, confidence and self-reliance play a key role in determining the ultimate outcome of that experience. Unfortunately, people are not only dependent on their technology but are products of a culture that has little need for individuals to be self-reliant on a daily basis. Self-reliance is developed through actual experience and dependence on one's self for everyday needs. There is no substitute for actually having performed a task that is designed to save lives.

The Necessities of Life

What does it take for a human being to stay alive for an indefinite period of time? Typical answers might include clothes, a house, a car, and three meals a day. However, several thousand years ago, humans did not have these conveniences, yet they still survived. By listing the necessities of life and asking how long a human can live without each item, it is possible to prioritize these necessities. The time factors involved with this type of analysis should be in terms of minutes, hours, days, and weeks. Although this approach may seem elementary, it provides a foundation for good judgment when dealing with all life-threatening emergencies (**TABLE 6-1**).

TABLE 6-1 Necessities of Life and Survival Time

Necessities of Life in Priority Order	Survival Time if Requirement Not Fulfilled
Positive mental attitude and will to live	Depends entirely on you
Oxygen in air	3 to 5 minutes
Body shelter from extreme temperatures	3 to 4 hours, depending on the environment
Rest (mental as well as physical)	30 hours in extremes
Water	3 days in extremes
Food	3 weeks or more

SEARCH AND RESCUE TIP

The necessities of life are:

1. Will to live/positive mental attitude (PMA)
2. Air/oxygen
3. Shelter/clothing, warmth
4. Rest
5. Signals (if you expect to be found)
6. Water
7. Food

Priority 1: Positive Mental Attitude

Air, shelter, rest, water, and food are presented in a logical order of their importance to human survival. However, an often overlooked but vital priority is a mental attitude that is positive in nature and appropriate in its perspective for a given situation. This is usually the result of a thorough background in the knowledge and skills necessary to preserve human life in a hostile environment.

An important part of emergency response from an individual's standpoint is the "whole person concept." An understanding of this basic proposition enables a person to better put into perspective the priorities of any emergency environment. The *whole person concept*, as it applies to one's reactions in an emergency, is a term that ties together both mental and physical body processes. Simply put, what affects a person physically also affects a person mentally, and whatever affects a person mentally will ultimately affect a person physically. Realization of this fact alone can have a tremendous impact on anyone's ability to cope with stressful environments.

If all other priorities have been maintained or procured, but an individual lacks the will to live or the ability to cope with the situation mentally because of physical condition, then all is lost. People are at the mercy of the elements and whatever luck might be thrown their way. The power of the mind must never be underestimated, especially as it relates to survival.

It is worth a note of caution here to emphasize that although a positive mental attitude (PMA) should be number one on the list of priorities, it is possible to take negative action even though your attitude is positive. Doing nothing to prevent or treat hypothermia will not save you from it, regardless of your attitude. Mental attitude must not be misconstrued as a cure-all for survival situations. PMA does very little to analyze the body's enemies, recognize a threat to life, or understand the counteractions necessary in an emergency situation. In most cases, it must be coupled with proper education, training, and experience.

Will to Live

To further clarify PMA, it is helpful to break the concept into two areas. The first is the *will to live*, which can be described as an overwhelming urge to survive no matter what the odds or circumstances. It has been debated extensively as to whether humans have a natural instinct for preservation. Numerous war accounts over the last century suggest that death often seems to be the easiest way out during periods of extreme physical and mental stress. People have the power to will themselves to die. Similarly, they also have the power to will themselves to live. To survive in a challenging situation, one must be able to focus on survival, visualize the future, and maintain a will to live, regardless of the circumstances.

Whole Person Concept

The second area of a PMA deals specifically with the whole person concept and a person's problem-solving ability. It is possible to be thoroughly knowledgeable, experienced, have a PMA commensurate with the situation, and still not operate at 100% of your capability.

Those with a PMA that is appropriate in its perspective for a given situation coupled with a strong will to live ultimately are in the best position to assess the situation realistically and prioritize what needs to be accomplished during any survival situation.

Priority 2: Air

Breathing is essential to maintain life on a minute-by-minute basis. Air, specifically its life-sustaining component, oxygen, must be the second priority. The average survival time without air is measured in minutes.

Priority 3: Shelter

Inherent to most survival situations is coping with inclement weather. Since human beings are designed to live naked only in areas where temperatures are very close to that of the body, environments outside this realm pose a variety of body protection problems. Anything that protects the body can be called shelter. Clothing is shelter in proximity to the body.

How to provide adequate shelter for a specific environmental situation is the dilemma. There are temperature extremes in the United States where inadequate shelter could cut survival time to a few hours, and in some cases, it could be reduced to one hour or less. Fire and warmth also can be considered under shelter because, by definition, they help maintain the body's temperature in a cold environment.

Priority 4: Rest

As mentioned earlier, energy levels within the body are vitally important and significantly impact the ability to cope with any given situation. There is a good possibility that it may not be possible to renew or increase energy levels during an emergency. In survival situations, it is imperative to conserve what is already present in the body. One of the most efficient ways of doing this is through adequate rest. The human body is a wonderful machine that can do amazing things when provided with proper care and maintenance. Timely periods of rest in stressful situations conserve energy for future use, and rest rids the body's tissues of carbon dioxide, lactic acid, and other body wastes. Taking a short time for rest also provides time for reflection and analysis of the situation. Mental rest is just as important as physical rest, if not more so. Extreme stress periods (both physical and mental) with no rest can significantly decrease survival time.

Priority 5: Signals

If you are lost or immobilized and become the subject of a search, it is important for searchers to be able to find you. In this situation, deploying some type of signal(s) could be helpful. Details on signaling are presented later in this chapter.

Priority 6: Water

It is generally accepted that water and its associated problems, such as dehydration and whether it is potable, are among the most pressing in any survival situation. The body comprises approximately two-thirds water that is stored within its tissues, circulatory system, and internal organs. Water is essential for body temperature regulation, waste elimination, and digestion of food. While at rest with no activities, the body uses approximately two quarts of water a day merely to carry on normal body functions. Consumption of any amount less than this results in dehydration. Activity of any kind drastically increases the body's requirements for water. Therefore, it is not the water that should be rationed but one's sweat and activity. A 2.5% water deficit can occur in as little as a few hours, and this can result in a 25% loss of efficiency. Extreme conditions without water could cut survival time to a matter of only a few days, even if methods of water conservation are used. Water is high on the list of priorities for maintaining life. (See Chapter 5, *Physiology and Fitness* for more information on hydration.)

Priority 7: Food

Contrary to popular belief, the human body does not require three meals a day to remain alive. Countless people across the world live on far less. Many have only one meal a day and some not even that. Records from survival experiences show numerous accounts of 40- to 70-day periods with no caloric intake. This fact, coupled with current records showing that most survival situations last a few days at the most, emphasizes that procurement of food in a survival situation should be *last* on the list of priorities.

Energy levels within the body play an important role in warmth and performance. High-energy snacks provide additional calories for heat production as well as movement. Although food would play a minor role under most circumstances, cold environments require many calories to maintain normal body temperature. As mentioned earlier, conservation of existing energy levels is the best strategy when survival is an issue.

SEARCH AND RESCUE TIP

Keep these challenges in mind and be prepared to deal with them.

- The same environment that caused another person problems can also cause difficulty for you.
- You can find yourself doing SAR work in unfamiliar terrain where all the potential hazards are unknown.
- You can become lost or disoriented in unfamiliar areas, especially if you are unprepared in the first place.
- Hazardous areas are some of the first areas to be searched. In your zeal to help others, you can also become a victim if you are not careful.
- "First Notice" information is often vague. The severity/magnitude of a SAR incident is often misrepresented or misjudged in the early stages. SAR personnel are often quick to venture into situations with less information than is necessary for safe operations.
- The incidence of injury in SAR operations is high. This may be due to poor preparation, adrenaline "poisoning," misdirection by incident managers, or a number of intrinsic problems related to SAR operations.

Mental Aspects of Emergency Response and Survival

A positive mental attitude, appropriate in its perspective for a given situation, ultimately assumes the highest of all priorities during any survival situation.

There is really no way to accurately predict any person's behavior or thought processes during sudden mental and physical stresses. Reactions to every situation will vary greatly with every circumstance and every individual. In general, there are two aspects of emergency response that should be considered by SAR personnel: (1) mental preparation for SAR operations, and (2) immediate response to an emergency situation.

SEARCH AND RESCUE TIP

Staying out of trouble is the name of the game in SAR operations. When SAR personnel become lost or injured, work efforts are often directed away from the original subject(s).

Mental Preparation

Mental preparation is vitally important to safe SAR operations. Anger, fear, frustration, depression, worry, and anxiety all affect a person's ability to concentrate. Anyone who brings their problems into SAR operations is easily distracted and less able to adjust to any kind of stress. The relationship between mental functions and physical capability has already been discussed.

An accurate prediction of how any one person may react in a life-threatening situation is nearly impossible. What is known is that under repeated stress situations, people will make more and more effective adjustments. There are many situations present in everyday life to provide indications of stress performance, but earlier reactions may be the most telling. We must learn to read these indicators and make necessary adjustments.

Response to Life-Threatening Situations

The theory of human evolution is based on the premise that some people will survive life-threatening events, which is why humans have over time adapted to respond to these situations in a beneficial way. In 1936, Hans Selye, an Austrian physician, discovered that his subjects demonstrated similar reactions to all types of life-threatening stimuli, which he generally referred to as *stress*. Selye collectively named these similar responses to stress *general adaption syndrome* or GAS (Selye, 1936). Researchers' thinking on this topic has evolved over the years, but the need for controlling the mind and thus one's actions in a stressful situation is widely recognized (Kemeny, 2003). A basic understanding of the stages of GAS may be useful so that SAR personnel can better understand how to effectively deal with, and mentally manage, a stressful situation.

The three stages of GAS are: alarm reaction, resistance, and exhaustion.

Stage 1: Alarm Reaction

The first stage of GAS—the alarm reaction—is an initial state of increased alertness that results from some stimulus or stress. This is where the body gears up for action. Almost simultaneously as the stimulus or stress is experienced, the amygdala, the part of the brain that contributes to emotional processing, sends a distress signal to another part of the brain called the hypothalamus. The hypothalamus acts like the command center of the brain and communicates with the rest of the body that "fight or flight" will be necessary (Harvard Health Publications, 2016). While all this is happening, anxiety increases as the entire body, both physically and mentally, starts to comprehend the possibility that something is going to happen that will impact it.

The following physical and physiological reactions occur in the first stage of GAS:

- Adrenaline (epinephrine) starts to circulate through the body and triggers the release of blood sugar (glucose) and fats from temporary storage sites, which supplies energy to all parts of the body.

- Breathing rate increases, and small airways in the lungs (bronchioles) dilate to allow more oxygen in, which is sent to the brain to increases alertness.
- Heart rate and blood pressure increase, pushing blood to the muscles, heart, and other vital organs.
- Sight, hearing, and other senses become sharper.
- Muscles tighten.

If allowed to progress uncontrolled, anxiety turns to overt fear. This may quickly progress to complete panic, characterized by frozen limbs and mind (including physical weakness, crying, trembling, nausea, or vomiting). An individual might turn and run, stand and do something positive, or merely stand there shaking. It must be understood that anxiety and fear are perfectly natural feelings that can and must be controlled.

This is the point at which training and/or experience can most impact subsequent events. If SAR personnel have practiced both standard procedures and a methodical approach to managing a problem, then it is likely that the response will be natural and positive. If the response requires involved thought or lengthy decision-making, chances are that anxiety and fear will increase and negatively influence one's actions. When appropriate action is required in an emergency, there is no substitute for practice and experience. The more you practice, the more likely you can react appropriately and automatically in high stress situations, but in preparing for survival, there is no substitute for having experienced adversity and hardship in your life and having overcome it (Siebert, 2010). Strength is gained in adversity, and overcoming significant challenges in life may well be the best preparation for survival in any situation, including SAR. As philosopher Friedrich Nietzsche said, "What does not destroy me, makes me stronger" (Nietzsche, 1990).

Stage 2: Resistance

The initial alarm reaction is hard for the body to sustain, and it eventually wants to return to a more balanced, normal, and stable state (i.e., homeostasis). Eventually, the body adjusts its physiological reaction to reduce the remaining threat. Although the glucose levels, pulse rate, blood pressure, and general arousal may still be elevated, the stress hormones begin to return to normal, and the body starts to replenish at least some of its resources. When the body recognizes that the alarm reaction may no longer be necessary, new hormones are released in the body that begin to counteract the adrenaline previously produced. This allows the body to transition from alertness to repair (Selye, 1936; Psychologist World, 2016; Nairne, 2006).

Stage 3: Exhaustion

At this stage, the stress has continued for some time, and the body's resistance to the stress may be collapsing. "The body just can't continue to maintain a high state of readiness for extended periods of time" (Nairne, 2006, p. 544). This final stage is where the body recognizes that it has depleted its resources after trying to repair itself in the previous stage. Eventually, the body just gives up, and irreversible damage, even death, becomes a real possibility.

This stage is inevitable and may manifest itself as a sharp emotional letdown after high-energy output. The one stressed is often physically and emotionally drained and may experience significant shock and symptoms of other serious medical maladies such as stroke and heart attack (Selye, 1936; Nairne, 2006).

Comfort Zones

Humans are basically creatures of habit and are dependent on routine, organization, and some degree of discipline. Once these habits are established, people become comfortable with their behavior and surroundings. People generally become skilled and proficient only after a period of slow, deliberate actions while learning what is expected of them. Everyone establishes these comfort zones both physically and mentally. It follows then that whenever a person is placed in a situation that forces use of the outer limits of his or her comfort zone, anxiety and stress are created.

Comfort zone limits vary with each individual in accordance with experience and knowledge. Everyone is unique in abilities, and since a human being is basically a creature of habit, most go outside of their comfort zones only rarely. Herein is the difficulty of functioning in any emergency environment. Very often, every decision is important, and there is little room for mistakes.

At best, decision-making is difficult, and this difficulty is amplified in times of emotional upset. The best way to prepare mentally is through self-discipline and practice during everyday routine. Look for opportunities to expand your comfort zone into areas that you may be unsure of now.

Are you a person who continually takes the easy way out, or do you tackle everyday problems with a positive attitude and direct approach? These questions can be applied to personal relationships and situations that develop. The answers may give you a good indication of your ability to react under stress. Good habits in training and everyday life pay off in an emergency.

SAFETY TIP

To make sound decisions in stressful situations, establish self-discipline and good habits in your daily training.

Controlling Fear

As any individual approaches comfort zone limits, an unconscious level of fear known as *anxiety* can be experienced. Anxiety is characterized by feelings of uneasiness, nervousness, and worry about something in the future with an uncertain outcome. These feelings can vary in intensity, duration, and recurrence. If this anxiety progresses, it may become overt fear—an unpleasant emotion that serves only to increase anxiety, which in turn increases fear. This can be a vicious cycle, which some have referred to as the "circle of fear" (Walter, 2011). Fear that is unchecked and reinforced by other thoughts or stimuli can quickly turn to panic that is accompanied by a complete loss of reasoning. Fearfulness turned to blind panic can cause an experienced person to injure or kill himself or herself—and perhaps others—in the intensity of terror. As philosopher Edmund Burke said, "No passion so effectively robs the mind of all its powers of acting and reasoning as fear" (Burke, 2001).

Training, including knowledge and experience gained in simulated emergencies, reduces the unknown and helps to control anxiety and fear. When fantasy distorts a moderate danger into a major catastrophe, behavior can become abnormal. If this happens, people may be reacting to feelings and imagination or past traumatic events rather than the actual problem at hand. In such cases, people tend to unconsciously force themselves to underestimate (rather than overestimate) the danger, which readily leads to reckless, even foolhardy, behavior.

There are many ways to fight fear, but one of the best may be to meet it head on. Recognize fear as a natural phenomenon. Try to establish just why it is that you are afraid and accept it as the defense mechanism that it is.

To best manage fear in an emergency, make sure you have the following:

- As much knowledge about the situation as possible
- The proper tools and/or equipment for the response
- The necessary physical fitness to meet the challenge
- A positive mental attitude (will to live)

Tell yourself that others have conquered the same situation. There are no clear-cut lines between recklessness and bravery or caution and panic. That is why it is essential to maintain proper mental control in an emergency.

Symptoms of Fear

Fear can manifest itself in both physical and mental signs and symptoms, which may include the following:

- Quickening of pulse, breathlessness
- Dilation of pupils
- Increased muscular tension and fatigue
- Perspiration of hands, feet, and armpits (diaphoresis)
- Frequent urination (polyuria)
- Dry mouth and throat, high-pitched voice with stammering
- "Butterflies" and faintness caused by empty stomach
- Nausea, vomiting, and diarrhea
- Irritability, increased hostility
- Talkative at early stages, later speechless (aphasia)
- Laughing or crying hysterically
- Confusion, forgetfulness, inability to concentrate
- Feeling of unreality, flight, panic, and sometimes stupor

Controlling Your Fear

Fear has several benefits. It can cause you to avoid something dangerous, it can improve your focus and provide clarity on what is most important, and it can force you to be open to receiving help from others, even when you might not otherwise do so. This last one is important in that fear often teaches us that we cannot survive on our own and that self-sufficiency is an illusion. This is one reason we are so much more powerful as part of a team than by ourselves.

Fear is also often imagined, not real. Both real and imagined fear can be managed and even relieved by following some suggestions and applying a few specific techniques:

- Keep yourself physically fit. Eat healthily, get regular exercise, and get plenty of rest through a regular sleep pattern. Avoid alcohol, unprescribed drugs, and junk food.
- Recognize that fear can be beneficial. When you feel fear, ask yourself what benefit it might be offering, or what you might learn from it.
- Do not try to physically or mentally run away from the situation. Recognize fear for what it is and accept it. Try to learn what your reactions are likely to be by looking at your daily habits.
- Learn how to make decisions quickly and logically by establishing good habits. Take positive action to take control of the situation instead of letting it control you.

- Develop self-confidence by continually expanding your comfort zone to encompass experiences that are unfamiliar. Define your fears and recognize them.
- Realize that "it can happen to me" and be prepared. Be properly equipped and prepared at all times. Always have several options in your plan. Prepare for the worst and hope for the best.
- Keep informed and increase your knowledge to reduce the unknown.
- Have procedures mapped out so that you will be busy—if not physically, then mentally.
- Set realistic goals. Rather than trying to achieve all your goals immediately, take baby steps and get there slowly.
- Realize that teamwork always accomplishes more than a one-person show.
- Replace negative self-talk with affirmative and coping self-talk. When you find yourself thinking negative ("I can't do this; it's too hard"), replace it with something more positive and helpful, like "This is hard, but I can get through it." Talk positively about your actions and your future.
- Use spiritual faith.
- Gather as much information about your situation as possible.
- Cultivate good survival-oriented attitudes. The main goal is survival with everything kept in perspective. The discomforts of the moment are only temporary.

SEARCH AND RESCUE TIP

Traits of a survivor include the following:

- Can make decisions
- Can improvise
- Can adapt and "make the best" of the situation
- Has patience—can keep cool, calm, and positive
- Is prepared—hopes for the best, but prepares for the worst
- Knows own special fears and worries, and most importantly, can control them

Controlling Fear in Others

Since teamwork is so important to SAR and survival, it should be no surprise that a situation could arise where you, your colleagues, and even a patient might benefit from supporting each other.

One example of this might be when fear strikes another, and his or her reaction is inconvenient and possibly hazardous. When this happens, you can help by first demonstrating a calm demeanor and practicing good leadership skills. Talk to them about your positive mental attitude and why it is important while being a model of composed professionalism. Accept their right to individual feelings, even if they differ from yours, and do not show resentment of their reactions. Accept their physical and emotional limitations and talk calmly and confidently to them without scolding or diminishing them or their feelings. Comfort them without encouraging them to feel sorry for themselves and involve them in simple tasks that can occupy their mind and body. These simple measures can reduce anxiety and prevent panic, even in overwhelming circumstances.

Mental Steps of Managing an Emergency

One way to find answers in a survival situation is to use the mnemonic STOP:

S: Stay/stop

T: Think

O: Observe

P: Plan/proceed

Stay/stop at the first sign of trouble. Rushing around only causes confusion. Stopping helps fight the emotions of anxiety and panic and greatly improves your chances of surviving. You got yourself into this situation, and you can get yourself out. Stop for a moment and be patient. If anyone needs medical assistance, administer first aid.

Think about immediate and future dangers. Analyze the weather, terrain, and available resources to sustain life. Look for recognizable landmarks or study a map for clues. If you are lost, how long ago did you know where you were? Can you return to that spot? Are there footprints or signs to guide you? Can you hear signs of civilization? Move slowly, and do not make hasty judgments. Think about what the correct future actions should be.

Observe and size up the situation. Look around for immediate hazards that may threaten you. How long until darkness? What is available to work with? Look for the best possible course of action.

Plan the best course of action before implementing any action. Be deliberate and practical. Your plan should be a blueprint based on the necessities and priorities of life. Then, once thinking, observing, and planning have taken place, you can *proceed.*

In a true survival situation, time often works against you. The environment, untreated injuries, decreasing nutrition, dehydration, fear, and other stressors can detrimentally affect your mind and thinking, which is why practicing this specific approach to managing an emergency is so important. As time progresses, your thinking can become increasingly diminished, so it is also important to make a plan (P in STOP) early, while your thinking is the clearest. Writing the plan can also have significant benefits. It gives your mind and body something on which to focus and provides a solid plan to follow that was created when your mind was sharp.

Individual Beliefs

Many adult fears and related misconceptions are based on stories and statements originating during early years of life from unenlightened sources. These thoughts, statements, and stories are stored in the subconscious. Survival and emergency preparedness training is important to balance reality and experience against illusion and raw instinct.

Negative feedback inadvertently given during childhood or during any learning process may have a profound effect on behavior and reaction. Negative reaction to fledgling attempts at independence and self-reliance are good examples of how to program them for poor performance in the future. The same principle holds true after a person reaches maturity and receives negative feedback for some type of performance. Negative self-talk has a dramatic negative effect on performance. All people must learn to program themselves and others more positively, remembering that individuals act or react in accordance with what each believes to be true.

The mind is constantly at work picking up information and skills, and the subconscious never erases whatever is intentionally or unintentionally placed there. In any situation, actions are a reflection of how an individual perceives the environment and the individual in it. In short, the subconscious mind mirrors self-image. If the self-image is strong, the individual will be strong. If the picture is of a weakling, the individual will be weak. More importantly, individuals who think they cannot survive probably will not even try.

Every Survivor Sets a Goal

Hundreds of accounts and personal interviews with those who have undergone trying mental and physical experiences reveal that nearly every survivor has set some type of goal. The goal may have been simply to live, or it may have been a combination of staying alive and accomplishing something else. Philosophically, life is composed of setting one goal after another and taking the trip in between. Many prisoners of war who were released after the Vietnam conflict related numerous self-set goals that gave meaning and purpose to staying alive.

The goal-setting process is vital and has been used extensively, but many cheat themselves of its full effect. It has been said that it is truly not the setting of personal goals but the journeys to reach those goals that makes living worthwhile. If this is true, then constantly learning to readjust goals provides incentive, not only to live, but to give purpose to existence. Likewise, a survivor must readjust goals to suit the situation. Many people have survived tremendously difficult ordeals after crashing a vehicle only to die just after being rescued. Their main goal could have been to be rescued. Perhaps they failed to look beyond that goal and establish new goals. They simply let down and gave up too soon.

We Choose Our Path

We as individuals have the ability to evaluate performance potential during a time of emergency or stress. We are creatures of habit and do things regularly that give good indications of how we will react to emergencies.

Nearly always, we choose the path to follow after the onset of an emergency. All of us have the ability to use our mind as a valuable tool or have it work against us as a feared enemy. It is never too late for changing our habits, values, and attitudes to ones that produce positive mental actions during emergencies.

Maintaining a PMA is the key to successful emergency response and better everyday living. A "can do" attitude is necessary for both survival and SAR work. Solve the problems as they arise, one at a time, and you can stay alive with comfort and safety. Problem solving is a test of your ability to analyze and act in an appropriate way. You must improvise with what you know and with what you have.

As an individual involved in SAR, be prepared. The physical answer to being prepared lies in the clothing and equipment that you carry. The mental answer of preparedness is the training, education, and variety of knowledge that you have filed away in your brain.

SEARCH AND RESCUE TIP

Surviving the unexpected short-term emergency is both a preparedness and a problem-solving test.

Defensive Living: A Preparedness Ethic

The emergency preparedness education philosophy of defensive living is best defined as the constant conscious thought process and behavior of an individual to identify or predict situations that affect his or her comfort or existence. This philosophy is not meant to be an obsession or extreme preoccupation but rather a conscious development of an individual preparedness attitude to avoid unnecessary emergency situations. Defensive living is the knowledge to recognize dangers, make the proper choices, and have the necessary skills, equipment, and knowledge to cope with adversity.

Defensive living develops self-responsibility to always:

- Reduce any risk factors
- Maintain optimum body efficiency
- Solve the immediate threat problem
- Maintain positive action
- Guard personal comfort

The goal of defensive living is to create in each of us the habits of forethought, awareness, preparedness, and alertness to cope with changing situations that threaten or affect our lives.

Improvisation

Solving the problem of staying alive in any life-threatening situation requires a basic understanding of several concepts. Survival is based on resilience, that is, the ability to overcome difficulties and disappointments. It also requires talent (skills), desire, and the optimism to overcome those difficulties and disappointments. It is essential to understand the nature of threats posed by the natural environment and the corresponding physiological effects on the body. With this knowledge should come an ability to assess the level of threat and establish a set of priorities. While there is no substitute for preparedness, there will always be situations where the right resource to do a job is simply not available. What is available must be adapted to meet the needs at hand. This adapting of one's surroundings to solve problems is called *improvisation*. Occasionally, procuring the necessities of life is not easily accomplished, and one must improvise to accomplish a goal or solve a problem. Being adaptable, or capable of improvising, is an important survival skill.

Survivors have used chunks of rotten log for building blocks and bark stripped from fallen trees for floors, walls, and roofs. There are stories of stormbound pioneers who wore bark slab clothing. Nothing is useless when survival is the issue. A car, a downed airplane, or any human-made object contains a potential source of needed materials.

Improvising means a person must reason, compare, analyze, and solve problems to accomplish an objective (**FIGURE 6-2**). It involves a basic knowledge of physics, chemistry, mechanics, and common sense to utilize what is available to accomplish the task. It may not be perfect, but it could be adequate for short-time emergency use. As soon as a problem is recognized, decide what is required, and then decide how to do it. Be positive, look around, and try to make what is needed from materials at hand. Prioritize needs using the necessities of life and the rules and principles of improvising.

The contents of a SAR ready pack (described in Chapter 9) were specifically designed to contain items with multiple uses, including many that can serve as the

SEARCH AND RESCUE TIP

While the ability to improvise is a useful skill in survival, it is not an excuse to be ill prepared. Carry what you need and have the knowledge to properly use all that you carry.

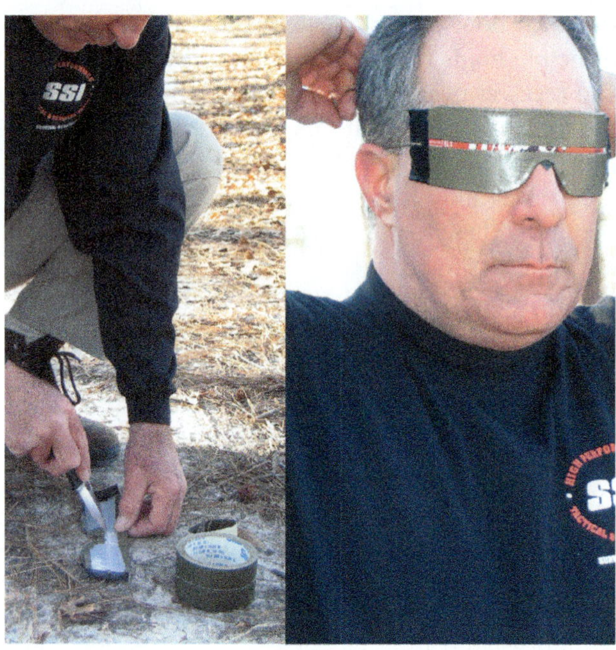

A B

FIGURE 6-2 Improvising means a person must reason, compare, analyze, and solve problems to accomplish an objective. Shown is a pair of "pinhole" goggles used to enhance or protect vision in the absence of eyeglasses or sunglasses. **A.** A knife is used to punch two rows of small holes in a piece of aluminum cut from a soda can. **B.** Completed glasses.

Courtesy of F. Wysocki, Survival Strategies, Inc.

basis for improvisation. For example, a cotton bandana can also be used as a sweatband, washcloth, dish towel, bandage, arm sling, towel, knee pad, tinder (unraveled threads), head cover, tourniquet, and many other uses limited only by one's imagination. A small tarp, with some imagination, can be used as shelter, patient litter, shade device, wind block, signaling device, rain catcher, and so much more. Just imagine what can be done with duct tape and plastic garbage bags.

Six simple steps can be followed to determine if what you need can be provided by what you have:

1. Size up the situation.
   - Determine your needs.
   - What is your priority? Shelter? Fire? Medical?
   - Is there a need that you must take care of first?
   - How was it done in early or primitive times?
2. Identify contingencies.
   - Could the situation get worse if I do not improvise something? If so, how bad could it get?
3. Determine your goal.
   - Exactly what do I need and what is the time frame?
4. Inventory your resources.
   - What materials and tools are available?
5. Build a plan.
   - Consider the alternatives: What can I use instead?
   - Keep it simple and think about simple machines.
   - Select the alternative providing the most efficient use of your materials, time, and energy.
6. Take action.
   - Make your product durable and safe.
   - Remember the real priorities and necessities of life.

Look at resources and materials as a primitive society would look at them: How can I use this piece of material to provide a basic need, or how can this resource be useful to accomplish a particular task? Think of an object that normally does the job. How is it constructed, what material is it made of, and what principles does it incorporate? Now, look around and see what is available. Can you construct it from what you have? Try it. Use failures as incentives to try again. Never quit trying.

Useful articles for improvising include the following:

- SAR ready pack
- Your clothing
- Contents of your pockets
- Other personal equipment
- Items in the natural environment (trees, vines, roots, plants, etc.)
- Garbage, litter, and rubbish
- Stalled transportation

High-Priority Needs

The necessities of life, described earlier, can serve as a priority list of what is needed to survive. When improvising, it is also important to address your most important needs first—that is, address what may kill you before concerning yourself with comfort (**TABLE 6-2**). For

TABLE 6-2 Improvising

Type of Materials	Possible Improvisation
First aid	▪ Bandages: clothing, belts or seat belts, sleeping bags, tents ▪ Splints: sticks and limbs, molding, seat foam, carpet ▪ Crutches: limbs and branches, ski poles, tent poles, skis, ice axe ▪ Neck support: foam rubber in seats, magazines, maps, sleeping pad
Clothing and shelter	▪ Protection: carpet, tent material, garbage bag, stuff sac, plastic tarp ▪ Cordage: wire, seat belt, belt, strips from plastic bag or clothes twisted together ▪ Insulation: upholstery padding, maps, newspaper, carpet, dry grass, pine needles ▪ Eye protection: side of soda can with pinholes, paper with pinholes, bark, t-shirt
Fire starting	▪ Spark: battery and wire, lighter striker ▪ Stove construction: Fill a container with fuel and oil mixed with sand, loamy soil, or dirt. As the fire dies down, stir the sand or soil, and the flame will flare back up.
Signaling	▪ Lights: battery, a light and some wire (stalled transportation), chemical lights, headlamps ▪ Fire: Oil, tires, foam rubber, and hoses all burn with black smoke. Also, upholstery in vehicle ▪ Ground signal: part of an aircraft, boughs, clothing, rocks, logs, shadow from sides of a shallow trench dug in the ground ▪ Signal mirror: reflectors, light lens, mirrors, glass, polished metal

SAFETY TIP

Garbage bags have many improvisational uses. When all else fails, they can be used as a shelter to help prevent hypothermia. Always carry one or two with you.

example, treating wounds and protecting yourself from a severe environment are likely priorities, but starting a fire (warmth, signal), calling for help (signal), and thinking about how you will procure water may be needed shortly after your highest priorities have been met.

Improvised water procurement materials include:

- Collectors: black plastic in winter, clear plastic in summer (transpiration bag); condensation on metal surfaces, deep hole in the right location
- Storage: zip-lock bags, sheet of plastic with tied opening, vehicle parts, rubber gloves, section of tarp, in clothing or shoe (boot)

Shelter

Shelter is anything that protects the body from temperature extremes, weather, insects, or any other life-threatening force or element. In fact, our clothing is the shelter we wear, and it constitutes the first line of defense in any environment. Without shelter (adequate protection from the elements and environment) in most places on Earth, humans can survive for only a short time. Without adequate clothing, a shelter is essential. Without adequate clothing and shelter on most of the Earth, a fire is essential. The ability to maintain the body's optimal temperature (98.6°F or 37°C) and the knowledge of how to apply body shelter concepts are essential for comfort and survival in the outdoors. In its simplest form, a shelter may or may not have a heat source, though in colder climates, some form of heat is desirable for additional comfort. In an emergency (severe weather, inadequate clothing, injured companion), it is important to find protection from the elements as soon as possible.

There are three basic types of shelters that can be utilized in an emergency (**FIGURE 6-3**). The first is called an *immediate action shelter* and can serve to protect an individual within minutes. This type of shelter normally consists of something carried by an individual that can be accessed and put into use very quickly. It serves as an immediate body protection mechanism and is generally small, compact, and lightweight. This type of shelter is commonly usable in water or on land and can be as simple as one or two leaf bags (taped together) or a heavy-duty, 55-gallon barrel liner. Many outdoorsmen prefer the heavy-duty, high-density polyethylene trash

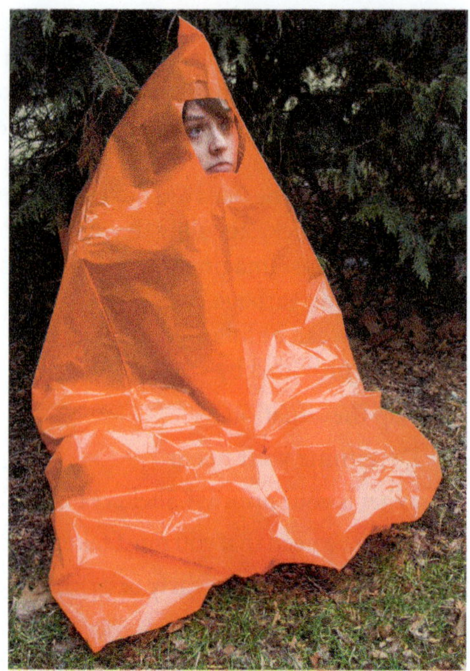

A

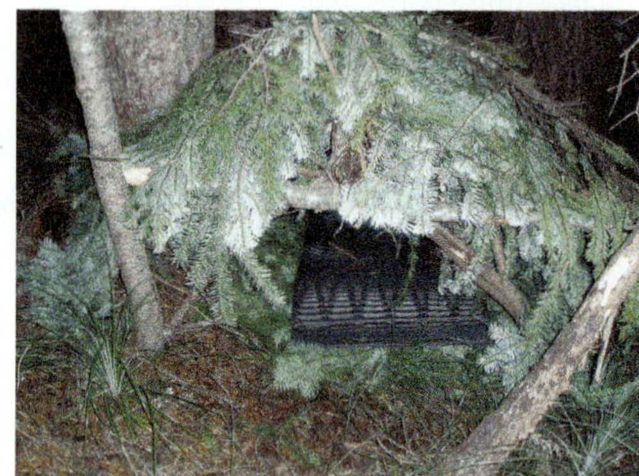

B

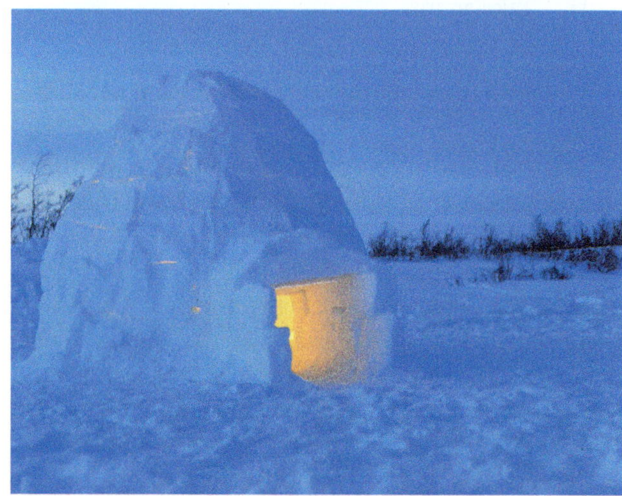

C

FIGURE 6-3 Three basic types of shelters can be utilized in an emergency. **A.** Immediate action shelter. **B.** Temporary shelter. **C.** Long-term shelter.

A: Courtesy of New York State Department of Environmental Conservation; **B:** Courtesy of John Carlson/Wind River SAR; **C:** © Stuart Westmorland/Index Stock Imagery/Photolibrary/Getty.

bags used by highway departments to pick up trash and other litter. Christmas tree bags, intended to dispose of Christmas trees after holiday use, also work well. These bags are large, inexpensive, made of polyethylene like other trash bags, widely available, and often bright white in color.

SAFETY TIP

Parts of any vehicle can be the fastest, most available resource for shelter and insulation.

Another type of immediate action shelter can be something that already exists, such as a cave or other naturally occurring phenomenon. Getting beneath the boughs of an evergreen, behind a downed tree, or inside a small outbuilding can provide immediate protection from the wind, sun, rain, heat, cold, or other environmental threats. In a survival situation, do not overlook that which already provides what you need.

A *temporary shelter* is a second type of shelter that can be accessed or built and utilized within 30 to 60 minutes. Minimal energy is expended to construct or access this survival-type shelter. It generally requires improvisation, some basic tools, and knowledge of shelter construction and design. Temporary shelters utilize existing resources from the environment, stalled transportation, personal items, or the contents of a SAR ready pack. In many cases, this can be a transition to the last type of shelter, which is more long term in nature.

As with an immediate action shelter, a temporary shelter is best built on something that already exists. Using a partially downed tree or building on existing trees or rocks as part of a shelter can save a great deal of time and energy.

The third type of shelter, commonly called a *long-term shelter*, is a structure designed to accommodate someone for 72 hours or more. This type of shelter requires substantially more resources and energy to build and incorporates more of what we would like to think of as "creature comforts." It is normally built only when an extended stay is anticipated, but in most cases, it would not be necessary.

SEARCH AND RESCUE TIP

There are three general types of shelter:

- Immediate action shelter: Can protect you within minutes.
- Temporary shelter: Can be accessed and utilized in 30 to 60 minutes.
- Long-term shelter: Designed and built to accommodate someone for 72 hours or more.

While some say, "do like the animals do" and seek shelter by burrowing under foliage or in a protected area, this advice must be qualified. It is virtually impossible to build a waterproof and windproof shelter from natural materials. You must be prepared! There is no substitute for good rain gear, tarps, tents, a good rain fly, and/or adequate clothing. Do not waste reserves of energy and body heat with futile unproductive efforts. Fire and light are pleasant, but starting a fire in rain or snow and/or high wind may be impossible and only serve to waste calories, get clothing wet, and expend resources that will be needed later.

Whenever a situation requires immediate body protection, a shelter can be improvised from what you have with you or around you. Your preparation and the materials at hand will determine a shelter's efficiency. Efficient shelters need little or no external headroom to maintain body warmth. Adequate body shelter can be improvised with the right materials and preparation.

Shelter is a supplement to clothing, and a properly built shelter should protect the body from wind, wet, cold, and insects. Through a lack of adequate body shelter or clothing, the already limited supplies of body heat, energy, and water are quickly lost. Remember, a sleeping bag is a shelter composed of two layers of relatively weatherproof fabric separated by insulating material. Heat produced by the body is retained inside the bag even when outside temperatures drop below freezing.

The efficiency of a sleeping bag is improved by added ground insulation (more trapped dead air space or thickness of material), extra insulating material fabricated in the bag itself, and overhead protection (tent or tarp) from wind and rain. Keep this sleeping bag principle in mind when building emergency shelters.

When building a shelter, be sure to:

- Keep it simple and small, no bigger than what is absolutely needed for body protection.
- Minimize expenditure of time, energy, and body water.
- Minimize body heat loss or gain through the primary mechanisms of temperature transfer in the body (conduction, convection, radiation, evaporation).

The usefulness and efficiency of a shelter is dependent on many factors, such as where it is built, what it is made from, and the environment in which it is built.

Shelter Location

It would be nice if there were always choices for ideal shelter locations. Sometimes circumstances dictate that we must "hole up" at whatever location or set of circumstances where the need exists. Stalled transportation provides the best source of immediate shelter needs, but many times a vehicle is not available.

If caught outside unexpectedly, a good first step is to get out of the wind and into the driest place possible. Move to the downwind side of a rock, ridge, or tree. Even just turning your back to the wind can make a difference by reducing or eliminating wind chill. A spot beneath fallen logs, a space under dense evergreens, or under a rocky overhang can not only protect from the wind, it can help keep you dry. Once you are wet and cold, it may be impossible to get warm and dry and again.

Next, check the area for possible dangers. Avoid areas such as dry streambeds in desert regions; avalanche chutes in steep, rocky, high country; rock fall areas; dead trees (snags) with large limbs; exposed mountain saddles or valley openings where strong winds tend to blow; low valley areas in winter or autumn, where cold air pockets and/or frost may accumulate; and thick, dense woods where moisture tends to accumulate and not dry out. Also, pay attention to insect or animal signs in the area; do not build a shelter on a well-worn game trail. Slow-flowing river edges with swampy areas tend to accumulate mosquitoes and other biting insects. Considering these potential problems ahead of time can eliminate a lot of grief.

Usable Materials

What a person carries is always the most easily accessible and the most dependable shelter material, and the SAR ready pack should be the best place to find what you need.

If it is necessary to build a temporary emergency shelter, first determine what type of shelter you need and what it is you need the shelter to protect you from. Do you need protection from cold, heat, rain, snow, insects, or something else? When building a shelter, function is always more important than shape or beauty.

From an energy expenditure point of view, it makes sense to look for already developed sites or easily convertible resources, such as a hollow tree trunk or a fallen tree, so that with little effort a site can be turned into a serviceable shelter. A good example of this would be an exposed root ball from a tree that has blown down or eroded at the roots and fallen. In areas with no trees, you may be forced to build a shelter with insulating (nonheat conducting) materials such as dirt, brush, sod or grass, and even leaves.

It is worth repeating that it is virtually impossible under typical emergency conditions to build a waterproof and windproof shelter from natural materials, which is exactly why the SAR ready pack includes plastic bags and a tarpaulin. If you do not have access to these important tools and you find it necessary to utilize boughs, leaves, or other natural materials, use them as they grow in nature. This may be one bough stacked upon another with the butts pointing in the same direction—up. Using any natural materials in this fashion, like shingles on a house, is the only hope for effective precipitation protection. However, it will be marginal at best. Make sure to build the shelter just big enough for you to stretch out underneath. Any bigger and you will spend too much time and energy building it and too much body heat keeping it warm.

SAFETY TIP

Shelters should always be kept small, dry, and well insulated. Less body heat will be needed to warm it, and warmth will be retained longer.

Basic principles of heat transfer (body heat loss or gain) and thermal conductivity (insulation) are the foundation for proper shelter building. *Thermal conductivity* is the measure of any substance's ability (or inability) to conduct heat. Comparisons of example substances are shown in **TABLE 6-3**, where a lower value indicates a better insulator. In terms of survival, remember that the human body loses or gains heat anytime it is in contact with a surface that is cooler or warmer than body temperature (conduction). Thus, to retain body heat, it is a good idea to insulate your body from whatever you are touching.

Insulation Sources

Any human-made or natural materials that provide dead air space between you and the ground or environment can be considered an insulation source. Although natural materials such as bark, deadwood, thick boughs, grass, or leaves do provide a measure of insulation, they are certainly not as efficient as most of the human-made products that could be available with any degree of preparation. In stalled transportation, any upholstery, carpet, foam rubber, or other padding material would be considered good improvised insulation. Many outdoorsmen prefer to carry a short section of insulated pad specifically for kneeling or sitting on when hiking in the outdoors. A small pad of this type can be a lifesaver in cold, wet, or snow conditions when used in conjunction with a plastic leaf or garbage bag.

TABLE 6-3 Thermal Conductivity of Various Materials/Substances

Material/Substance	Conductivity
Vacuum	0
Air	0.024
Foamed plastic (insulation materials)	0.03
Feathers	0.034
Cotton, felt insulation, fiberglass, wool blanket	0.04
Paper	0.05
Snow (temp < 0 degrees C)	0.05 – 0.25
Cork	0.07
Sawdust	0.08
Soft woods (fir, pine)	0.12
Hardwoods (oak or maple)	0.16
Sand (dry)	0.15 – 0.25
Cellulose, cotton, wood pulp (dry)	0.23
Concrete (medium density)	0.4 – 0.7
Ground or Soil (dry)	0.5
Ground or Soil (clay)	1.1
Ground or Soil (very moist)	1.4
Rock (solid)	2–7
Ice	2.18
Stainless steel	16
Lead	35
Steel, carbon 1%	43
Aluminum	205
Gold	310
Copper	401
Diamond	1000

Note: Measured at 25°C. SI: W/(m K); Imperial: Btu/(hr ft °F). The lower the value, the better the insulator. The higher the number, the better the conductor. Trapped air is considered good insulation and is, therefore, a poor conductor.
Data from Engineering Tool Box. (2016). Thermal conductivity of materials and gases. Retrieved from http://www.engineeringtoolbox.com/thermal-conductivity-d_429.html.

Do not overlook your SAR ready pack or spare clothing items laid on the ground with some type of vegetation stuffed inside as insulation. Coiled rescue rope with a stuff sac filled with leaves or grass on top have been used successfully as an insulator from the ground.

Provided you have adequate protection directly from the surface, snow is a great source of insulation in bitter cold winter environments. Snow can measurably enhance the efficiency of any natural material shelter by blocking the wind and adding dead air space to the walls of a shelter.

Fuel Sources

Gathering fuel for a fire and keeping it stoked costs energy and usually requires extended exposure to the elements. There may not be enough readily available fuels to warrant the effort to maintain a fire. A few hard and fast questions must be answered quickly: Are there adequate fuels? Should any shelter that I build be constructed to allow a fire inside or near the opening? Fire is a great morale builder, but is a fire really needed? A small, cramped, slightly uncomfortable shelter may be better with no fire.

If a fire is needed, consider selecting or building a shelter near a source of wood for fuel, and make sure to assess the wind direction before building a fire near a shelter. This is not only important for fire safety; it may prevent you from having to relocate due to smoke being blown into your shelter.

Wind Direction

Check wind direction and exposure. Wind generally blows down drainages at night and up during the day. If possible, a shelter entrance should be 90 degrees to the prevailing wind, so it blows across the opening and not into it.

Water Sources

While having water available near a shelter may seem convenient, it also has its drawbacks. Shelters right next to creeks, rivers, lakes, etc., will be damper and cooler in general and, in most cases, much more prone to flying insects such as mosquitoes and no-see-ums. At certain times of the year, this can be particularly annoying or even dangerous. Moving water such as streams and rivers can also be noisy and mask other sounds that might indicate rescue, such as someone yelling your name or the sound of an aircraft. Thus, sources of drinking water, while convenient, should not really be a determining factor for shelter placement in any environment except extreme desert conditions.

General Considerations

The best shelter material and resources are the ones you carry with you. Natural materials can enhance and make any shelter more efficient, but do not count on utilizing natural materials exclusively. They may be in short supply when you most need them. Think and improvise more insulation materials to improve what you brought in your SAR ready pack.

Improve on what is already there in nature. Enlarge a natural opening so it is possible to get in and out easily. Try to make enough room to stretch your legs, but this is not necessarily a prerequisite to an effective shelter.

Dirt and grass can be used for filling cracks or making the wall base. Snow can be used in the winter on a tarp or a tent as an insulating cover, but this may require supportive pieces of wood, poles, or skis for the structure.

In hot weather, consider the following when building a shelter:

- Shade from the sun is the most important daytime shelter requirement. Materials or objects that produce shade are a valuable resource.
- Moving air (convection) is helpful. Beware of pockets or locations where there is little air movement.
- Putting a shelter floor 12 to 18 inches (30.4 to 45.7 cm) above or below the ground level during the day reduces the temperature in the shelter substantially. However, the very real issues of energy expenditure, availability of digging and construction tools, and the capability to dig if injured or while caring for another may make this impractical.
- Keep clothes on, head covered, and sleeves rolled down to protect against sunburn.
- Do not stay in closed metal structures such as a vehicle without adequate ventilation. Temperatures can become intolerable and can cause heat-related injuries.
- At night, when the air cools considerably, a better shelter and a fire might be needed. Work during cooler periods to improve shelter and general situations.
- Insects, snakes, scorpions, and the like are active at night. Protect your sleeping area, shelter, clothes, and shoes from easy access by these critters. Shake out clothing and shoes before putting them on again.

In cold weather, consider the following when building a shelter:

- Forested areas can provide overhead shelter, fuel for fires, and materials for insulation. A downed tree shelter can be the easiest natural shelter of all to exploit. It may already have a roof, floor, and one or both sides. If there is snow, a tree pit shelter (digging into the space beneath the boughs of an evergreen) may be a very real option and readily available.
- Scrape out a trench in the snow or ground on wind-blown prairies or exposed ridges. Pile rocks or other materials for a windbreak. Line the trench with limbs, grass, bark, stalled transportation materials, extra clothes, or anything that provides insulation. Put snow or dirt on top of a framework, crawl in, and close up.
- Make a signal visible from the air, especially if you are using a shelter covered with snow or otherwise invisible from the air.
- Snow at specific temperature gradients is a good insulator and gives good wind protection if used properly. However, it is hard to work with, requires a degree of practice and skill, and takes considerable energy. Digging a snow cave takes a long time and requires a tool. A large snow cave is not considered an immediate action survival shelter. Digging into a snow bank may use less energy. Work at a pace to minimize sweating and try to keep clothes dry by utilizing plastic bags, tarps, or some type of ground cloth material. Snow shelters must have adequate ventilation, especially with two or more people. A candle provides light, some heat, and is also an excellent indicator that oxygen is running out (you need to provide better ventilation).
- Avoid overheating the inside a snow shelter, and as a precaution against getting wet, round and smooth inside surfaces so that any moisture will run down the sides. If it melts, you may get wet.
- Protracted use of a snow shelter can cause the walls and ceiling to thaw and freeze into ice. Ice that builds up on the walls is not as good an insulator as snow because ice has less air trapped in it.

Firecraft

It is said by some that the ability to light a fire under a variety of conditions is among the most valuable of all survival skills. A number of years ago, in the forested high-country wilderness of Oregon, two teenage girls undergoing an Outward Bound experience got into trouble in a bad storm. Though they repeatedly tried to start a fire, they were not successful, and the two young women died of hypothermia. In this case, the ability to start a fire may have literally made the difference between life and death.

Fire building is a skill that is mastered only by practicing in a wide spectrum of conditions with different materials. Proficiency requires a basic knowledge of how a fire burns and which tinders and fuels are best.

If for no other reason, fire plays a vitally important psychological role in survival. Once having started a fire in difficult or emergency conditions, it provides a sense of achievement that to some extent replicates some of the most important elements of everyday life: the ability to cook or heat liquids to drink, to feel warm in the worst of conditions, and most of all, the ability to see in the dark. Fire can also provide dry clothing, a signal, a big boost to morale, and it can also be used to purify water (boiling).

If your clothing is inadequate, you will need a shelter. If your clothing and your shelter are inadequate, then you will definitely need a fire. Steep terrain, ground cover, availability of fuel, environmental conditions, and even time can all have an adverse impact on your capability to start a fire. Ask, "Is it worth the cost of energy expended to build and maintain a fire?" This is a realistic hard and fast decision that may have to be made. The smaller, drier, and better insulated your shelter is, the less heat is lost and the less need you have for fire.

Location of a Fire

Look for a location that is open and away from trees or other ground cover. Sandy or gravelly soil without grass or roots is best. The area should be protected from the wind, near water if possible, and near additional fuel supplies.

In forested or brushy areas, insure that the fire cannot spread out of control. In dry summer forest conditions, or even in dry grassy or low vegetation areas, it is a good idea to clear a fire circle that is about 5–6 feet in diameter on sandy or gravelly soil and scraped down to mineral earth that is free of duff, grass, and roots.

A circle of dry rocks can contain the fire and is helpful for cooking and expanding the heat source. *Caution:* Do not use river rocks, as they contain moisture and can explode when heated.

Never build a fire:

- Near dry, combustible materials
- In very dry grassland
- Under overhanging branches
- In a very resinous (pitch-smelling), dry forest
- Under a snow-laden tree
- Directly on the snow
- On or near wet rocks

Fire Making Sources

Here we will consider two primary types of fire-starting devices: friction (including wooden matches) and spark/heat-producing (**FIGURE 6-4**).

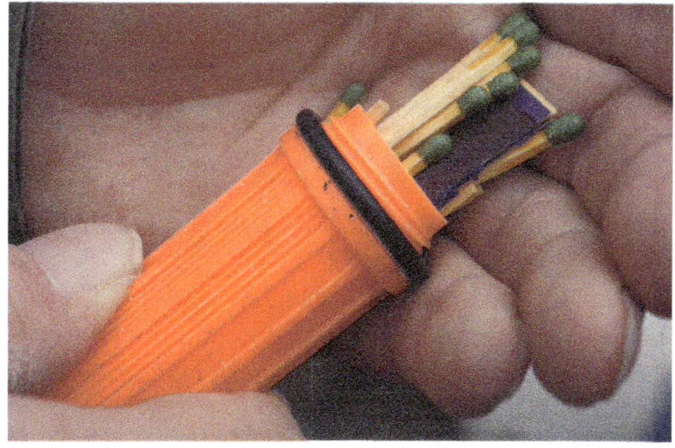

A

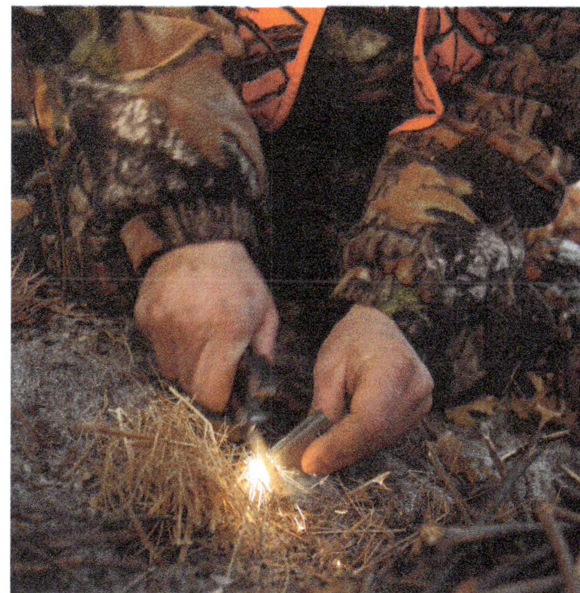

B

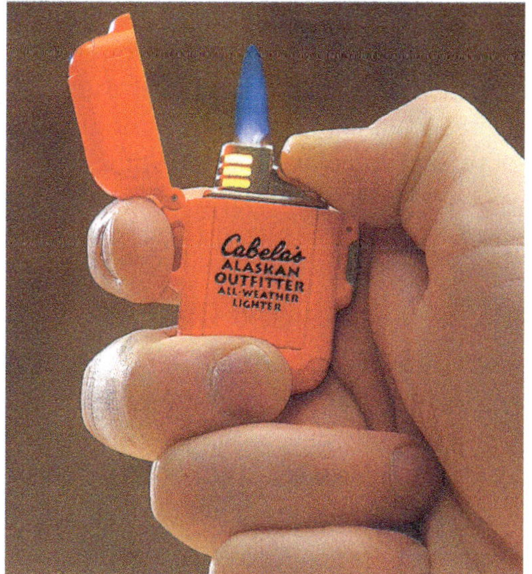

C

FIGURE 6-4 Any emergency survival kit should contain several methods of fire starting. **A.** Matches and striker in a waterproof container. **B.** A magnesium bar and steel knife. **C.** A specialized survival lighter.

A: © 2016 Howard Paul, Photography for Communication and Commerce; **B:** © Design Pics Inc/Alamy; **C:** Courtesy of Cabela's, Inc.

Friction and Matches

There are many ways to start fires using friction, but the match is the most available, least expensive, and easiest to use. Wood matches carried in a waterproof container with a striking pad (strip of the striker attached to the match box) are one of the best and most reliable methods of starting a fire.

The "strike anywhere" matches (two-tone heads) are not generally good for extended outdoor situations because they are significantly affected by moisture and, regardless of their name, must be struck on just the right type of surface to cause ignition. Although some people have developed the ability to ignite these with a thumbnail, on a zipper, across the backside of trousers, and even on their teeth, these matches are generally unreliable for use in a survival situation.

Coating a match with shellac, varnish, or other similar waterproofing material that hardens often makes the match more difficult to light. Waterproofing a match with wax or paraffin tends to be much more reliable. Practical field trials and personal experience show that the best type of match to have in an emergency is the Storm Proof Matches, which come in a vinyl pouch with multiple strikers in waterproof packets (Bowman and Kummerfeldt, 2017). They are reliable, readily available, and waterproof, and they work incredibly well.

Primitive skill methods for starting fires with friction—such as bow and drill, hand drill, fire saw, plow board, fire thong, or South-Seas fire plunger—are all methods developed in specific environments with specialized resources, and all require a high degree of skill and practice to accomplish. It is unrealistic to think that SAR volunteers or the average outdoors person could depend on these methods as reliable and effective under adverse conditions. Acquiring primitive skills using friction takes a lot of time, practice, and energy. While some of these more primitive methods are great confidence builders, it is far better to carry matches in a waterproof container.

Spark/Heat-Producing Devices

One of the best backup systems to have as a fire starter is a metal match (spark-producing ferrocerium rod with a steel striker). Although not as easy to use as a wooden match, this device is second only to the wooden match as a reliable means of starting a fire, especially with the right tinder.

Using alternatives to matches and friction to start a fire generally requires good tinder (such as petroleum jelly [e.g., Vaseline™] and cotton balls) to capture the heat and/or spark produced, ignite the tinder, and subsequently ignite kindling. Unlike the use of matches and friction devices, using spark- and heat-producing devices is almost always reliable despite the presence of damp or wet conditions; they just take more practice to be effective. Examples of these devices include the following:

- Flint and steel (chert, a form of quartz that produces a spark when struck by steel)
- Vehicle battery (shorting the terminals or live wires produces a spark; vehicle cigarette lighter produces heat)
- Zippo lighter (liquid fuel, wick, flint, and steel produce both spark and flame from the wick)
- BIC lighter (liquid fuel, flint, and steel produce spark and flame from ignited gas—must keep finger depressing trigger)
- Piezo lighter (liquid fuel, piezo igniter [piezoelectricity], spark and flame from ignited gas)
- Metal match (ferrocerium [e.g., mischmetal and Auermetall] rod and steel striker produce spark)
- Magnesium fire starter (metal match with attached magnesium block from which one can scrape shavings to use as tinder)
- Chemicals/exothermic reaction (e.g., combine a small amount of potassium permanganate powder and liquid glycerin to produce enough heat to ignite tinder)

Sporting goods and recreation stores often carry many types of spark/heat-producing fire starters. Any emergency survival kit, and SAR ready pack, should contain several methods of fire starting, but stormproof matches in a waterproof container with a striker pad, and a metal match as a backup, are great choices for SAR work.

Fire Materials

Fire materials should be gathered before attempting to start a fire. Try to use the driest possible materials that may be obtained from hollow logs, dead stumps, dead limbs on living trees, or dead twigs and limbs found away from the damp ground.

In very wet weather, dry wood can be found in the center of old stumps and the center of dead standing trees. Dry twigs can usually be found near the trunks of larger trees. Old burned-out or broken-off stumps (and any spires sticking out of the stump) usually indicate high pitch concentrations ideal for building fires. Carefully plan, collect, and protect from the elements all necessary components: tinder, kindling, and sustaining fuel.

Tinder

Tinder is anything that ignites at a very low temperature, with a spark, small flame, or other heat source. It must be dry. Remember to start small and work up to larger combustible materials.

Consider the following for tinder:

- Petroleum jelly-impregnated cotton balls (this is the best; carry it in a small film canister)
- Dry grass, crushed
- Cotton or scraped cloth (not synthetic material)
- Fine, dry wood shavings
- Dry cattail fuzz
- Bird down
- Pitch wood, fine shavings or powdered wood
- Petroleum products
- Dry, reddish pine needles
- Seed down
- Shaved sticks
- Paper (shredded or rolled and tied into a knot)
- Inner bark of cedar or birch
- Dried moss or lichen
- Candle
- Oil- or gas-soaked cloth
- Flares or other pyrotechnics
- Birch bark

Kindling

The initial fuel stage is **kindling**. Find something that ignites easily from the tinder. It needs to be relatively easy to burn material such as small-diameter sticks and twigs, broken wood splinters, split or shaved pieces of wood to increase surface area and flammability, or it can simply be a material such as congealed pitch that provides the increased heat to start larger sustaining fuel. Dry kindling can be split from larger pieces of dry wood using a knife and another piece of wood as a mallet.

Consider the following for kindling:

- Finely split wood
- Fuzz stick, carved with knife
- Small dry, dead branches and twigs
- Dry grasses twisted into bunches
- Congealed pitch that bleeds from conifers

Sustaining Fuel

Sustaining fuel is anything that will burn for an extended period of time. Generally, it does not burn from the initial flame or spark and requires high temperatures for continued burning.

Consider the following for sustaining fuel:

- Dead wood (standing or recently fallen trees or shrubs)
- Dry peat
- Dried dung
- Rubber
- Green wood that is split
- Animal oil or fat
- Bundles of grass
- Pitch
- Petroleum or fuel, oil, and soil mixture for improvised stove

Be cautious and do not use human-made products (e.g., plastics, upholstery, carpet), as many emit poisonous gases when burned, and some may explode.

Building the Fire

It is a good idea under virtually all conditions to start with a small platform of sticks or logs. This elevates the tinder off the damp ground, vegetation, snow, or other less than desirable base material. Place a bigger log, larger-diameter branch, or stick at one side of this small platform. This base serves as the foundation structure and lends itself to the fire-starting process (**FIGURE 6-5**).

Tinder should be arranged on the platform right next to the larger branch or log on the side. Kindling is then placed over the top of the tinder so that it rests against the larger log or branch, much like the roof on a lean-to shelter. This ensures adequate oxygen flow to the tinder and can also allow maximum heat from the tinder or flame to rise through the greatest amount of kindling. When the kindling begins to burn well, add larger pieces of fuel. The platform provides several key functions. First, depending on which side of the platform the larger log or branch is placed, it provides a windbreak. It also provides elevation from the ground dampness, better oxygen flow to the tinder and kindling, and an excellent base for adding sustaining fuels. Be patient and do not smother the kindling flames with larger material until the flame has reached a good, hot temperature. The second mistake often made in fire building is cutting off the flow of air (oxygen) to the flame by adding too much fuel too quickly.

All combustible components (tinder, kindling, and sustaining fuel) must be gathered before attempting to build a fire. Keep all materials as dry as possible. Remember that the heat from each successive stage in the process should rise through the maximum amount of material stacked neatly on top in the next stage. Properly built, a fire should gradually and steadily build in intensity throughout the entire process.

Fire Without Wood Fuel

A metal can, container, or improvised container such as a headlight holder or battery box can serve as an emergency

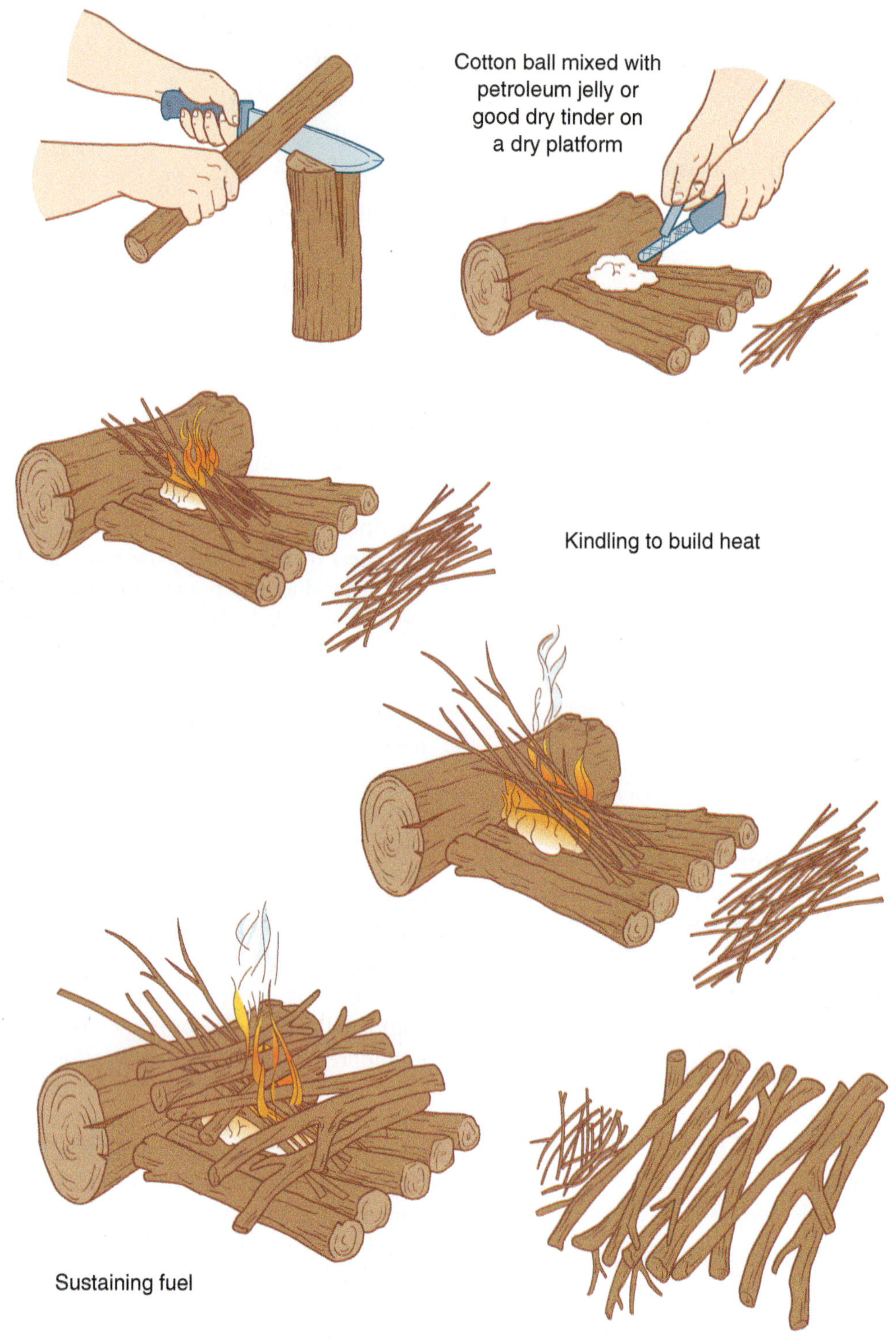

FIGURE 6-5 The process of building a fire.
Adapted from Emergency Response International.

stove with a mixture of oil, gasoline, and a cloth wick. Oil-soaked rags or shredded upholstery in a shallow pan of oil will also burn. Fill a container one-third full of dry dirt or sand. Although it improves the draft to make small holes on the sides, it really isn't necessary. Saturate the soil with a mixture of one part oil to two parts gasoline or diesel. Wait a few minutes, and then ignite it with a match or spark. Stir occasionally when the flames die down. The wicking action up through the soil pulls the gas–oil mixture up to the surface. Be very careful anytime you are using flammable fuels, such as gasoline, around a source of ignition, such as matches or a spark.

SEARCH AND RESCUE TIP

Keep in mind the following firecraft tips:

- Conserve matches whenever possible by lighting a candle or fuzzy stick.
- Green wood burns if finely split.
- Find dry wood for fire starting in the center of standing dead trees or large undergrowth. Small, dry twigs are often available near the base of green trees.
- If you have no cutting tool sufficient for splitting wood, whittle a hard wood wedge, and drive it into weathering cracks in the end of the wood. A good knife and a wooden mallet (branch from a tree at least 2–3 inches in diameter) can serve as a good improvised splitting tool (see Figure 6-5).
- A reflector (metal, rock, wood) on one side of a fire makes it more efficient. For a fire site with a large rock surface on one side or at the base of a cliff, do not use the rock as a reflector. Build the fire far enough away from the rock so that you can sleep between the two. The rock provides warmth on one side, while the fire warms the other.
- Fire supplements the body's heat-producing mechanism. In colder weather, several small fires built around you heat better than a single, larger fire.
- Cooking fires should be walled-in to concentrate the heat.
- If a fire must be built in deep snow, build it on a platform of green logs. Two layers of green logs 3 to 4 inches in diameter stacked in opposing directions will usually suffice to keep the fire from sinking for a good number of hours. Obviously, any platform of green wood prolongs a fire from sinking in these conditions. The thickness of the wood is the determining factor on time.

Signaling

Emergency signaling is intended to make a person or persons more visible and most often implies distress of one form or another. Individuals and small groups are difficult to spot from either the ground or air, especially when visibility is limited. When individuals or groups want to be seen, they must find a way to "make themselves big," as children are taught in The National Association For Search And Rescue's Hug-a-Tree® program, and this can be done in many ways. The time it takes to be rescued depends largely on how effective distress signals are and how fast they can be deployed. In a distress situation, the sooner you effectively signal, the sooner you will receive assistance.

In general, electronic devices or beacons are reliable and easily activated when they are used correctly. There are several types, most of which include some type of global positioning system (GPS) location technology: Emergency locator transmitters (ELTs) carried on aircraft, emergency position indicating radio beacons (EPIRBs) carried on watercraft, personal locator beacons (PLBs) carried by an individual in any environment, proprietary satellite devices (e.g., SPOT), satellite phones, and mobile phones using cellular technology. The use and operation of these devices is discussed in Chapter 2, *Search and Rescue Systems*.

One would think that having and using a mobile phone is enough when the need arises to communicate distress. Unfortunately, phone batteries do not work well in very cold or very hot weather, their battery life has severe limitations, they can be rendered inoperable when wetted or dropped, and they can be simply lost or forgotten. Even if a mobile phone is available and working when needed, its effective use often requires the user to be able to describe his or her correct location, which history has shown is not always possible. Integrated GPS technology in mobile phones has helped get rescuers close, but this, too, is not always effective depending on several factors that are out of the control of the user. Mobile phones should not be depended on as the sole source of signaling distress.

Signaling, in the context of survival, is about more than communicating your distress; it is also about how to make yourself heard by and visible to rescuers already aware of your distress. This can be accomplished by several methods ranging from just wearing brightly colored clothing to employing pyrotechnics.

Sight and sound are the senses most involved in perceiving a signal. Blowing a whistle or making a loud noise can help attract attention of ground searchers, especially when the sound is not one that is found in nature (think whistle), but the value of sound as a signal is reduced or removed when the searchers are in an aircraft or are far away, or when ambient noise (e.g., moving water, wind, etc.) covers the sound signal.

A visual signal works better when searchers are visually looking for evidence of your location, such as searching from an aircraft or from a position far away. In this situation, contrast and motion can be used to maximize a signal's effectiveness and serve as visual cues that attract searchers' eyes (Ngo and Spence, 2010).

Contrast is the difference in **luminance** (intensity of light emitted from a surface) and/or color that makes an object visually distinguishable. A dark shadow from a shallow trench dug in the ground contrasts with the surrounding ground awash in bright sunlight. With the sun at the right angle, stamping footprints in deep snow can have a similar effect, especially if done in a long, straight line, which is rarely found in nature. A slurry of red mud on white snow, brightly colored clothing strewn on the ground, or any number of imaginative applications of this concept can all effectively attract the eye of a searcher.

Motion is particularly effective in attracting the human eye, especially when it is used in combination with something that contrasts with the environment. Waving a high-visibility vest on a stick, or the rising white smoke from a fire, both might contrast well with a surrounding conifer forest or background of green grass. Waving a brightly colored tarp over your head and flashing a light from a strobe or signal mirror both combine high contrast with perceived motion, which is why they both would work well as signals. Combining both contrast and movement can be an effective way to attract the attention of searchers and thus becomes a fundamental principle of all visual signaling.

Good signaling is really the application of common sense about what to use, when to use it, and how to use available resources. Be ingenious, follow the basic principles of signaling, and your chances of being seen or discovered will be greatly enhanced. The more signals you make, the better your chances of being seen. The more isolated your environment and the less likely rescuers know of your situation and location, the more important signals become.

Although various types of flares and smoke-generating devices (pyrotechnics) make excellent signals, they are heavy, require training in their safe use, can be dangerous, and are not generally recommended as part of a SAR ready pack. The following signals are recommended for use by SAR personnel, so SAR personnel should know how to generate and use them:

- Fire (smoke and light)
- Mirror (preferably glass, not metal)
- Loud whistle, such as Fox 40® or Lifesaver #1® (very loud)
- Colored signaling panels (tarpaulins or clothing)

Standard Signals

The international distress designation is a series of three repetitions of any signal, such as three loud sounds, three fires, three flares, three piles of rocks, three whistle blasts, or three flashes of light, all followed by a one-minute pause and repeated until a response is received. Voice distress is *Mayday, Mayday, Mayday* or *S.O.S.* Acknowledgment by rescuers is two repetitions of the distress signal.

Smoke Signals

To be effective, smoke signals need to contrast with the environment, such as dark smoke against a light background, white smoke against a dark background, dark smoke against light skies, or light smoke against clear skies.

For black smoke, add the following to a fire:

- Engine oil
- Rags soaked in oil
- Pieces of any rubber product
- Plastic or synthetic material (polyester, nylon, polypropylene, etc.)
- Pitch (tree sap)
- Pitch wood

For white smoke, add the following to a fire:

- Green leaves or grass
- Moss, ferns, or other wet vegetation
- Green tree boughs
- A limited amount of water or wet cotton clothes

In some environments, an evergreen torch can be an extremely effective signal. Select a small evergreen tree with dense foliage, cut it down, and move it to the center of a large clearing or some other location where fire is not likely to get out of control. Place dry tinder and kindling material in the lower branches of the cut tree, and secure it either by burying the butt of the tree in the soil or with a smaller stake driven into the ground. If an aircraft or ground searchers are heard or seen, ignite the tree. In most low-wind situations, this signal can punch smoke to over 1000 feet (305 meters) above the ground.

Signal Mirror

Practice mirror-signaling techniques in advance because aircraft pass over very quickly, and even distant rescuers on the ground will move out of a direct line of sight if surrounded by vegetation (**FIGURE 6-6**). Prepare and be ready, as the opportunity may pass quickly without anyone seeing the signal.

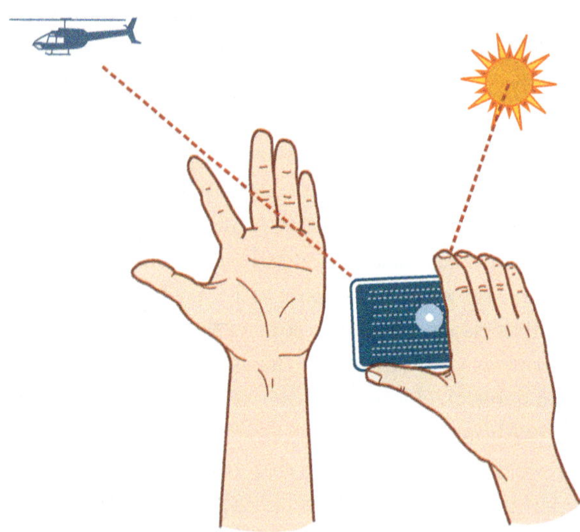

FIGURE 6-6 Aiming a signal mirror.

Mirror flashes or reflections off shiny objects have saved many lives. Use all the mirror or small parts of it, a piece of shiny metal, or improvise a mirror from a food tin, belt buckle, or aluminum foil. A compact disc also works. Use your extended hand with two fingers held up, similar to a rifle sight, as an aiming device. Find the reflected sunlight on the ground from the mirror or shiny object, and then position the mirror or object so that the reflected light passes across your extended two fingers. Now, keeping the reflected light on your two fingers, move your arm so that your target (aircraft or rescue team) is centered between your fingers. Move the mirror or shiny object's reflected light back and forth across your fingers while keeping the target centered between them. It may be a good idea to continue sweeping the horizon even though no aircraft are visible. Mirror flashes can often be seen for many miles, even on hazy days.

Shadows on Ground Signals

Shadows enhance and define ground signal formations, making them bigger and easier to see. Use the sun to cast shadows from raised portions of the signal or into depressions in the ground. The signal should have the right directional orientation if optimum shadow effect is to be utilized. Near the equator, a north-south line gives a shadow at any time except noon. Further north or south, that same north-south line will also give the best results. Brush, foliage, rocks, or snow blocks piled in a line are effective methods of increasing the shadow size and emphasis. There are very few straight lines and right angles in nature, and the goal is to get someone's attention.

Color Signals

During daylight (photopic vision; plenty of ambient light and higher visual acuity), some colors contrast with their background and are visually conspicuous. On the other hand, in the same light conditions, white clothing on snow or green outer garments in forests are nearly impossible to see. SAR personnel should always wear high-visibility clothing or accessories. Searchers can best see bright colors that contrast with their background, such as fluorescent yellow and orange, royal blue, and bright white against green vegetation. Clothing technology today now includes reflective ink and glass micro beads, both of which make the wearer highly visible when even a small amount of light is shone onto them. The visual attractiveness of these items can be enhanced even further by introducing motion (i.e., waving the clothing over your head).

If you want to be seen and are wearing dark clothes, change to a high-contrast color in a forested area. Use white underclothes as flags or change the color of any clothing by turning it inside out. Small signal panels or flags are more visible when moved slowly or waved; movement increases visual conspicuousness.

With some planning, the contents of a SAR ready pack—or the pack itself—can be used as a signal or to enhance the visibility of a signal. Bright- or fluorescent-colored articles of clothing, tarps, plastic bags, trail tape, and even duct tape can be included and used when you want to be more visually conspicuous.

Other Signaling Methods

Repeated sounds coming from unusual places and at set times attract attention. Whistles, drums, gunshots, or anything audible, such as using a big stick to bang on a tree or hollow log, can carry a vital message. If a whistle is not available, one can be improvised from a sapling or piece of metal (practice this). Yelling or shouting is effective only when a ground party is nearby. If searchers are looking, change your surrounding landscape. In brush, cut conspicuous patterns in the vegetation. In snow, tramp large side trenches or pile brush or rocks to spell out a message such as SOS or HELP. Place trenches or piles so the sun creates shadows to make obvious contrast to the normal scene.

In the woods, spread colored tarps over treetops, or hoist a large white or colored flag on a pole lashed to the top of a tall tree.

At night, use flashlights, strobe lights, recognition lights, or vehicle lights and flashers. Light can be seen several miles over water on a clear night.

A Cyalume or chemical glow stick can be tied to the end of a string or rope and twirled around to make a large signal called a "buzz saw." This can be extraordinarily visible from the air.

A whistle at night or in a fog can attract surface vessels, people on shore, or locate another separated raft.

The basic principles of signaling include the following:

- In SAR work, carry a loud whistle and a small signal mirror.
- In a survival situation, have signals ready for immediate use.
- Pyrotechnics should be used only in a manner that does not threaten safety, and they are generally not recommended for use by SAR personnel.
- Use a ratio of 6:1 on letters or ground marks used. (Example: 3 feet wide and 18 feet long.)
- Fires are usually very visible at night or in reduced light.
- For maximum efficiency, place signal fires in open areas. Trees tend to disperse smoke.
- White or black smoke (depending on the surrounding/background terrain and vegetation) can be very visible when they contrast with their background.

- Moving or flashing lights attract attention in virtually any terrain.
- Shadows define, emphasize, and enlarge any ground-to-air signal.
- Combine high contrast (color and luminance) with movement whenever possible; they are key to effective visual signals.
- Colored flags, ground cloths, high-visibility vests, or bright clothing that contrast against the natural terrain, used with movement, are very visible. Fluorescent, high-visibility colors such as green-yellow and orange, or reflective materials such as 3M™ Scotchlite™, are visually conspicuous in nearly all environments.
- There are very few straight lines and right angles in nature. Therefore, they attract attention.
- Out-of-place formations, structures, vegetation, or colors attract attention. Do everything possible to disturb the natural look of the environment.
- Bigger is better if you want to be seen.
- Choose a spot for signaling that is visible from 360 degrees, such as high ground, clearing, ridge, etc.
- Stay with your stalled or crashed transportation. If you must travel, leave a note and signs of your direction of travel.

Successful signaling can speed rescue and eliminate the possibility of a long, uncomfortable ordeal. Signals make you effectively larger and are an important survival technique.

Improvising Time and Direction

A situation may arise where SAR personnel may wish to roughly estimate the time of day or orient themselves relative to north. Although many methods exist for accomplishing this, only a few of the easiest and most reliable options are described.

During the Day

Under normal circumstances, directional orientation and time can be established and monitored with a compass, GPS, and a wristwatch. However, there may be circumstances where it is necessary to improvise navigation and estimate time without such tools. In these circumstances, observing natural phenomena such as the position of the stars or sun, or even how a shadow falls, can provide valuable information.

You can use the sun to find north (and any other direction, once north has been located) using a branch or stick placed in the ground to cast a shadow (**FIGURE 6-7**). With a fairly straight stick about 18 to 24 inches long, follow these steps:

1. Find a fairly level, brush- or vegetation-free spot. Push the stick into the ground, inclining it to get a longer, bigger shadow if necessary.
2. Mark the tip of the shadow with the stick, stone, etc. Wait until the shadow tip moves a few inches (10 to 15 minutes with an 18-inch stick).
3. Mark the position of the new shadow tip.
4. Draw a straight line from the first marker (shadow tip) through, and about a foot past, the second marker.
5. The line just drawn is an east-west line. The first mark made was toward the west end of the line. The last mark made is toward the east end of the line. A line perpendicular to the drawn east-west line is a north-south line.

This system works because the sun always travels precisely east to west, even though it might not rise and set at exactly 90 degrees and 270 degrees. The shadow tip moves in the opposite direction, so the first shadow tip mark is always west of the second, anywhere on Earth. Keep in mind that these improvised methods

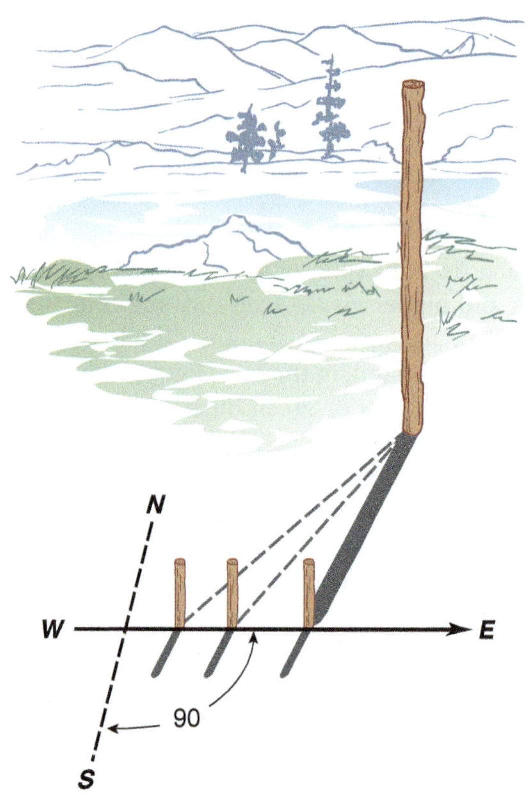

FIGURE 6-7 Stick-and-shadow method of determining direction.
United States Air Force. (1985a). Search and Rescue Survival Training. AF Regulation 64-4. Washington, D.C.: Department of the Air Force.

of determining direction are fraught with factors that reduce accuracy. They are only general indicators and are far from providing the accuracy of a compass or GPS. However, they can provide enough data to confirm what the tools are telling you or to roughly estimate direction in the absence of these tools.

An alternate method also uses a 3-foot stick, this time pushed into the ground so it points directly at the sun, casting no shadow on the ground at the base of the stick. Wait 10 or 15 minutes and check the direction in which the shadow falls. A line drawn through the tip of the shadow and the base of the stick is an east-west line. The narrower the stick is at the top, the easier it is to determine general direction.

The shadow tip method used for finding direction can also determine approximate time of day:

1. After drawing an east-west line, draw an intersecting, perpendicular north-south line. Push a stick into the ground at the intersection. The west part of the line indicates the position of the stick's shadow at sunrise (arbitrarily 0600 hours). The east part of the line indicates shadow position at sunset (1800 hours). The north-south line indicates shadow position at noon.
2. The shadow of the stick becomes the hour hand of your clock, and you can estimate time using the noon and 6-o'clock lines as guides.
3. The shadow clock is not even close to being as accurate as a watch. However, it divides the day into 12 unequal hours, with sunrise always 0600 and sunset always 1800.
4. Twelve o'clock shadow time is always true midday, but spacing of other hours varies somewhat with location and time of year.

Drawing a clock face on the ground that reflects the current time, or using an analog wrist watch, can help establish direction (**FIGURE 6-8**). Point the hour hand at the sun or draw the face of a clock on the ground that shows the current time with the hour hand pointing at the sun and determine the halfway point between the hour hand and 12 o'clock or 1 o'clock (daylight savings time), and that will indicate a north-south line (south in the northern hemisphere and north in the southern hemisphere). On cloudy days, hold a small stick at the center of the watch or drawing on the ground so its shadow falls along the hour hand. A line drawn halfway between the shadow and 12 o'clock (on the side of the dial that contains the smaller numbers, 1 to 6) indicates north in this hemisphere.

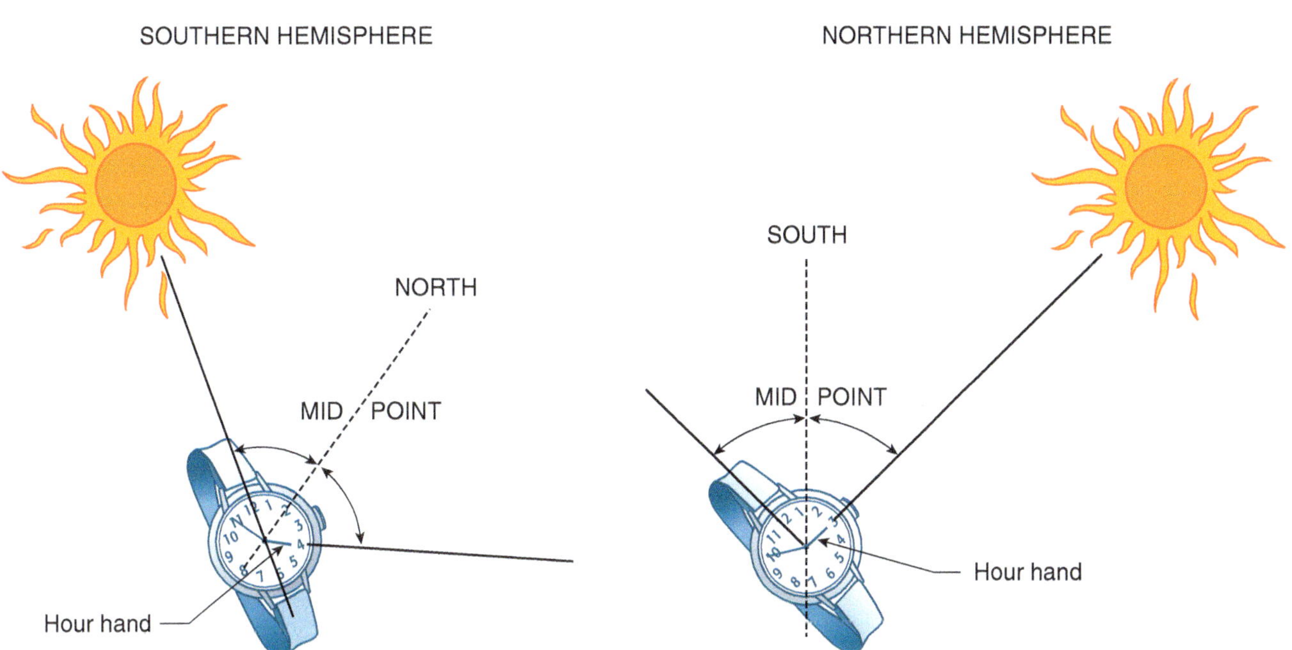

FIGURE 6-8 Finding directions using a wristwatch.
United States Air Force. (1985a). Search and Rescue Survival Training. AF Regulation 64-4. Washington, D.C.: Department of the Air Force.

At Night

Determining direction at night takes a little knowledge of the constellations (**FIGURE 6-9**). On a clear evening in the northern hemisphere, you can find the North Star by locating the Big Dipper. The two stars forming the end of the bowl are "pointers." Visualize a straight line drawn through the "pointer stars." Along this line, approximately five times the distance between the pointers, is the North Star (Polaris), which is located above the Dipper lip. The Big Dipper rotates around the North Star and is not always at the same position in the sky. When the Dipper is low in the sky and is obscured by trees or high ground, the constellation Cassiopeia (The Queen's Chair)—a group of five bright stars shaped like a lopsided "M" (or "W" when low in the sky)—can be used. The North Star is straight out from the middle star in Cassiopeia, at about the same distance as from the Dipper lip. A straight line from the middle star in Cassiopeia through the North Star intersects the first star up the handle of the Big Dipper. Since Cassiopeia is almost directly opposite the Dipper, one constellation will generally be observable for finding the North Star.

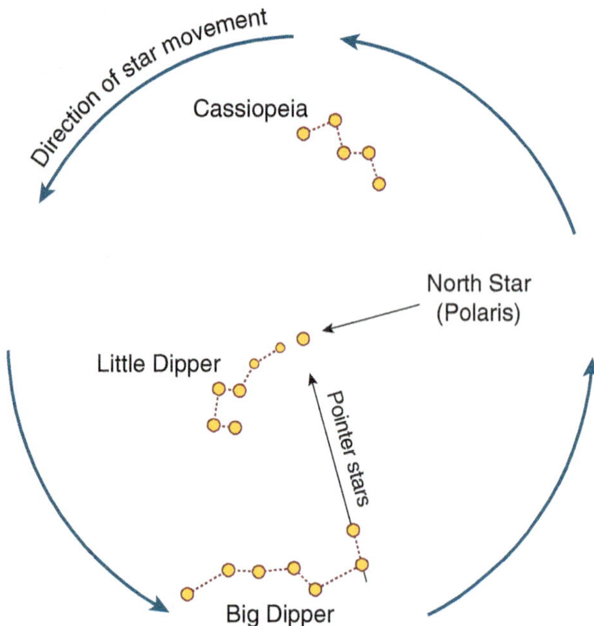

FIGURE 6-9 The relationship between the Big Dipper, Polaris, and Cassiopeia. In the Northern Hemisphere, a line drawn straight down from the North Star (Polaris) will be within 1° of true north. Find the North Star by locating the Big Dipper or Cassiopeia. The two stars on the outer edge of the Big Dipper point almost directly to the North Star. If the pointers are obscured by clouds, Polaris can be identified by its relationship to the constellation Cassiopeia.

United States Air Force. (1985a). Search and Rescue Survival Training. AF Regulation 64-4. Washington, D.C.: Department of the Air Force.

Direction from Orion

The constellation of Orion consists of seven stars (**FIGURE 6-10**). The three central stars close together are called the Belt of Orion. The star through which the north-south line passes is exactly on the celestial equator. No matter where on Earth you are, this star rises due east of you and sets due west.

Water Procurement and Treatment

The daily intake and output of liquids and certain chemicals by the body are essential for life processes and normal functions of vital organs. As mentioned in Chapter 5, the body itself is approximately two-thirds water, and the general recommendation for total daily water intake—from all beverages and foods—ranges from approximately 2.7 liters (91 ounces) for women to 3.7 liters (125 ounces) for men. An average inactive person might require less, but stress, physical exertion, and high humidity can easily double these requirements. Thus, water can be critical in an emergency, and in harsh desert terrain, your life depends upon your water supply and how well you manage and conserve your body water. Always carry enough water, or when water is plentiful, carry the means by which you can render water for safe consumption (Institute of Medicine, 2005).

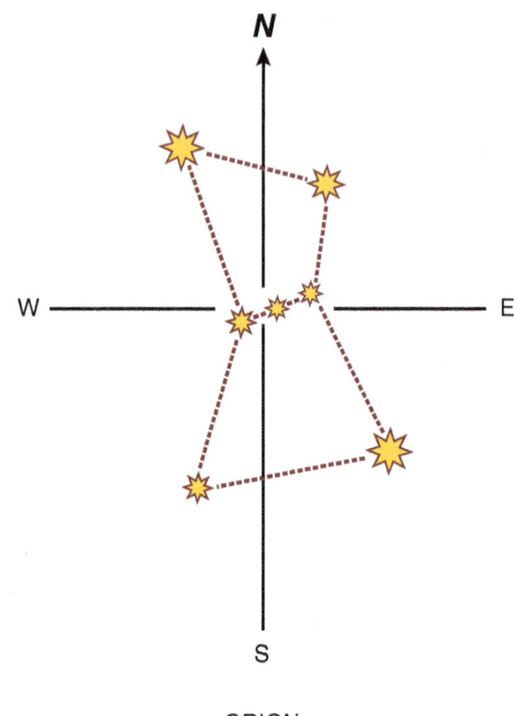

FIGURE 6-10 Direction to north from Orion.

United States Air Force. (1985a). Search and Rescue Survival Training. AF Regulation 64-4. Washington, D.C.: Department of the Air Force.

Improvised methods of water procurement, such as transpiration bags, stills, catch basins, or seepage holes, are really survival situation sources. They are usually marginal at best and should never be relied upon to supply enough water for field operations.

Along the Seashore

Along coasts, fresh water may be found in dunes above the beach, or in the beach itself, well above the high tide line (**FIGURE 6-11**). Check hollows between dunes for visible water. Dig if the sand is moist. Otherwise, along the seashore on sandy beaches, dig a hole just over the first sand dune that is directly adjacent to the water. A damp area in a depression is a good place to dig. This is where rainwater and drainage from the local water tables collect. Dig until the hole begins to fill with muddy water; a deep hole is not necessary. (If you dig too deep, you may reach saltwater, which is unfit to drink.) Shore up the sides of the hole with beach wood or brush. Let the impurities and suspended particles settle and the water clarify. Make the water safe by some purification method.

Desert or Arid Lands

Assess your water requirements. Can you expect rescue within 12 to 24 hours? It may be wisest to sit and conserve body water while awaiting assistance. Efforts to find water by searching and digging consume energy and water and increase your water requirements.

Do not rely on the sensation of thirst to indicate how much water you need. Drink plenty of water anytime it is available, particularly when you are eating. Do not eat if you cannot drink water. The best way to conserve your total body water is to control the amount you perspire. In other words, conserve your sweat, not your drinking water.

Take the following steps to control perspiration and conserve body water:

- Keep your clothes on. Clothing helps control sweating by not letting perspiration evaporate so fast. Clothing also prevents sunburn.
- Wear a hat and cover your neck with a neck cloth.
- Light-colored clothing reflects light and heat.
- Stay in the shade and rest during the day.

SAFETY TIP

Never drink seawater or urine. The chemical makeup actually causes dehydration and even toxicity.

Where to Look for Water

Water is more abundant and easier to find in loose sediment than in rocks. Look for springs along valley floors. Flat benches or terraces of land above river valleys may have springs or seepages along their bases, even when streams are dry. Signs of damp sand along the bottom of a canyon or base of a hill can be dug in as described in the previous seashore section. Dry streambeds may have water just below the surface. Try

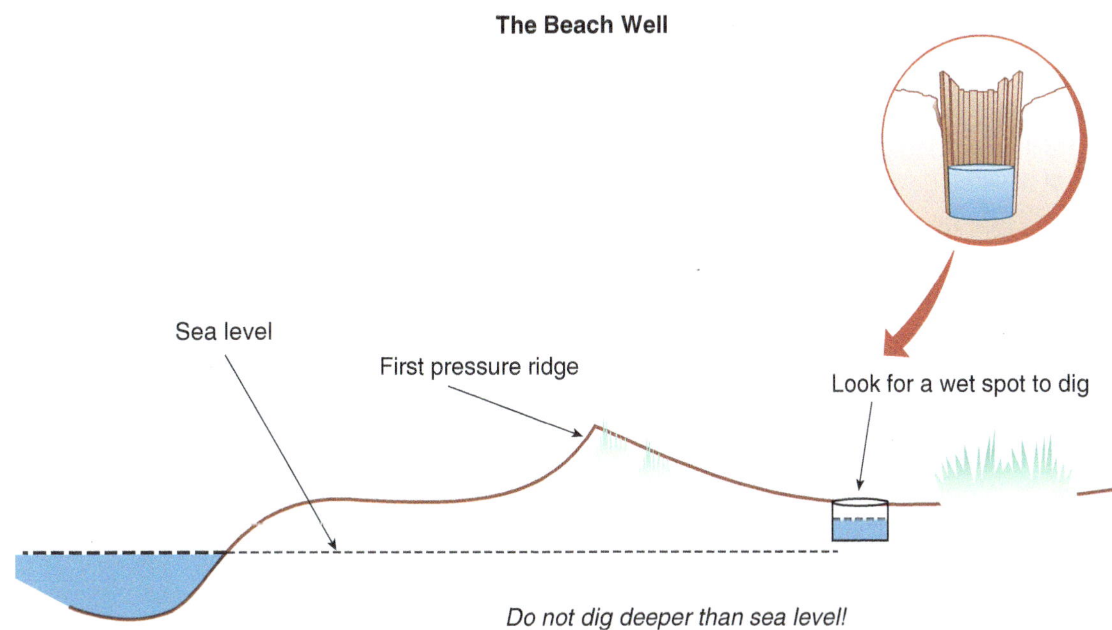

FIGURE 6-11 Water from a beach well.
United States Air Force. (1985a). Search and Rescue Survival Training. AF Regulation 64-4. Washington, D.C.: Department of the Air Force.

digging at the lowest point on the outside of a bend in the streambed channel.

Animal trail forks often point toward a source of water. As the animals move from their various habitats, they progressively converge as they approach water. Watch for animals and birds moving in the early morning or late evening. They are probably moving toward water.

SAFETY TIP

Ration your sweat, not your water.

Contrary to popular belief, the water found in the pulp of the barrel cactus and other similar plants is not suitable for human consumption. The moisture is far too alkaline. Furthermore, the law protects many of these fragile cacti. The pulp may be productive in a vegetation bag still (see next section), but the effort to get at the pulp from a cactus usually outweighs the benefit.

Vegetation Bag Water Still

Vegetation bag water stills are a relatively new innovation that appears to be superior to traditional desert solar stills (**FIGURE 6-12**). Water produced through vegetation bag stills tastes much like the plants used, but the idea is sound when poisonous plants are avoided.

Follow these steps to build a vegetation bag still:

1. Cut foliage from trees or leafy plants.
2. Shake the branches thoroughly to eliminate dust, bird droppings, and insects because these can taint the water source.
3. Seal them in a large, clear, plastic bag. Do not completely fill the bag.
4. Set the sealed bag in the sun to extract the fluids contained within.
5. If available, insert a piece of surgical tubing into the water reservoir so that the bag does not have to be opened to get at the water.

If a large, clear plastic bag is used and filled with approximately 1 cubic yard of foliage, the bag should yield a little less than a pint per day. Do not use poisonous or irritating plants.

Water produced by this method is normally bitter to taste, which is caused by biological breakdown of the leaves as they lie in the water produced and are heated in the moist "hot house" environment.

Water Transpiration Bag

One of the most efficient and easily constructed water sources in both desert and mountainous regions is the water transpiration bag (**FIGURE 6-13**). It is efficient because it capitalizes on a plant's capability to pull water from the ground. It also requires very little energy to construct and is easy to tap into.

Follow these steps to construct a transpiration bag:

1. Place a plastic bag over a living limb of a medium-sized tree or large shrub. (Do this after shaking the branches thoroughly to eliminate dust, bird droppings, and insects because these would taint the water source. If available, a tube can be used to suck the water from the bag so it does not have to be opened.)
2. Seal the bag opening at the branch and tie the limb down to allow collected water to flow to the corner of the bag.

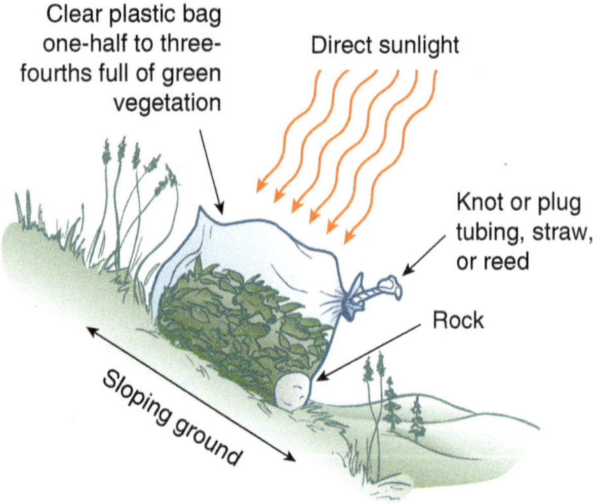

FIGURE 6-12 Vegetation bag water still.
Larsen, M. U.S. Army Survival Handbook, Revised. Figure 6-6, p. 89. Morris Book Publishing, LLC: 2009. Reprinted with permission.

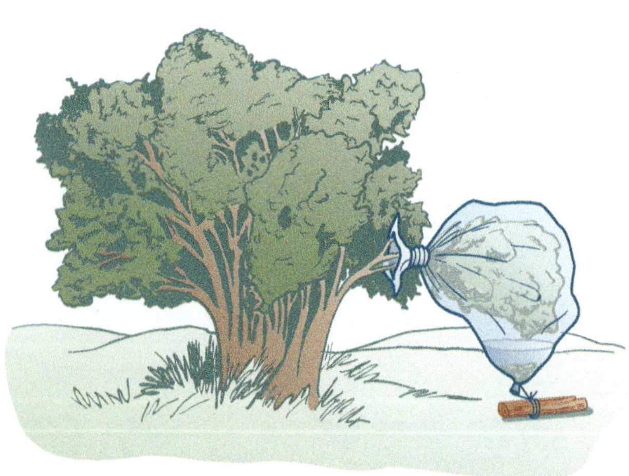

FIGURE 6-13 Water transpiration bag.
United States Air Force. (1985a). Search and Rescue Survival Training. AF Regulation 64-4. Washington, D.C.: Department of the Air Force.

The amount of water collected, and the taste of the water procured by this method, depends on the species of trees and shrubs used. The water transpiration bag method often surpasses other methods (vegetation bag or solar still) in yield and ease of construction, but it will likely still take multiple transpiration bags to provide enough water for one person.

Conventional Desert Solar Water Still

Even though this method is portrayed in most survival books as a viable source in desert conditions, do not waste your time. This method is very costly in terms of energy, and hundreds if not thousands of outdoor "experts" have tried in vain to make this method work effectively. Again, the prevailing advice is: don't waste your time with this method.

Mountains

A mountainous area is often the easiest geographic environment in which to locate water. The amount of difficulty depends on elevation, vegetation type in the area, geologic structure of the mountains, and annual precipitation.

Most canyons have streams, springs, or intermittent run-off flow during all or part of the year. Look in the very bottom of the canyon floor near catch pools and depressions of streambeds. Look for changes in vegetation, which are clues leading to a seep spring. If there is no water visible, often a small amount of digging will uncover water.

Look for large rock formations with green moss or lush vegetation and seek water at the base. Small clumps of isolated green vegetation in arid mountains is a good sign of a spring. You can also collect dew from leaves, plastic sheets, metal of the stalled transportation, or any wet surface. Sponge the water off with an absorbent cloth. Improvised rainwater collectors can be made from plastic sheets or waterproof clothing. *Caution:* Avoid water holes with few or no tracks nearby and no plants in or around them.

Arctic and/or Extreme Winter Conditions

Water procurement and dehydration (lowering of the body's water content) are as great a problem in cold conditions as in the desert. In arctic conditions, all the available water is frozen, and the extremely low humidity saps your body of water through respiration and perspiration.

In cold weather environments, water might be found in the following ways:

- Frozen streams and lakes may cover water.
- If the sun is shining, you can melt snow on black or dark-colored plastic, a dark tarp, metal surfaces of any stalled transportation, or any surface that absorbs the sun's heat. Arrange the surface so that it tilts slightly, or any fluid on the surface will run to a low spot and perhaps refreeze. The melted water can be directed to drain into a hollow or container at the edge of the surface.
- Whenever possible, melt ice rather than snow for water. You get more water for the volume with less heat and time.

If planning on flying over or traveling through arctic or winter environments, your emergency preparedness kit should contain a stove and pot to melt ice and snow. Do not eat ice or snow. A day or two of eating ice or snow results in swollen, raw mucous membranes in the mouth. Also, the expenditure of body heat and energy to melt the snow may be more detrimental to your health than the lack of water.

Preparation of Water Under Emergency Conditions

Water is heavy; 1 gallon (3.78 liters) of fresh water weighs 8.34 pounds (3.78 kilograms). Because of this, carrying enough water to operate in a SAR environment can be problematic. In addition, all water found in nature should be considered contaminated regardless of how clear or clean it appears (White, 1992; Gerba and Rose, 1990). These two reasons are why it is prudent to supplement the water in your SAR ready pack with one or more methods of treating water found in the environment.

Going without water, especially while working hard, can lead to dehydration and death within a few days. Drinking contaminated water can cause nausea, vomiting, diarrhea, fever, and fatigue. If not managed properly, any of these can also lead to more serious illness, such as dehydration and even death. Under emergency conditions, to prevent dehydration, it might be necessary to treat muddy, stagnant, or otherwise contaminated water so you can drink it. This type of water may not seem palatable, but if treated properly, it can be made harmless enough to save your life.

Clarification is the act of removing or filtering sediment (dirt, debris, etc.) from your water and should be done before attempting **purification**, which is the removal of pathogenic (disease causing) microorganisms in the water, such as bacteria, viruses, and parasites. Mechanical devices (filters) have been developed for outdoor use to filter some impurities from water. Other devices combine a filter (clarification) with chemical treatment of water (purification) to make what is called a water purifier.

Clarification

There are four general methods of clarifying water: sedimentation, coagulation–flocculation, activated carbon (charcoal), and filtration. *Sedimentation* is simply allowing gravity to settle large particles to the bottom of a container before decanting the clear water off it. *Coagulation–flocculation* removes small suspended particles (colloids), most microorganisms, and some dissolved substances from the water by sedimentation after introducing specific chemicals (e.g., aluminum salts [alum], iron, or lime [alkaline chemicals mostly containing calcium or magnesium and oxygen]) that bind with the contaminants. *Charcoal*, usually in a filter, absorbs dissolved compounds such as toxic organic and inorganic chemicals, removes radioactive contamination, and improves odor and taste. *Filtration* uses one or more filter media to stop contaminants from passing through (Backer, 2012). Each of these methods has its respective pros and cons, but regardless of the specific technique chosen, ". . .all [clarification] methods will greatly reduce the load of microorganisms and reduce the risk for illness" (Backer, 2012, p. 1348).

In most SAR environments, sedimentation and filtration are the most accessible options for water clarification. Sedimentation takes only patience, waiting for the sediment to settle out of water in a container before carefully decanting or filtering off the water on the top. Filtration, on the other hand, requires additional materials/equipment and some prior planning. The good news is that many relatively small, packable water filters, including simple coffee filters for removing turbidity (cloudiness), are commercially available.

The size of a microorganism is the primary determinant of its susceptibility to filtration, and the effectiveness of the filter depends primarily on the pore sizes in the filter media. The smaller the pore size, the more particles and microorganisms are removed. However, smaller pores clog faster, which then requires more pressure to push the water through the filter. More pressure increases the chances of forcing contaminants through the filter and increases the amount of time it takes to filter a quantity of water. Filtering water through a coffee filter or even a clean cloth (e.g., bandana, shirt sleeve) to remove turbidity before using a mechanical filter can help reduce clogging and extend the life of the filter media. Mechanical filters can also be expensive, may require field maintenance or repair (e.g., replacing or cleaning a clogged filter), and are subject to mechanical damage and damage from freezing. Including a lightweight filter in a SAR ready pack for use in an emergency is a reasonable option, keeping in mind that carrying enough clean water for normal use is also an important part of a SAR ready pack.

For natural water found in wilderness areas outside of developing countries where humans and domestic animals are not a significant source of contamination, one reliable source suggests that the primary health concerns are protozoa (e.g., Giardia, Cryptosporidium, Cyclospora) and enteric (intestinal) bacteria such as *Escherichia coli* (Backer, 2012). A microfiltration filter with a pore size of 0.1 micron (1 micron = one millionth of a meter) effectively filters out protozoa, but it removes only some bacteria. An ultrafiltration filter with much smaller pores (0.01 micron) is required to effectively remove both bacteria and protozoa from water. Neither of these filters removes viruses or chemicals from water, and neither is likely to remove odor (CDC, 2014). Because clarification may not remove enough contaminants from water to make it safe to drink, purification is recommended after clarification for all water procured in the field.

Purification

Heat is one of the oldest methods of purifying water. **Sterilization** is one method that involves raising the temperature of water high enough, and for long enough, to completely remove or destroy all living microorganisms (Rao, 2008). Sterilization is usually far more than is needed to make water safe to drink. **Disinfection** refers to the removal or destruction of harmful microorganisms in water. **Pasteurization** is applying enough heat to water ($<$ boiling point) to reduce the number of surviving microorganisms in the water to such a low level that they are unlikely to cause illness or disease. Death of these microorganisms occurs quicker at higher temperatures, while lower temperatures can be effective with longer contact time (Backer, 2012). Where heat is used to purify water, the higher the temperature and longer the exposure time, the more disinfection occurs.

Solar water disinfection (SODIS) involves the combined use of solar energy to heat water and exposure to ultraviolet (UV) light to kill pathogens (Cervantes and Xanet, 2003; Conroy et al., 2001; Oates et al., 2003; Sobsey, 2003). This is usually accomplished by putting the water in clear containers and placing them in bright, direct sunlight for many hours. Cloudy water can take much longer, up to several days, because the opacity inhibits the UV effects (Joyce et al., 1996). In SAR situations, this method may only be useful in long-term survival situations, but the point is that exposing water to UV light (bright sunlight) and heating it to moderately warm temperatures (i.e., far less than boiling) for long periods of time can significantly reduce the pathogens in water. These facts may be useful to SAR personnel should they be forced to improvise water procurement.

UV light from artificial sources can also purify water, and many commercial devices use this approach. One example is the SteriPEN® Adventurer Opti handheld UV water purifier (**FIGURE 6-14**). This device weighs 3.8 ounces (108 grams) and uses two CR123 batteries to power a flashlight-like device, the lamp of which is inserted into a liter-sized bottle of water. The manufacturer of the SteriPEN claims that exposure of a liter of water to the UV light for 90 seconds purifies the water enough to drink, and that the lamp purifies up to 8000 liters of water. UV light leaves no taste in the water, requires no chemicals, and if the water is overdosed, unlike with other methods, the result is beneficial. The down side to this purification method is that it can be expensive, requires power—in the form of batteries in the example given—and the UV lamp has a limited useful life.

In all but the very highest altitudes, heating water until it boils and then letting it cool can be an effective purification method. Any water brought to a boil, even for a few seconds, is adequately disinfected (Sobsey, 2003; Backer, 2012). However, the U.S. Centers for Disease Control and Prevention (CDC) recommends boiling water for one minute to make it safe to drink (CDC, 2013). Although this method may be effective, it takes time, fuel, and possibly equipment (e.g., stove) that may not be available in all situations. In a SAR environment, having the ability to make a fire or light a stove to boil water is a reasonable alternative—or backup—to carrying other means of clarifying and purifying water, but it should not be the only method of water purification carried into a SAR environment.

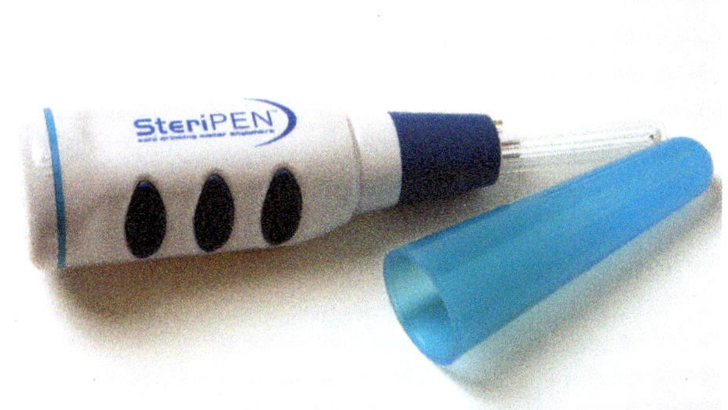

FIGURE 6-14 Example of a lightweight UV water purifier. These purifiers are typically 3 to 4 ounces (85 to 113 grams), powered by disposable batteries, and work in containers with 1 to 2 inch (25 to 51 mm) diameter openings.

The use of halogens (chlorine and iodine) to disinfect water is also effective and has the additional benefit of being relatively inexpensive and easy to use. Several commercial products are available (e.g., Oasis Plus® Water Purification Tablets, Potable Aqua® [chlorine dioxide tablets and tetraglycine hydroperiodide tablets], Coghlan's Emergency Drinking Water Germicidal Tablets, Chlor-Floc®, Globaline™, and Aquamira®) that require dropping a tablet or two—or a few drops—into the water, stirring, and letting it sit. At least one small electronic product, which comes with an attached solar panel, uses salt and a small electric charge to produce a disinfectant—chlorine liquid that is poured into your water container (Potable Aqua Pure® device). Regardless of the product or device used, make sure to follow the manufacturer's instructions exactly.

Commercial laundry bleach (8.25% hypochlorite) and iodine can also be used to purify water, but they must be handled very carefully since both are poisonous in high concentrations and can permanently stain anything they touch.

TABLE 6-4 shows the amount of commercial bleach solution (8.25% hypochlorite) to add to water for purification. Add the chlorine solution to the water, stir, and let it stand for at least 30 minutes. After this length of time, the water should have a distinct taste or smell of chlorine. If not, then add several more drops of chlorine, stir, and let the mixture stand for another 15 minutes. The slight taste or smell of chlorine in the water is a sign of safety. (Note: several drops of hydrogen peroxide removes the smell of chlorine from the water, making it more palatable.)

A 2% tincture of iodine can purify water by adding four drops to each quart of clear water or eight drops to each quart of cloudy water. For a gallon, add 12 drops for clear water or 24 drops for cloudy water. Stir thoroughly and let it sit for at least 30 minutes. Be careful, though, as iodine is a potent poison. Too much—and any amount of solid iodine crystals—can be toxic if ingested. Although rare, some people are allergic to iodine and could have a serious or fatal (anaphylactic)

TABLE 6-4 Use of an 8.25% Sodium Hypochlorite Solution (Commercial Bleach) to Purify Water

Amount of Water	Amount of Bleach to Add to Clear Water[1]
1 quart/liter (1/4 gallon)	2 drops
1 gallon	6 drops
2 gallons	12 drops (1/8 teaspoon)
4 gallons	1/4 teaspoon
8 gallons	1/2 teaspoon

Note 1: Stir and let stand for 30 minutes. Double the amount of bleach for water that is cloudy, colored, or very cold.

Reproduced from U.S. Environmental Protection Agency [EPA]. (2016). Ground water and drinking water: Emergency disinfection of drinking water. Retrieved from https://www.epa.gov/ground-water-and-drinking-water/emergency-disinfection-drinking-water.

reaction to ingesting it, and certain medical problems can be exacerbated by the ingestion of even a small amount of iodine. Because of these potential problems, iodine should not be the first or only method of water purification in one's SAR ready pack.

Recommendations for SAR

Although many methods can be effective, at a minimum, the following water treatment methods are recommended for SAR personnel. Because "...removal of turbidity and particulates may be important in preventing chemical or infectious illness" (Backer, 2012, p. 1332), carry several paper coffee filters to pre-filter cloudy, contaminated water. These filters can serve other purposes in your SAR ready pack (e.g., fire tinder, dressings, and note paper), and they are light, inexpensive, readily available, and ideal for reducing turbidity and removing sediment in water procured in the field. A bandana, gauze, or other close-weaved cloth can also serve the purpose.

Carry a lightweight microfiltration water filter (0.1-micron pore size or smaller) with enough capacity for one or two people; for example, the Sawyer® Mini, which weighs less than 3 ounces (0.09 kilograms) and costs less than $30. Know how to use, and be familiar with, any device you carry in your SAR ready pack.

Carry a halogen that can be used to purify water after it is filtered. A commercial product works, as does a small amount of chlorine bleach or iodine. Become familiar with the instructions from the manufacturer on any commercial product carried in your SAR ready pack and follow the instructions precisely when using the product. A small, lightweight, portable UV water purifier is an excellent alternative to carrying chemicals for purification.

Carry in your SAR ready pack that which is necessary to heat water to boiling. This is not a primary water purification option, but having this capability as a backup could be helpful. To treat water in the field, follow these steps:

1. Filter it first with a coffee filter or cloth to remove sediment and turbidity.
2. Use a microfiltration water filter to remove protozoa and some bacteria.
3. Apply a halogen to the water, stir, and let it sit for at least 30 minutes to disinfect it further before consuming (longer for cold or cloudy water; see Table 6-4).
4. Alternatively, use a small, portable, commercial UV water purifier for at least 90 seconds.
5. If microfiltration, halogen treatment, or UV water purification is not available, or if there is any doubt as to any remaining contamination of the water, heat the water to boiling, then let it cool before consuming.

Taking these precautions may not completely prevent water-related illness, but it can minimize the hazard and reduce the statistical likelihood of an illness to an acceptable level (Backer, 2017).

Another important point on this topic is that submerging a water bottle in a stream, river, or lake to collect water for treatment covers both the inside and the outside of the container with contaminated water. Thus, if you drink from the container, even after clarifying and purifying the water on the inside, contaminated water from the outside of the bottle can still be ingested and cause illness. Be sure to wipe clean or use purified water to rinse the parts of the water bottle that touch your mouth and lips before use. Carry at least two water bottles so that one can be used to store water that is being purified and the other can be used for drinking.

If questionable water must be consumed in an emergency, seek medical attention as soon as possible.

Personal Waste Disposal

Preparations for an overnight stay, planned or unplanned, should include arrangements for waste disposal. Do not urinate directly on green vegetation or in or near bodies of water. If you are alone or your group is small (no more than three to four) and staying only a night or two at one location, each of you can dig a "cat-hole" to dispose of human waste. A cat-hole is approximately 18 inches (46 cm) deep, or as close as you can get with the available tools; anything shallower is likely to be dug up by animals. It should be about 6 inches (15 cm) wide and dug at least 200 feet (60 meters or about 80 steps) downhill from where you will sleep, any trail, any water sources, or snow that is to be melted for water (Bowman and Kummerfeldt, 2017; U.S. Army, Navy, and Air Force, 1999). Choose a location that is not likely to be visited by others and dig the hole with the heel of your boot or a sharp stick. After use, cover the hole completely with dirt or snow.

Bury nothing in a cat-hole except human waste. Animals dig up buried garbage and scatter it around the forest, and materials such as plastic, glass, metal, and cardboard take years to decompose (**TABLE 6-5**). When possible, carry all rubbish out of the field with you for appropriate disposal. Except for emergencies, if you packed it in, you must pack it out.

TABLE 6-5 How Long Litter Lasts

Item	Time to Decompose
Styrofoam	Indefinitely
Plastic bottle	Indefinitely
Glass bottle	1 million years
Plastic six-pack holder	100 years
Aluminum cans/tabs	80 to 100 years
Tin can	50 years
Leather	Up to 50 years
Nylon fabric	30 to 40 years
Plastic film container	20 to 30 years
Plastic bag	20 to 30 years
Plastic coated paper	5 years
Cigarette butts	1 to 5 years
Wool socks	1 to 5 years
Orange/banana peel	2 weeks to 5 months

Data from U.S. Department of the Interior National Park Service [NPS]. (2016). How long does litter last? Retrieved from https://www.nps.gov/tuma/learn/kidsyouth/upload/ HowLongDoesLitterLast.pdf.

Personal Cleanliness

Good hygiene and cleanliness are essential in the outdoors. They safeguard good health by minimizing the potential for internal and external infections as well as infestation by parasites such as fleas and lice. The smallest abrasion of an unclean body can easily become infected and present a major survival obstacle.

It is very important to wash feet only after the day's travel is done. Do not rinse feet at travel breaks. It significantly softens them and makes them more prone to blisters and injury.

Make sure to keep hands as clean as possible by washing them with soap and water regularly, and do not forget to clean under the fingernails. Wash your face, underarms, groin, and feet at least once each day. This is especially important after urinating or defecating and before treating a wound. Keep the perineum (the area between the anus and scrotum or vulva) and perianal (the area around the anus) areas particularly clean to prevent uncomfortable and inconvenient rashes and itching. Carry and use toilet paper and wipes, and a light coating of petroleum jelly (fire starter in SAR ready pack) can help prevent chafing (Hawkins, Millin, and Smith, 2017). While you probably will not wash as frequently as you do at home, frequent bathing is strongly encouraged in the field. However, do not simply douse yourself in the nearest lake or pond. The best approach environmentally involves taking water away from natural water sources, washing, and then disposing of the wastewater in a cat-hole. All soap used should be biodegradable, but friction often works as well. Water for bathing is best taken from rapidly moving water sources as opposed to stagnant ponds or lakes, which helps avoid bacterial problems and limits involvement with leeches and other parasites. Water used for brushing teeth, gargling, or rinsing your mouth or eyes should be purified and safe for drinking.

When washing in water is impossible, "air" baths are better than none. To take an air bath, simply remove clothing, especially underwear, and allow air to circulate over the bare skin. This can help prevent chaffing and some skin problems. Regularly exposing the bare skin briefly to direct sunlight can also have health benefits, but be careful to avoid sunburn.

Special Considerations

For most people, discussing personal physical problems with others can be disconcerting and difficult. However, no one involved in SAR should hesitate to communicate unusual discomfort, pain, or malaise to coworkers because the result may affect both the outcome of the incident and the safety of others.

The responsibility for communicating relevant personal health information is shared by all SAR team members. In addition, SAR leadership involves kind and often discrete inquiry into any individual team member's difficulties. Responsible leadership includes the ability to deal with problems appropriately without exaggeration or overreaction. Situations unique to women are no exception to this rule.

SAR leaders should make it understood that any individual with problems that affect the team's effectiveness and/or safety will be treated sympathetically, knowledgeably, and confidentially without undue embarrassment. If anxiety is involved, SAR leaders should be nonjudgmental and sympathetic. If rest is required, the group should adjust, just as it would for a team member with a blister.

Special Considerations for Women

The physical and mental stress related to search and rescue challenges, long-term heavy physical exercise, or even the reduction of fat in the blood may all induce changes in a woman's menstrual cycle. Like many athletes in training, some women experience temporary amenorrhea, in which menstruation stops completely.

It is important to note that medical research indicates that women's strength and endurance are in no way diminished during menstruation. However, SAR leaders should know about and be willing to openly discuss these topics. For instance, women between menstrual periods, during ovulation, sometimes experience cramping on either or both sides of the abdomen and/or lower back. However, most women who experience it can adequately identify and deal with it.

Vaginal infections can be particularly problematic in the field and are often caused by stress, the use of oral contraceptives, and because of excessive sugar intake. Therefore, SAR leaders and female SAR personnel should be aware that, to avoid these infections during extended field operations, women should be encouraged to wear loose-fitting cotton underpants, drink sufficient water, and, when possible, keep their sugar and carbohydrate intake down.

High altitudes increase the risk of blood clotting for both men and women. Women who take oral contraceptives are already at a higher risk of clotting, so a woman who takes oral contraceptives and expects to spend much time above 12,000 feet (4000 meters) should discuss the risks with her doctor. Also, due to the possibility of unrecognized or undiagnosed complications, a woman with a recently inserted intrauterine device may be advised to wait a month or so before traveling deep into the backcountry or to high altitude (Salas and Anderson, 2017).

Any SAR team member who is pregnant should advise her team leader. In addition, a pregnant woman should consider consulting her physician prior to participating in SAR operations so that both understand the extent and the requirements of her involvement. Some physicians might suggest that pregnant women consider not participating in the more vigorous field aspects of SAR during their third trimester. However, the same physicians are also likely to suggest that a woman's participation in SAR, or any vigorous activity, be limited by her comfort and health, keeping in mind the importance of nutrition and hydration during pregnancy.

Pregnant women in isolated, outdoor environments are at high risk for miscarriage. A miscarriage or ectopic pregnancy is possible in a woman who does not believe she is pregnant and can be a true emergency (Salas and Anderson, 2017). Vaginal bleeding can be an early sign of these and other serious problems and so should be monitored, especially if the bleeding differs in quantity and/or duration from normal menses.

Iron deficiency is common and can cause anemia, which makes one more susceptible to illness and infection. Pregnant women are particularly susceptible to anemia, but anyone with iron deficiency or anemia may wish to include in their diets some foods that are high in iron. Foods that meet this criterion and are easily carried in the field include dried prunes, dried peaches, raisins, dates, sesame seeds, pumpkin seeds, and wheat germ (Mayo Clinic, 2016). It should also be noted that some of these foods, when eaten in quantity could cause constipation, so their intake in the field should be carefully monitored.

In the field, feminine hygiene supplies such as pads and tampons have multiple improvisational uses such as tinder, water filter, cordage, dressings, and bandages. They are particularly effective when used to pad or cushion an injury. Several alternative menstrual products exist that are lightweight, environmentally friendly, safe, convenient, economical, and do not require packing out consumable supplies after use. Two examples are the DivaCup® and the Mooncup®; small, soft, silicone devices that can be cleaned and reused for many years.

Used tampons and pads must either be burned in a very hot fire or carried out. Female SAR personnel should be sure to add small plastic bags to their packs for this purpose. Crushing a few aspirin and placing them in the bag, or wrapping the tampons in fragrant leaves, can help eliminate the problem of odor. Extra care should be taken to keep a pack containing used pads or tampons out of the reach of animals. The odor of these items is particularly attractive to many animals and can lead to unwanted confrontations (McConnell, 2016).

Wrap-Up

READY FOR REVIEW

- In terms of SAR, survival is about rescuers being able to take care of themselves, and perhaps one another, in harsh, challenging, or less than optimal circumstances.
- The necessities of life, in order of priority, are a will to live (positive mental attitude), air/oxygen, shelter/clothing/warmth, rest, signals, water, and food.
- In general, there are two aspects of emergency response that should be considered by SAR personnel: (1) mental preparation for SAR operations, and (2) immediate response to an emergency situation.
- Survival is based on resilience and requires talent (skills), desire, and the optimism to overcome difficulties and disappointments.
- Shelter is anything that protects the body from temperature, weather, insects, or any other life-threatening force or element. In fact, our clothing is the shelter we wear, and it constitutes the first line of defense in any environment.
- Fire building is a skill that is mastered only by practicing in a wide spectrum of conditions with different materials.
- Emergency signaling is intended to make a person or persons more visible and most often implies distress of one form or another. The time it takes to be rescued depends largely on how effective distress signals are and how fast they can be deployed.
- Under normal circumstances, directional orientation and time can be established and monitored with a compass, GPS, and a wristwatch. However, there may be circumstances where it is necessary to improvise navigation and estimate time without such tools.
- The daily intake and output of liquids and certain chemicals by the body are essential for life processes and normal functions of vital organs. Always carry enough water, or when water is plentiful, carry the means by which you can render water for safe consumption.
- It is prudent to supplement the water in your SAR ready pack with one or more methods of treating water found in the environment.
- Preparations for an overnight stay, planned or unplanned, should include arrangements for waste disposal.
- Good hygiene and cleanliness are essential in the outdoors. They safeguard good health by minimizing the potential for internal and external infections as well as infestation by parasites such as fleas and lice.
- Do not hesitate to communicate unusual discomfort, pain, or malaise to coworkers because the result may affect both the outcome of the incident and the safety of others.

SEARCH AND RESCUE TERMS

Clarification For water, the act of removing or filtering sediment and debris from water to make it clearer.

Comfort zone Any area of human existence, based on a state of physical ease and freedom from pain or constraints, with which people become accustomed (habit) and from which people do not wish to deviate.

Contrast The difference in luminance (intensity of light) or color that makes an object visually distinguishable.

Disinfection For water, the removal or destruction of harmful microorganisms in drinking water.

Kindling The initial fuel stage of a fire; used to ignite sustaining fuel.

Luminance The intensity of light emitted from a surface per unit of area in a given direction.

Pasteurization For water, applying enough heat to water (< boiling point) to reduce the number of surviving microorganisms in the water to such a low level that they are unlikely to cause illness or disease.

Purification For water, the removal of pathogenic (disease causing) microorganisms in the water such as bacteria, viruses, and parasites.

Sterilization For water, raising the temperature of water high enough, and for long enough, to completely remove or destroy all living microorganisms.

Sustaining fuel Anything that burns for an extended period of time.

Tinder Anything that ignites at a very low temperature, with a spark, small flame, or other heat source.

REFERENCES AND SUGGESTED READING

Auerbach, Paul S., editor. 2017. *Wilderness Medicine*, 7th edition. Philadelphia, PA: Elsevier.

Auerbach, Paul. 2013. *Field guide to wilderness medicine*, 4th edition. St. Louis, MO: Mosby, Inc.

Backer, Howard D. 2012. Field water disinfection. In *Wilderness Medicine*, 6th edition, edited by Paul S. Auerbach, pp. 1324–1359. St. Louis, MO: Mosby, Inc.

Backer, Howard D. 2017. Field water disinfection. In *Wilderness Medicine*, 7th edition, edited by Paul S. Auerbach, pp. 1985–2030. Philadelphia, PA: Elsevier.

Bowman, Warren Jr., and Peter Kummerfeldt. 2017. Essential of wilderness survival. In *Wilderness Medicine*, Seventh Edition, edited by Paul S. Auerbach. pp. 1327–1357. Philadelphia, PA: Elsevier.

Burke, Edmund. 2001. *On the Sublime and Beautiful*. Vol. XXIV, Part 2. The Harvard Classics. New York: P.F. Collier & Son.

Campbell, John. 2013. *The Complete Survival in the Southwest: Guide to Desert Survival*. CreateSpace Independent Publishing Platform, On-Demand Publishing LLC.

Centers for Disease Control and Prevention. 2013. Resources for travelers: Water disinfection, heat. https://wwwnc.cdc.gov/travel/page/water-disinfection.

Centers for Disease Control and Prevention. 2014. Drinking water: A guide to drinking water treatment technologies for household use. http://www.cdc.gov/healthywater/drinking/home-water-treatment/household_water_treatment.html.

Cervantes, Flores and Déborah Xanat. 2003. Feasibility of semi-continuous solar disinfection system for developing countries at a household level. Master's thesis. Boston, MA: Massachusetts Institute of Technology.

Conroy, Ronán, Michael Meegan, Tina Joyce, Kevin McGuigan, and Joseph Barnes. 2001. Solar disinfection of drinking water protects against cholera in children under 6 years of age. *Archives of Disease in Childhood* 85, no. 4 (2001): 293–295.

Engineering Tool Box. 2016. Thermal conductivity of materials and gases. http://www.engineeringtoolbox.com/thermal-conductivity-d_429.html.

Fears, J. Wayne. 2000. *The Complete Book of Outdoor Survival*. Revised edition. Fairfield, OH: Krause Publications.

Gerba, Charles, and Joan B. Rose. 1990. Viruses in source and drinking water. In *Drinking Water Microbiology*. New York, NY: Springer-Verlag.

Harvard Health Publications, Harvard Medical School. 2016. Understanding the stress response. http://www.health.harvard.edu/staying-healthy/understanding-the-stress-response.

Hawkins, Seth C., Michael G. Millin, and Will Smith. 2017. Wilderness emergency medical services and response systems. In *Wilderness Medicine*, 7th edition, edited by Paul S. Auerbach. pp. 1200–1212. Philadelphia, PA: Elsevier.

Institute of Medicine of the National Academies. 2005. *Dietary Reference Intakes for Water, Potassium, Sodium, Chloride, and Sulfate*. Washington, DC: The National Academies Press.

Johnson, Mark. 2003. *The Ultimate Desert Handbook: A Manual for Desert Hikers, Campers, and Travelers*. New York: Ragged Mountain Press/McGraw Hill.

Joyce, Tina, Kevin McGuigan, Michael Elmore-Meegan, and Ronán M. Conroy. 1996. Inactivation of fecal bacteria in drinking water by solar heating. *Applied and Environmental Microbiology* 62, no. 2 (1996): 399–402.

Kemeny, Margaret E. 2003. The psychology of stress. *Current Direction in Psychological Science* 12, no. 4 (2003): 124–129.

Lindin, Cody. 2003. *98.6 Degrees: The Art of Keeping Your Ass Alive*. Layton, UT: Gibbs Smith.

Manning, Harvey, and Bob Cram. 1986. *Backpacking: One Step at a Time*, 4th edition. New York: Vintage Books.

Mayo Clinic. 2016. Diseases and conditions: Iron deficiency anemia – prevention. http://www.mayoclinic.org/diseases-conditions/iron-deficiency-anemia/basics/prevention/con-20019327.

McConnell, Ruby. 2016. *A Woman's Guide to the Wild: Your Complete Outdoor Handbook*. Seattle, WA: Sasquatch Books

Mears, Ray. 2003. *Bushcraft: An Inspired Guide to Surviving in the Wilderness*. New York: Hodder & Stoughton.

Nairne, James S. 2006. *Psychology: The Adaptive Mind*. Belmont, CA: Thomson Wadsworth.

Ngo, Mary Kim, and Charles Spence. 2010. Auditory, tactile, and multisensory cues facilitate search for dynamic visual stimuli. *Attention, Perception, & Psychophysics*. 72, no. 6, 1654–1655. doi:10.3758/APP.72.6.1654.

Nietzsche, Friedrich W. 1990. *The Twilight of the Idols and the Anti-Christ: Or How to Philosophize with a Hammer*. New York, NY: Penguin Classics.

Oates Peter M., Peter Shanahan, and Martin F. Polz. 2003. Solar disinfection (SODIS): Simulation of solar radiation for global assessment and application for point-of-use water treatment in Haiti. *Water Research* 37, no. 1.

Petzoldt, Paul. 1974. *The Wilderness Handbook*. New York: W.W. Norton & Company, Inc.

Psychologist World. 2016. General adaption syndrome: How your body copes with stressful situations and adapts to survive them. https://www.psychologistworld.com/stress/general-adaptation-syndrome.php.

Rao, Sridhar. 2008. Sterilization and disinfection. http://www.2ndchance.info/Salmonella-Rao2008.pdf.

Salas, Renee and Anderson, Susan. 2017. Women in the wilderness. In *Wilderness Medicine*, 7th edition, edited by Paul S. Auerbach, pp. 2118–2148. Philadelphia, PA: Elsevier.

Schlangenhauf, Patricia, Lin H. Chen, Mary E. Wilson, David O. Freedman, David Tcheng, et al. 2010. Sex and gender differences in travel-associated disease. *Clinical infectious diseases* 50, no. 6, 826–832.

Selye, Hans. 1936. A syndrome produced by diverse nocuous agents. *Nature,* 138, no. 3479, 32.

Siebert, Al. 2010. *The Survivor Personality: Why Some People Are Stronger, Smarter and More Skillful at Handling Life's Difficulties . . . and How You Can Be, Too*. New York: Berkley/Perigee Publishing.

Sobsey, Mark. 2003. Managing water in the home: Accelerated health gains from improved water supply. Geneva, Switzerland: World Health Organization, WHO/SDE/WSH.

U.S. Air Force. 1985a. *Search and Rescue Survival Training*. AF Regulation 64-4. Washington, DC.: Department of the Air Force.

U.S. Air Force. 1985b. *Aircrew Survival*. U.S. Air Force Pamphlet 64-5. Washington, DC.: U.S. Department of the Air Force.

U.S. Army, Marine Corps, Navy, Air Force. 1999. *Survival, Evasion, and Recovery: Multiservice Procedures for Survival, Evasion, and Recovery*. U.S. Army Regulation FM 21-76-1, U.S. Marine Corps Regulation MCRP 3-02H, U.S. Navy Regulation NWP 3-50.3, U.S. Air Force Regulation AFTTP(I)3-2.26. Washington, D.C.: Air Land Sea Application Center.

U.S. Army, Navy, and Air Force. 1999. Sanitary control and surveillance of field water supplies, TB Med 577; Navmed P-5010-9, AFOSH Standard 48-47. May 1, 1999. Washington, DC: Departments of Army, Navy and Air Force.

U.S. Department of the Interior National Park Service. 2016. How long does litter last? https://www.nps.gov/tuma/learn/kidsyouth/upload/HowLongDoesLitterLast.pdf.

U.S. Department of the Army. 2002. *U.S. Army Survival Handbook*. Guilford, CT: The Lyons Press.

U.S. Environmental Protection Agency. 2016. Ground water and drinking water: Emergency disinfection of drinking water. https://www.epa.gov/ground-water-and-drinking-water/emergency-disinfection-drinking-water.

Walter, Linda. 2011. Life without anxiety: To fear or not to fear, you're in control. *Psychology Today*, Blog. https://www.psychologytoday.com/blog/life-without-anxiety/201108/fear-or-not-fear-you-re-in-control.

White, George. 1992. *Handbook of Chlorination*. 3rd edition. New York, NY: Van Nostrand Reinhold.

Wiseman, John. 2014. *SAS Survival Handbook: The Ultimate Guide to Surviving Anywhere*. New York, NY: William Morrow Paperbacks.

Chapter Opener: Courtesy of NASAR; Backpack with external metal frame: © Hemera/Thinkstock/Getty; Small campfire: © Emil Ivanov/Alamy.

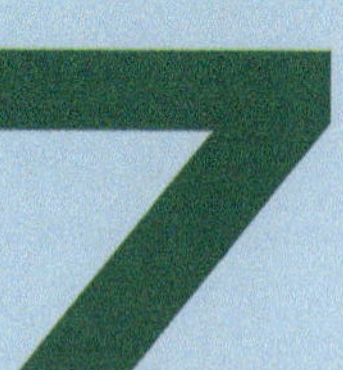

CHAPTER 7

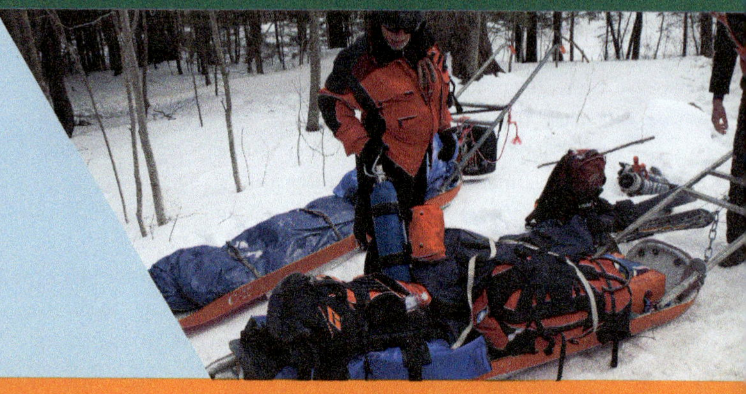

Search and Rescue Clothing

OBJECTIVES

Upon completion of this chapter and the related course activities, the student will be able to meet the following objectives:

- Describe the primary function of each of the following clothing layers:
  - Wicking
  - Insulation
  - Protective
- Describe at least three basic considerations when choosing clothing for the outdoors to protect the head, neck, hands, and feet.
- Discuss the positive and negative characteristics of the following materials used in clothing for the outdoors:
  - Cotton
  - Wool
  - Silk
  - Down
  - Synthetic
- Describe the basic characteristics of the different levels of waterproof and water-resistant fabrics.
- Discuss conduction, convection, radiation, and evaporation and how each relates to search and rescue (SAR) clothing.
- Explain the concept of layering in maintaining a comfortable body temperature.
- List at least three survival tips for SAR clothing.

Dress for the Occasion

Search and rescue (SAR) operations pose unique clothing challenges for SAR personnel. History shows that lightly dressed SAR responders often become accustomed to working hard and traveling through varied environments with no thought of their clothing needs should they suddenly be forced to spend an undetermined amount of time in harsh conditions. Many do not carry or wear the clothes needed to survive. A simple rule before starting out is to ask, "Is what I plan to wear and carry adequate for the expected weather and environments in which I will be working? What about carrying a bit more, just in case?"

In general, there is no need to reinvent the wheel when it comes to state-of-the-art clothing. Since many outdoor sports use new materials and technology in their sport-specific clothing systems, SAR personnel could easily borrow from others' experience by exploring clothing systems designed for use in sports such as climbing, backpacking, hunting, kayaking, cycling, mountain biking, mountaineering, skiing (Nordic and cross country), and adventure racing.

Understanding clothing and clothing systems is essential for SAR personnel. To be comfortable, effective, and safe in a variety of environments, an understanding of clothing materials, designs, and systems is necessary.

Clothing Materials

Fibers that comprise clothing may be either found in nature (natural) or be human-made (synthetic). In addition, each of these natural and synthetic fibers has its own unique characteristics. These fibers may be hollow, oily, chambered, scaled, porous, long, short, thick, curly, straight, **hydrophobic** (repel water), **hydrophilic** (absorb water), or any combination of these, depending on the material from which they are made. Enlightened textile and clothing manufacturers use the inherent characteristics of specific fibers to construct clothes that meet specialized needs. Durability, breathability, waterproofness, ability to wick moisture, insulation value when wet, and resistance to burning or melting are all variables that are manipulated using various fibers. Understanding the characteristics of a wide variety of fibers provides a foundation for understanding the principles of building a clothing system for SAR work.

Natural Fiber Materials

Natural fibers are those derived from plants or animals. Cotton comes from the cotton plant, wool from the shorn fleece of sheep, silk from the web of the silkworm, and down from the feathers of waterfowl.

Cotton

Cotton is the most common natural fiber and is often used in nontechnical clothing such as T-shirts and blue jeans. Cotton readily absorbs moisture (hydrophilic), but it does not easily release moisture to external clothing layers for evaporation. In fact, once cotton gets wet, it rapidly loses up to 90% of its insulative value, which is why it is generally not recommended as an insulating layer when one is trying to keep warm (Dow, 2017). Conversely, in warm or moderate climates, cotton provides excellent properties for protection because it helps keep the body cool through conduction and convection.

Since SAR operations usually involve physical labor, perspiration is always wetting one's clothing from the inside, and the environment is often wetting it from the outside. Thus, the SAR mantra, "cotton kills," refers to when cotton is worn inappropriately in cold environments (**FIGURE 7-1**).

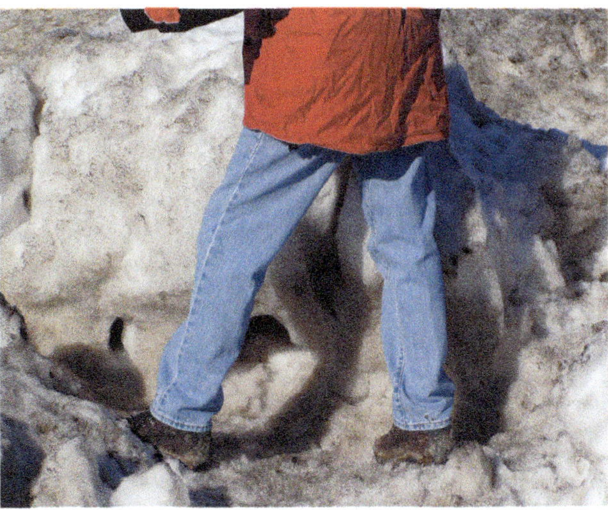

FIGURE 7-1 When kept dry, cotton affords excellent insulation against cold. However, when it gets wet from rain, snow, or perspiration, its insulation value drops to almost nothing. Thus, the SAR mantra "cotton kills" refers to when cotton is worn inappropriately in cold environments. Cotton jeans are usually not well suited for field SAR operations.
Courtesy of Donald Cooper.

Some types of cotton are better suited for use in SAR operations. Canvas, for example, is heavyweight cotton used for items that require strength and durability. Other strong, durable cottons include denim, duck, and poplin. When tightly woven, these fabrics are abrasion resistant, and when treated for water repellency, they can protect against light wind and rain.

Additional properties of cotton include the following:

- It burns easily but does not melt.
- It can be heavy, especially when wet.
- Light-colored, thin cotton is excellent for hot, dry climates because of its breathability and high ability to absorb water.
- Generally, it abrades easily (not very durable) unless blended with tougher synthetics or woven tightly and heavily
- It rots under continued wet or hot and sunny conditions.
- Thick cotton dries slowly from the outside, which is beneficial in hot, dry weather and detrimental in cold weather.
- Tightly woven cotton makes a good windbreak and may be water resistant, but it can also be heavy.
- It can freeze solid when wet in extreme cold.
- When cut or torn into strips, it can be used as a bandage, cravat, sling, or fire starter, and has multiple other uses.

Wool

True wool is spun from the fleece of sheep, but other fibers—also referred to as wool but actually from alpacas and llamas (camelids), and goats (cashmere)—have similar characteristics and are often softer and more expensive. Merino wool comes from Merino sheep and is prized for its softer feel. Cashmere and camelid fibers are frequently combined with Merino and true wool to produce a soft, durable weave that can be used in clothing designed to be worn against the skin.

The principal advantage of wool over many other fabrics is its ability to insulate even when wet. The fibers are naturally curly and trap air in tiny pockets between them. Wool in its raw, unprocessed state also contains lanolin, a wax secreted by the sebaceous glands of wool-bearing animals, which repels water. Processing and washing over time removes these natural oils, and dry cleaning does so even faster. To keep wool garments more water resistant and comfortable, they should not be laundered often, and when they are laundered, it should be with mild soap specially designed for use with wool.

In the past, wool was often scratchy and uncomfortable to wear against the skin because of the short, irritating, barb-like structures in the outer layer of the fiber (epicuticle). In fact, some individuals are especially sensitive to wool, thus SAR personnel should be mindful when using wool in patient packaging materials (e.g., wool blankets) that might come in direct contact with a patient's skin. Today, modern textile manufacturing processes have overcome the scratchiness problem by using softer blends (e.g., Merino, camelids, cashmere, synthetics), by marrying the wool to a layer of softer material, or by otherwise using special wool treatments to render the material extra soft and comfortable.

Wool remains one of the best insulating natural fibers, even when wet, and so it has been a primary choice of outdoor users for hundreds of years (**FIGURE 7-2**).

SAFETY TIP

Any clothing will lose its insulation qualities when dirty. Clean material maximizes dead air space. Keep clothing clean, especially in cold environments.

Research shows that people dressed in wool are more apt to survive in an outdoor environment than those dressed in cotton (Nyerges, 2014). However, the loose weave of some woolen fabrics does little to stop the wind. A close-weave, windproof shell is essential over this type of wool in cold weather where wind is a factor.

Additional properties of wool include the following:

- When wet, it generally does not freeze solid in extreme cold.
- It burns very slowly and is very resilient, breathable, and durable.
- In its pure form, it tears easily, so it is usually blended with other, stronger materials.
- It may give off an unpleasant odor when wet.

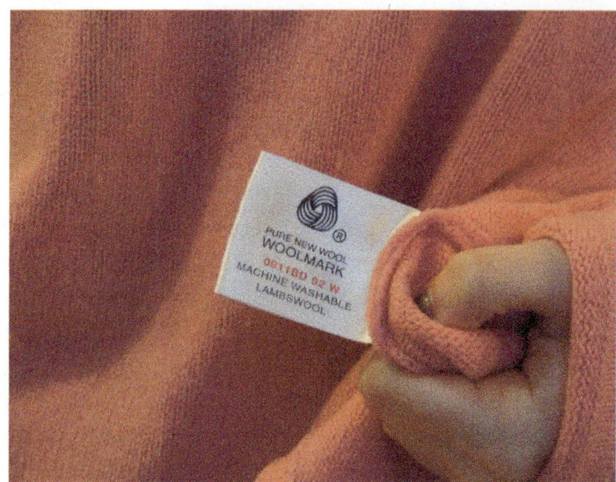

FIGURE 7-2 Wool remains one of the best insulating materials, even when wet, and so it has been a primary choice of outdoor users for hundreds of years.
Courtesy of Donald Cooper.

Silk

Silk is a natural fiber long recognized for its value in cold weather. It is the lightest, strongest, and softest of all natural fibers. It has hollow fibers that absorb and transport moisture away from the skin, making it a good insulator and useful as an underwear layer. Silk is noted for its comfort and higher relative cost, but the price has come down over the past few years. Silk blends are also now available that are more competitively priced and are often as comfortable as pure silk.

Silk can be used alone or combined with synthetics or wool. It comes in several forms, the most common of which is spun filament silk consisting of several strands of monofilament fibers twisted around one another. Spun filament silk is heavier, softer, and even warmer than monofilament silk.

Additional properties of silk include the following:

- Silk is very comfortable against the skin, traps much air, and is very light.
- It is relatively expensive and tends to hold odors and stains.
- Silk is damaged by a hot iron, inorganic acids, sunlight, perspiration, strong soaps, and alkaline substances.

Down

Down is the soft, fine type of feather found beneath the larger, tougher feathers of a duck or a goose. It is an excellent form of insulation when dry because of its ability to trap vast amounts of air in the clusters or plumes it forms when the fine feathers clump together. It is also lightweight and very compressible.

Virtually no other insulation traps as much dead air spaces pound for pound, and thus, it is one of the best insulators available when it is clean and dry. This dead air space trapped in the plumes provides loft, which in turn traps air that prevents heat loss. Down is used in bedding (duvets), pillows, sleeping bags, parkas, sweaters, vests, booties, pants, hats, and gloves.

According to the IDFL Institute and Laboratory, international developers of standards regarding textile fills, *down* refers to a mix of down clusters, feather fibers, feathers, and residue. To be labeled down, however, more than 75% of the mix must be down and down fibers, and less than 25% of the mix should be feather fiber, quill feathers, landfowl feathers and fibers, damaged and broken feathers, and residue. A label claiming "100% down" is not permitted by the standards (IDFL.com, 2016).

The textile industry refers to *fill power* as the number of cubic inches displaced by 1 ounce of down. The higher the fill power, the more air an ounce of down can trap. Standard entry level for the industry is 550 fill power down, which means that 1 ounce of down fills 550 cubic inches. The highest quality (usually goose) down commercially available is 900 fill down, and generally costs much more than lower fill power items. The advantage of higher fill power is obvious: greater loft for less weight.

As a type of insulation added to clothing being worn in extremely dry, cold conditions, down is superior to almost everything else. However, when wet, down loses nearly all its insulation properties and becomes virtually useless. To avoid this problem, some manufacturers have treated the down clusters with a water-repellant, polymer coating, which prevents the absorption of water (i.e., hydrophobic). This allows the clusters of down to stay dry longer, loft better, and dry faster than untreated down. Brands that include this or similar technologies include DriDown™, DownTek™, and Nikwax Hydrophobic Down™. Each of these items usually requires periodic treatment to maintain its hydrophobic characteristics.

Down must be sandwiched between layers of materials to stabilize it, that is, keep it from shifting to one corner of the garment. Therefore, some mention needs to be made of the quality of the material from which a down garment is made: the stabilizing fabric. When this material is very thin (read, "cheap"), and low-grade down is used, tiny feather quills can punch through the material and cause irritation of the wearer and loss of the down. This is undesirable but should be expected to some extent with most down garments.

Since SAR personnel frequently store gear for long periods of time, it should be noted that down-filled garments and gear (e.g., sleeping bags, overshoes, hats) should be stored uncompressed. That is, items with down in them should not be compressed during storage. They should be hung or laid out so that they are stored as close to full size as possible. Storing them with all the air squeezed out tends to reduce the loft of the garment and thus its insulation power over time.

Additional properties of down include the following:

- It clumps up with moisture and dampness.
- It absorbs and retains odors and will mildew when damp.
- Some people are allergic to down, but the associated dust mites and molds are more often the actual cause of down-related allergies (Kilpio et al., 1998).

Synthetic Fiber Materials

Synthetic materials are not found in nature; they are made from fibers that are produced by chemical synthesis. A wide variety of chemical compositions and fiber designs allow synthetic fibers to be an outstanding basis for materials used in outdoor clothing.

Polyester

Developed by DuPont in the 1940s, polyester is the generic term for any petroleum-based fiber, and it is used in the production of everything from seat belts to pillows (Dow, 2017). Today, it is also the most common material used in outdoor clothing. It is strong, durable, and inexpensive, and it is now used to produce some of our most versatile outdoor garments.

Fabrics made from polyester fibers are washable, durable, and softer than other synthetic fabrics, giving them a softer, more comfortable feel in clothing. Polyester fibers can be manufactured in almost any thickness and design, can be molded with a hollow core for added insulation, and are hydrophobic. However, polyester is better at wicking moisture than many other synthetics. Polyester fibers move moisture away from the skin by wicking it along the fibers to the surface of the fabric, where it evaporates.

Loosely woven polyester fleece traps air and is very warm for its weight but allows wind to pass through it easily. Tightly woven polyester can resist wind and water but loses much of the insulative value of fleece. However, the two can also be combined to provide the benefits of both. One example is W.L. Gore's Windstopper® fabric, which is completely windproof, somewhat water resistant, and can be built into fleece or a shell.

Polyester insulation evaporates water readily and has high **moisture regain**, but it is not as compressible as down. Time, repeated use, prolonged compression, and multiple washings break down polyester fibers, which leads to loss of loft and insulative value. Thus, like down, polyester insulation should not be compressed in storage.

Some examples of popular polyester insulation materials include Polartec®, PolarGuard™ (Delta), Primaloft®, Thinsulate™ (mixture of polypropylene and polyethylene terephthalate [PET], thinner than polyester fibers), and Climashield® (Apex).

Polypropylene

Polypropylene fiber was one of the first synthetic fibers used in undergarments and wicking layers (Dow, 2017). It is durable, dries rapidly, insulates when wet, and wicks moisture well. It is hydrophobic and has the lowest thermal conductivity and highest insulation power of any synthetic fiber; however, it also stains easily, melts at relatively low temperatures, and retains odors, which is why it has been largely replaced by newer synthetic materials like Capilene®, Coolmax®, and Polartec®.

Nylon

Nylon, like polyester, is a polymer filament fiber and is stronger than cotton for an equivalent weight. It is also abrasion resistant, quick drying, long wearing, and nylon threads are almost completely impervious to penetration by both water and water-repelling compounds. This presents difficulty in two respects. First, perspiration stays on the surface and does not easily pass through the fabric. Thus, if nylon is worn as underwear, perspiration remains against the skin and is not wicked away. Second, waterproofing compounds do not unite with the nylon fibers as in cotton, and therefore must be "painted" onto the nylon material to fill in between threads.

One high-quality type of nylon, called *ripstop*, is alternately stitched with thin and thick threads, giving it a checkerboard appearance. If torn, the tear allegedly stops at the thicker cross thread—thus, the name ripstop. Ripstop nylon is generally wind and abrasion resistant and is often used to make pants, shirts, and windproof shells.

Another variety of nylon, Cordura® (also developed by DuPont), is an abrasion-resistant, lightweight, and durable fiber available in various deniers (a measure of stitches per unit area). As examples, a lightweight version of the material (160-denier Cordura) is perfect for active and performance outerwear, and a heavyweight version (1000-denier Cordura) is more suited for backpacks or boots. Many styles of alpine/outdoor technical outerwear also use high denier Cordura in high-impact areas such as knees, elbows, and around the ankles to help resist abrasion.

Nylon is manufactured into a variety of products, including parachutes and rope. It is also commonly used in conjunction with a waterproofing coating or membrane to make an excellent shell. Nylon is also used in various blends (e.g., polyester/nylon) to make garments with characteristics of both materials.

The wide variety of colors in which nylon is available makes it easy for the wearer to be very visible (e.g., bright blue or orange), or very invisible (e.g., camouflage). The preference for SAR personnel is always to be more visible, so camouflage and darker colors for outer layers should be avoided, used only when brighter colors are not available, or supplemented with a high visibility vest, hat, etc.

In general, nylon exhibits the following characteristics:

- Retains high strength when wet
- Resists alkali, mildew, and insect damage well
- Resists abrasion well
- Washes and dries easily
- Blends well with other fibers
- Does not absorb much moisture
- Can be damaged by sunlight
- Has a melting point of 263°C (505°F) but may become malformed (in a hot dryer or near a fire) well below that temperature
- Absorbs and holds perspiration and body oils (between fibers)
- Can be easily damaged (holes and melting) from fire sparks and embers

Blends

Blends of natural and synthetic fabrics are also available, and the combinations have properties of all fibers they incorporate. For example, polyester is often blended with wool to make socks that provide outstanding insulation, stretch, durability, and better retain their shape than wool alone. Polyester shrinks less than cotton, so polyester is often added to a cotton shirt to reduce shrinkage.

Waterproof and Breathable Fabrics

Waterproof and breathable fabrics are designed to allow moisture in the form of water vapor to pass through the fabric while repelling water in the form of droplets. This allows evaporating perspiration (vapor) to pass through to the outside while preventing rain from penetrating to the inside. Fabrics are made waterproof and breathable through the application of coatings, laminates, and durable water-repellent finishes.

Laminates. Laminated fabrics are manufactured by bonding a waterproof and breathable membrane to the inside of a durable fabric, usually nylon (fabric backer). The laminate is most often combined with a second, durable, water-resistant outer layer (face fabric) or sandwiched between a durable, water-resistant outer layer (two-ply) and an inner liner (three-ply). The latter is more durable and comfortable but also a bit heavier.

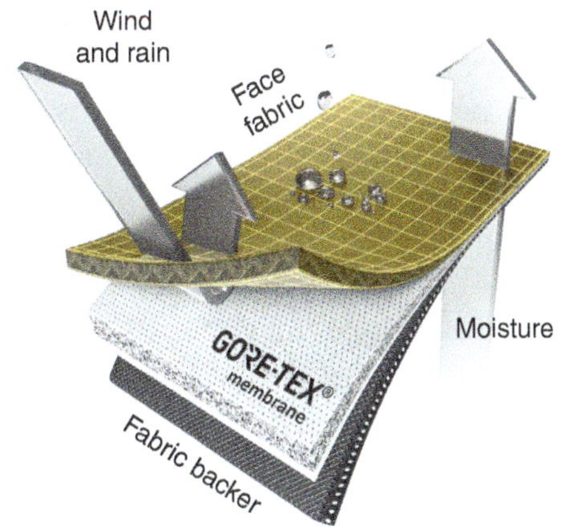

FIGURE 7-3 Gore-Tex® fabric and how it works.
Courtesy of W.L. Gore & Associates, Inc.

W.L. Gore and Associates developed the first waterproof and breathable laminate membrane (Gore-Tex®), but today there are many manufacturers of similar products (**FIGURE 7-3**). The technology is based on a synthetic membrane that is stretched to cause small (micro) tears in the laminate that allow water vapor from perspiration to pass through, making it breathable, while preventing water droplets from entering from the outside, making it water resistant. Note that such a laminate is technically not waterproof. Water under pressure can be pushed through the membrane, and if the material is dirty or contaminated, the membrane can leak, allowing water to pass through. Some manufacturers—Gore and eVent® being the most predominant—further treat or coat the laminate to reduce contamination and thus leaking, keeping it breathable under a wide variety of conditions.

SEARCH AND RESCUE TIP

Waterproof: Material is impermeable to water, even water under pressure.

Water-repellent: Sheds water that is not under pressure; however, falling or wind-blown rain may penetrate the fabric.

Water-resistant: The material temporarily resists water under pressure.

Waterproof and breathable: Material is nearly impermeable to water droplets (waterproof) but allows water vapor to pass (breathable).

Coated Fabrics. The material in a garment can be coated with a liquid, such as polyurethane, that is further treated so that it dries leaving cracks (**micropores**) that are big enough to allow water vapor to escape but too small to allow water droplets to penetrate. This type of coating is both breathable and waterproof, although less so than a laminate. If the polyurethane is applied thicker or without the specialized treatment that causes micropores, the coated material is not breathable at all. In fact, a heavier coating of polyurethane can be applied to nylon to produce rubberized garments that are useful in marine environments where waterproofness is necessary but the accumulation of sweat is not an issue. It is also a good method of waterproofing nylon tarpaulins and rain flies.

Coated fabrics are generally less breathable and durable than laminates, but they are also much less expensive and usually more compressible.

Soft Shell Fabrics. Soft shell fabrics use soft, flexible, and tightly woven outer layers to provide moderate water and wind resistance while remaining very breathable. To enhance these characteristics, some manufacturers add a water- and wind-resistant laminate layer, and a durable water-repellent (DWR) finish. These garments can simultaneously serve as a warm insulation layer while providing an outer layer that offers moderate protection from wind and precipitation, which is why these garments are popular with those participating in highly aerobic activities where rain is not a significant concern, much like many SAR situations.

Durable Water-Repellent Finish. After the manufacturer constructs a waterproof and breathable garment, a durable water-repellent finish is applied. This enhances water resistance but does not reduce breathability. The finish works by adhering to the fibers and not the pores. This causes water droplets to bead up and roll off the exterior of the garment rather than penetrate (**FIGURE 7-4**). The DWR finish can wear off

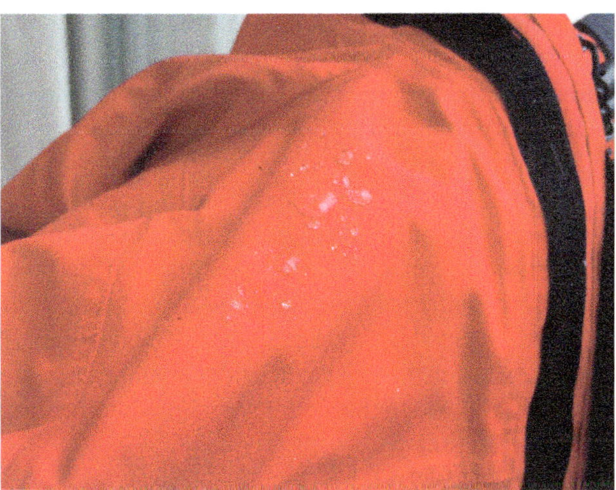

FIGURE 7-4 After the manufacturer constructs a waterproof and breathable garment, a durable water-repellent (DWR) finish is applied. This enhances water resistance without reducing breathability and causes water droplets to bead up and roll off the exterior of the garment rather than penetrate.
Courtesy of Donald Cooper.

over time, and its water repellency can be detrimentally affected by smoke and the buildup of dirt and contaminants. Thus, manufacturers usually recommend that their waterproof and breathable garments be washed periodically—one recommendation is at least yearly (Dow, 2017). The finish may also be restored by placing the clean garment in a dryer on a low setting for 10 to 15 minutes. If water no longer beads up on the outside layer of a garment, the DWR finish can be reapplied either by a spray-on product (when the garment includes a laminate layer) or a wash-in product (when the garment does not have a laminate layer). Examples of these aftermarket products include NikWax® Soft Shell Spray, NikWax® TX.Direct, and Gear Aid ReviveX®.

Heat Loss and Garment Features

Heat Transfer

The rate of heat transfer through clothing depends on three factors. First is quantity and thickness of dead air spaces trapped within the clothing and its layers. In addition, if the skin touches clothing, heat may be lost through conduction. For cold, still air conditions, thick layers of dead air spaces—such as those found in dry down—or other fiber-filled clothing are needed for warmth.

Second is the amount of air that passes through a material: the more air that passes through the clothing, the greater the heat loss through convection and evaporation. Layered clothing traps air between layers and against the skin. The body warms this trapped air, which keeps the body warm. If air moves through the clothing, this warm air is replaced with colder air, which robs the body of warmth. Large knit, wool sweaters and fleece jackets are fine in still air but may allow rapid heat loss in even moderate winds.

Third is water and moisture, which increase heat loss mostly through conduction. Heat loss through wet clothing is generally very rapid since thermal conductivity of water is 24 times greater than still air. This means that wet clothing can extract body heat nearly 200 times faster than dry clothing, depending on the material from which the clothing is made (Engineering Tool Box, 2016).

Garment Closures

Closures can be problems if they are not designed or applied properly. When choosing a closure, consider the environment in which it will be used. Most zippers offer little insulation or protection from the wind and necessitate some type of covering or at least some additional consideration. A covering or flap over the zipper usually does the job for wind and warmth, but the result is not waterproof. Zippers are available that provide a waterproof and windproof barrier on the outer (shell) layer (**FIGURE 7-5A**). Snaps are hard to work while wearing gloves and can get clogged with dirt or snow, but if they can be set without having to be adjusted in the field, they can work well. Buttons can be an annoyance and even painful if something applies pressure to them against the skin, which is why they are usually reserved for insulation layers and more fashionable outerwear. Hook-and-loop closures (e.g., Velcro®) are often used to close sleeves and storm flaps on outer layer jackets and parkas (**FIGURE 7-5B**). Although not waterproof, hook-and-loop closures generally offer complete closure and versatility, are easily adjusted in the field, and offer moderate protection against water and wind (**FIGURE 7-5C**). However, loosely woven fabrics (e.g., fleece, wool, etc.) can get stuck to the hooks, causing some annoyance, and mud and wet snow can clog the hooks and loops and prevent them from operating properly.

Seams can be a problem, especially if waterproofness is important. During garment design, seams can be placed in a different area of a garment to help minimize the potential for water penetration, for example, away from the top of the shoulder in rain gear. Seams can also be taped and sealed to prevent leakage in waterproof garments (**FIGURE 7-5D**).

Vents may also be included in higher quality insulation and protective layer garments. These features are usually located in high heat and perspiration areas to allow moisture and heat to escape quickly without having to remove the garment. Locations of vents are usually such that, even when open, the waterproof characteristics of the garment can be maintained (**FIGURE 7-6**).

In SAR, having quick and easy access to pocket items is a convenience that borders on necessity. Since many otherwise useful outer layers are designed for recreation and not work, pockets are often missing altogether, minimally sized, or inappropriately placed. It is highly recommended that the placement and size of externally accessible pockets be a primary consideration when selecting and purchasing clothes for SAR work. Some thought must also be given to where pockets, zippers, and other closures fall when a pack is worn.

SAR personnel may also benefit from clothing specifically designed for active outdoor sports. As an example, trousers designed for snowboarding are often durable, loose-fitting, comfortable, warm, waterproof, and contain numerous pockets. Some have zip-off legs, and their loose fit allows for additional layers underneath.

Many useful types, styles, and materials have been developed to help cross-country runners run in a wide

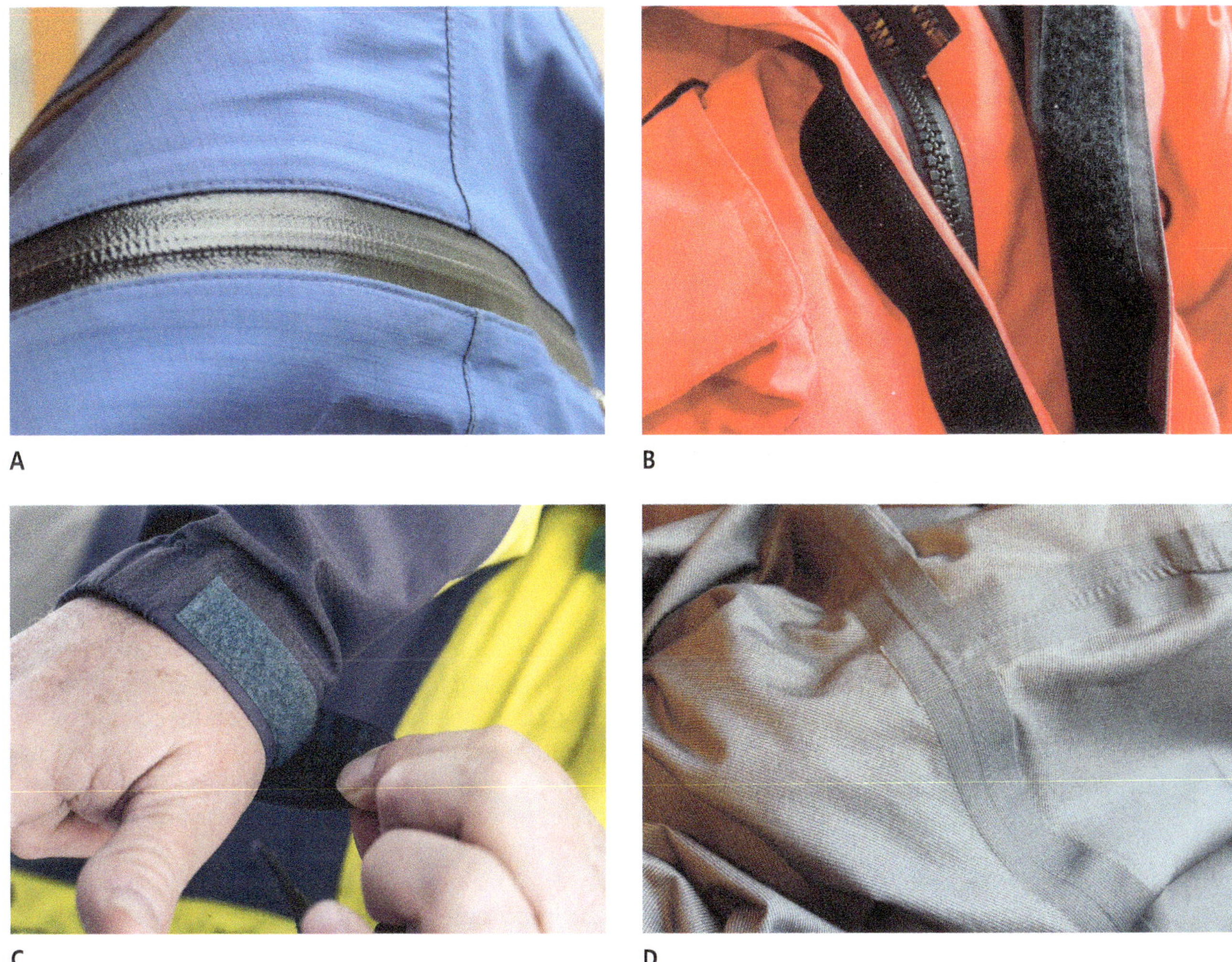

FIGURE 7-5 **A.** Zippers are available that provide a waterproof and windproof barrier on the outer (shell) layer. **B.** Hook-and-loop closure over zipper. Although not waterproof, hook-and-loop closures generally offer complete closure and versatility, are easily adjusted in the field, and offer moderate protection against water and wind. **C.** Hook-and-loop closure around wrist. **D.** Seams can be taped and sealed to prevent leakage in waterproof garments. Shown are taped seams inside a waterproof jacket.

A, B and **D:** Courtesy of Donald Cooper; **C:** © 2016 Howard Paul, Photography for Communication and Commerce.

variety of weather conditions. Lightweight, warm, long-sleeved shirts are common and wick moisture away from the skin while providing some wind and thermal protection. Of course, the same items are also available for the lower body. Some shirts have glove attachments to help protect the wrists and backs of the hands from sun, wind, and weather. Hats have been developed to block/reflect the sun while allowing perspiration to easily escape and evaporate. Many of these features make garments expensive, but just knowing that these types of garments and features exist could be beneficial to SAR personnel.

Layering

Each of us is a heat-producing, homeothermic organism (able to maintain a constant body temperature) that depends on clothing to protect us from environmental extremes. However, each of us also has a different tolerance level or comfort zone for deviations from the body's normal temperature, so a system of protecting one's body is needed that is versatile enough to work for different people in different conditions and portable enough to fit into a SAR pack. One way to accomplish this has been termed the *layering system* and involves the use of multiple, adjustable layers of garments that can easily be added or removed to suit the environment, conditions, and desired level of heat loss. Multiple layers are used in lieu of one heavy layer to allow for fine-tuning of one's comfort.

As physical exertion or the outside temperature increases, layers can be removed to facilitate heat loss and the movement of evaporating perspiration away from the body. As exertion decreases or the outside

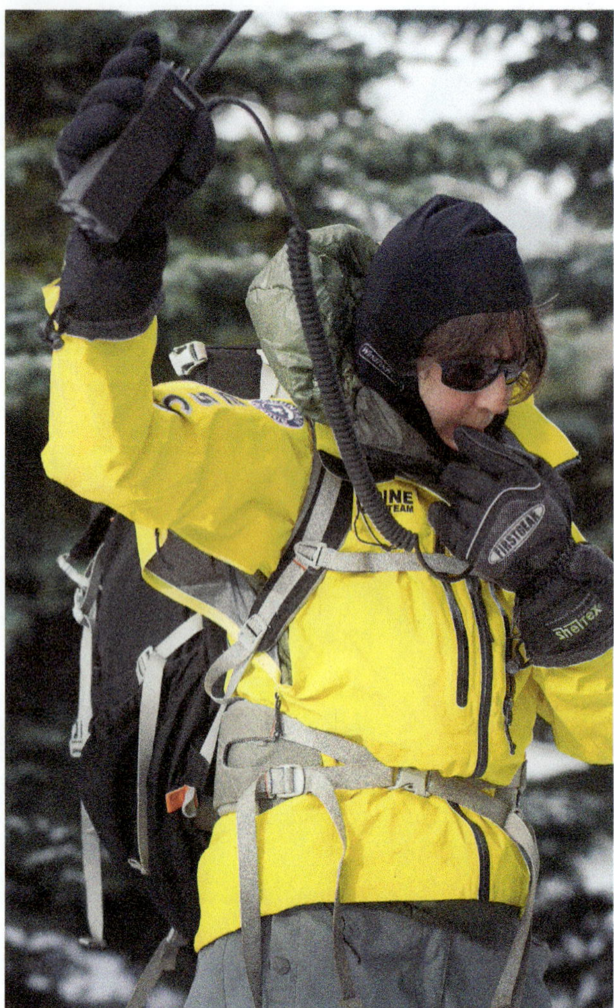

FIGURE 7-6 Vents are often integrated into higher quality shells to allow moisture and heat to escape without having to remove the garment.

temperature drops, layers can be added to reduce heat loss. A primary principle of the layering method is that several thin layers of clothing trap more air between them, and thus provide more insulation, than one massively thick layer. The ideal layering system seeks to establish a balance between breathability, wicking (movement of moisture away from the skin), quick drying, insulation, durability, wind resistance, and water repellence while remaining lightweight and offering freedom of movement with a minimum amount of bulk.

The system suggested for SAR consists of a wicking layer, an insulation layer, and a protective layer, and the fit of each layer is important. The wicking layer must be snug but not be too tight or confining. The insulation layer must fit comfortably over the wicking layer, adding warmth without restricting movement. The protective layer must fit over the insulation layer without compressing the insulation, which would reduce the amount of trapped air and thus insulation, without constricting the wrists and ankles. The intended combination of all the layers should be tested prior to going into the field to check for points of pressure and abrasion from things such as seams, belts, zippers, harnesses, boots, **gaiters**, and pack straps.

Generally, clothes for SAR operations should meet the BUBU criteria, meaning that they should be **b**ig (able to fit additional layer beneath), **u**nconstricting (not tight, especially at the ankles and wrists), **b**aggy (loose-fitting to allow freedom of movement), and **u**gly (meaning high-visibility and function are more important than fashion).

Wicking Layer—Moisture Management

The wicking layer is worn against the skin and helps regulate body temperature by moving moisture, including perspiration, away from the skin. This layer should be snug enough to avoid wrinkles in the fabric that may cause irritation by belts, harnesses, pack straps, or outer layers, but not too snug to restrict movement or blood flow. The seams should also fall where they do not cause irritation or annoyance.

For hygiene, discretion, and sometimes comfort, many prefer to wear undergarments such as briefs, boxers, a bra, panties, or an undershirt against the skin. These are often made of cotton for ease of cleaning, comfort, and low cost. In cold weather, cotton can hold moisture against the skin, does not wick moisture away, loses insulation value when wet, and may impede the performance of other clothing layers. Some people, therefore, prefer not to wear underwear at all. This is especially prevalent in hot environments where perspiration would quickly wet a cotton garment and hold it damp against the skin. Unfortunately, over long periods, this could cause chaffing, irritation, and even injury. The option to wear this layer is, of course, up to the wearer, but, overall, undergarments of the appropriate material (usually quick-drying synthetics) are recommended if for no other reason than to extend the usable life of other clothing that would normally be worn over this layer.

Although the wicking layer provides some insulation, its primary function is to control moisture and provide comfort against the skin. Functionally, the outer layers should pull moisture away from both the skin and the wicking (inner) layer to the outside of the garments where it can evaporate. If moisture is not wicked away, it remains on the skin and in the clothing, which can reduce comfort and potentially lead to either **hypothermia** (in cold weather) or **hyperthermia** (in hot weather).

Most modern cold weather garments that qualify as a wicking layer (or underwear) come in ultra-lightweight, lightweight, mid-weight, and expedition weight. Heavier weight equates to thicker material and increased insulation.

Since it is not easy to adjust this layer once donned, only the lightest or thinnest of these garments necessary to maintain comfort should be worn. A zipped top is one way to add versatility to the wicking layer in that it can be unzipped to allow ventilation or zipped to provide protection.

In cool weather, the warmth of dry, snug-fitting garments worn against the skin is often preferred. Although thin silk or wool may work fine, fabrics such as variations of polyester (e.g., Capilene®, Coolmax®, and Polartec®) are excellent at passing moisture from the skin to outer layers for evaporation. Many of these now have the additional benefit of odor control that stops the growth of odor-causing bacteria on fabrics. For maximum performance, synthetic underwear layers should be thin and in close contact with the skin so that perspiration moisture can easily pass through it to outer layers. Therefore, a synthetic insulation layer is often recommended over its natural fiber counterpart when physical exertion is expected (e.g., skiing, SAR operations).

In hot weather, moisture-laden clothing close to the skin can prevent evaporation and reduce the body's ability to control its temperature—two bad things for the SAR worker. Thus, many prefer to wear loose absorbent clothing with minimal or no underwear so that air can flow freely next to the skin and promote evaporation, drying, and cooling. Thin cotton, silk, and even fine grades of wool work well as a loose layer and may feel comfortable in the heat. Whatever the material, wearing very baggy clothing in hot environments promotes the "bellows effect" and keeps the body cool. The same wind that can kill in a cold environment can save a life in very hot environments.

Socks and Feet

Socks deserve more than just superficial consideration. Socks should not clump up against the feet or cause constriction or abrasion. They should provide comfort, promote circulation, wick moisture away from the skin, and provide insulation in cold weather. Cotton socks, like cotton underwear, are generally not recommended for strenuous backcountry travel in any weather but are especially poor in cold weather. They are poor insulators when wet, absorb and retain perspiration readily, stay wet, and hold the moisture against the skin, which softens the skin and makes it more susceptible to blisters and abrasions. For constant, strenuous activities, including walking long distances, two pairs of socks are recommended: one thin, smooth, wicking layer against the skin (e.g., silk, polyester, nylon) to wick away moisture, and one wool or wool blend insulating layer (thickness dependent on environment) for warmth and cushioning.

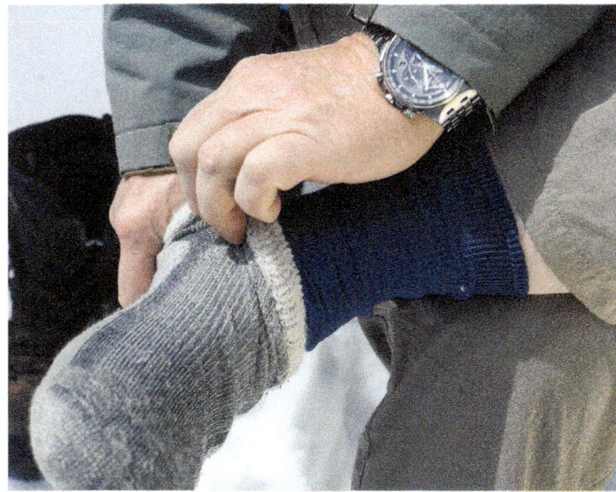

FIGURE 7-7 Wearing two pairs of socks (one thin layer against the skin and one insulating layer, as needed) helps keep the feet dry and minimizes mechanical friction against the skin that leads to blisters.

This helps keep the feet dry and warm (as necessary) and minimizes the mechanical friction on the skin of the feet that leads to blisters (**FIGURE 7-7**).

SAR work requires that the feet be monitored and cared for constantly. Completely wash and massage the feet at the end of every day and let them dry thoroughly. During the same day or operational period, do not rinse or wash the feet between long field exercises or assignments. This causes the skin on the feet to soften and become more prone to abrasion and injury. Wait until the end of the travel day to wash the feet, and change into clean socks at least daily. A preferable alternative to submerging the feet in water during SAR operations might be to use a damp towel or disposable towelette to wipe off the feet without getting them soaking wet. During long field operations when washing one's feet is not a simple option, changing into clean socks at least once per day should work in the short term.

Insulation Layer

The insulation layer includes garments worn over the wicking layer and under the protective or shell layer. The purpose of the insulation layer is, well, insulation, and it may include multiple garments, each of which should fit comfortably without being constricting, dry quickly, and provide insulation (**FIGURE 7-8**). Multiple closures in this layer offer alternative methods of ventilation without actually removing the entire layer. For example, unbutton some buttons or unzip a zipper (partially or all the way). In moderate conditions, where an outer, protective

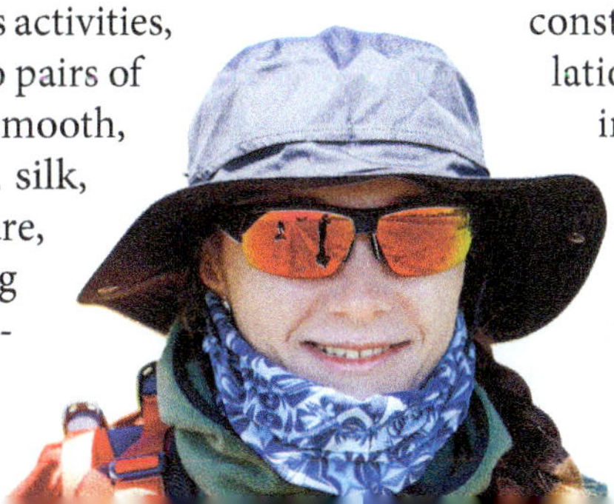

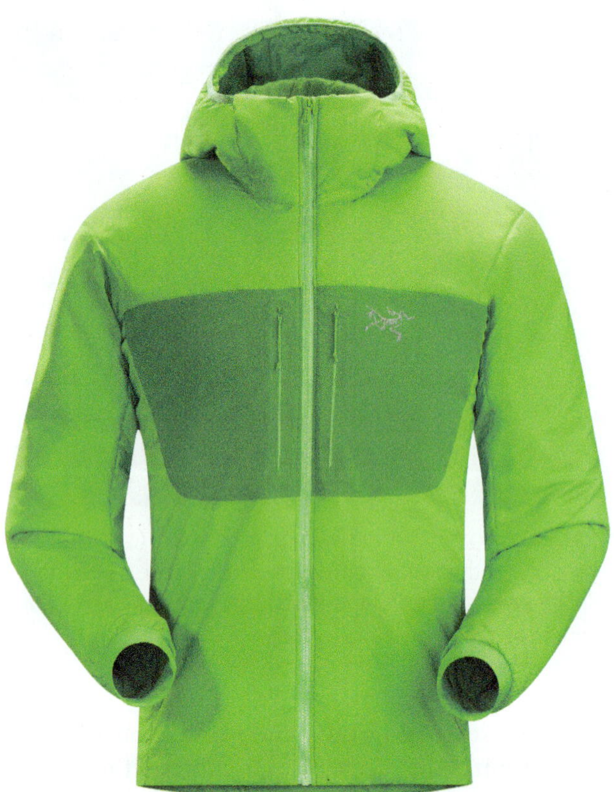

FIGURE 7-8 An example of an insulation layer: a water-resistant, wind-resistant, air-permeable, insulating jacket designed to be worn beneath a waterproof, breathable outer, protective layer. It allows air to pass through to prevent vapor accumulation.
Courtesy of Arc'teryx.

layer is not worn and the insulation layer is exposed to the environment, durability and snag/tear resistance should also be considered. This might also be a good place for a water-resistant, soft shell fabric garment used as an outer layer.

With very few exceptions, material thickness equates to insulation and warmth, but insulation is better achieved through multiple thin layers than one thick layer. Examples of garments that might work well as insulation layers include sweaters, fiber pile jackets and trousers, parkas, insulated vests, coveralls, mittens, face masks, or anything that might help prevent heat loss. The use of cotton in the insulation layer may be acceptable in dry conditions where little activity is expected, but in cold temperatures where clothes are likely to get wet, cotton is not a good choice and should be replaced with a wool or light/midweight synthetic shirt, sweater, or fleece.

The style of the insulating garment is also important. Pullover, button-down, full-zip, and integrated systems (insulation that zips into a shell) are some of the options. Whatever style is chosen, the closure systems should be varied between layers for best results. For example, if front zippers are present in both insulation and shell layers, a relatively unprotected area exists in the center of the chest where the zippers overlap. Alternating the location of closures between layers can prevent this type of problem.

Many garment manufacturers suggest synthetic insulation layers because they retain much of their insulating ability when wet, wick better, and dry more quickly than natural fibers. Polyester fleece has become very popular for good reason. Besides being soft and lightweight, polyester fleece fibers trap dead air well and are hydrophobic. Also popular are down-like, synthetic fill materials such as Primaloft®, PolarGuard®, Thermolite®, Quallofil®, and Thermoloft®, all of which are moisture resistant, nonallergenic, and quick drying.

Generally, when dry, polyester fleece and batting, goose down, and wool all have similar insulation values for the same thickness. The exceptions to this rule include some high-density foams and synthetics such as Thinsulate®, which provides nearly twice the insulation per unit of thickness. If insulation comparisons are made by weight only, however, dry, clean, high-quality goose down is unparalleled.

Insulation capability when wet is especially important when considering usefulness of a garment over a broad spectrum of environmental conditions. In this regard, synthetics are superior to all-natural materials (e.g., down, wool, and cotton) because they retain more of their loft and insulation while absorbing less—and being less effected by—water.

Insulation of the torso is most important and may be accomplished with a fleece vest or jacket. Extremities—including legs, arms, hands, feet, face, and head—are also important areas to protect from heat loss (covered further below). The insulation provided should be adequate for all climatic conditions the wearer may encounter, and, again, multiple thin layers are more versatile than one thick layer.

Multilayer garments are available that serve as both an insulation and protective layer. Soft shell garments with tightly woven fabrics and a DWR finish are common examples of this and may be useful when a separate protective, outer layer is not needed, such as when rain and extreme cold are not expected. Manufacturers also produce garments that combine a soft insulation layer with a waterproof outer layer. These types of garments may be useful in conditions that are wet but not extreme and where vigorous exercise is not expected.

Technology also offers an interesting twist on garments that could be used in the insulation layer. Several manufacturers offer battery-powered, electric jackets, trousers, vests, socks, and gloves. Unlike the electric blankets of the past that have the visible wires running through them to produce heat, these garments use lightweight batteries to conduct heat through imbedded microfibers. In many of these garments, the fibers are flexible, washable, and as soft as the fabric through which they are woven. This technology may be expensive and not always appropriate for SAR work, but it is another great example of how technology can positively impact outdoor wear.

Protective Outer Layer

The protective layer is the layer that protects the wearer from dirt, wind, sun, sand, rain, and snow. At a minimum, it should cover and protect the head, neck, torso, legs, and arms. The protective layer should fit easily and loosely over any insulation layers without compressing them. It should also avoid too much bulk that could cause problems with packs or other gear. Multiple pockets are also desirable, especially in SAR work, and they must be roomy, accessible while wearing gloves, and include a cover flap or zipper to secure any contents. Zippers anywhere in the protective layer must be easy to operate while wearing gloves and must be as waterproof as the rest of the garment (**FIGURE 7-9**).

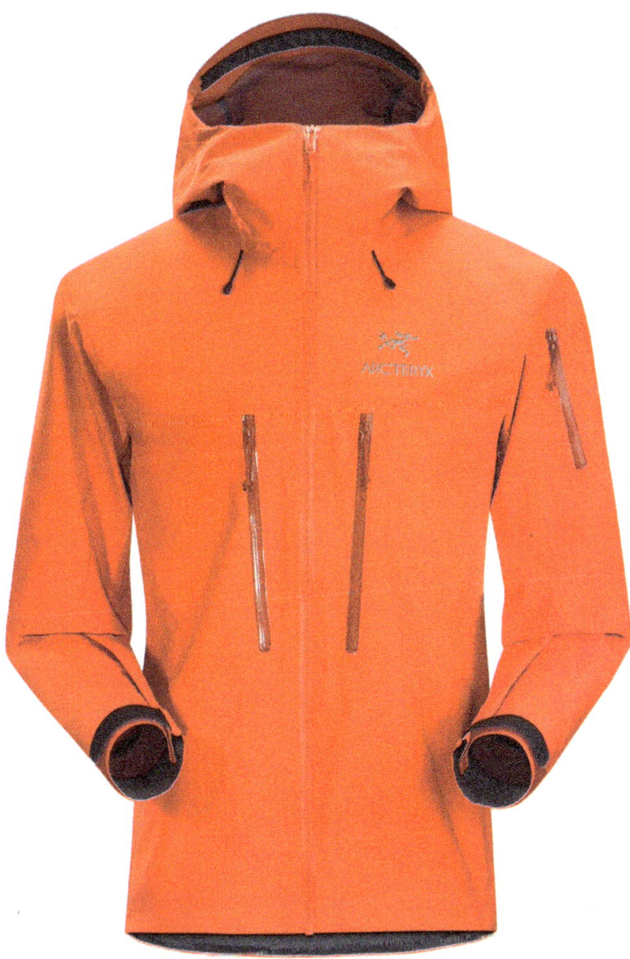

FIGURE 7-9 An example of a high-performance protective layer jacket designed for extended activities (such as SAR operations) in severe alpine environments. It is waterproof, windproof, breathable, abrasion resistant, and includes waterproof zippers throughout.
Courtesy of Arc'teryx.

Effectiveness in the protective layer is dependent on the tightness of the weave of the fabric rather than its thickness. However, as the weave gets tighter, the garment becomes less breathable, allowing less moisture to escape from within. Tight weave produces a durable, abrasion-resistant shell but must be balanced with the need for breathability. This is often achieved through the integration of a laminate layer rather than just a tight weave. Excessive exercise and perspiration can overwhelm the breathability of a protective layer, so additional ventilation is often incorporated into protective layers through vent flaps and armpit zippers (see Figure 7-6).

Protective-layer garments range from light, water-resistant pullovers and wind shells to full-zip, hooded, heavy parkas. They may be lined, insulated, waterproof, water-resistant, or have many other characteristics. Their length may vary from short, waist-length (for ease of movement), to mid-thigh length (for improved wind and thermal protection). Some of these garments include hoods (highly recommended), which also come in many styles ranging from detachable with zipper or hook and loop to permanent, and/or styles that can be tucked away. Hoods must be adjustable, able to fit over a helmet if necessary, and able to completely cover the head. Pull strings and hook-and-loop connectors can help prevent the entry of rain and snow, but all adjustments must allow full movement of the head and at least 180 degrees of forward vision.

At lower altitudes in dry weather, heavy-duty, reinforced cotton or blend trousers, such as Army fatigues, are frequently used in the protective layer because of their loose, roomy fit and their multiple utility pockets. Brush pants with reinforcing material at the knees, seat, and leg fronts, are commonly used by bird hunters to handle thick, wet underbrush. These, too, can make excellent trousers for SAR operations in cool weather.

Thin, inexpensive, waterproof, plastic or vinyl emergency rain gear is available but not recommended for SAR operations. They may offer limited protection from wet weather, but they are generally too flimsy to withstand the rigors of nearly any SAR environment. They may also include elastic at the wrists, hood, and/or waist. Elastic can cause a constriction problem and should generally be avoided in outdoor clothing worn in SAR work. Because of their material, these garments may also become brittle and tear easily in cold weather. Next to footwear, purchasing high-quality protective layer garments may be the best investment made by SAR personnel interested in warmth and comfort, especially during extended SAR missions (**FIGURE 7-10**).

No waterproof material or garment is suitable in all outdoor environments. When working hard outside in the pouring rain, you will get wet no matter what is worn, from both the inside and the outside. Even if it

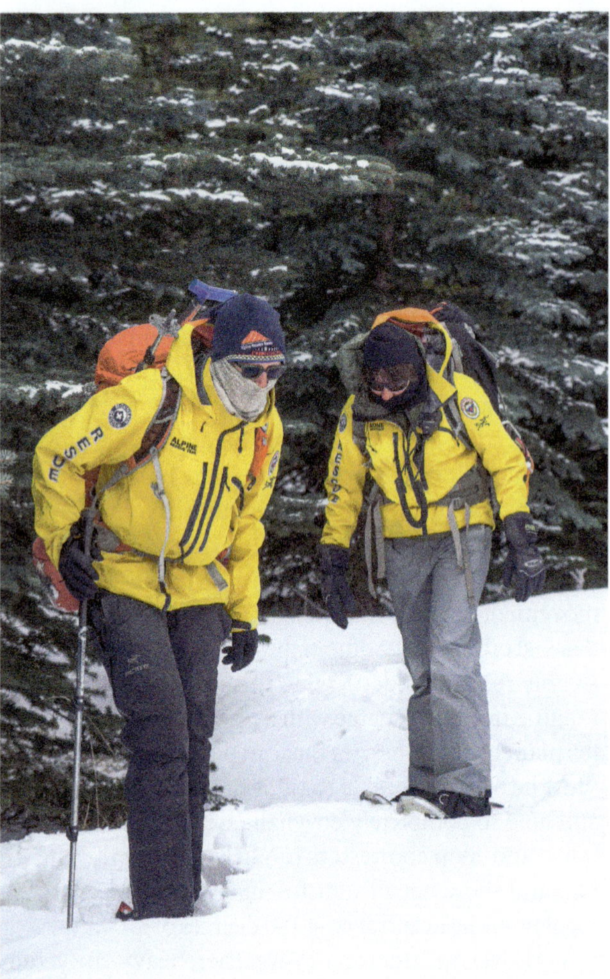

FIGURE 7-10 Next to footwear, purchasing high-quality protective, outer garments may be the best investment made by SAR personnel interested in warmth and comfort, especially during extended SAR missions.

is impossible to keep dry, it is possible to remain fairly comfortable by picking the right system to begin with and properly adjusting the layers as necessary.

Short pants may work in some limited circumstances, but they are generally not recommended for SAR work. Cotton blue jeans, although popular and fashionable in the United States, are usually constrictive and possess all the limitations of cotton (cold when wet, absorb and hold water, etc.). Therefore, cotton jeans are not well suited for field SAR operations.

Accessories and Additional Clothing Considerations

When dressing for the outdoors, certain parts of the body require special attention. There are also special considerations for clothing systems and SAR operations that are often overlooked.

Protective Layer Color

The color of the protective, outer layer is important, especially in SAR. Dark colors absorb the heat of the sun and are generally a better choice in cold climates, especially with snow in the background, but dark colors are hard to see at night and in wooded or dark environments. Lighter colors, on the other hand, reflect more of the sun's radiant heat, are preferable in warmer climates, and are usually easier to see in environments that present dark backgrounds.

Besides controlling temperature, colorful clothing has other benefits. SAR personnel wearing colors that contrast with the environment are easier to see, and SAR personnel need to be seen. Bright colors such as fluorescents or colors not commonly found in the outdoors should be worn during SAR field operations. Royal blue is probably the least occurring color in nature. It also contrasts with many environments and is easily seen in most outdoor settings, but modern technology now offers a wide variety of highly visible colors for outer layers, including various fluorescent colors that are hard to miss in any environment. Camouflage clothing is also available but should be avoided in SAR work.

High-visibility, lightweight vests can also be worn over any protective layer to increase visibility and easily identify their wearers as part of a SAR operation. These vests are inexpensive, integrate retroreflective materials (a surface that reflects light back to its source), and may be a good alternative to expensive, highly visible protective layer garments such as parkas. ANSI 107 standard provides design guidelines and specific light reflective requirements for garments and headwear to enhance the visibility of workers. When working around moving vehicular traffic, Type "R" Class 2 or 3 high-visibility apparel are required by the U.S. Occupational Safety and Health Administration (OSHA) (3M, 2016). These vests are also useful during SAR operations when visibility of individuals is desirable or necessary for safety.

During SAR field operations, it is also helpful to clearly display some indication of your affiliation with a SAR organization. An emblem, logo, or patch will work, as would the words "search and rescue" or "SAR" painted or affixed to your protective, outer garment.

Head

The unprotected head can be responsible for more than half of the body's heat loss in cold environments and a similar amount of heat gain in hot environments, mostly by radiation. Since the head has relatively little insulation of its own, head covering of some type should be worn in virtually all environments: in cold weather to protect from heat loss (**FIGURE 7-11**) and in hot weather to keep from overheating (**FIGURE 7-12**).

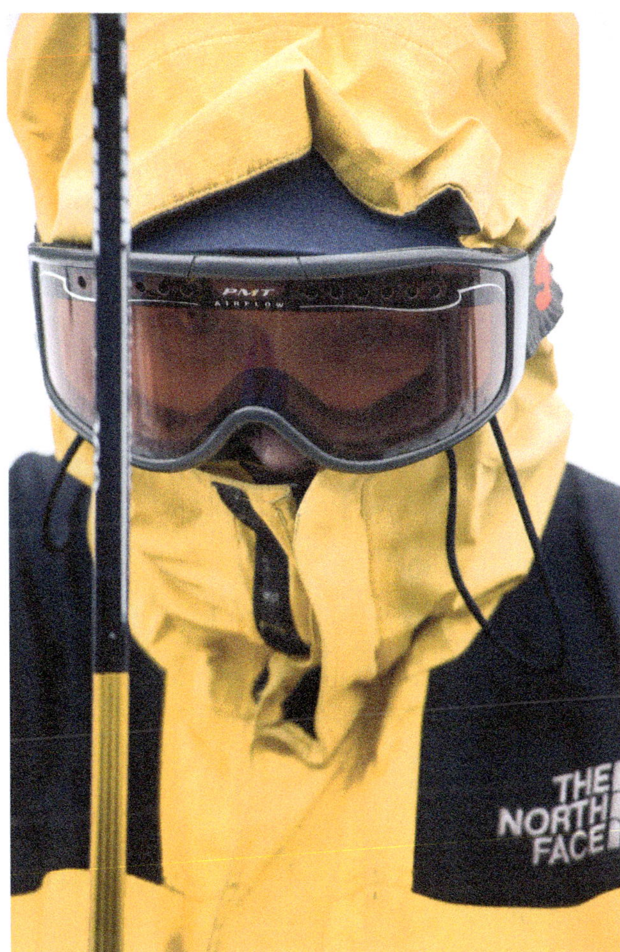

FIGURE 7-11 Balaclavas, face-mask type headwear, and hoods are great for protecting the entire face and head. In addition, do not overlook the importance of protecting the eyes in cold weather.
© 2016 Howard Paul, Photography for Communication and Commerce.

A brimmed hat may also be needed to protect the face, ears, and neck from the sun, and it must have a brim wide enough to protect all the necessary areas.

As with all protective, outer layer garments, the level of activity, expected environment, and exposure duration should be considered when choosing headgear. Headgear must be snug enough to stay on while moving, be comfortable while worn, and provide the desired protection from the environment (wind block, water resistance, insulation, etc.). Be careful that no part of the headgear interferes with your pack or other outer layer garments. If a helmet will be worn, it may require a specific type of winter liner to be worn with it to work properly. Do not wear a hat beneath a helmet if that hat has not been approved by the manufacturer for use with the helmet (OSHA, 2017).

In colder conditions, fleece or wool work well. Choose a fiber that is hydrophobic and wicks moisture away from the head and face. Protecting the entire face and head is important in cold weather. Balaclavas and face-mask type headgear are great for this task (FIGURE 7-13). Ear bands protect the ears but leave the top of the head—a major source of heat loss—exposed and uninsulated. In milder temperatures, lighter hats with a brim or vented ball caps allow air to circulate near the head while shading the head, face, and eyes from the sun. Waterproof hats can even be used as improvised water containers.

In desert environments, the head still needs protection, but from external heat, not heat loss. To promote cooling, wear a light-colored, light-material hat with a wide brim

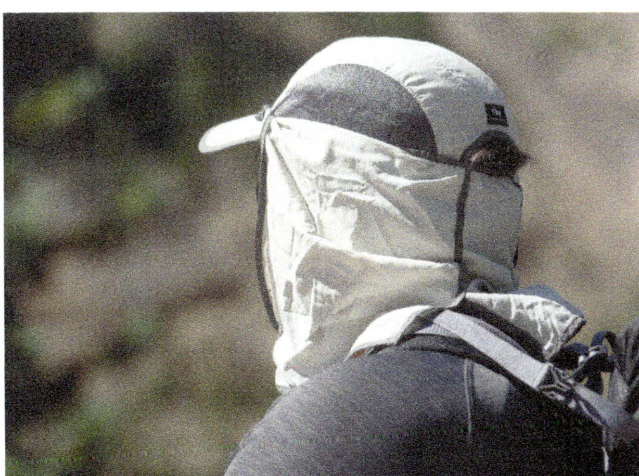

FIGURE 7-12 In hot weather, wear a light-colored, light material hat with a wide brim and plenty of ventilation. As a minimum, it should shade the head, face, and neck from the sun.
© 2016 Howard Paul, Photography for Communication and Commerce.

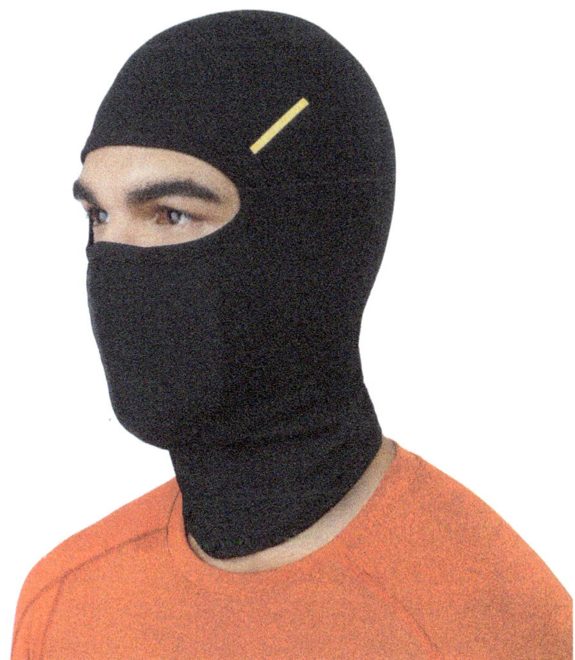

FIGURE 7-13 An example of a balaclava made of breathable, moisture-wicking material that provides thermal protection for the head, neck, and face.
Courtesy of Arc'teryx.

and plenty of ventilation. The idea is to reflect the sun's radiant heat away from the head, provide as much shade as possible, and promote the circulation of air beneath the hat so that perspiration evaporates quickly. Hats with extended bills, mesh sides (for ventilation), drawstrings (to hold them on), and drapes to cover the neck have been specifically designed for desert use (see Figure 7-12).

Many do not realize that constriction can also be a problem with headgear. This can lead to impeded blood flow to the ears and scalp, be uncomfortable, and predispose one to cold injuries. Make sure that whatever type of headgear worn is not too tight, remove it periodically, and massage the scalp when possible and safe to promote circulation.

Many recognize that sunblock and sunglasses (high UV protection) should be used to protect the skin and eyes in sunny and high-altitude environments. However, the need for eye protection from flying debris, small tree limbs, brush, and other hazards is often overlooked. Walking through a wooded area, especially at night, is a serious hazard to the eyes. High winds, especially in sandy, dry environments, can also be a significant problem. Glasses may be needed to protect not only from the sun's rays but also from hazards in the environment, and simple eye glasses may not be enough. Not only should sunglasses be worn in sunny and high-altitude environments, but clear safety glasses may be needed in wooded environments, especially at night, and goggles may be needed in high-wind situations. Since vision is the primary search sensor used by humans, serious consideration should be given to the effect any glasses, including sunglasses, might have on a searcher's ability to see in the search environment.

Neck

Scarves are what usually come to mind when one thinks of neck protection. A scarf can be configured to protect the entire head, including the face and neck, but depending on the length and material, it can catch in hook-and-loop fasteners, be bulky and cumbersome, and become entangled in hardware. In a hot, desert environment, a thin, cotton scarf can be wrapped around the head and face to provide protection from the sun and keep sand and dust off the face. In a cold environment, a scarf can protect bare neck skin that might be otherwise exposed. A neck gaiter is a scarf alternative that is essentially a tube of soft material such as fleece or wool that is pulled over the head to surround the neck. It protects the neck like a scarf but is not as bulky or, unfortunately, as versatile. Like a hat, a neck gaiter should fit comfortably and not be too snug.

Balaclavas are knit hats that can be unfolded to cover the head, neck, and most of the face. They are versatile in that they can be worn as a hat or pulled down in cold weather to cover the face and neck. One variation on this theme combines a windproof, longer, fleece neck gaiter with a hood to provide excellent protection for the head and neck. It is pulled over the head, like a neck gaiter, to encircle the neck, but it has an attached hood that can be pulled up and cinched around the face with a drawstring. A variety of similar garments are available and should be investigated for superior cold weather protection.

Hands

The fingers are very often affected by extreme cold and, therefore, deserve special attention in such climates. Since SAR work often necessitates dexterity, the hands are important tools. Mittens generally keep the hands warmer than gloves do, but they usually impair dexterity. Overmits (a second, larger pair of mittens worn over other gloves or mittens) may be necessary in very cold environments or where snow or slush might be encountered, but they further detrimentally affect dexterity.

Leather gloves may be required in SAR work, but they should not be exclusively depended upon for warmth in very cold environments, as leather tends to absorb water and offers minimal insulation by itself. Leather does a great job of protecting the hands from abrasions and wind while improving traction and grip. In cold weather where leather gloves are needed, consider wearing larger ones with wool or fleece gloves underneath, or wearing leather gloves lined with a suitable insulating material.

Fingerless gloves can also be useful where fine finger dexterity is required (**FIGURE 7-14**). Also, do not forget to protect the wrists. A great deal of heat can be lost in cold weather through wrists exposed to the wind, rain, snow, and cold, and the wrists are vulnerable to cold injuries just like any exposed skin. Generally, make sure to overlap all adjacent garments in cold weather (e.g., gloves and jacket, jacket and trousers, jacket and headwear) to prevent the exposure of bare skin (**FIGURE 7-15**).

Following the principles of layering, wearing a thin pair of gloves under mittens can keep the hands warmer in extreme cold. Thin gloves (polyester, silk, nylon),

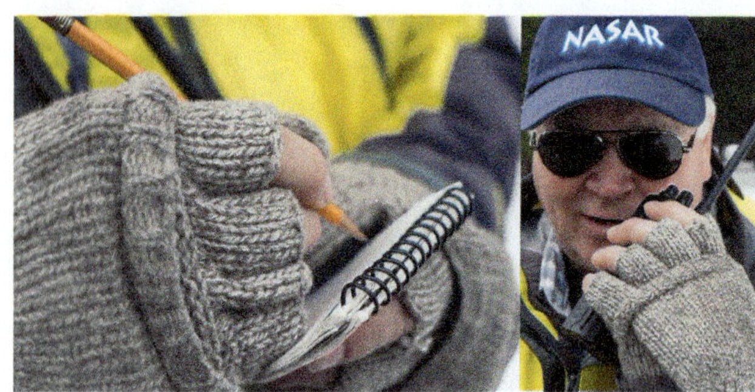

FIGURE 7-14 Fingerless gloves can be useful where fine finger dexterity is required.

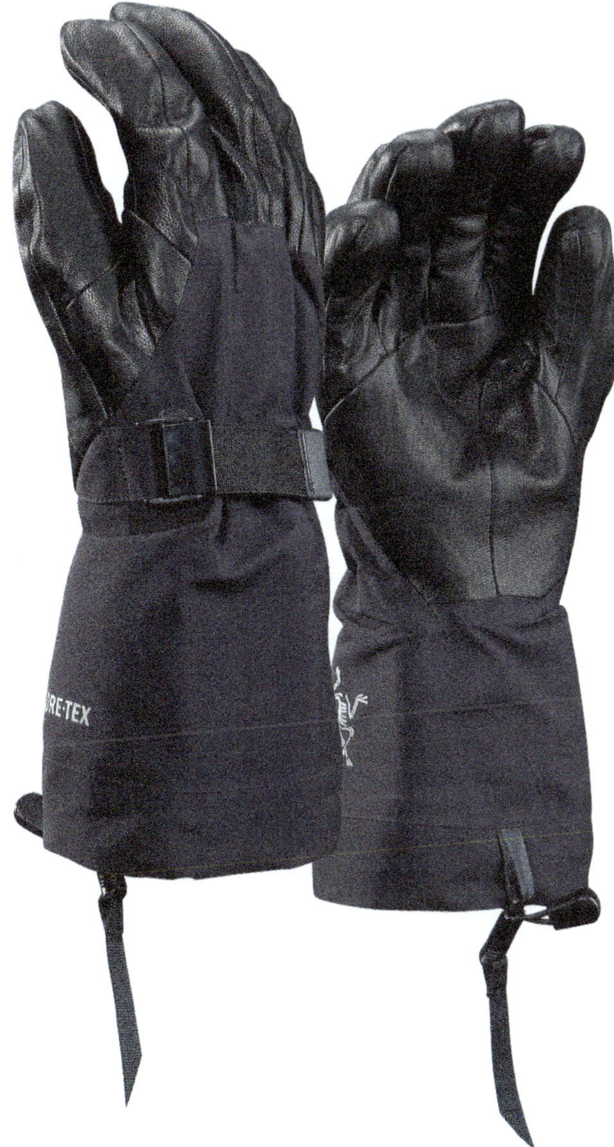

FIGURE 7-15 An example of cold weather gloves designed for winter and alpine activities. These gloves are waterproof, windproof, breathable, heavily insulated, and durable, which makes them well suited for SAR operations in severe weather.
Courtesy of Arc'teryx.

sometimes called *glove liners*, allow the heat from the fingers to warm each other inside a mitten. These thin gloves provide some protection should the mittens have to be removed briefly in extreme cold, and also allow perspiration to pass through the gloves into the insulating mittens to keep the hands drier and, in turn, warmer. Antiperspirant applied to the hands and feet can also reduce perspiration in those areas and, thus, keep hands and feet warmer in cold environments.

Where bodily fluids or biohazards may be encountered, latex or vinyl gloves (some people are allergic to latex) should be worn for protection. If additional gloves are also necessary for protection from abrasion or cold, latex or vinyl gloves can be worn underneath to keep them from being damaged during use.

SAFETY TIP

SAR personnel should consider removing all jewelry before operating in the field. In cold weather, metal jewelry can be dangerous because the metal can be cooled to a temperature that can cause a localized cold injury to the skin. In any type of weather, dangling jewelry from the ears, wrists, or neck can become entangled and cause traumatic injuries.

Feet and Footwear

In ground SAR operations, the feet are in constant contact with the environment, and foot problems can incapacitate SAR personnel. Therefore, both the feet and footwear require special attention. Preventative maintenance is half the battle to having comfortable feet. In terms of foot care, here are some suggestions:

- Examine the feet at the end of every day and clean them thoroughly.
- Tend to any hot spots immediately. (A hot spot is a reddened, slightly tender area on the skin of the foot that is evidence of rubbing or pressure from footwear and is an early sign of an impending blister.)
- Massage the feet regularly.
- Always wear clean, dry socks.
- Consider wearing two pairs of socks for field work (the inner one thin).
- Avoid folds in socks while they are in use and prevent seams from causing pressure on the feet.
- Air dry the feet often, but do not soak or rinse them until the end of the day.
- Keep toenails trimmed but not too short.
- Tighten footgear on inclines and loosen them a bit on flat ground.
- Have footgear properly sized by a professional.
- Keep the feet dry.

Important factors when selecting footwear for SAR work are fit, comfort, stability, support, durability, traction, and protection from the elements.

Proper fit is the most important aspect of any footwear. Something as seemingly insignificant as a blister from ill-fitting footwear can eventually incapacitate an individual to the point of not being able to travel, a potentially dangerous situation in many environments. In addition, SAR personnel can hardly be effective when their feet hurt.

Boot technology and fit have improved significantly over the past years. Fitting boots properly is a science and can include the use of customized **orthotic** shoe inserts and molded boot liners. Varying lengths of **shank** in the sole can be used to increase stability on uneven surfaces, and the materials from which boots are made include rubberized polymers, silicone-impregnated leather, dense synthetic insulation, waterproof and breathable laminates, and other durable synthetic materials that are crafted to meet the needs of the wearer.

Fit is directly related to comfort, and properly fitted footwear by definition is comfortable. There should be plenty of room for the toes without the foot slipping forward or back during uphill and downhill travel. There should be no heel rise when walking, and there should be no pressure points. Because of the many subtleties of properly fitting footwear and the high cost of making a mistake, having footwear properly sized and fitted by a professional is highly recommended. In fact, many believe that being fitted by someone who knows exactly how to do it may be the most important aspect of buying new footwear.

Before seeking a professional, however, a buyer should be familiar with the terminology of the shoe trade. Terms like *upper*, *lower*, *mid-sole*, *tanning*, *gusseted tongue*, *bellows tongue*, *shank*, and *welt* (different types) will likely be used. One should also be familiar with the various types of footwear before venturing into the marketplace. These include running, trail running, hiking, light hikers, mountaineering, rock climbing, walking, tennis, cowboy, arctic, snow, cross trainers, and many more. The best choice depends on the types of specific environments and SAR operations one is likely to encounter, and one pair of footwear is unlikely to meet all of your needs. A boot designed for use in the mountainous terrain of Colorado may not be suitable for the desert terrain of south Texas. Similarly, an insulated, waterproof boot may be desirable in Maine in autumn, but the same boot may not be suitable for use in Georgia in July. Even though a pair of cowboy boots may be quite appropriate for a mounted search team in California, and deck (boat) shoes may be perfect for use by a water rescue team in Florida, neither type of footwear may be safe in mountainous terrain.

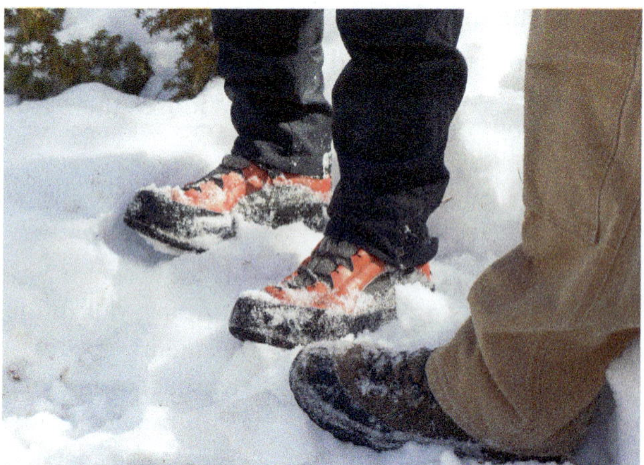

FIGURE 7-16 For most SAR operations, mid-height, light hikers or light mountaineering boots should be adequate. However, in technical terrain (e.g., high altitude, vertical rock, snow/ice), specialized footwear should be worn after seeking professional advice.

Footwear for SAR work must also provide stability and support. That is, it must neither allow one's ankle to turn easily in rough terrain nor allow the wearer to feel the rough terrain through the sole. It must also be durable enough to withstand many uses (without damage) and offer a superior return on investment. Traction is also a consideration. The sole of the footwear must provide adequate traction in the terrain in which it will be used without causing undue damage to the environment or the wearer.

Footwear must also protect the wearer from the elements (**FIGURE 7-16**). Automatically putting on additional socks in cold weather is not always a good idea because it may constrict the feet (more than when they were sized), impede blood flow, and cause the feet to get cold. Wear two pairs at all times (see the wicking layer section for more about socks). An adequate amount of insulation should be integrated into the footwear to protect the wearer from temperature extremes, but one pair of boots is unlikely to be adequate for year-round use. Footwear needs to be chosen based on the environment in which it will be used with thoughtful consideration given to several issues, such as the level of waterproofness and/or breathability desired, insulation desired, ankle support required, and characteristics of the environment. In cold weather, insulation can also be added to the outside of the footwear (e.g., mukluks, overboots) as long as the feet do not get constricted, but this may adversely affect safe foot travel during SAR operations.

For most SAR operations, high-top, mid-height hiking shoes or light mountaineering boots should be adequate (**FIGURE 7-17**). However, in technical terrain (e.g., high altitude, vertical rock, snow/ice) specialized footwear should be worn after seeking professional advice.

Properly cared for, expensive boots like those often necessary for SAR should last for many years. To help assure longevity, clean and dry them after every use, and then store them in a cool, dry place away from sunlight, insects, and vermin. Never dry boots over or near a fire or in a tumble dryer. Overheating can damage the material and weaken stitching. Boots should be dried at room temperature but may be placed near a radiator or forced air heating vent. Highly effective commercial boot dryers are available that gently dry from the inside. This is the best method of drying boots, but improvising

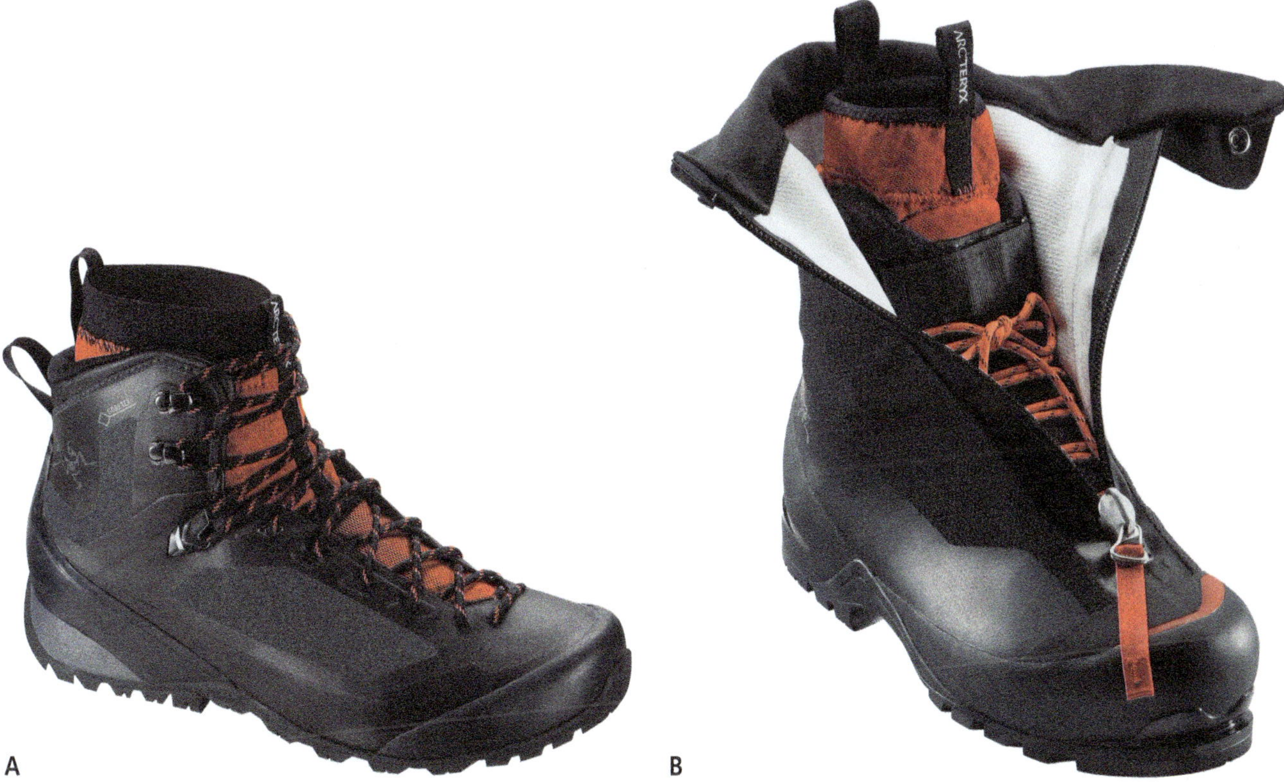

A B

FIGURE 7-17 **A.** An example of a high-quality leather hiking boot that is well suited for most SAR field work. This example includes a Gore-Tex® boot liner. **B.** An example of high-end mountaineering boots specifically designed for mountaineering, ice, and mixed climbing. They are a light, durable, and low-profile insulated double boot with integrated boot liners and overboots. A high-performance boot like this would be appropriate for SAR operations in an extreme alpine environment.

Courtesy of Arc'teryx.

by placing a couple air-activated hand warmers in the boots overnight can also help dry them from the inside.

Applying conditioners and/or sealers to boots may also help protect them. Products such as mink oil (leather protector), Sno-Seal® (leather treatment), Seam Seal (a waterproofing liquid by Aquaseal®), silicone spray, and beeswax all provide some level of protection for leather and rubber products but should be applied only if suggested by the boot's manufacturer. Be aware that using these and many similar products may damage existing sealed seams, eliminate breathability, and void the warranty on the footwear. For best results, instructions provided by the manufacturer for boot care should be followed.

Once the purchase is made, break in any footwear before wearing it into the field. While wearing the same socks that will be used outdoors, wear them around the house, walk stairs, and test their fit. If there is a problem, some manufacturers may exchange boots that were worn only inside for replacements. However, the best reason to break them in is to work out any problems—including pressure points, arch support, and the like—before going into the field.

Footwear should be worn snug, but not tight, during travel on tracks, trails, and level ground. When walking uphill or downhill, tighten the laces a bit to remove any possibility of movement of the footwear. Loosen them again once back on flat ground. Overly snug footwear is a primary cause of cold feet among outdoor travelers. Keep footwear only as tight at necessary to maintain comfort, minimize blisters, and promote safety.

Generally, when hands and feet are cold, one should check for constriction problems and then put on a hat. Much of the body's heat is lost through the head and neck, so when the feet and hands are cold, it could be because the blood flowing to them is not being warmed enough due to heat loss elsewhere. Use the BUBU approach to dressing for the outdoors: big, unconstricting, baggy, and ugly.

Gaiters

Gaiters applied to the lower legs prevent and protect against dirt, debris, snow, ticks, and chiggers from getting in the boots and on the legs. They can also keep snow and water from wetting the trousers and subsequently promoting heat loss in cold environments. Snow can melt quickly in the trousers and wet the garment. Walking through dew-covered grass or weeds can wet the lower trousers very quickly.

Gaiters usually attach with a small hook to a lower lace toward the toe of the shoe or boot. Some boots provide

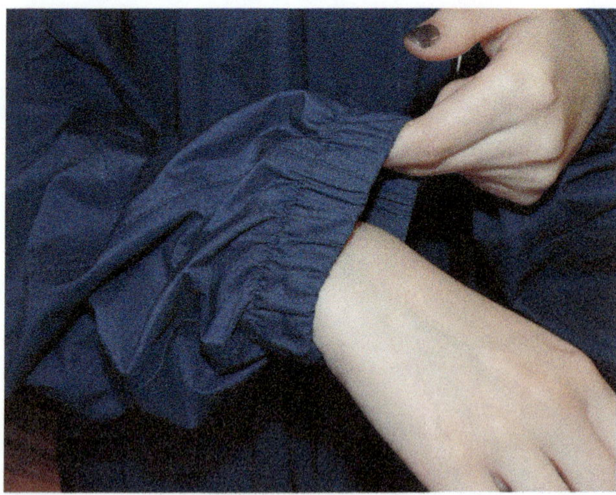

FIGURE 7-18 Elastic should generally be avoided in outdoor clothing; use a strap to hold on a hat, suspenders instead of a belt, and—bottom line—avoid all tight and constricting clothing of any kind.
Courtesy of Donald Cooper.

a small hook for this purpose. Some gaiters connect to the boot by a tight, wide rubber band that is especially designed to adhere to the welt of the boot (perimeter of the sole). All also have some method of attaching around the lower leg.

Gaiters are usually constructed with a durable synthetic material that resists abrasion. Most are coated or treated with a waterproofing agent or incorporate a waterproof and breathable laminate into its design. They may use hook-and-loop closures, zippers, snaps, or any combination of these. There are many lengths of gaiters. A shorter length, 6 inches or so, primarily protects and prevents entry of foreign matter into the boot. It simply wraps around the ankle/collar of the boot. The longer versions can run the length of the shin up to the knee and provide a broader range of protection. It attaches underneath the boot with strap and buckle or cordage and is usually used in conjunction with elastic or a small strap to keep secure on the shin. Not only does the longer gaiter protect against foreign object entry, it may also help as a windbreak, and it protects the lower leg against abrasion, insects, plants, and even snakes. Use them with caution, though. Constriction can be a problem, especially if worn improperly, and waterproof gaiters can cause the same problems as a vapor barrier; that is, condensation under the layer can wet the garments underneath and hold water against the skin.

Constriction

Elastic at the wrists, ankles, waist, head, or feet can cause a problem with blood flow. These constriction problems impede the flow of the blood that warms the extremities. As the blood flow decreases to the extremities, the risk of cold injuries increases.

From these considerations, some general guidelines can be derived: elastic should generally be avoided in outdoor clothing; use a strap to hold on a hat, suspenders instead of a belt, and—bottom line—avoid all tight and constricting clothing of any kind (**FIGURE 7-18**).

Care and Storage

Properly cleaning and storing clothing used in SAR extends its life and helps retain its important characteristics such as waterproofness, breathability, and insulation value. However, if it is done improperly, significant damage can result.

Generally, soil, soot, grease, body oils, and contaminants such as sunscreen on clothing detrimentally affect the desirable characteristics of the garment. Soiled synthetic fabrics are more susceptible to abrasion, which leads to fraying of the material, sometimes called pilling, which attracts more soil and leads to further fraying. **DEET**, a common ingredient in insect repellants, can cause physical damage to certain plastics and fabrics such as rayon and spandex (Petherick, 2008; Dow, 2017), but it does not damage wool or cotton (Dow, 2017).

For specialized clothing, manufacturers' guidelines should be followed for the laundering of each garment. This usually includes emptying pockets and closing all zippers, snaps, and other closures before washing, and carefully selecting the correct cleaning solution. Turning the garment inside out before washing reduces abrasion on the garment's exterior, and using a front-loading washing machine prevents abrasion from an agitator.

Most commercially available laundry detergents leave a residue that reduces the effectiveness of a DWR finish, the waterproofness and breathability of laminate layers, and the wicking ability of a fabric. Thus, only a cleaning solution that is compatible with the specific garment being washed should be used. Also, do not use fabric softeners during washing or drying (dryer sheets). Softeners also leave residues that impair effectiveness.

Outdoor garments should generally be dried by hanging in a cool, dry room out of direct sunlight. Some manufacturers allow drying in a tumble dryer on a low heat setting, but be careful. The drum in a tumble dryer can get hot enough to damage some synthetic fabrics. The garment must be removed immediately after drying and not allowed to sit in a hot machine. Air drying also reduces shrinkage, which can be excessive in a tumble dry machine for certain materials like wool and cotton.

DWR finishes are applied to all waterproof and breathable fabrics and are a special case when it comes to washing. Any contamination or soiling, including soot and smoke from a fire, can affect DWR finishes, so most manufacturers suggest washing these garments regularly and often with a manufacturer-approved cleaning solution.

Clothing used for SAR should be stored uncompressed in a dry place out of direct sunlight. Moisture leads to mold, which damages clothing. Thus, damp basements or garages are not good storage choices. Fiber-filled and down-filled garments may lose their loft, and thus insulation value, if stored in a compressed condition, so store them uncompressed and in a dry location. Insects can also damage stored clothing and are drawn to food sources such as food crumbs, lint, pet hair, and human hair. To prevent infestations, clean and thoroughly dry the clothing and store it uncompressed in airtight containers. The fumes from mothballs can be hazardous, and cedar chips or blocks just do not repel clothes moths (Sorensen, 2011).

Survival Tips on Clothing

There are some fundamental guidelines/issues concerning dressing for the outdoors that must not be overlooked:

- When your feet are cold, put on a hat.
- Do not overheat so that clothing becomes wet by perspiration. If clothing becomes wet from perspiration, remove and/or replace the wet layer and slow your pace.
- Use the layering system; add layers when cold and remove layers when hot.
- When sleeping in harsh, cold conditions, arrange dry, spare clothing around the neck and shoulders with padding and insulation added to each kidney region, as these areas are more susceptible to cold. Also, wear a knit stocking cap because if your head is warm, chances are your feet will be, too.
- Dry wet clothing by allowing it to freeze and then beating ice crystals from the fabric.
- Wearing darker clothing in winter to absorb the sun's heat energy may be a good idea, but beware of not being visible enough. SAR personnel must be highly visible.
- Clean clothing allows proper ventilation through clothing layers. Dirty clothing inhibits ventilation and causes moisture buildup on clothing layers. Wear clean clothes.
- Light-colored clothing reflects the sun and heat in warm weather.
- In hot weather, wear clothing that promotes circulation of air beneath garments.

Suggestions for Outdoor Clothing Purchases

One of the first questions asked in basic SAR skills classes is, "Where/how do I purchase appropriate outdoor clothing without spending a lot of money?" Indeed, it is possible to find inexpensive, quality clothing that will provide you with the protection and comfort needed for SAR. Here are some suggestions:

- Plan ahead and buy winter/outdoor clothes/items during spring and winter clearance sales.
- Using this same "reverse season" purchasing thought process, check various stores/catalogs/Internet sources other than the stereotyped label of "outdoor stores" to purchase clothes and all sorts of equipment that can be used for SAR. Consider the following (catalogs and stores):
  - Ski shops for winter gear, waterproof pants, gloves, eyewear, undergarments, etc.
  - Cross-country running specialty stores for lightweight breathable clothes, layers that wick, water bottles, socks, hats, etc.
  - Snowboarding specialty stores for waterproof pants, socks, eyewear, gloves, undergarments, neck gaiters, face fleece, etc.
  - Parachute supply houses for socks, gloves, eyewear, pouches that can be attached to packs, wrist altimeters, etc.
  - Recreational vehicle stores for environmentally biodegradable toilet paper, glow sticks, 12-volt portable water heater, folding tables, 12-volt lights, etc.
  - Rafting supply stores for waterproof bags and containers, lightweight tarps, folding tables, folding cots, etc.
  - Forestry supply stores for colored flagging tape, high-visibility vests with pockets, compass kits, reflective tape, etc.
- Try the clearance sales offered by name brand outdoor shops and websites.
- Some stores specialize in selling seconds from all sorts of companies.
- Use the "reverse season" thought process when checking at the local Salvation Army or other secondhand stores.
- Even though the military surplus stores really do not have an off season, it may be fruitful to rummage around in the store periodically just to see what is available.
- Consider repurposing existing clothing items such as wool dress pants or wool sweaters to enhance the insulation layer.

Wrap-Up

READY FOR REVIEW

- A simple rule before starting out is to ask, "Is what I plan to wear and carry adequate for the expected weather and environments in which I will be working? What about carrying a bit more, just in case?"
- Textile and clothing manufacturers use the inherent characteristics of specific fibers to construct clothes that meet specialized needs. Durability, breathability, waterproofness, ability to wick moisture, insulation value when wet, and resistance to burning or melting are all variables that are manipulated using various fibers.
- The rate of heat transfer through clothing depends on three factors:
  - Quantity and thickness of dead air spaces trapped within the clothing and its layers (radiation)
  - Amount of air that passes through a material (convection)
  - Water and moisture (conduction and evaporation)
- As physical exertion or the outside temperature increases, layers can be removed to facilitate heat loss and the movement of evaporating perspiration away from the body. As exertion decreases or the outside temperature drops, layers can be added to reduce heat loss.
- When dressing for the outdoors, certain parts of the body require special attention. There are also special considerations for clothing systems and SAR operations that are often overlooked.

SEARCH AND RESCUE TERMS

DEET Abbreviation for *N,N*-diethyl-3-methylbenzamide—also called *N,N*-Diethyl-m-toluamide or diethyltoluamide—a common and effective ingredient in many insect repellants.

Gaiters Garments worn over the shoe and/or lower leg that protect the wearer from abrasion, dirt, debris, snow, moisture, insects, snakes, and other foreign objects.

Hydrophilic Refers to fabric that absorbs water.

Hydrophobic Refers to fabric that repels and does not absorb water.

Hyperthermia Condition or illness caused by the body's core temperature being significantly higher than normal (normal is 98.5°F/37°C).

Hypothermia Condition or illness caused by the body's core temperature being significantly lower than normal (normal is 98.5°F/37°C).

Micropores Pores with a diameter less than 2 nanometers.

Moisture regain The amount of water a completely dry fiber absorbs from the air at a standard condition of 70° F and a relative humidity of 65%, expressed as a percentage of the dry fiber weight (textileglossary.com, 2016).

Orthotic An artificial support, brace, or splint used to support, align, or correct the function of movable parts of the body. Shoe inserts are orthotics that are intended to correct an abnormal or irregular walking pattern by altering slightly the angles at which the foot strikes a walking or running surface (MedicineNet.com, 2017).

Shank In a boot or a shoe, a part of the supportive structure between the insole and the outsole traditionally made of steel but often made from polymer materials.

Waterproof Material that is impermeable to water, even water under pressure.

Waterproof and breathable Material that is nearly impermeable to water droplets (waterproof) and yet allows water vapor to pass (breathable).

Water-repellent Sheds water that is not under pressure; however, falling or wind-blown rain may penetrate the fabric.

Water-resistant The material temporarily resists water under pressure.

REFERENCES AND SUGGESTED READING

3M. 2016. Regulatory Update, Standard Update #34: ANSI/ISEA 107-2015 Made Easy. http://multimedia.3m.com/mws/media/638577O/ansi-107-2015-made-easier-high-visibility-apparel.pdf.

Dow, Jennifer. 2017. Outdoor clothing for the wilderness professional. In *Wilderness Medicine*, 7th ed., Volume 2, edited by Paul S. Auerbach, pp. 2396–2408. St. Louis, MO: Mosby, Inc.

Engineering Tool Box. 2016. Thermal conductivity of materials and gases. http://www.engineeringtoolbox.com/thermal-conductivity-d_429.html.

IDFL.com. 2016. USA down and feather apparel labeling requirements. http://beta.idfl.com/en/articles/standards/usa-down-feather-apparel-labeling-requirements/.

Johnson, G. Mark. 2003. *The Ultimate Desert Handbook: A Manual for Desert Hikers, Campers, and Travelers*. New York: Ragged Mountain Press/McGraw Hill.

Kilpiö, Katriina, Soili Mäkinen–Kiljunen, Tari Haahtela, and Matti Hannuksela. February 1998. Allergy to feathers. *Allergy* 53, no. 2: 159–164.

Lanza, Michael. 2003. Winter Hiking and Camping: Managing Cold for Comfort & Safety. New York: Mountaineers Books.

Linxweiler, Eric, and Mike Maude, Editors. 2017. *Mountaineering: Freedom of the Hills*, 9th ed. New York: Mountaineers Books.

Manning, Harvey. 1986. *Backpacking: One Step at a Time*, 4th edition. New York: Vintage Books.

McManners, Hugh. 2007. *The Complete Wilderness Training Manual*. 2nd rev. ed. New York: DK Publishing.

MedicineNet.com. 2017. Definition of orthotic. http://www.medicinenet.com/script/main/art.asp?articlekey=40206.

Nyerges, Christopher. 2014. *How to Survive Anywhere: A Guide for Urban, Suburban, Rural, and Wilderness Environments*. 2nd edition. Mechanicsburg, PA: Stackpole Books.

Petherick, Anna. 2008. How DEET jams insects' smell sensors. *Nature News*. http://www.nature.com/news/2008/080313/full/news.2008.672.html.

Petzoldt, Paul. 1974. *The Wilderness Handbook*, 1st ed. New York: W.W. Norton & Company, Inc.

Rawlins, Chip, and Colin Fletcher. 2002. *The Complete Walker IV*, revised edition. New York: Alfred A. Knopf, Inc.

Sorensen, Janelle. 2011. Healthy begins here: Are mothballs safe? http://blogs.webmd.com/health-ehome/2011/02/are-mothballs-safe.html#.

Textileglossary.com. 2016. http://www.textileglossary.com/terms.

Townsend, Chris. 1994. Clothing for the Snow. *Wilderness Skiing and Winter Camping*. Camden, ME: Ragged Mountain Press.

U.S. Department of Labor, Occupational Safety and Health Administration. 2017. Interpretation letter, 29 CFR 1926.31 and 1926.100. https://www.osha.gov/pls/oshaweb/owadisp.show_document?p_table=INTERPRETATIONS&p_id=25336.

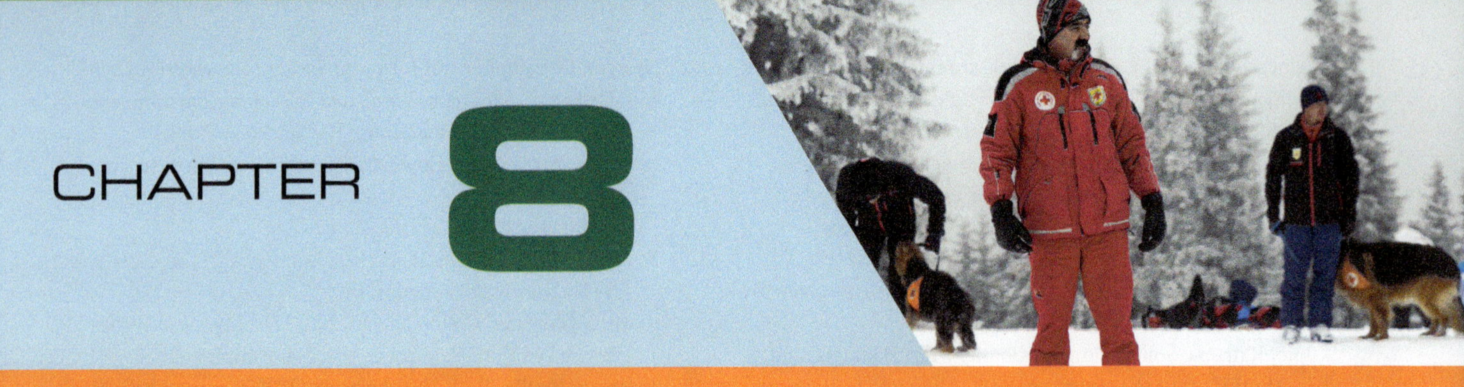

CHAPTER 8

Safety in SAR Environments

OBJECTIVES

Upon completion of this chapter and the related course activities, the student will be able to meet the following objectives:

- List, in priority order, the five primary hazard controls.
- Describe the hazard control that is the last resort and explain why.
- Explain what is meant by a "safety culture."
- Identify at least three of the standard precautions in health care and describe their importance in a search and rescue (SAR) environment.
- List at least three general safety rules that should be followed during SAR operations.
- Discuss safety considerations for SAR personnel regarding lightning.
- Describe the signs and symptoms of hypothermia.
- Describe three types of cold injuries and their respective signs and symptoms.
- Describe three types of heat injuries and their respective signs and symptoms.
- Explain why ascending too quickly to above 8,000 feet (2438 meters) without taking time to acclimate is a problem.
- Describe at least three ways to prevent tick bites.
- Describe the top three priorities in SAR.

Safety Basics

A **hazard** is something that has the potential for harm. For example, when walking on a frozen pond during an ice rescue, the ice is a hazard for several reasons. It is slippery—you may fall and become injured—and thin ice may break and plunge you into very cold water. **Hazard mitigation** is any sustained action taken to reduce or eliminate the long-term risk to people and property from hazards and their effects (Mitigation Planning, 2009). Wearing some type of cleat on your boots every time you walk on ice would be a mitigating action, although it does not entirely reduce or eliminate all hazards related to walking on ice.

Hazards are generally caused by one of three things: nature (e.g., terrain, weather, earthquake, pandemic), humans (e.g., vehicle crashes, intentional acts, entrapments, hazardous materials, terrorism), or technology (e.g., information technology failures, utility interruptions and outages, transportation interruptions). In search and rescue (SAR) specifically, hazards may include environmental dangers (e.g., extreme cold or heat, high winds, insects), severe weather, difficult terrain, animals that may injure or harm, equipment failures and loss, injury, getting lost, and other threats to SAR personnel and operations. These types of hazards must first be recognized before they can be mitigated or managed.

Risk is an estimate of the probability of a hazard-related incident or exposure occurring (ANSI/ASSE, 2016). When walking on thin ice, there is some risk that you might slip, fall, hit your head on the ice, and become injured, but there could be a higher probability—a greater risk—with more serious consequences, that you may break through the thin ice and find yourself in very cold water fighting hypothermia—a life-threatening situation.

Before walking on thin ice (hazard), you might consider that there is a high probability (risk) that you may fall through, and that, if you do fall through, the consequences are significant in that hypothermia may quickly threaten your life. This mental process of considering the risk and its impact would likely force you to rethink your actions, whether you should proceed at all, and, if you do decide to proceed, how best to do it safely. The process of identifying hazards, evaluating operational risk, mitigating hazards, and controlling them is called **risk assessment**: an important tool that can be used by an individual or team to effectively mitigate and manage risks to an acceptable level (ANSI/ASSE, 2011b). As part of this risk assessment process, you would also likely implement several **hazard controls**, which are procedures adopted to minimize injury, reduce adverse health effects, and control damage to property (ANSI/ASSE, 2016).

SAFETY TIP

The process of identifying hazards, evaluating operational risk, mitigating hazards, and controlling them is called *risk assessment*: an important tool that can be used by an individual or team to effectively mitigate and manage risks to an acceptable level. Use procedures approved by the authority having jurisdiction (AHJ) to evaluate the hazards and determine the safest response.

Risk assessment may be as simple and informal as mentally noting what could go wrong and preventing or preparing for it, as in the ice rescue example, and as you very likely do every time you engage in any SAR activity. It can also be formalized in writing by listing any potential hazards; noting their likelihood and consequences; calculating a level of total risk; then identifying and describing mitigation, prevention, and control measures for each hazard. In the United States, risk assessment is usually relegated to the less formal approach, but in many parts of the world (the United Kingdom, for example), a formal written risk assessment is often required when workers undertake potentially dangerous activities (Management of Health and Safety at Work Regulations [MHSWR], 1999). Although not every hazard can necessarily be identified and mitigated in SAR operations, the purpose of mentioning it here is to emphasize the life-saving benefits gained from the process of identifying and managing hazards that might be encountered. In SAR, the principles of risk assessment should be applied to all activities where the safety of personnel and/or the mission may be compromised.

Safety is simply being free from unreasonable risk and is a goal of every search and rescue operation. To achieve this goal, risk assessments are performed. In the ice rescue scenario, after a risk assessment, we would quickly conclude that the only absolute position of safety with regard to the ice is to stay off it. If complete avoidance or elimination of the hazard is not possible, there are other things we can do to reduce the potential risk of any identified hazards as much as reasonably possible (ANSI/ASSE, 2016).

Controlling exposures to operational hazards is the fundamental method of protecting SAR personnel. A **hierarchy of hazard controls** has been used as a means of determining how to implement feasible and effective control solutions (CDC/NIOSH, 2017). The options for controlling hazards are generally applied in order of most effective to least effective (**FIGURE 8-1**). The idea behind this hierarchy is that the control methods at the top of Figure 8-1 are potentially more effective, protective, and less expensive than those at the bottom. Following this hierarchy normally leads to the implementation of inherently safer systems, where the risk of illness or injury has been substantially reduced (CDC/NIOSH, 2017).

The most effective hazard control is elimination, which means to physically remove the hazard or to design a plan that does not involve it at all. In the ice rescue scenario, this would mean staying off the ice, thus eliminating the ice as a hazard. If this were not possible, the next best approach would be to substitute something else or replace the hazard. For example, if the use of a single, aluminum, nonlocking carabiner represents a hazard in a particular rescue system, replacing it with a stronger, steel, locking carabiner would be a substitution control.

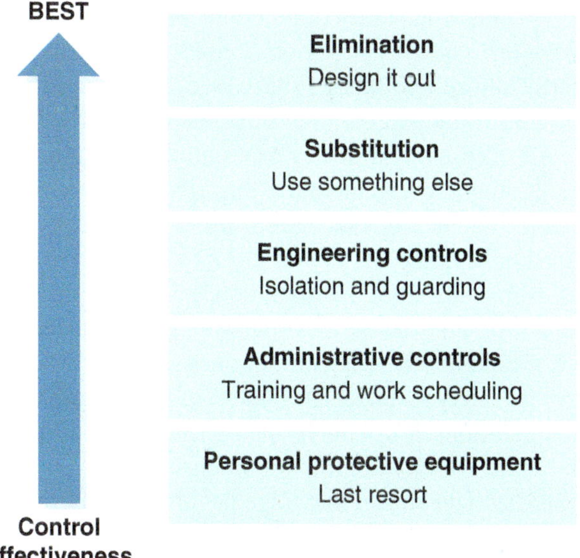

FIGURE 8-1 Hierarchy of hazard control. Effectiveness decreases as you move down the list, and personal protective equipment is the last resort.

The third most effective hazard control is an engineering control. This does not eliminate or replace the hazard; it isolates or protects people from it. Improvising shade in a desert search to get out of the sun (hazard) while resting and being belayed while working near a dangerous edge (hazard), might be considered engineering controls.

The fourth most effective hazard control is administrative. This usually involves training personnel or putting policies and/or procedures in place to help assure operations are conducted safely. Of the hazard controls described, the least effective is personal protective equipment (PPE). Although we often consider PPE such as helmets and gloves essential and mandatory—and they are—PPE is the last barrier between the hazard and us. In the realm of risk management, all other methods of controlling the hazards should be attempted before PPE comes into play, or said a different way, all other methods of controlling the hazards should be undertaken while everyone is also wearing their PPE.

Safety Culture

A widely respected anthropologist once defined organizational culture this way:

> Organizational culture is a pattern of shared basic assumptions that the group learned as it solved its problems of external adaptation and internal integration, that has worked well enough to be considered valid and, therefore, to be taught to new members as the correct way you perceive, think, and feel in relation to those problems (Schein and Schein, 2016).

Similarly, a **safety culture** is the attitude, beliefs, perceptions, and values that people, usually in one industry or in one organization, share in relationship to safety. Culture, and safety culture, is learned and, simply put, is the way you conduct business (Cooper, 2017). In SAR, like in any industry or organization, culture is usually taught to new members through formal training, but informal methods such as stories, myths, rituals, and shared behavior generally do more to teach personnel how things are done (Jordan, 2003). The importance and role of safety in SAR is conveyed in the same way. If no one talks about safety, emphasizes safety, acts safely, enforces safety rules, teaches safety, or integrates safety into operations, it will not be part of the culture and will not be integrated into how we do business.

Studies have shown that tragedies are often the result of both a breakdown of procedures and policies designed to promote and ensure safety and inadequate attention being paid to safety issues (Schein and Schein, 2016). To prevent such breakdowns, safety must be part of every discussion, every plan, and every operation. Safety is not merely a task to be performed; it must be a deeper part of our thinking. It must be part of SAR culture.

In SAR, a safety culture is important and depends mostly on a philosophy of personal responsibility, personal preparedness, and **situational awareness** (Cooper and Finley, 2013).

Personal Responsibility for Safety

In SAR, safety is the responsibility of everyone who participates. Although there may be a safety officer assigned and many crew leaders and supervisors watching every task performed, in the end, every single person involved in the operation has a personal responsibility for his or her own safety; the safety of colleagues; and the safety of the injured victim, patient, and/or lost subject. In SAR, safety is never delegated to another. Everyone possesses and retains a personal obligation to encourage, monitor, and enforce safe practices (**FIGURE 8-2**).

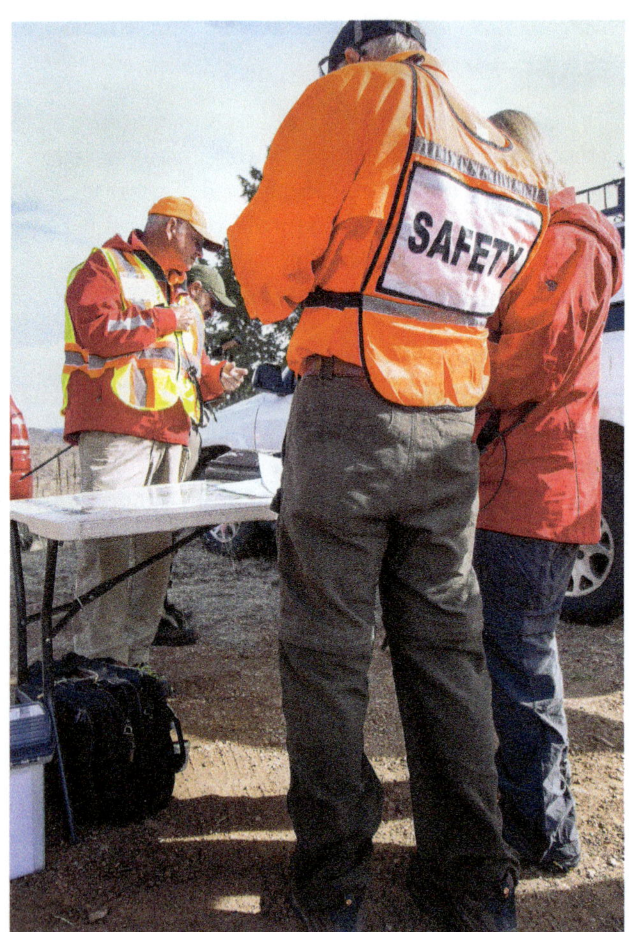

FIGURE 8-2 Although there may be a safety officer assigned and many crew leaders and supervisors watching every task performed, every single person involved in a SAR operation bears a personal responsibility for his or her own safety.

Personal Preparedness

Being prepared for field operations starts with personnel being well nourished, hydrated, and fit. This serves as a solid foundation but is not enough on its own. Operational training is necessary to build competence and confidence, and relevant skills practice is necessary to build muscle memory (the consolidation of a specific task into memory through repetition) so that correct and appropriate actions become automatic, even under stress. Finally, an essential part of being prepared is an understanding of the basic principles of risk assessment, which is necessary to evaluate an activity to determine how best to mitigate, avoid, and/or effectively deal with any associated hazards.

Situational Awareness

Operational safety cannot be achieved without at least an understanding and awareness that hazards exist in any SAR environment. Therefore, ASTM F2890 (2012a), *Standard Guide for Hazard Awareness for Search and Rescue Personnel,* was written and offers suggestions on some hazardous situations with which SAR personnel may be confronted.

Operationally, safety begins with information gathering and surveying the environment in which operations will take place. Thus, information is a valuable commodity when it comes to safety. Knowing what and where the hazards are, what to expect, and what is happening around you is invaluable when trying to stay safe. In other words, situational awareness is key (**FIGURE 8-3**). Although situational awareness was originally a military term describing a soldier's understanding of his or her surroundings and its effect on decision making, today the term has broad applications that can also be useful in search and rescue.

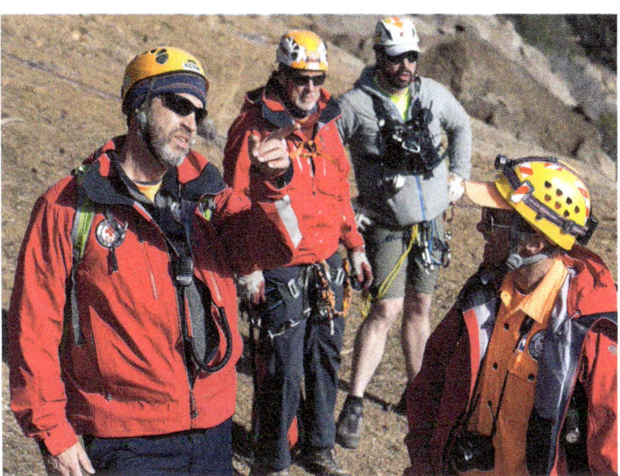

FIGURE 8-3 Knowing what and where the hazards are, what to expect, and what is happening around you is invaluable when trying to stay safe. In other words, situational awareness is key.

The late Colonel J. Cooper, a noted military author, emphasized situational awareness in a color-coded system he devised to help soldiers gauge their mindset and readiness in combat situations (Rosenberg, 2011). This approach is also useful to SAR personnel who are attempting to operate in a safe manner, often in an unforgiving, stressful environment. The system involves four colors, each used to represent a person's potential state of awareness and focus in a stressful situation: condition white, condition yellow, condition orange, and condition red.

Condition white represents a situation in which an individual is completely unaware of his or her surroundings. If something bad happens, the individual is caught completely off guard and is unable to adequately respond. **Condition yellow** represents a relaxed, heightened situational awareness where no threat exists, but the individual is alert, observant, aware of his or her surroundings, and ready to respond to a problem or threat. Condition orange exists when a specific threat is identified, and the individual verifies the threat and prepares to respond (e.g., recognizing an immediate hazard, smelling smoke, seeing an injured person). Condition red represents a verified, specific threat that demands immediate action. This situation exists, for example, when a searcher first sees a missing subject, when a person in the water is recognized as drowning, and when an injured subject is first known to require technical rescue.

This color-coded system teaches us that SAR personnel must continuously operate in condition yellow. SAR personnel must remain vigilant, aware of their surroundings, and prepared to respond to a rapidly changing environment or immediate safety threat. This persistent situational awareness is necessary for SAR personnel to stay ready to recognize and respond to unsafe situations, and it is key to safe SAR operations.

SAFETY TIP

SAR personnel must continuously operate in condition yellow and remain vigilant, aware of their surroundings, and prepared to respond to a rapidly changing environment or immediate safety threat.

Operating in condition yellow—always being cautious, alert, observant, and ready to act—also helps prevent **normalcy bias**, the tendency of an individual to underestimate the possibility of something bad happening. Normalcy bias causes people to believe that since a disaster has never happened, it never will. It therefore leaves one unprepared to deal with a hazard or threat, preventing him or her from reacting appropriately. An ongoing, full understanding of one's situation and surroundings (i.e., situational awareness) must replace normalcy bias if safety is the goal.

One simple way to achieve situational awareness is by frequently asking yourself a series of questions about your surroundings: What is going on? How are we doing? Does everything look right? What is my role and what are the hazards in my area of operation? Answering these questions helps you recognize and identify a problem that is developing, which in turn allows you to intervene and do something about it should it be necessary. In addition, several things can work against situational awareness, such as fatigue, drugs/alcohol, and complacency. If situational awareness is key to safety, then these activities should be recognized as direct threats to safety that must be avoided.

Standard Precautions

In the field of health care, it is widely accepted that all human bodily fluids and tissue must be treated as if they were known to be infected with **bloodborne pathogens**. To address this, what are known in the healthcare field as **standard precautions** are hazard control measures that must be applied in SAR situations when personal contact is made with a subject (patient) during the provision of medical care. Standard precautions include two general types of control measures: (1) the use of personal protective healthcare equipment such as gloves (e.g., latex, nitrile, or vinyl), facemasks/face shields (e.g., surgical), eye protection (e.g., eye visor or goggles), and gowns (e.g., clothing covers), and (2) other practices, such as hand hygiene and respiratory hygiene/cough etiquette, that mitigate the risk of exposure to the transmission of infectious agents (CDC, 2017).

According to the World Health Organization (2007), standard precautions should include the following. Although they may be difficult or impossible to accomplish in the field during SAR operations, SAR personnel should know what standard precautions are and that they are appropriate in a SAR environment—to the extent they can be accomplished—because the standard applies when providing medical care to a patient.

- *Hand hygiene.* Hand washing (40–60 seconds): wet hands and apply soap; rub all surfaces; rinse hands and dry thoroughly with a single-use towel; use the towel to turn off the faucet. Alcohol-based hand rub (20–30 seconds): rinse/wipe mud and dirt from hands; apply enough product to cover all areas of the hands; rub hands until dry.
- *Gloves.* Wear when touching blood, body fluids, secretions, excretions, mucous membranes, and nonintact skin. Latex, nitrile, or vinyl gloves can be worn under work gloves. Change gloves between tasks and procedures on the same patient after contact with potentially infectious material. Remove after use, before touching noncontaminated items and surfaces, and before going to another patient. Perform hand hygiene immediately after removal.
- *Facial protection.* Wear (1) a surgical or procedure mask and eye protection (eye visor, goggles) or (2) a face shield to protect mucous membranes of the eyes, nose, and mouth during activities that are likely to generate splashes or sprays of blood, body fluids, secretions, and excretions. If this equipment is not available, protecting the eyes and mucous membranes from body fluids in any reasonable way (glasses, balaclava, etc.) may be helpful.
- *Clothing cover (gown).* Wear to protect skin and prevent soiling of clothing during activities that are likely to generate splashes or sprays of blood, body fluids, secretions, or excretions. Remove soiled clothing or covering as soon as possible, and perform hand hygiene.
- *Respiratory hygiene and cough etiquette.* Cover the patient's nose and mouth when coughing/sneezing with a tissue or mask, dispose of used tissues and masks, and perform hand hygiene after contact with respiratory secretions.
- *Environmental cleaning.* Use adequate procedures for the routine cleaning and disinfection of environmental and other frequently touched surfaces.
- *Clothing.* Handle, transport, and process these in a manner that both prevents skin and mucous membrane exposures and contamination and avoids transfer of pathogens to other patients/personnel and/or the environment.
- *Waste disposal.* Ensure safe waste management. Treat waste contaminated with blood, body fluids, secretions and excretions as clinical waste, in accordance with local regulations. Discard single-use items properly.
- Patient care equipment. Handle equipment soiled with blood, body fluids, secretions, and excretions in a manner that prevents skin and mucous membrane exposures, contamination of clothing, and transfer of pathogens to other patients or the environment. Clean, disinfect, and reprocess reusable equipment appropriately before use with another patient.

When SAR personnel come in direct contact with an injured or ill patient, they have a **duty of care** to equip themselves, know how, and be prepared to use standard precautions.

Special SAR Environments

Search and rescue teams throughout the world are called upon frequently to solve complex problems in many diverse environments. Search and rescue personnel, whether at the end of a long search or responding directly to a person in distress, should realize that most SAR incidents are solved by well-trained, highly specialized—not just well meaning—responders.

Because of the critical and sometimes dangerous nature of these specialized skills, any responder must be able to recognize when the special abilities required to resolve a situation exceed his or her personal skillset. Knowing when to call someone else to help because the situation calls for more than what your skillset provides is itself a specialized skill on which life and death may depend. For those responders trained to NFPA 1006, *Standard for Technical Rescue Personnel Professional Qualifications*, this may mean calling for rescue at the technician level if the situation is beyond the capabilities of operations level rescuers. Deciding to ask for help and having the personal courage and maturity to do so may be the most important decision one can make in a SAR situation—for both the subject and the responders.

Some of the specialized environments and associated problems that SAR team members may have to deal with are included in **TABLE 8-1**.

Regardless of the type of rescue environment involved, following guidelines common to all can be helpful:

- Technical personnel should be used for technical rescue.
- If the subject is deceased, evacuate only if and when there is no risk to fellow team members, or at least when the hazards have been assessed and justified.
- Stabilize the subject before evacuating, if possible; continue stabilization procedures during transport.
- Decide on the easiest route before traveling.
- Appoint someone to serve as route-finder, who with a radio and markers can report potential hazards, problems, etc.
- Litter teams of at least six to eight personnel (three teams preferred) should be used in no more than 20-minute shifts. Others may also be required to carry equipment.
- Use accepted procedures to care for and protect the subject.
- A radio operator should follow the litter team.
- If using a helicopter for evacuation, make sure that:
  - The subject is informed and briefed about what he or she may experience.
  - The subject is protected from wind and noise.
  - Someone goes with the subject who knows what has been done medically for the patient.
- Sworn law enforcement and fire service personnel should be easily identified as such in the field (e.g., wear uniform or clearly marked clothing). SAR personnel should be identifiable as such but must not be dressed so as to be mistaken as sworn public safety personnel.

TABLE 8-1 Specialized SAR Environments and Challenges

Mountain, alpine	Air shaft
Vertical rock	White-water river
Vertical ice	Coastal white-water surf
Flat ice	Flash flood
Avalanche	Slow rising flood
Crevasse	High wind
Cave	Sea and lake
Mine	Snow and blizzard
Well	Booby traps
Hazardous material dump	Confined space
Urban/city	Trench

Specialized SAR environments bring a diverse set of problems and potential complications for rendering aid to injured and/or stranded subjects. Each environment holds its own set of obstacles to increase the complexity and difficulty of a particular mission.

Technical Rock Rescue

The popularity of mountaineering, rock climbing, and casual scrambling have created the need for specialized SAR expertise (**FIGURE 8-4**). Individuals and groups involved in this type of rescue have refined and developed techniques for most situations. The hallmark of a technical rock rescuer is the ability to improvise and modify tools or techniques to meet any crisis. He or she must be comfortable using climbing gear and working at heights.

Once an individual has been located in this environment and the situation surveyed, it becomes necessary to gain access to the subject. Local climbing or mountaineering groups familiar with the area likely have already solved

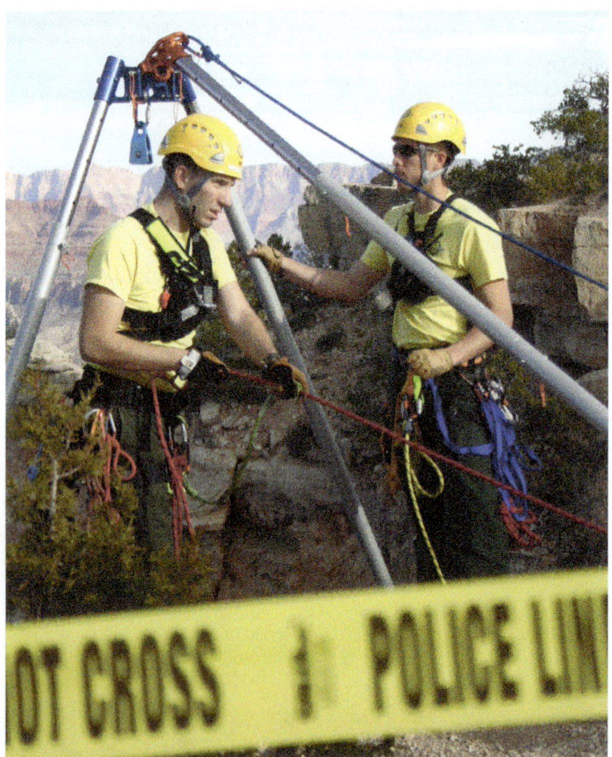

FIGURE 8-4 Specialized SAR expertise is necessary for technical rock rescue in mountainous terrain.
Courtesy of Ken Phillips.

this problem. The solution may involve either climbing or descending to the subject. Safety for all persons involved is paramount because an accident during a rescue can be catastrophic. Climbing up to the subject requires knowledge of climbing techniques, possession of the proper equipment, and familiarity with its use. Local clubs or mountaineering stores can be contacted for more detailed assistance. Specialized technical rescue teams, such as those accredited by the Mountain Rescue Association, routinely practice climbing techniques and the solving of vertical rescue problems.

The decision to go up, down, or sideways to reach a subject depends on ease of access to both the top and the bottom. Fast-moving water at the bottom, for example, may preclude an approach from below. Conversely, a brush-filled approach to the top may preclude a topside approach. Helicopter availability, adequate landing sites, suitable anchors, and ease of climbing are also considerations when deciding whether to approach from the top or bottom.

Descending necessitates good technique and proper anchors. Rappelling, or descending via rope, allows more control by the descending rescuer, but "ties up" his or her hands. Because of this, the incident commander may elect to lower the rescuer rather than allow him or her to rappel. Lowering necessitates greater communication between the top and the rescuer but allows the rescuer's hands to be free. Lowering also usually takes more rescuers to perform.

If the subject can assist himself or herself, self-rescue may be possible. On the other hand, if the subject needs to be placed in a litter, the assistance of additional rescuers and equipment may be required.

Steep inclines, cliffs, bluffs, and similar terrain features that involve elevation differential may require specialized skills and equipment to ascend and/or descend. SAR personnel should not attempt traveling over this type of terrain without expert guidance and the proper equipment and training. When these are not available, SAR personnel should travel around the area, note it, and describe it when debriefed. During a search, it may also be prudent to determine if the subject fell in the hazardous terrain by carefully searching likely landing spots if they can be safely accessed.

ASTM F1773, *Standard Terminology Relating to Climbing, Mountaineering, Search and Rescue Equipment and Practices*, defines many terms that would be helpful in communicating in and about these types of rescues.

Cave and Mine Rescue

Standard obstacles in the underground environment include poor communications; difficulty in lighting; and cramped, wet spaces. In addition, reduced visibility often mandates lighting the rescue scene beyond the normal limits of a flashlight or headlamp (**FIGURE 8-5**).

Most caves involve moisture ranging from a bit of mud to fast-moving rivers. In the United States, western caves are generally drier than eastern caves. However, humidity, wetness, and cold temperature create a potential for hypothermia greatly underestimated by the average caver. Flooding is often a great problem, and many cavers have died because of inattention to the weather on the outside. Caves become natural drains for streams during heavy rains and thus can provide

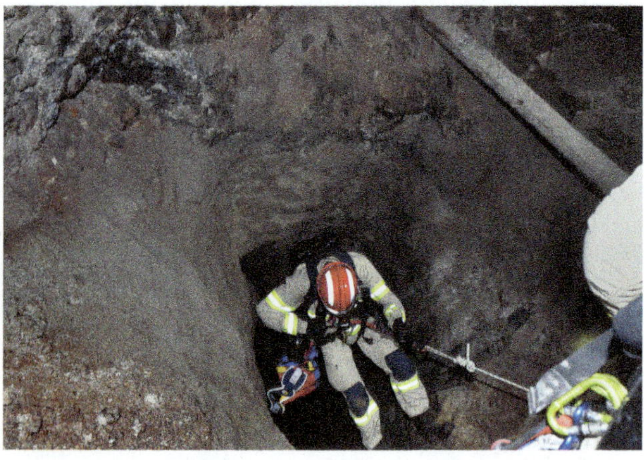

FIGURE 8-5 Standard obstacles in the underground environment include poor communications; difficulty in lighting; and cramped, wet spaces.
© 2016 Howard Paul, Photography for Communication and Commerce.

problems for both caver and rescuer. Wind and temperature are other underestimated problems associated with cave and mine emergencies. Extreme movements of air often develop along passages, which, like in any environment, intensifies convective air chilling.

Confined passages, low crawls, and squeezes pose unique problems for the rescue of injured cavers. The use of standard items such as litters, backboards, and splints may not be possible in such places. Confined passages with varying, often toxic, constituent gases can also lead to difficulties for victims and rescuers alike. Occasionally, self-contained breathing apparatus (SCBA), surface-supplied air, and/or self-contained underwater breathing apparatus (SCUBA) may be required. The potential for toxic gases justifies extensive and constant atmospheric monitoring while operating in the subterranean environment.

It is important to note that SCUBA diving, especially in a cave or similar confined space, is a very specialized skill that requires unique equipment and training. A standard recreational diving certificate (sport diving) by itself does not qualify an individual to conduct or participate in diving operations in a cave, under ice, or in contaminated water, among other hazardous environments. A public safety diving certificate with specialty training in the environment involved (e.g., cave, ice, contaminated) is recommended, as is a basic open water certification. Public safety divers are trained in diving in black water (zero visibility) and in various hazardous environments. Public safety diving is conducted by public safety agencies such as fire and police department dive teams, and several high-quality training programs exist, many of which meet NFPA training standards relevant to public safety diving (NFPA, 2017a; NFPA, 2017b). More information about safe cave diving is available through the National Speleological Society Cave Diving Section (NSSCDS, 2017) and the National Association of Cave Diving (NACD, 2016), both not-for-profit organizations long dedicated to safe diving in caves.

An essential part of any cave and mine rescue operation involves a thorough orientation to the specific hazards known to be associated with a particular underground area. This involves pinpointing the locations of pits, waterfalls, siphons, canyons, and other difficult formations that may pose extrication, search, or safety problems. Many caves have been mapped by the National Speleological Society (specifically, the Survey and Cartography Section of the NSS) and the National Park Service. Eleven U.S. states, each with numerous caves, also have cave survey organizations that provide a source for printed and electronic maps (SACS NSS, 2017). The National Cave Rescue Commission (NCRC) offers excellent cave rescue-related training in the areas of incident management, patient medical care underground, rope skills, technical ropes and anchors, leadership, practical cave rescue skills, and more (NCRC NSS, 2017). Anyone interested in cave SAR should take advantage of this training

The Federal Mine Safety and Health Act of 1977 (Public Law 95-164) can be found in the U.S. Code under Title 30, Mineral Lands and Mining, Chapter 22, Mine Safety and Health, and established the Mine Safety and Health Administration (MSHA) within the U.S. Department of Labor. The Mine Act requires that every operator of an underground mine assure the availability of mine rescue teams for purposes of emergency rescue and recovery of trapped or injured miners (**FIGURE 8-6**). Rescue teams must receive adequate training in accordance with 30 CFR Part 49.8 for underground mines and 30 CFR Part 49.18 for underground coal mines (MSHA, 2017). In-person courses are held regularly at the National Mine Health and Safety Academy in Beaver, West Virginia, and can also be scheduled at other locations upon request. No team should attempt a rescue in a mine without personnel trained to meet these national standards.

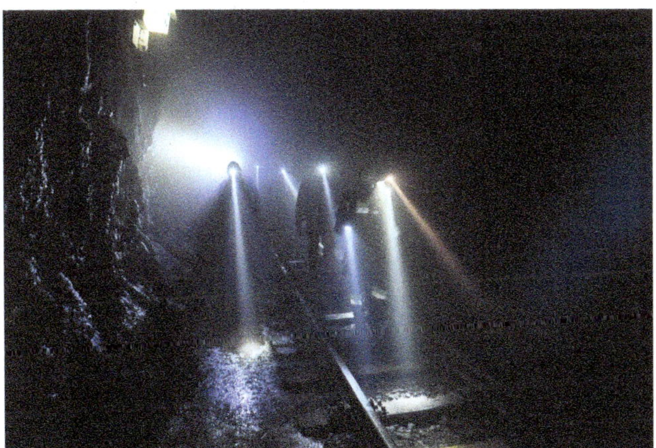

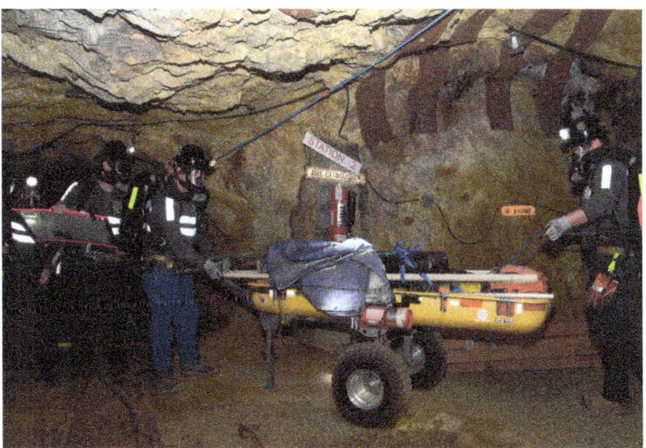

FIGURE 8-6 Once a subject has been located in a cave or mine, the goal is to move that person rapidly and comfortably to the surface, but without practice underground, that task will be virtually impossible.

Once a subject has been located in a cave or mine, the real difficulties may begin. The goal is to move that person rapidly and comfortably to the surface, but without practice underground, that task will be virtually impossible. Neoprene exposure bags similar to body bags have been used for this purpose and serve well to keep the individual dry and protected during what may be a very long and slow evacuation.

From a medical aid standpoint, procedures must be performed smoothly in dark, cold, and muddy conditions. Experienced cave rescuers agree that repackaging supplies and equipment for underground use is essential. Streamlining kits, packs, and containers is a must for unobstructed passage through crawlways and tight spaces in the cold, damp conditions.

Team members often carry a minimum of 24 hours of light in a helmet-mounted lamp, two additional sources of light with spare bulbs and batteries, and waterproof matches and candles. Other equipment needed in this environment might include:

- High-quality helmet with chinstrap and headlamp attachment
- Sturdy, warm clothes, including gloves, for damp, dirty conditions for up to 24 hours (i.e., wool material, fit that allows good mobility)
- Lug-soled boots that are light, warm, inexpensive, and drain water
- Nonstretch (static), specialized caving rope that is highly resistant to abrasion
- Neil Robertson-style wraparound litter that can aid in dragging an injured person through small passages. A common Stokes litter may work fine.
- Wetsuits for longer missions in extremely wet caves
- Durable harnesses and slings that are resistant to both chemicals and water
- Plastic sheeting to divert water and waterfall around a subject during evacuation
- Small portable pumps, siphon hose, and plastic to divert, dam, or pump water around areas during operations
- Warm food and drink carried in thermally insulated containers

Essential caving skills include all the capabilities and proficiencies that exist in rock climbing, including vertical rope technique, ascending, rappelling, belaying, and being comfortable while working at the end of a rope. All of these must be practiced until they can be done well in cold, wet, and dark confined spaces. Team practices should be conducted both on the surface and underground with participants being forced to work in mud, suffocating tight squeezes, soaking waterfalls, and occasional blinding darkness. Under these conditions, all team members should be aware of the possibility of hypothermia during training.

SEARCH AND RESCUE TIP

Essential caving skills must be practiced repeatedly until they can be done well in cold, wet, and dark confined spaces.

If a cave or mine is found in one's assigned search segment, the following guidelines should be followed:

1. Examine the area near the opening for evidence of the entry of others (e.g., tracks, sign).
2. Do not enter the cave or mine beyond the natural light zone near the opening. Safely going past this area requires specialized equipment and skills.
3. Note the cave or mine on a map and make sure to mention it, along with the likelihood someone would/could have entered it, at the debriefing.

Exploring newly discovered caves, especially ones that are unattended, is dangerous. Never enter a cave alone or without the company of knowledgeable and experienced cavers.

NFPA 1670, *Standard on Operations and Training for Technical Search and Rescue Incidents*, and NFPA 1006 include standards relevant to cave and mine search and rescue. Reviewing and becoming familiar with these documents is recommended for SAR personnel who may operate in or around caves and mines.

River and White-Water Rescue

There are dozens of potentially dangerous situations that can arise when operating in and around **swift water**. Log and debris piles at various points in the river can become a **strainer** and death trap to both the victim and the would-be rescuer. The banks of the waterway may be deeply undercut with treacherous overhanging debris and snags that can catch on clothing, equipment, and flesh. These factors combine with muddy and rapidly moving and rising water to render river rescue difficult, unpredictable, and treacherous.

In fast-moving water, the single greatest problem associated with the environment is that responders too often underestimate the power and threat of moving water (**FIGURE 8-7**). Foolhardy heroics and overzealous enthusiasm frequently lead to further tragedy. Cold water coupled with wind and cold temperatures may predispose anyone to hypothermia. Then, wet clothing, darkness, and injury may add to the danger. Noise associated with moving water is often significant and may obviate clear communications. Poor contact between the victim and rescuers, or between rescuers and their colleagues, can be both confusing and hazardous.

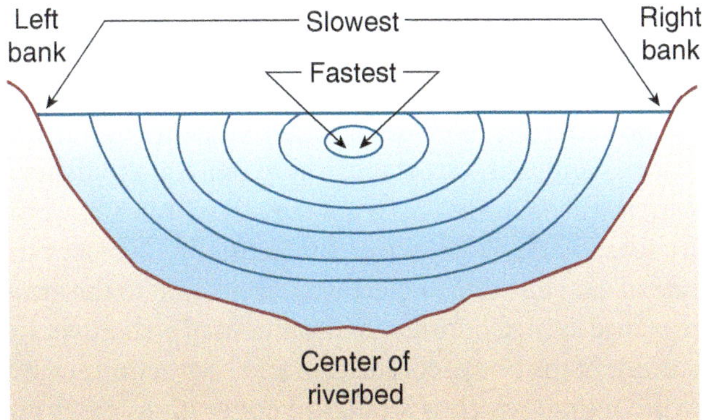

FIGURE 8-7 The cross section of a river, showing the relative velocity of moving water.

All potential responders in this environment must know how to read the water for dangerous phenomena such as hydraulics, strainers, and floating debris. A **hydraulic** formed by a **low head dam**, collapsed bridge, or other submerged object or debris (e.g., strainers) can be a drowning machine for unsuspecting individuals. Rescue team members must know how to protect themselves at all times in and around fast-moving water. Mandatory skills in this environment include good judgment, strong swimming skills, knowledge of all types of technical systems and equipment used in rope rescue, and a thorough understanding of river dynamics and hydraulic influences.

Swift water rescue is a very specialized subject that requires specialized equipment and skills. Entering the swift water environment, including walking near moving water, should be attempted by specially trained and equipped personnel only. If properly trained and equipped personnel are not available, the river/moving water environment should be carefully avoided. SAR personnel without specialized training who come across moving water during a search should note or confirm the location on the map, be careful not to approach too closely, and make sure to mention the water during the debrief. Do not attempt to cross moving water deeper than midthigh, and crossing swiftly water moving (greater than 1 knot [1 nautical mile per hour]) should not be attempted. Chapter 12, *Foot Travel for SAR Personnel*, contains more information on how to cross moving water.

The following standards include water search and rescue requirements and are recommended reading for SAR personnel who may be involved in water rescue:

- NFPA 1670, *Standard on Operations and Training for Technical Search and Rescue Incidents* (NFPA, 2017a)
- NFPA 1006, *Standard for Technical Rescue Personnel Professional Qualifications* (NFPA, 2017b)
- ASTM F1730, *Standard Guide for Throwing a Water Rescue Throwbag*
- ASTM F1739, *Standard Guide for Performance of a Water Rescuer–Level I*
- ASTM F1824, *Standard Guide for Performance of a Water Rescuer–Level II*

General Water Precautions

A fundamental understanding of certain techniques and hazards is important in all water rescue situations. Survival swimming is a technique that may be useful in relatively warm water, and an understanding of immersion hypothermia will be useful if you find yourself in cold water.

Survival Swimming

Most swimmers do not realize that if they are injured but conscious, even without a personal flotation device (PFD), they can survive in all but the coldest and roughest seas. A simple technique called *survival floating* or *drown proofing* was developed during World War II. The technique is based on two principles: (1) Almost everyone will float while their lungs are full of air, and (2) it is much easier to float vertically than horizontally.

To perform the survival float, first take a deep breath, then float vertically with your hands limply held at your sides, allowing your body to relax in the water with your chin tucked to your chest. As the need to breathe arises, exhale slowly through your nose while raising your arms and crossing them in front of your face. Now, extend your arms as if parting a curtain, and push downward with cupped hands and fingers held tightly together. At the same time, tilt the head back and, as your mouth comes out of the water, take a breath, lower the head, and relax again. If you can control your anxiety and stay relaxed with this technique, you can also alternately switch between a slow, horizontal movement toward shore and the survival float. Even with a cramp, it is possible to stay afloat and relax the muscle by slowly massaging it between breaths of air. The only place where survival floating is not recommended, and indeed may be dangerous, is in cold water where hypothermia is a factor.

Immersion Hypothermia

All people who play or work on or near water should appreciate the factors that determine the body's cooling rate while immersed. Properly used, this vital water safety knowledge can extend survival time from minutes to hours. In terms of rescue, this could be the difference between life and death.

As discussed in the section on survival physiology, hypothermia is cooling of the body's inner core. In immersion hypothermia, this rate of cooling is greatly accelerated because, submerged in water, the skin and peripheral areas cool very rapidly due to the increased surface area in direct contact with cold water.

Sea water freezes at around 28° to 29° Fahrenheit (F) (−2.2° to −1.7° Celsius [C]) and fresh water at about 32°F (0°C), but a high level of impurities lowers the freezing point of both. Depending on clothing worn, a person suddenly immersed in water at or near freezing quickly exhales uncontrollably, shivers violently, and contracts into a fetal position with hands and knees under the chin, usually with little to no control of skeletal muscles.

A body immersed in water near its freezing point cools very rapidly. Upon submersion, reflex contractions of smaller blood vessels give a fleeting increase in blood pressure and heart rate, but subsequently both reduce to near death levels.

As the body starts to cool in water, vasoconstriction (narrowing of blood vessels) occurs in the peripheral blood vessels of the limbs and skin. This decreases blood flow to the extremities to preserve heat in the core, thereby protecting the vital organs but allowing the periphery to cool. Exercise increases body temperature by burning calories and is an acceptable way to maintain body temperature in open air. This is not the case in water, however. Increased activity in water substantially increases the rate of heat loss due to increased circulation to the arms, legs, and skin. Continuous movement of water over the surface of the body (conduction and convection) causes this cooling, which is similar to convection losses due to wind but much more severe. In the coldest water, it takes most adults more than 30 minutes to become even mildly hypothermic (Giesbrecht, 2011). Subjects finding themselves immersed in cold water should consider how long it would take to swim to safety and compare it to the benefits of waiting for rescue while preserving body heat through special positioning (see following sections), especially if wearing a PFD, or finding a way of getting out of the water (e.g., onto flotsam).

Survival Time

Survival time in cold water is affected by several variables including the temperature of the water, length of exposure, activity levels, metabolic rate, body fat, physical size, age, gender, and type of clothing worn. **TABLE 8-2** shows general survival times for an average adult holding still in water of varying temperatures while wearing a standard PFD and light clothing.

Personal Flotation Devices

A **personal flotation device (PFD)** is designed to serve one primary purpose: to help keep the wearer's head above water. Because no PFD is capable of keeping one's head above the water in all situations, some compromises usually have to be made in terms of mobility, comfort, and flotation for a particular application. It is critical that all rescuers wear PFDs when working

TABLE 8-2 Effects of Immersion on the Average Adult Holding Still in Water While Wearing a PFD

Water Temperature	Effects of Immersion	
Degrees F (°C)	**Exhaustion or Unconsciousness**	**Expected Time of Survival**
32.5° (0.3°)	Under 15 minutes	15–45 minutes
36.5–40° (0.3–4.5°)	15–30 minutes	30–90 minutes
40–50° (4.5–10°)	30–60 minutes	1–3 hours
50–60° (10–15.5°)	1–2 hours	1–6 hours
60–70° (15.5–21°)	2–7 hours	2–40 hours
70–80° (21–26.5°)	2–12 hours	3 hours to indefinite
Over 80° (Over 26.5°)	Indefinite	Indefinite

Data from United States Coast Guard [USCG]. (2017). PFD Selection, Use, Wear & Care: Cold Water Survival. Retrieved from http://www.dco.uscg.mil/CG-ENG-4/PFDSel/.

near or on the water to guard against the hazards of hypothermia and drowning.

PFDs should always conform to standards set by the appropriate national regulatory authority, which is the U.S. Coast Guard (USCG) in the United States. In addition, a PFD used for SAR should:

- Be highly visible
- Provide adequate flotation for the individual using it and the specific situation in which it is used
- Be adequately fitted for the individual who will be wearing it
- Offer unrestricted mobility
- Allow for impact protection for the wearer using foam panels
- Offer protection from hypothermia and heat illness associated with use
- Provide multiple closure devices for a secure fit (ASTM, 2012b)

In addition to these performance requirements, PFDs used in SAR should have a loud whistle (for signaling) attached. A small knife in a sheath may also be attached to the PFD for if cutting line becomes necessary. River rescue personnel often attach a length of webbing or Prusik loop with one or two carabiners, which can be useful in several ways, including rolling a canoe or kayak off a rock.

In the United States, OSHA requires that PFDs be worn when there is a chance of a worker falling into water, such as working near unguarded edges, boarding or leaving small boats, or working on floats. OSHA also requires that PFDs be inspected for defects before each use and that they be worn and fastened properly (OSHA, 2017b).

There are five types of USCG-approved PFDs in the United States, and each type is designated with a Roman numeral (**TABLE 8-3**).

Type I PFDs are required on commercial vessels and provide the maximum **buoyancy** (**FIGURE 8-8**). They are brightly colored and designed for use in rough water where they should turn an unconscious person into the face-up position. Because they tend to be large, bulky, cumbersome, and come in only two sizes (adult and child), they are usually not recommended for most SAR work. However, where rough waters are anticipated, and maximum flotation is required, a Type I PFD may be the best tool for the job.

Type II PFDs are the relatively inexpensive "horse collar" style devices that are made to be donned easily in an emergency (**FIGURE 8-9**). Although not as effective as the Type I, the Type II is also designed to turn an unconscious person to the face-up position. Its relatively low cost, and other features, cause it to be best suited for general boating and quick rescue activities.

TABLE 8-3 Types of U.S. Coast Guard Approved Personal Flotation Devices

Type	Description
I	Maximum buoyancy, bulky, turns an unconscious wearer face up. Minimum adult buoyancy 22 pounds.
II	Horse-collar type, easily donned, turns an unconscious wearer face up. Minimum adult buoyancy 15.5 pounds.
III	Minimum safe buoyancy, comfortable, does NOT turn unconscious wearer face up but keeps conscious wearer upright. Minimum adult buoyancy 15.5 pounds.
IV	Throwable devices, designed for grasping and holding, not for wearing. Minimum adult buoyancy 16.5 (ring buoy) and 18 pounds (boat cushion).
V	Specific activity or hybrid (inflatable) class; turns unconscious wearer face up. Minimum adult buoyancy for special use inflatable, 22 to 34 pounds; hybrid inflatable, 7.5 pounds (deflated) to 22 pounds (inflated); and special use noninflatable (buoyant), 15.5 to 22 pounds.

Data from United States Coast Guard [USCG]. (2017). PFD Selection, Use, Wear & Care. Retrieved from http://www.dco.uscg.mil/CG-ENG-4/PFDSel/.

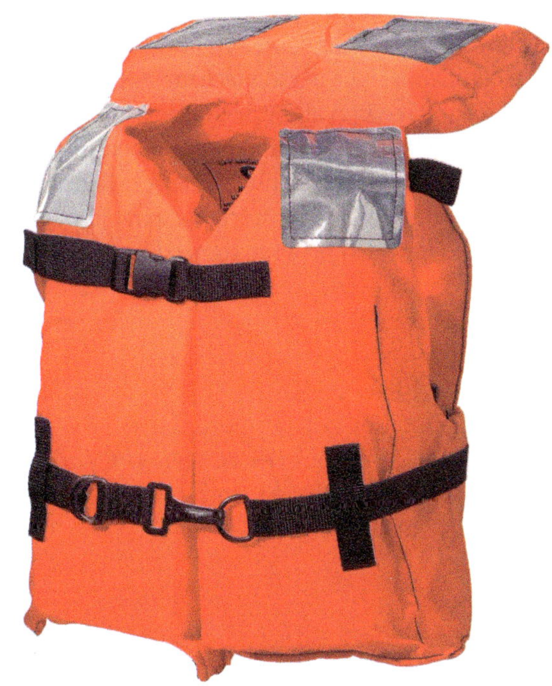

FIGURE 8-8 Example of a Type I PFD.

Courtesy of Onyx Outdoor.

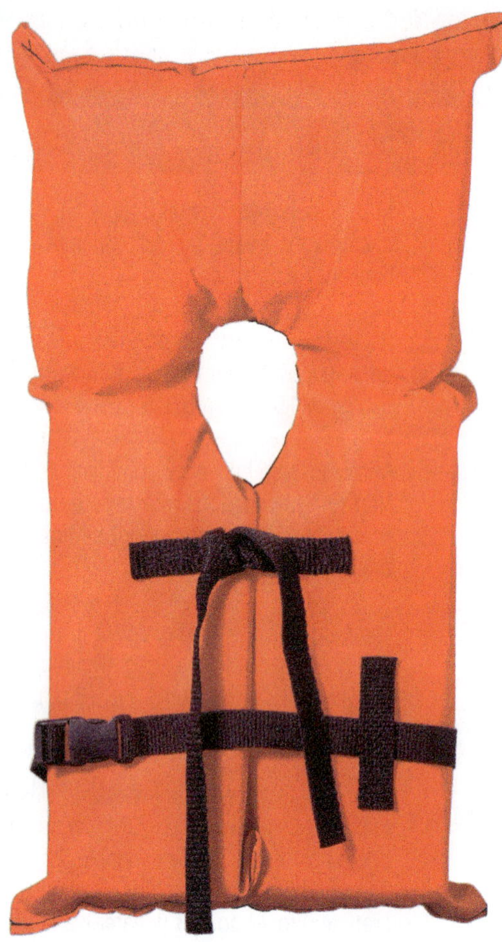

FIGURE 8-9 Example of a USCG-approved Type II PFD.
Courtesy of Onyx Outdoor.

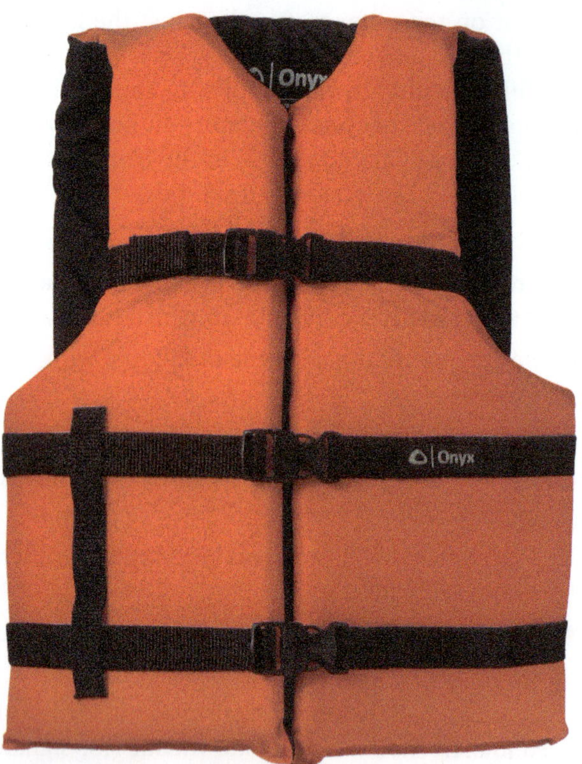

FIGURE 8-10 Example of a USCG-approved Type III PFD.
Courtesy of Onyx Outdoor.

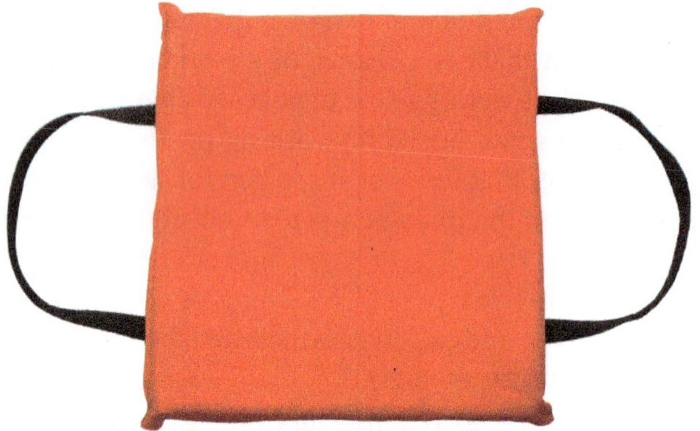

FIGURE 8-11 Example of a USCG-approved Type IV PFD.
Courtesy of Onyx Outdoor.

Type III PFDs contain the minimum amount of buoyancy required for safety, usually maintain a conscious person in an upright position, but do not necessarily turn an unconscious person face up (**FIGURE 8-10**). These characteristics allow flexibility in design to match the needs of specialized and general boating activities such as fishing, skiing, canoeing, and kayaking. In general, these devices are comfortable, pliable, and easy to swim in. They also provide some thermal protection, are brightly colored, come in various sizes, combine both zippers and torso straps, and provide an excellent choice for most water rescue activities.

Type IV PFDs are throwable devices such as ring buoys and flotation seat cushions that have a minimum of 16 pounds' buoyancy (**FIGURE 8-11**). These devices are not designed to be worn but grasped and held in the water until rescue.

SEARCH AND RESCUE TIP

To provide protection, a PFD must be *worn*.

Type V PFDs are divided into two classes: specific activity and hybrid (**FIGURE 8-12**). The specific activity devices are designed and restricted to the specific applications indicated on the label. Examples include water skiing, board sailing, work vests, and commercial white-water rafting. The hybrid class of Type V PFD, on the other hand, is **inflatable** and contains a minimum of 7.5 pounds' buoyancy when uninflated and 22 pounds' buoyancy when inflated. These devices have an oral inflation tube, often have an automatic carbon dioxide (CO_2) inflation cartridge, and are designed to turn an unconscious person face up, the same as a Type I or II. For USCG acceptability, however, these hybrid PFDs

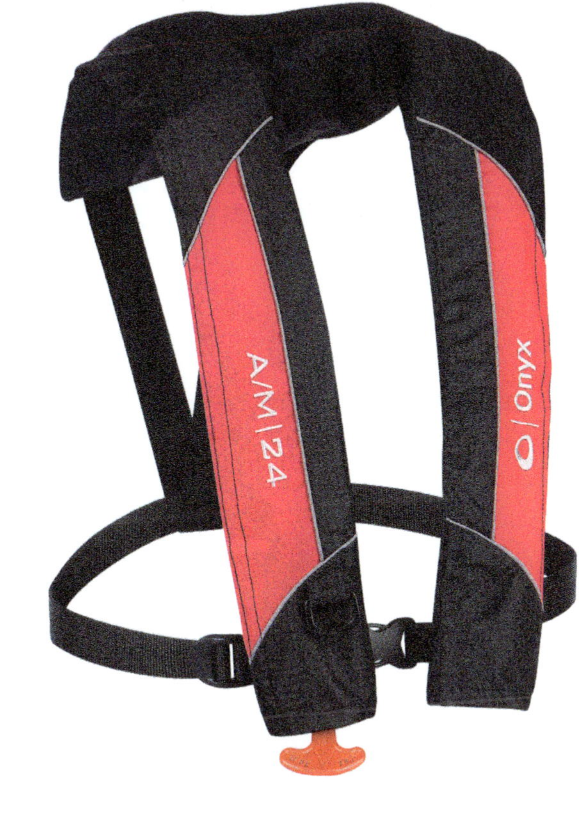

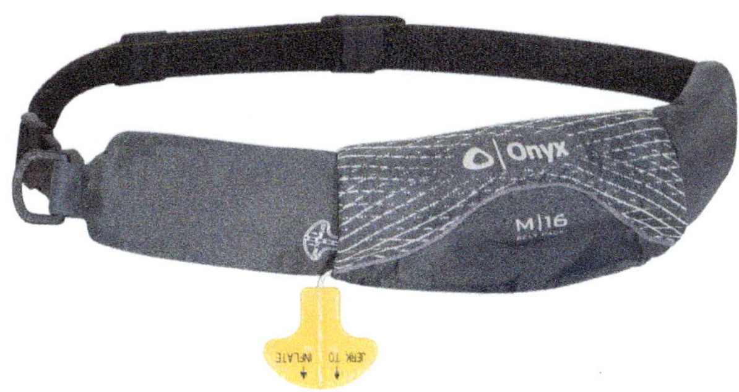

FIGURE 8-12 Example of a USCG-approved Type V PFD (specific activity hybrid class shown).
Courtesy of Onyx Outdoor.

must be worn (except when the vessel is not underway or when the user is in an enclosed space).

In summary, USCG-approved Type I PFDs are best suited where rough waters are expected and maximum flotation is required (e.g., rescue on the open sea). Type II PFDs are useful where ease of donning is important and a quick rescue is anticipated (e.g., flat water rescue or sudden boating accident). Type III PFDs are best suited where comfort and mobility are important, but where maximum flotation is not (e.g., river rescue). Type IV PFDs are useful for throwing to a victim during a rescue but should not be worn as flotation to effect a rescue. Type V specific activity PFDs are appropriate when the particular device has been specifically designed for its intended use. Type V hybrid PFDs, on the other hand, should be used as flotation only in an emergency.

PFDs offer more than just flotation; they also act as a cushion to protect the user from a fall, debris in the water (rocks, logs, etc.), or other trauma. In addition, they provide a layer of thermal protection. For instance, Type I and Type II PFDs offer limited thermal protection, but well-designed Type III and Type V PFDs may offer 50–75% increases in the predicted survival time. In the end, one point needs to be emphasized: A PFD must be worn to offer protection.

Dry suits (neoprene suits that trap air against the skin, providing both warmth and buoyancy) are generally expensive and may be bulky; however, they are useful in many cold water or ice situations where hypothermia is a primary concern. The "Gumby" suit is an example of a type of dry suit that is designed for use where a clothed rescuer could quickly don the suit and effect a surface rescue in cold water. The Gumby suit is an oversized, one-piece garment built from 1/4-inch (6.35-mm) neoprene, which offers substantial buoyancy. It has an integrated hood and booties with rubber seals at the wrists and face that prevent the entrance of water. An insulating clothing layer can be worn beneath it, which contributes to its bulk but enhances its warmth. Other thinner, less bulky types of dry suits are better choices when greater dexterity is needed, such as in moving water rescues. Regardless of the increased buoyancy a dry suit provides, a PFD should always be worn over it during a water rescue.

Three options are open to a person in cold water without a life jacket: swim to safety, survival float, or tread water.

With the first option, swimming, the time spent swimming, or the swimming distance, is the primary consideration, especially if the water is very cold. If there is no refuge within a safe swimming distance, or the water temperature is too cold to swim for it, only survival floating or treading water remain as choices. If the drown proofing (survival floating) method of conserving energy and staying afloat is used, the primary heat-radiating area of the body—the head—is repeatedly immersed and the body cools much faster. Therefore, drown proofing is considered dangerous in cold water (Tawrell, 2006). The third option, treading water, loses body heat much faster than floating motionless in a PFD but not as fast as while drown proofing. Treading water slowly, therefore, is likely the better choice when a PFD or other flotation is not available.

Increasing Survival Time

The body's primary heat loss areas are the head, neck, sides of the chest/underarms, groin area, sternum, and wrists (**FIGURE 8-13**). Therefore, it makes sense to concentrate primarily on protecting these areas from

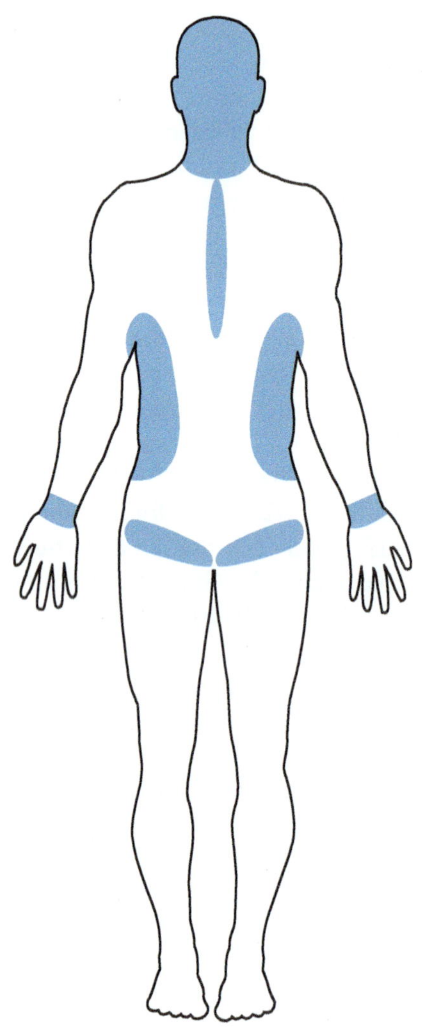

FIGURE 8-13 Body zones of heat loss. Shaded regions depict areas of greatest heat loss in the body.

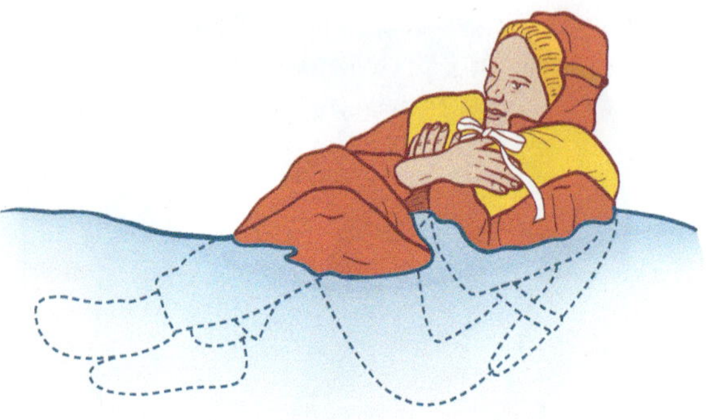

FIGURE 8-14 Curl into the fetal position with legs and arms crossed to keep yourself warm in cold water.

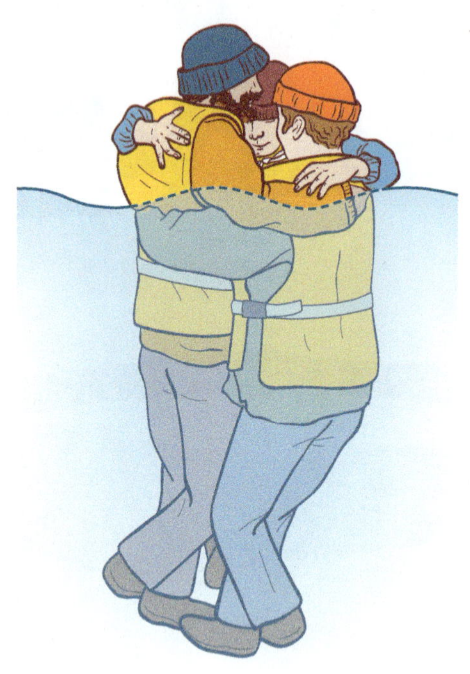

FIGURE 8-15 Huddle position for keeping more than one person warm in cold water.

heat loss if immersed in cold water. To do so, pull your knees toward your chest, cross your ankles, and cross your arms at your chest. Doing so helps reduce heat loss from your core (ASTM, 2014a). This position can double survival time in cold water compared to treading water (**FIGURE 8-14**) (University of Minnesota, 2015).

If more than one person is immersed, they can all extend survival time by huddling together, arms linked. This positioning allows the group members to share body heat (ASTM, 2014b) (**FIGURE 8-15**).

Cold, Snow, and Ice SAR

Perhaps no other type of SAR environment requires a more diverse and broad-based foundation of personal and team skills than those that involve cold, snow, and ice. The skills required might include downhill and/or cross-country skiing, snowshoeing, technical climbing, winter survival, and a good understanding of snow and ice physics. Unlike climbing on rock, snow and ice conditions change on a frequent—even minute-to-minute—basis. The effects of gravity, wind, temperature, slope, heat exchange, load factors, and avalanche continually impose problems for missions. Technical and nontechnical SAR problems in snow and ice environments are longer, more taxing, technical, and complex. Combined with shorter days, extremes in weather, and the ever-present threat of hypothermia and cold injuries, technical missions of this type can be prohibitively hazardous for all but the most experienced team members.

Versatility and improvisation are essential components of the overall strategy that must be used in snow and ice. Transportation of the patient is often one of the most difficult problems, and it can be all but resolved through detailed planning. Innovations such as covering a litter with a tarp or improvising an attachment to cross-country skis provide some clever solutions to common winter problems. Commercial products like the Sked® litter have streamlined the laborious task of transporting injured people in snow and ice conditions.

Ice Safety

There are many specific types of ice, each with distinctive characteristics. Knowing the difference between them can mean the difference between a successful rescue and a tragedy.

The first type of ice to form is called **frazil ice**. Frazil ice is formed by the collection of disk-shaped crystals suspended in water, forming a thin, opaque film that floats to the surface. As the temperature drops, these crystals combine to form a solid sheet. **Frazil slush** is a soft collection of frazil crystals that forms in moving water where a current prevents a solid freeze. **Clear ice** is new ice formed by a long, hard freeze. It often reflects the color of water beneath and can be many colors. It is considered the strongest ice. **Snow ice** is opaque or milky-colored ice that is formed from the freezing of water-soaked snow. This low-density ice is porous and is very weak. **Layered ice** has a striped appearance and is formed from many layers of frozen and refrozen snow. **Candle ice** forms into finger-like structures in an ice surface as it rots or disintegrates. Candle ice resembles many candles bundled together and is commonly found in late winter or early spring. **Rotten ice** is old ice that is honeycombed with pockets of air bubbles that in advanced stages of disintegration looks black as it becomes saturated with water. Old rotten ice may appear to be quite thick but may crumble under the slightest pressure.

Ice thickness is only one factor that determines its strength. Weather, water depth, size of the body of water, and obstructions all affect the strength of ice. For instance, pure water freezes faster and deeper than water containing chemicals or pollutants, and large, deep lakes take longer to freeze but are slower to decay. New ice is usually stronger than old ice, and a light wind tends to speed up ice formation while a heavy wind slows it down. Water rising through cracks in the ice, warm temperatures, and rain can all cause slush to form on ice. Ice covered with slush should be avoided because it is a sign that ice is no longer freezing from below, and water or slush on ice erodes it. River ice is generally considered weaker than lake ice due to the current, and smooth, straight stretches of river ice are stronger than ice at river bends where the current is faster and undercuts the ice. Obstructions such as rocks, logs, decomposing vegetation, and piers produce heat, which slows ice formation. Thus, numerous objects protruding through ice usually indicate that it is weaker. Waterfowl and fish can also hinder ice formation. Waterfowl often gather to try to keep an area of open water for feeding. If they leave, the area will have far less ice over it than surrounding areas.

> **SAFETY TIP**
>
> The only absolute regarding ice safety is to stay off it.

The only absolute regarding ice safety is to *stay off it*. To be properly equipped to judge ice dangers and potential rescue techniques, one must possess knowledge of how ice is formed, the many types of ice, and factors affecting its strength. However, as a general guide to indicate what kinds of activities good, clear, solid ice can support, use the following:

2 inches = walking

4 inches = fishing

5 inches = snowmobiles

8–12 inches = vehicles

Ice Self-Rescue

Large sections of the United States lie in latitudes far enough north for low temperatures to freeze most still bodies of water. Every year, unsuspecting travelers and outdoor enthusiasts fall through ice and drown or die from hypothermia. Unfortunately, this happens to unprepared rescuers, too. While it is impossible to detail all conditions or indicators for safety on ice, there are basic techniques that could save a life when someone finds himself or herself swimming in an ice hole.

The first reaction after going through any ice is panicky groping and grasping at the edge of the ice to get out. There are often no handholds, and victims often exhaust themselves without making headway toward escape. A normal person may not have the energy to break ice all the way to shore unless the distance is very small and the ice very thin. Without tools, the best way to escape is to fully extend your arms and hands as far and as wide as possible up onto the ice, then kick your feet up and extend them horizontally to the rear, as if swimming. Continue until you slowly work yourself onto the ice. Anything sharp such as a knife, keys, belt buckle, or pen, may help get a hold on the ice. The key is to distribute your weight over the widest possible area and to move slowly and deliberately—avoiding quick, panicky moves. Once solid ice is reached, roll away from the weak areas as far as possible before trying to crawl or stand. If ice cracks or starts to give way, lie down quickly, spread out, and roll away from the area.

If you carry ice awls (sharp spikes with handles) on a string over your shoulders while walking on ice, they can be used to self-rescue. If you fall through the ice, strike the awl against the top of the ice and use it as an anchor by which you can pull yourself onto the ice surface in a horizontal position, distributing your weight to avoid re-immersion (ASTM, 2014c).

A similar self-rescue procedure can be performed using an ice staff (a stick or pole with a sharp spike on one end) in the same way ice awls are used to pull yourself away from an ice hole (ASTM, 2014d). An ice staff can also be used to prevent breaking through thin ice by tapping/testing the ice in front of you while walking.

Ice Rescue for Others

As with all water- and ice-related rescues, the phrase "Teach, Reach, Throw, Row, Go" should be used to indicate the order in which various types of rescues should be attempted. "Teach" means that the rescuer attempts to talk the victim into self-rescue. When dealing with ice, the first four options (teach, reach, throw, and row) are often ineffective, especially if the victim has become hypothermic. However, they should still be attempted. Before attempting a "go" rescue on ice, a rescuer must be completely familiar with self-rescue, hypothermia, and the various techniques (along with their associated hazards) for ice rescue. Traveling onto the ice to effect a rescue can be extremely dangerous and should not be attempted without proper training and equipment.

After removing the subject from the ice/water, beware of hypothermia. If snow conditions are dry, a wet subject can be rolled in the powder to absorb as much moisture as possible. If there is no snow or other way to absorb moisture, wet clothing should be removed and replaced with dry as soon as possible. Hypothermia associated with sudden immersion can incapacitate a subject rapidly. Rescuers should therefore improvise a shelter, build a fire, or share clothing with others to protect the subject from further heat loss. In such a situation, immediate decisions and utilization of resources could mean the difference between life and death.

Many high-quality ice rescue training programs exist. In addition to the self-rescue training mentioned previously, however, rescuers should endeavor to be trained to the relevant standards that address ice rescue, including the latest versions of the following:

- ASTM F1739, *Guide for Performance of a Water Rescuer—Level I*
- ASTM F1783, *Standard Guide for Performance of an Ice Rescuer—Level II*
- ASTM F1730, *Standard Guide for Throwing a Water Rescue Throwbag*
- NFPA 1670, *Standard on Operations and Training for Technical Search and Rescue Incidents* (Chapter 19)
- NFPA 1006, *Standard for Technical Rescue Personnel Professional Qualifications* (Chapter 19)

SEARCH AND RESCUE TIP

As with all water- and ice-related rescues, the phrase "Teach, Reach, Throw, Row, Go" should be used to indicate the order in which various types of rescues should be attempted.

Avalanche

Although they represent one of the most catastrophic forces of nature, avalanches are not well understood. Basic avalanche ingredients—snow and slope—exist in mountains all over the world. Every year, hundreds of thousands—possibly millions—of avalanches occur. While most have no direct effect on human activity, the remainder constitute a significant threat to life and property.

SAR in potential avalanche areas can be hazardous because it requires that SAR personnel be able to recognize and identify avalanche hazards. This is a specialized skill that requires additional training above and beyond conventional SAR training. Although this section is not intended to serve as a comprehensive description of avalanched hazards and rescue, selected information is provided to illustrate some of the important issues involved.

Causes and Types

Snow undergoes very little change at constant cold temperatures and, therefore, usually remains unstable under these conditions. It settles and stabilizes rapidly when temperatures are near or just above freezing. Stabilization is a metamorphic change dependent on many variables, with temperature being the leading factor. However, storms starting with low temperatures and dry snow, followed by rising temperatures, are more likely to cause avalanches than continued constant cold. Rapid weather changes cause snow pack adjustments that may affect stability of snow and cause an avalanche.

The two principal types of avalanche are loose snow and slab. Loose snow avalanches, also called point-release avalanches, usually start at a point and spread in a fan shape or inverted "V" down a slope. They grow bigger, and the quantity of snow increases as they descend. Loose snow moves as a formless mass with little internal cohesion. Slab avalanches, on the other hand, start when a large, cohesive area of stronger snow begins to slide over a layer of weaker snow, breaking away over a wide area. There is a well-defined fracture line where moving snow has broken away from stable snow, and large, angular blocks or chunks of snow may be involved. Slab avalanches can involve a very large amount of snow. Ninety-five percent of avalanche fatalities in the United States are from dry slab avalanches (Grissom et al., 2017).

With ice avalanches, the principles and practical aspects are significantly different from snow avalanches. However, both kinds of avalanche occur in glacier-clad mountains and threaten human activities, including SAR. On some steep mountain flanks, both snow and ice avalanches fall from the same slopes.

Ice avalanches occur when material is released abruptly from perennial ice deposits, usually mountain glaciers, above steep slopes. Massive blocks of ice break free and fall down the mountainside, sometimes touching off secondary rock and earth slides.

Winds of 15 miles per hour (7 meters/second) are sufficient to move freshly fallen snow into drifts and **avalanche starting zones**. Higher wind velocities can move older snow with the same result (Grissom et al., 2017). Snow plumes (cornices) from ridges and peaks indicate that snow is being moved onto leeward slopes, which can create dangerous conditions (**FIGURE 8-16**).

When Can They Happen?

Newly fallen snow is what most often leads to avalanche, thus about 80% of avalanches occur during and shortly after storms. The risk of avalanche increases as more snow falls, although snowfalls of less than 6 inches (15 centimeters) rarely cause avalanches (Grissom et al., 2017). Snow depth may be the most obvious indicator of avalanche hazard; the deeper and newer the snow, the greater the hazard.

Snowfall rates of 1 inch (2.5 centimeters) per hour or more, especially over sustained periods, increase avalanche danger. Small crystals comprising needles and pellets are more dangerous than the more common, star-shaped snow crystals. Moist, dense snow settles rapidly but during windy periods can be dangerous.

Slope location, steepness, and shape are significant factors in avalanche formation. During spring, slopes facing the noon sun receive the most energy and begin to melt first, thereby increasing snow avalanche activity. Shaded slopes are more subject to dry snow avalanche activity.

Dangerous slab avalanches are more likely to occur on convex slopes but may also occur on concave slopes. Short slopes may be as dangerous as long slopes (**FIGURE 8-17**).

Humans and animals are very effective avalanche triggers. Severe ground vibrations, such as earth tremors or explosions, are powerful avalanche starting agents. Loud noises from explosions and supersonic booms can also start snow slides.

Where Can They Happen?

Avalanches most frequently occur on slopes of 30 to 45 degrees (60–100%), but avalanches, usually of the dry variety, have occurred on slopes as low as 22 degrees (**FIGURE 8-18**) (Grissom et al., 2017). An avalanche need not be spectacular to kill. People have been killed by local, very small slides, including roof-top slides.

Avalanches are prone to recur in the same locations. Pushed-over small trees and those with limbs broken off may indicate old slide paths. The nature of the slide path or track affects direction, speed, breadth, and density of an avalanche. Large rocks, trees, and heavy brush help anchor snow. Smooth, grassy slopes are more avalanche prone. Leeward slopes (the side sheltered from the wind) can create hollow-sounding slabs where

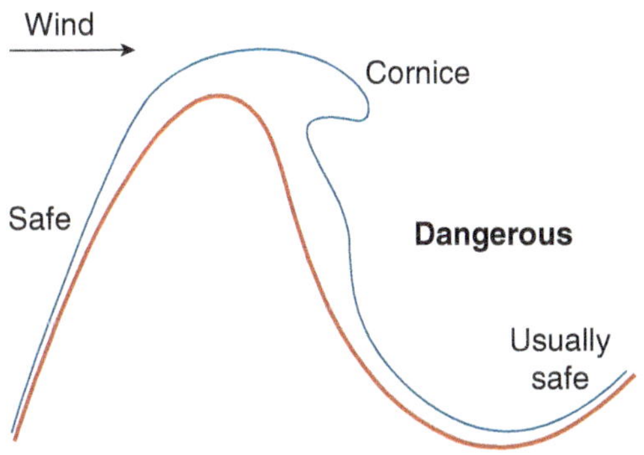

FIGURE 8-16 Avoid disturbing cornices from below or above. Gain ridge tops by detouring around cornice areas.

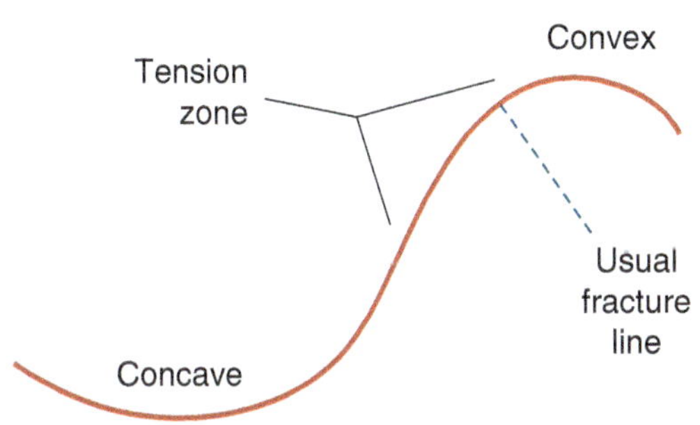

FIGURE 8-17 Slope profile. Dangerous slab avalanches are more likely to occur on convex slopes but may also occur on concave slopes. Short slopes may be as dangerous as long slopes.

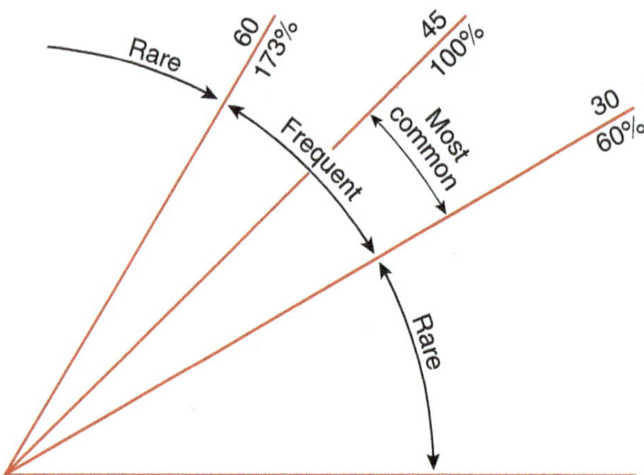

FIGURE 8-18 Avalanche slope angles and their effects. Avalanches occur most frequently on slopes of 30 to 45 degrees but have occurred on slopes as low as 22 degrees. The diagram shows the slopes where avalanches are most common.

avalanche danger is present. Windward slopes (facing the wind) are usually strong enough to resist movement.

Old snow surface is important. Rough surfaces aid stability; smooth surfaces are unstable. A loose underlying snow layer is more dangerous than a compacted one.

Specific Dangers

Although snow avalanches can occur wherever there are deep accumulations of snow on steep slopes, they are only a problem if they occur in proximity to people or property. For centuries mountain dwellers have stubbornly built and rebuilt in an **avalanche path**, and even added to their peril by cutting protective forests. The deadliest avalanche in U.S. history occurred on March 1, 1910, in Wellington, Washington. After days of swirling winds and drifting snow, it began to rain. A huge wall of snow broke loose and slammed into two trains that were stuck on the tracks in snow drifts. The train cars were swept 150 feet into the Tye River gorge in the high Cascades, causing 96 deaths (Mapes, 2010).

Catastrophic ice avalanches may descend unexpectedly from glacier tongues long considered stable. On January 10, 1962, in Peru, the greatest avalanche on record occurred when 6 million tons of ice broke from a hanging glacier near the summit of 22,000-foot (6706 meter) Mount Huascaran in the Andes Mountains. Falling over 3000-foot cliffs, ice tore out great chunks of rock and touched off secondary avalanches as it bombarded a lower glacier. The avalanche destroyed nine villages, killing 4,000 people and 10,000 farm animals, and traveled nearly 10 miles in only 7 minutes (History.com, 2017).

When an avalanche stops moving (**runout zone**), the snow sets up very hard. If you are buried in it, your chest may be unable to expand to take a breath, especially if buried at some depth (Stalsberg, 1989). If you are caught in the avalanche after it stops moving, it is often impossible to dig yourself out, even if you are close to the surface. Once buried, as your warm breath melts the snow around your mouth and nose, the moisture on the surface of the snow freezes into an ice layer that prevents air from moving through the snow, thus contributing to the rate of asphyxiation. This potential hazard is the reason some have taken to carrying and using a snorkel-type device like the Black Diamond AvaLung® that allows you, should you become buried, to breathe residual air trapped in your clothing and redirect exhaled breath away from your face and mouth (more about this in the following section).

Safety Procedures and Actions to Take

Everyone traveling in the backcountry where avalanches are a hazard should carry appropriate avalanche safety equipment. This equipment should include at least a sturdy shovel, avalanche transceiver, and probe (Grissom et al., 2017). Although a probe can be improvised with a ski pole or tree limb, a proper 10- to 12-foot (3- to 4-meter) folding avalanche probe is light, easy to carry, and the best choice when traveling in avalanche country. Light, foldable shovels are also available at mountaineering shops, and since avalanche snow is virtually impossible to move by hand, carrying a shovel is not optional in avalanche country.

In a frequently visited backcountry region, such as a ski area, several methods are used to monitor and manage avalanche activity, including the use of explosives. Avalanches are rare in these well-monitored and managed areas. However, avalanche management is not

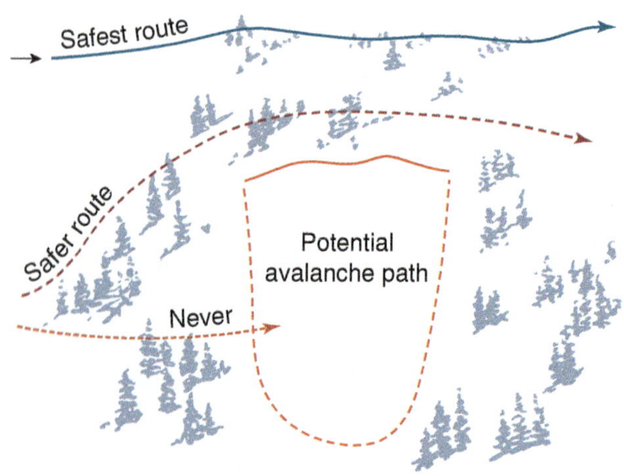

FIGURE 8-19 Potential avalanche path and safer routes of travel in relationship to it.

an exact science, and many isolated areas in which SAR is needed are outside these regions.

Backcountry skiing should be practiced only in groups and when avalanche conditions are considered stable. The safest routes are in valleys far from the bottom of slopes. If dangerous slopes must be crossed, stay high and near the top, and avoid avalanche fracture lines (**FIGURE 8-19**). If it is necessary to ascend or descend a dangerous slope, proceed straight up or down and not back and forth across the slope. Snowmobiles should not cross the lower part of slopes.

People caught in an avalanche can, immediately upon feeling the snow move, try to get out of the slide path or to catch hold of trees, shrubs, or other anchors in an attempt to let the force of the avalanche pass them by. If escape is impossible, skis or other impediments should be jettisoned so they do not cause injuries. Although it may not be easy, your backpack should be retained because it may make it more likely that you will stay close to the surface of the flow. Although some question its effectiveness, many survivors claim that "swimming" in the flow helped them stay on or near the surface (Grissom et al., 2017). It may be possible to get clear of the slide path by escaping to the sides, but the chances of directly outrunning an avalanche are poor to none. Avalanche victims are usually either carried away by the slide from its starting zone or hit by the front of a developed descending avalanche. If you are on a snowmobile, stay with it. You are twice as likely to be buried if you are separated from the machine (Grissom et al., 2017).

If caught in an avalanche, shout "Avalanche!" to warn others, then breathe through your nose and close your mouth to prevent it from filling with snow. As the motion begins to slow, place your hands in front of your face to make an air pocket. Do this sooner rather than later because the motion may stop suddenly, and you may not be able to move at all (Grissom et al., 2017).

If your companion is caught in an avalanche, call for help immediately (radio, mobile phone). Visually note the point where he or she was last seen (point last seen) using fixed objects in the terrain to help triangulate the location (e.g., rock outcrops, distant peaks, trees outside of the avalanche path). This point will be very important to searchers. Next, assess the situation for further slides, and, if deemed safe, physically mark the point last seen with trail tape or a highly visible piece of equipment so that it can be seen from both up and down slope. Initiate a search for clues to help narrow down the position of the victim, and turn your transceiver to receive with its volume turned up all the way (for now). A fully buried victim without a transceiver is unlikely to survive (Grissom et al., 2017). Begin a transceiver search and use spot probing with an avalanche probe where clues lead to likely burial spots. Likely spots should include bends, benches in the slope where snow and debris pile up, depressions, and uphill and downhill sides of rocks and trees. Where snow and avalanche debris pile up is often where victims are found (Grissom et al., 2017).

Survival during avalanche burial depends on the following:

- *Depth of the burial and whether complete burial, including the head, is involved (i.e., critical burial).* In a critical burial, asphyxiation is likely. Deeper burial reduces survival due to longer rescue times and less air trapped in the snow, which hastens asphyxia.
- *Amount and type of trauma.* Severe injuries can cause bleeding or airway obstruction and can significantly reduce survival. Up to 25% of all avalanche deaths are caused by trauma, usually of the head and neck (Hohlrieder et al., 2007; McIntosh et al., 2007).

SAFETY TIP

If it is necessary to ascend or descend a dangerous slope, proceed straight up or down and not back and forth across the slope.

- *Burial time.* Longer burial time increases the likelihood of asphyxia and hypothermia. Although nearly 75% of avalanche deaths are due to asphyxia, only a few are from hypothermia (Boyd et al., 2009; McIntosh et al., 2007).

The process of **granular convection**, or inverse segregation, is the reason avalanche air bags and wearing a pack might keep someone caught in an avalanche closer to the surface. Shaking a bowl of mixed nuts, which causes the larger ones to rise to the top, easily demonstrates this effect. A moving avalanche comprises many sizes of particles that tend to move in layers, with the larger ones rising to the surface. A person caught in the flow of an avalanche may be a small particle compared to moving slabs or large chunks of ice, which can cause burial, but using an airbag device or wearing a backpack may add enough surface area to cause you to be treated like a large particle and driven to the surface.

Avalanche airbag devices, such as the Mammut® Pro Removable Airbag Backpack, Black Diamond® Jet Force, and the Arc'teryx® Voltair, among others, combine a variably sized backpack (18–50 liters) with an avalanche airbag system (**FIGURE 8-20**). When deployed, the airbags fill by either a compressed gas cartridge (some of which are user-refillable) or a battery-operated, high-speed fan (which can be used multiple times on one battery charge). The compressed gas cartridges can

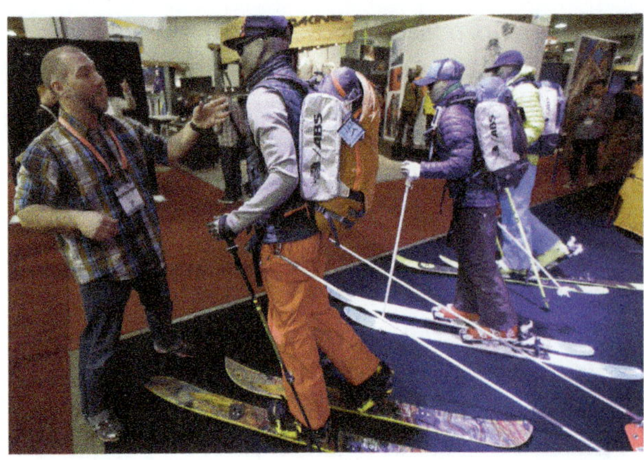

A

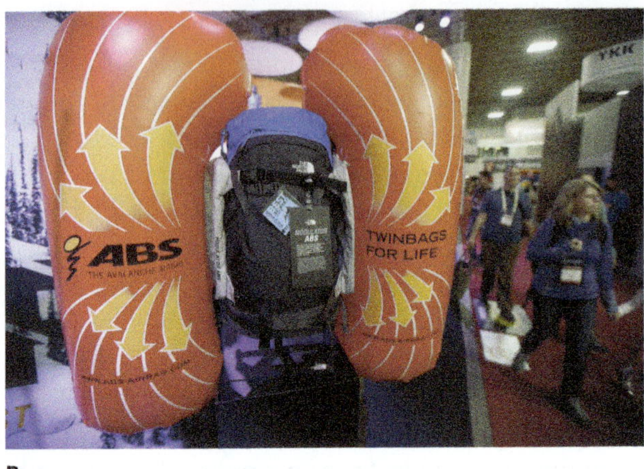

B

FIGURE 8-20 An example of an avalanche backpack airbag. **A.** Backpack before airbag deployment. **B.** Backpack with airbag deployment.

be a problem carrying on commercial airlines in the United States because compressed gas cartridges must be carried empty, but the battery-powered fan and refillable cartridge types do not present such challenges. The fan-activated types also allow for multiple uses on one battery charge, which permits practice in its use prior to going into the backcountry. Several manufacturers offer the option of moving their airbag mechanisms between different sized backpacks, allowing you to choose the best backpack for the situation. These are often more expensive but may be worth the cost.

Research shows that about 20% of the time an avalanche airbag system does not inflate when needed, usually due to failure by the user, but if it deploys and operates properly, mortality (death rate) is cut in half (Haegeli et al., 2014), which is undoubtedly why the popularity of these devices has increased over the past few years.

Another device that has been contributing to avalanche survival is the AvaLung by Black Diamond® Equipment. The AvaLung consists of a diminutive mouthpiece and hoses that are kept near the face while in avalanche country. The device is usually held in place by, and integrated into, the straps of a backpack so that the mouthpiece can quickly be inserted in the mouth should the wearer be caught in an avalanche. When in use, the device separates inhaled air from exhaled air and can extend survival time by slowing asphyxiation. Inhaled air is drawn in from the space surrounding the wearer, which is drawn directly through the snowpack, and the exhaled air, containing unwanted carbon dioxide (CO_2), is routed to the wearer's back and away from the inhaled air. The AvaLung prevents rebreathing exhaled air, which is a major contributor to asphyxiation from avalanche burial (Grissom et al., 2000), and survival using the device has been reported in many cases after complete avalanche burial (Radwin and Grissom, 2002).

Avalanche Search

Avalanche search is a discipline involving several specialized techniques that must be learned and practiced. Although some relevant issues are discussed here, many excellent resources exist that describe the technical details for searching in this three-dimensional environment. When SAR is necessary in environments in which avalanches threaten, additional training and specialized equipment are required. SAR personnel should be aware of this and seek specialized training before entering the backcountry.

Like any search, an avalanche search starts by looking for clues. Scan the **avalanche track** for equipment, a glove, a ski, an avalanche cord, or other objects that might have come from the victim. Once the area has been determined to be safe, mark the point last seen, if known, or a last known position based on clues. Immediately commence a shallow probe search around any obvious clue (spot probing). Call for the necessary assistance and equipment, deploy avalanche dogs if available, and organize and begin a beacon and/or probe search near and just downslope from the point last seen or the last known position and in other likely spots (e.g., bends, benches in the slope where snow and debris pile up, depressions, and uphill and downhill sides of rocks and trees).

The use of avalanche beacons or transceivers is common around the world and is usually considered one of the best ways to quickly find people buried in an avalanche. The battery-powered device works by emitting a pulse radio signal on the international standard frequency of 457 kHz. Transceivers are effective only if they are carried as the manufacturer recommends, which usually means they must be worn underneath the outer layer of clothing but not in a pack. While the group is traveling on the snow, each transceiver is set to transmit mode. In this mode, each device is continuously transmitting. If one gets buried in an avalanche, all other transceivers are set to receive this signal to help locate the buried subject. The signal usually carries about 100–150 feet (30–46 meters).

Because speed is of the essence when someone is buried in an avalanche, it is imperative that everyone involved in the search knows exactly how to use his or her transceiver. In actual practice, the use of avalanche beacons to locate a buried victim is difficult and takes practice. Experienced and skilled practitioners can often find a victim in a matter of minutes if they are properly prepared, but this takes training, familiarity with the specific device in use, and regular practice *before* entering the backcountry.

Transceivers come in analog and digital versions. Both are compatible with each other and transmit on the same international standard frequency. The analog versions are older technology, work at greater ranges from a source signal, take a bit more practice to use effectively, are generally being replaced by the digital versions, and cost less than their digital counterparts. Digital avalanche beacons incorporate a processing chip that converts the raw data into easier-to-understand directional arrows, distance numbers, and signal strength. Digital beacons are generally easier to learn how to use, have a smaller range than analog beacons, and are usually more expensive, depending on the specific features included. How each type of beacon is used to search most effectively is beyond the scope of this text, but users should closely follow and practice the manufacturer's recommendations regarding the use of any avalanche transceiver intended to be used in a search.

An electronic avalanche rescue system has been developed by RECCO®. It consists of two parts: reflectors and detectors. One or more small, unpowered, passive reflectors are permanently affixed to clothing or equipment such as outerwear, helmets, boots, or safety gear. The reflector weighs less than 3 grams (0.1 ounce), is about 3 inches long, requires no maintenance or batteries, and has an unlimited lifespan. The detector, about the size of a schoolbook, uses radar technology to locate the reflector within about 200 meters (656 feet) through air and 30 meters (98 feet) through snow. It can be used by a rescue team on the surface or even by a helicopter flying overhead to quickly search a large area that would otherwise be dangerous to search. SAR personnel may be involved in using the RECCO system and should be aware of its existence.

A trained avalanche dog and handler can be very helpful in avalanche search. Although few buried avalanche victims have been recovered alive by dogs in the United States, the probability seems to be the greatest when burial depths are less than 6 feet (1.8 meters) (Atkins, 2015). Trained dog teams are becoming increasingly prevalent in SAR and law enforcement agencies, and avalanche dogs are common in ski areas in the United States. Dogs do not find people, per se; they scan for human scent (i.e., shed human skin cells floating up through the snow pack), which can be affected by several factors, including wind/weather; snow density; contamination of the debris field by gasoline, urine, and other aromatic pollutants; and length of burial. Dogs have found bodies buried in snow at a depth of 33 feet (10 meters), but they have also missed bodies buried just under the surface. Trained avalanche dogs are far from infallible, but they can cover much more area in less time than human searchers. One source suggests that one trained dog and handler can search more effectively in 30 minutes than 20 searchers can in 4 hours using course probing (Grissom et al., 2017).

A probe search, albeit slow, may be run concurrently with other search methods or when other methods are unavailable or en route (**FIGURE 8-21**). Techniques for an avalanche probe search have evolved over the years, and the current best practice was suggested by computer modeling (Ballard et al., 2004). This approach includes the use of companions or onlookers, ideally trained in the technique, formed into a probe line and each equipped with a sturdy, light shovel, and a light, collapsible, avalanche probe pole (6–12 feet [1.8–3.5 meters] in length). After assessing the continued avalanche risk and posting an avalanche guard (one continuously monitoring the avalanche threat), the group can form

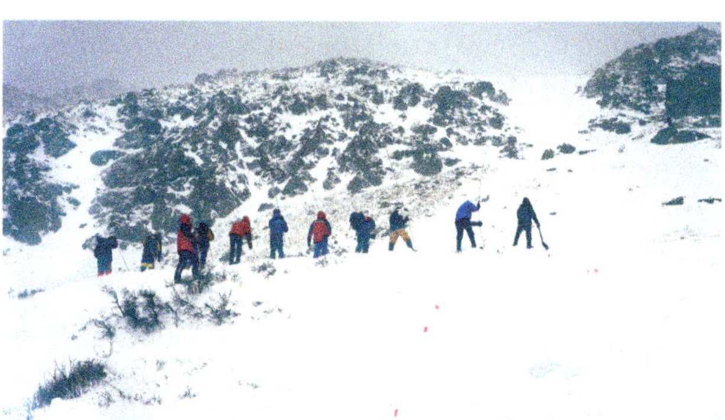

FIGURE 8-21 An avalanche probe search, albeit slow, may be run concurrently with other search methods or when other methods are unavailable or en route.

a "scuff line"—a single row of people standing about 2 feet (61 centimeters) (arms' length) apart—near where the subject is thought to be buried. Each person on the line then begins to probe once in front of them, once 20 inches (50 centimeters) to the right, and once 20 inches (50 centimeters) to the left. A probe line "guidon cord" (thin rope with marks or knots at 20-inch [50-centimeter] intervals) can be used to maintain the proper spacing across a probe line. The line then moves forward a step (20 inches [50 centimeters]) and repeats the process, eventually covering an area with a grid of probes with no more than 20 inches (50 centimeters) between them.

This approach is thought to provide the best combination of probability of detection and fast search time, and it can be repeated to increase the cumulative probability of detection (Grissom et al., 2017). While probing, anyone striking a possible subject should leave the probe in place and shout for some colleagues to start shoveling—approaching the subject from the side or downhill, not from above—while the probe line continues to march across the area. Since the chances of death increase with depth of burial, it is generally thought that a live rescue is more likely if more areas are probed, or areas are probed again, rather than probing deeper than about 6 feet (1.8 meters), which takes longer.

Avalanche cords, around 50 feet (15.2 meters) long, were once common pieces of equipment that skiers attached to their belts and let trail behind them in hopes that, should they become buried in an avalanche, the cord, or some portion of it, would come to rest on the surface. Then, rescuers could follow the cord to find the victim. The problem with the cord idea is that, although they have worked, they may not work all the time and may end up completely buried. Whether they work or not, SAR personnel should be aware that avalanche cords may be visible, and therefore useful, at an avalanche search.

Lightning

Lightning is a release of light and energy produced by discharge of atmospheric electricity. This discharge may occur within a cloud, between clouds, or between cloud and ground. This last form of lightning poses the greatest threat to humans. On a very minor scale, it is easy to produce our own lightning by walking across a rug or carpet and reaching out to touch something. The flash of light, spark, and pain that result are similar to what happens when lightning occurs.

Each year, lightning strikes in the United States about 25 million times and kills an average of 49 people while injuring hundreds more (NOAA NWS, 2017). From 2006 to 2015, two-thirds of these deaths occurred to people who had been enjoying outdoor leisure activities—mostly fishing (11%), on the beach (6%), camping (5%), and boating (4%)—and during the months of June, July, and August (Jensenius, 2016). Although most lightning occurs in the summer, people can be struck at any time of year.

Lightning powerful enough produces a distinct crackling, explosive sound called thunder. Thunder is sound caused by expansion of air heated by the intensity of the lightning stroke. Thunder can tell us approximately how far the lightning flash was from us. We can estimate distance in miles to the lightning by counting the number of seconds between lightning and thunder and dividing by 5. For example, if we see a stroke of lightning and count to 10 before hearing the thunder, the lightning flash was about 2 miles away.

The U.S. National Weather Service (NWS) suggests that when you see lightning or hear thunder you should immediately seek safe shelter, which they consider only (1) a building with electricity and/or plumbing or (2) a metal-topped vehicle with closed windows. The NWS does not consider tents, picnic shelters, dugouts, or small buildings without plumbing or electricity to be safe shelters (NOAA NWS, 2014). Unfortunately, a building or vehicle may not be accessible during SAR operations.

Protecting Yourself

Lightning is one of the most underrated severe weather hazards, ranking as one of the top weather-related killers around the world (**FIGURE 8-22**). The seemingly random nature of thunderstorms cannot guarantee the individual or group absolute protection from lightning strikes; however, being aware of, and following, proven lightning safety guidelines can greatly reduce the risk of injury or death.

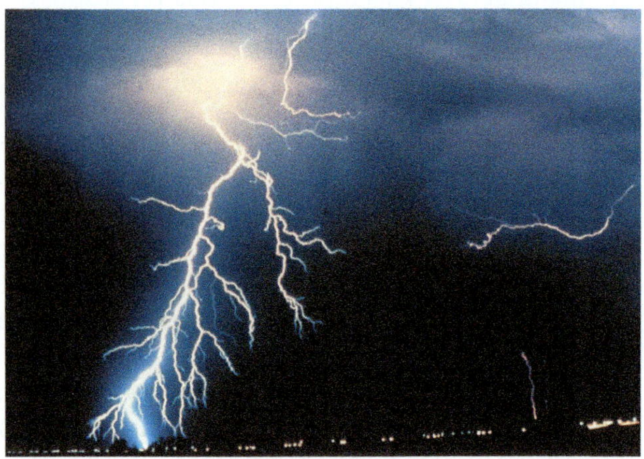

FIGURE 8-22 Lightning is one of the most underrated severe weather hazards. It ranks as one of the top weather killers in the United States.

NOAA Photo Library, NOAA Central Library; OAR/ERL/National Severe Storms Laboratory (NSSL), C. Clark.

Safer Locations and Locations to Avoid

No place is absolutely safe from the lightning threat; however, some places are safer than others:

- Large enclosed structures (substantially constructed buildings) tend to be much safer than smaller or open structures. The risk for lightning injury depends on whether the structure incorporates lightning protection, construction materials used, and the size of the structure.
- In general, fully enclosed metal vehicles—such as cars, trucks, buses, vans, fully enclosed farm vehicles, etc.—with the windows rolled up provide good shelter from lightning. Avoid contact with metal or conducting surfaces outside or inside the vehicle. This includes avoiding handling radio equipment inside a vehicle, especially equipment with large antennae.
- Avoid being in or near high places and open fields, isolated trees, unprotected gazebos, rain or picnic shelters, baseball dugouts, communications towers, flagpoles, light poles, bleachers (metal or wood), metal fences, convertibles (vehicles), golf carts, and water (ocean, lakes, swimming pools, rivers, etc.).
- When inside a building, avoid using the telephone; taking a shower; washing your hands; doing dishes; or having any contact with conductive surfaces with exposure to the outside, such as metal door or window frames, electrical wiring, telephone wiring, cable TV wiring, and plumbing.
- Tents, even the largest of them, are not a safe shelter from lightning.
- A natural cave can provide adequate shelter from lightning, but make sure to go in well past the entrance. Rock is a conductor of electricity, which means the cave provides a safe haven only if you are far enough into the cave to avoid the light zone—the area toward the front of the cave where natural light can be seen. Avoid a cave that is shallow, was an old mine, or has metal nearby (Kithil, 1998).
- If you must maintain a stationary position, such as in a tent or improvised shelter, and moving to a safer position is impractical, assume the "lightning position" by crouching with your feet together, ideally on an insulated pad, with only your feet touching the pad and no part of your body touching anything else (Gookin, 2010).
- There is no such thing as a surprise storm, so plan field operations after considering the possibility of threatening weather and move to safer terrain (avoid peaks/ridges and open ground, move away from tall trees and wet ground, move into a dry ravine, etc.) ahead of a storm.

Lightning Safety Guidelines

If you can see lightning and/or hear thunder, you are already at risk. Louder or more frequent thunder indicates that lightning activity is approaching, increasing the risk for lightning injury or death.

High winds, rainfall, and cloud cover often act as precursors to actual cloud-to-ground strikes, notifying individuals to take action. Many lightning casualties occur in the beginning, as the storm approaches, because people ignore these precursors. Also, many lightning casualties occur before there is a perceived threat or after the perceived threat has passed. Generally, the lightning threat diminishes with time after the last sound of thunder but may persist for more than 30 minutes. When thunderstorms are in the area but not overhead, a lightning threat exists, even when it is sunny, not raining, or when clear sky is visible.

When available, pay attention to weather warning devices such as National Oceanic and Atmospheric Administration (NOAA) weather radio and/or credible lightning detection systems; however, do not let this information override good common sense. Before conducting SAR operations, get a weather briefing from a competent source and do not bet your life on an app on your phone. An action plan or protocol must be in place and conveyed in advance to all SAR personnel.

Environmental Challenges

It has already been established that mental and physical functions of the body are virtually inseparable. Both can impact our ability to deal with the emergency environment effectively. Although injury is the greatest and most immediate physical concern, environmental stresses can produce equally dangerous but more subtle, insidious results.

This section is not a complete instructional manual on wilderness medicine at any level, nor is the information meant to replace field training by competent medical instructors, or to replace actual experience in treating and managing injuries and illness. It is recommended that all SAR personnel attend competent, prehospital medical training relevant to the environments in which operations are expected.

Training in specialized, prehospital medical issues should be undertaken by all SAR personnel. Several organizations specializing in this type of training offer outstanding programs in wilderness medicine and first aid.

Hypothermia

Hypothermia is defined as a medical condition or illness that is caused by the body's core temperature

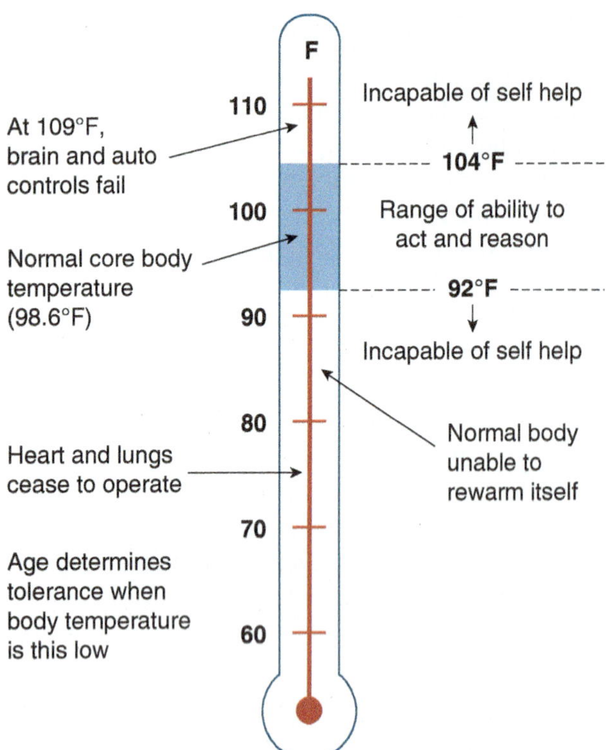

FIGURE 8-23 The temperature range for normal operation of the human body is between 92° (33.3°C) and 104°F (40°C), although the extremes of the range can be tolerated for relatively short periods of time only.

being lowered below its normal temperature of 98.6°F (37°C) oral/99.7°F (37.6°C) rectal (**FIGURE 8-23**).

Hypothermia is sometimes called *exposure*, although exposure is actually the method by which an individual becomes hypothermic. Hypothermia is also often called "the killer of the outdoors" because it has been established as a major cause of death among outdoor travelers. Factors contributing to hypothermia include falling into cold water (immersion hypothermia), traveling in cold weather while wet, alcoholic beverage consumption, drug use, improper dress, and even lack of funds for payment of utility bills (urban hypothermia). For SAR personnel and the subjects of their toil, hypothermia should be considered the most potentially important outdoor danger that is likely to be encountered.

A person can be considered hypothermic when their core temperature is found to be below 95°F (35°C). External (environmental) causes are related to the four primary ways in which heat can be transferred: radiation, conduction, evaporation, and convection (see Chapter 7, *Search and Rescue Clothing*, for definitions and details). Internal causes are usually related to the body's ability to produce heat required to maintain a constant body temperature. Heat is produced by movement of muscles (voluntary or involuntary), metabolism, and food. A failure or impairment in any of these sources can lead to hypothermia.

Hydration also plays a significant role in temperature regulation, as a small amount of dehydration (decrease in body water) can cause a decrease in thermal control. Dehydration occurs at a faster rate in cold and dry environments and at elevation. Other topics that play an important part in thermoregulation include physiological control of body temperature and nutrition. These topics are not specifically addressed here but deserve study by all SAR personnel.

A special low-reading thermometer is ideal in diagnosing hypothermia. Regular oral and rectal thermometers do not register low enough. Since these special thermometers are not always available and attempting to use a thermometer in the wilderness is not necessarily recommended, other methods of field diagnosis should be used.

Mild hypothermia should be handled immediately so that it does not progress into severe hypothermia, which has a much worse prognosis. A mildly hypothermic person (core temperature of 97° to 91°F [36.1° to 33.8°C]) may show the following signs and symptoms (Danzl and Huecker, 2017):

- Complaining of feeling cold with extremities showing "goose bumps."
- Frequently wet from rain, snow, or other sources.
- Usually shivering to some extent, which may become intense. This may not be apparent while walking.
- As hypothermia progresses, the patient may develop problems with muscular coordination, most often beginning with clumsiness in detailed hand movements.
- An inability to keep up with others in the party, later followed by stumbling and clumsiness.
- Approaching 90°F (32.2°C) core temperature, they may have difficulty in speaking, sluggish thinking, amnesia, or signs of depression.

Some suggest that an un-intoxicated person who is unable to walk a 30-foot (9.1-meter) line heel to toe as in a sobriety test should be presumed to be significantly hypothermic until proven otherwise (Forgey, 1989; Bacpacker.com, 2008; Curtis, 2010).

As hypothermia becomes more severe (core temperature of 90°F [32.2°C] and below), the subject becomes careless about protecting himself or herself, eventually stops shivering, and becomes increasingly confused, incoherent, and irrational. At 83°F (28.3°C) (severe hypothermia), unconsciousness occurs, heartbeat and respirations are erratic, and the pulse may seem absent. At 68°F (20°C) (profound hypothermia), ventricular fibrillation is likely, and at 64°F (17.8°C), the heart will stop beating altogether (asystole) (Danzl and Huecker, 2017).

If a subject is unable to protect himself or herself from the cold or understand the gravity of the situation, and certainly if the individual is unconscious, the core temperature is probably below 90°F (32.2°C), and the situation should be considered an emergency. Because of hypothermia's ability to so precisely mimic death, no one should be considered dead until they are warm and dead (Hilmo et al., 2014).

Before treatment can be rendered to the hypothermic patient, mild hypothermia must be distinguished from severe hypothermia. Severe hypothermia is a medical emergency that necessitates advanced medical intervention as soon as possible. Do not try to rewarm a victim of severe hypothermia in the field. Evacuate them as soon as possible, jostling them as little as possible, and gently transport. Remove wet clothes during this procedure but do so gently (**FIGURE 8-24**).

Mild hypothermia is treated primarily by preventing further heat loss. To do this, one must understand how heat is transferred and how to minimize these effects in the field. Remove wet clothes and replace with dry. Place

ASSESS COLD PATIENT

1. From outside ring to centre: assess Consciousness, Movement, Shivering, Alertness
2. Assess whether normal function, or impaired or no function
3. Treat according to appropriate result-quadrant
4. Treat all traumatized cold patients with active warming to upper trunk

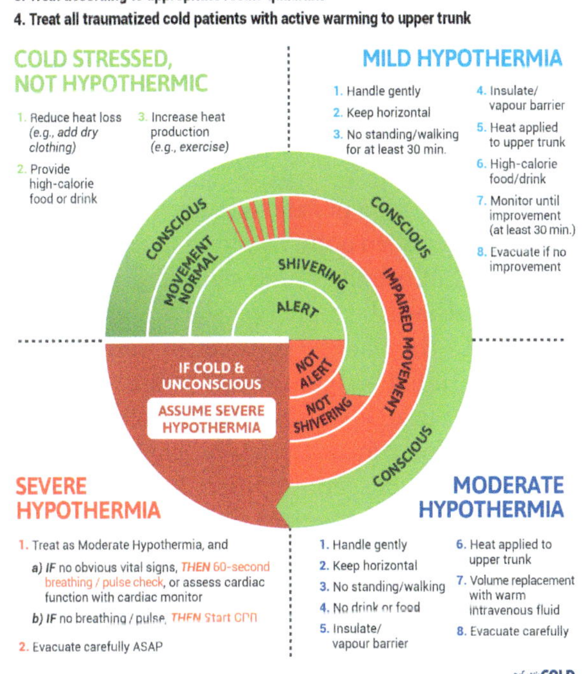

Canada BICOrescue.com Baby It's COLD OUTSIDE

FIGURE 8-24 Assessing a cold patient: A summary graphic from the Canadian *Baby Its Cold Outside* training program.

CARE FOR COLD PATIENT

SUGGESTED SUPPLIES FOR SEARCH/RESPONSE TEAMS IN COLD ENVIRONMENTS:

- 1 - Tarp or plastic sheet for vapour barrier outside sleeping bag
- 1 - Insulated ground pad
- 1 - Hooded sleeping bag (or equivalent)
- 1 - Plastic or foil sheet (2 x 3 m) for vapour barrier placed inside sleeping bag
- 1 - Source of heat **for each team member** (e.g., chemical heating pads, or warm water in a bottle or hydration bladder), or **each team** (e.g., charcoal heater, chemical / electrical heating blanket, or military style Hypothermia Prevention and Management Kit [HPMK])

INSTRUCTIONS FOR HYPOTHERMIA WRAP "The Burrito"

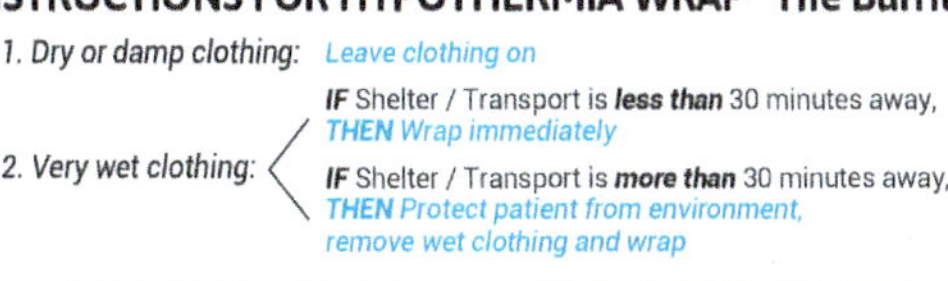

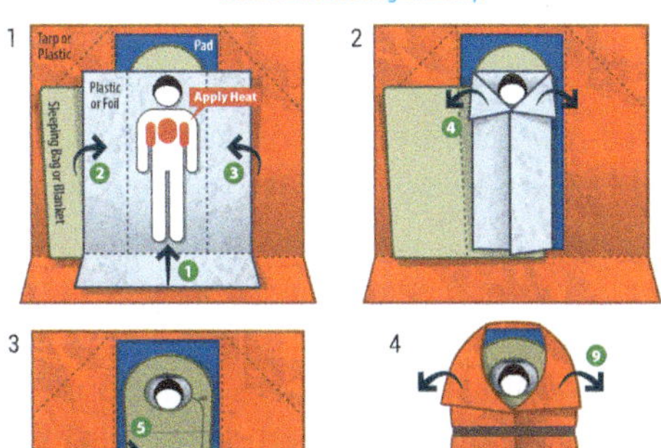

Sources: BICOrescue.com; Zafren, Giesbrecht, Danzl et al. Wilderness Environ Med. 2014, 25:S66-85.

FIGURE 8-25 Care for a cold patient: A summary graphic from the Canadian *Baby Its Cold Outside* training program.

the victim in a warm environment, if available (e.g., tent, near a campfire, in a vehicle, in a sleeping bag with another person). Add dry insulation to the victim's clothing system. Make the person more comfortable. Consider a hypothermia or "burrito" wrap (**FIGURE 8-25**).

When treating hypothermia patients, watch for core temperature afterdrop. This phenomenon is defined as the continued decline in the core temperature of a hypothermia patient after removal from a cold environment. As cool blood in the extremities returns to the core, the core temperature may continue to drop, even after treatment has begun (Giesbrecht and Bristow, 1997). It may look like the patient is not reacting positively to treatment of hypothermia, but continue to prevent heat loss and warm the core, as needed.

Prevention of hypothermia is directed toward reducing heat loss and increasing heat production, both or either as needed. Reducing heat loss can be achieved almost entirely by appropriate dress (see sections on clothing in Chapter 7). Proper nutrition and hydration are also important to staying warm. Beware of caffeine, alcohol, and "downer" types of drugs that may promote hypothermia. Hypothermia is much easier to prevent than treat, so know how to prevent it.

Treatment of severe and profound hypothermia is a true emergency and should involve gently transporting the patient to an appropriate medical facility.

Cold Injuries

Localized cold injuries include: **frostbite**, which is the general term used for frozen tissue; **frostnip**, a superficial skin injury; **trench foot** (immersion foot), caused by exposure of tissue to wet, cold conditions; and **chilblains** (pernio, kibe, chimetlon), caused by the exposure of dry skin to cool or cold temperatures in a damp environment.

Frostbite and Frostnip

Frostbite is the true freezing of flesh. Frostnip is a superficial version associated with severe constriction of blood vessels that occurs on the ears, the tip of the nose, and cheeks. Many argue that frostnip is not an injury at all since tissue damage and tissue loss does not occur.

Like burn injuries, frostbite is commonly classified in degrees, although other methods of describing it do exist. First-degree frostbite involves numbness, redness, and swelling of the involved area, but there is no tissue loss. Second-degree frostbite involves fluid-filled blisters, redness of the skin, and swelling. Third-degree frostbite shows deeper, blood-filled blisters that are often purple in color. Fourth-degree frostbite involves full-depth frozen flesh that often involves muscle and bones (Freer et al., 2017).

Toes are most often affected by frostbite, but fingers and hands are also common sites. Pain in the associated tissues is the earliest symptom of frostbite. As the tissue freezes, the pain disappears, and the only symptom that may be apparent is numbness in the area. Affected tissue may turn pale or white, but usually it is not recognized because clothing normally covers the areas. Frostbitten tissues may also be cold and hard.

In the field, frostnip can be readily rewarmed, but a person with frostbite should be evacuated before rewarming is attempted. Rewarming frostbitten tissue and allowing it to refreeze can cause much more damage than simply leaving it frozen. The general treatment considerations for frostbite include:

1. Remove all constricting clothing to promote circulation to the injured area.
2. Do not allow a frostbite patient to walk on a frostbitten foot or to use a frostbitten hand.
3. Insulate and protect the affected area from further damage.
4. Elevate the injured area during transport.
5. Smoking and alcohol use are strictly forbidden for frostbite patients.

Nonfreezing Cold-Induced Injury

Immersion or "trench" foot is a nonfreezing injury that usually strikes the feet after being immersed in cold water for an extended period. It usually presents as redness of the skin that eventually leads to swelling and blisters. It may also extend to the legs, knees, and thighs (Imray et al., 2017). Numbness and pain may also be present. Treatment includes removing the involved area from the environment that caused the injury, rewarming it in warm water (100–108°F [37.8–42.2°C]), drying the area, and keeping it dry. Mild analgesics may help alleviate the pain.

Chilblains (Pernio) involve bluish-red skin lesions that are a result of an abnormal reaction to a damp, cold environment, even after as little as 30 minutes of exposure (Imray et al., 2017). Chilblains are uncomfortable but usually cause little impairment. Affected skin may be red, tender, warm, swollen, and itchy. Treatment is the same as for trench foot: remove from the cold environment and warm the area.

All cold injuries can be prevented by proper nutrition, hydration, and clothing. Never touch metal outside when the temperature is below freezing. Avoid direct exposure to organic liquids (gasoline, solvents, alcohol, etc.) in cold environments, as they can immediately cause frostbite upon contact with the skin.

Heat-Related Problems

Heat injuries important to SAR personnel include heat exhaustion and heatstroke. Heat cramps are often considered a heat-related injury but, in fact, they are a localized muscle soreness resulting from vigorous exercise that usually resolves without intervention or damage.

It is unusual for a person to suffer only one of these maladies. They often occur in a continuum that includes a great deal of overlap of the signs and symptoms of each. Sometimes, heat cramps signal imminent heat injuries, but they can be completely unrelated. Heat exhaustion, if not recognized and treated, can lead to heatstroke, but one is usually not stricken with just heatstroke. Heat exhaustion has probably been present and may still be to a certain extent. It is important that these problems be recognized and treated immediately or, better yet, prevented.

Heat Cramps

Heat cramps are muscle pains that may occur when an individual exercises vigorously to the point of profuse sweating (fluid loss) and electrolyte (salt) depletion. An otherwise healthy person may complain of sudden cramping in their lower extremities, abdomen, or both.

They probably will be sweating and most likely have been working hard in a warm environment. Treatment is aimed at eliminating the exposure and replenishing the lost water and salts. Immediately remove the affected person from the exposure (i.e., stop working, get out of the hot environment). Salt tablets should be avoided, but sports-type electrolyte drinks can be helpful, especially if diluted with water. Rest, water, and electrolyte replacement usually allow for a quick recovery.

Heat Exhaustion

Heat exhaustion (sometimes called *heat prostration*) is characterized by high core body temperature, weakness, fatigue, dizziness, nausea, vomiting, headache, malaise (general feeling of discomfort), low blood pressure, fast heart rate (tachycardia), and the potential for collapse. It can occur with or without exertion and may lead to more severe heat-related injury if not treated (Winkenwerder and Sawka, 2007). Heat exhaustion, like heat cramps, is also related to water and electrolyte loss. Heat cramps are a local (single area) affliction, whereas heat exhaustion is a generalized (whole body) problem. Heat exhaustion is more likely to have associated dehydration and may be first apparent by sudden unconsciousness. A person with heat exhaustion is usually sweating profusely, and the skin is cool to the touch. This coolness of the skin is evidence of the body's evaporative heat transfer mechanism at work. If heat exhaustion is minor and has just occurred, the treatment is the same as for heat cramps. If heat exhaustion is more severe, intravenous (IV) fluids may be required, which means advanced medical care. In the field, keep the person supine (lying down on the back), comfortable, and cool while evacuating.

Heatstroke

Heatstroke is caused by a severe disturbance in the body's heat regulating mechanism and is considered a life-threatening emergency. Generally, the sweating mechanism, one of the primary methods with which the body cools itself, fails in heatstroke and the body temperature increases. The temperature of the body can reach 106°F (41.1°C) and higher within minutes. If the situation is not corrected quickly, then serious damage can occur to the vulnerable cells of the brain and central nervous system. When heatstroke occurs, someone has probably ignored the warning signs.

Heatstroke is recognized by three primary symptoms. The first is high body temperature, usually greater than 104°F (40°C). The second is dysfunction of the central nervous system, which usually includes delirium, combativeness, seizures, and eventually unconsciousness. The third is exposure to a hot and humid environment and/or vigorous physical exertion (Winkenwerder and Sawka, 2007).

The skin is hot and red in heatstroke, as opposed to cool, moist, and often pale in heat exhaustion. In addition, this person will probably have a strong, full pulse. A person with heatstroke may experience headache, dizziness, and dry mouth, and may lapse into a coma and have seizures. This person may be aware of the heat but then quickly becomes confused, uncoordinated, delirious, or unconscious. The body temperature would be high, probably very high, and should be treated immediately. Almost all untreated cases of heatstroke lead to brain damage and eventually death.

SEARCH AND RESCUE TIP

Heatstroke, caused by a severe disturbance in the body's heat-regulating mechanism, is considered a life-threatening emergency.

Treatment is aimed at lowering the body temperature as soon as possible by immersing the body in cool water, making sure not to cause shivering, or applying cold packs to pulse points until the core temperature drops to normal. Remove clothing immediately, and place the patient in a cool area with low humidity, if possible. Massaging the extremities during the cooling process may help. Sprinkling or spraying cool water onto the patient while fanning is an easy way to cool a person quickly. Avoid causing shivering while cooling. A person suspected of experiencing heatstroke, even if his or her temperature is brought back into normal ranges, should be seen immediately at a medical facility.

Prevention of nearly all heat injuries can be assured by knowledge of the body and how it works in hot environments. Clothing systems appropriate for the environment must be used. The body should always be covered when in direct sunlight, and this includes the head. Generally, in a hot environment, the clothing should be very loose, thin, and light colored.

Solar Injuries

Sunlight helps warm the Earth, helps plants produce oxygen through photosynthesis, triggers the release of the hormone serotonin in the body (boosts mood and helps a person feel calm and focused), and causes a person's skin to create vitamin D, which provides many health benefits. However, too much ultraviolet (UV) light from the sun can damage the skin and lead to skin cancer, elastin breakdown (wrinkles, skin sagging), and injuries taking longer to heal (WebMD, 2017). When one may be exposed to the sun for long periods of time, as is often required in SAR work, preventing, recognizing, and treating some common injuries from the sun can save a great deal of pain and suffering. Sunburn and snow blindness are problems for SAR personnel caused by exposure to UV light.

Sunburn

Sunburn is a first-degree burn (superficial, thermal burn) that causes reddening and pain of the skin after being exposed to sunlight. Swelling might accompany the reddening, and more prolonged exposure to sunlight might cause severe pain and blistering. Chills, fever, and headache may also develop, and if the lips are sunburned, cold sores (herpes simplex) can occur. Everyone has a different sensitivity to sunlight; in general, blue-eyed redheads and blondes are more susceptible to sunburn than brunettes, and children are more susceptible than adults.

Use of some drugs, soaps, creams, cosmetics, and even ingestion of certain vegetables can vary one's ability to fight off the damaging rays of the sun. Ultraviolet light from the sun is the cause of sunburn and can cause burns even on cloudy days. The sun's effects can be intensified by increasing altitude, low latitude, highly reflective environments, wind, and lack of clouds. However, none of these are necessary to receive a burn. Cold, wet dressings may relieve the pain of sunburn, and soothing lotions such as those containing aloe vera may ease discomfort. Preventing further exposure and pain relief is the basic treatment plan. A physician should evaluate severe sunburn that affects a large portion of the body; include blisters; or involve the face, groin, hands, or feet.

Covering exposed skin with clothing when you are in the sun best prevents sunburn. This should include covering the entire body and head. Sunscreen preparations are available that can block the harmful rays of the sun, but these must be reapplied frequently and may reduce the body's natural ability to regulate heat (sweating). Covering exposed skin with clothing is therefore preferred. If sunscreen is used, preference should be given to preparations that block as much of the sun's rays as possible—usually those labeled **sun protection factor (SPF)** 30 or higher.

Snow Blindness

Snow blindness (photokeratitis) could be thought of as sunburn of the eyes. Symptoms may not occur for many hours after the injury, and at first, it may feel like the eyes are simply irritated and dry. A sunburned face and red eyes also often accompany these symptoms, and the discomfort may persist for 24 to 48 hours (Pavan-Langston, 1996). After the initial symptoms, the sensation of a foreign body or sand in the eyes may develop with associated pain when the eyes are moved or opened. Sensitivity to light (photophobia) is also common. Eyes will look red, the eyelids may swell, and excessive tearing is probable. Cool, moist coverings for the eyes might relieve some discomfort, but the condition should clear up within a few days if the eyes are allowed to rest while kept closed. A physician's care should be sought in case medication is needed to prevent infection or relieve pain.

Protecting the eyes from the sun with sunglasses, goggles, or a wide-brimmed hat can prevent this condition. Sunglasses for everyday use may not be suitable for use in the mountains, especially while you are surrounded by snow and ice. Sunglasses worn at altitude and in a reflective environment should block all UV radiation, have side shields, and limit the amount of visible light that is transmitted through them to the 5–10% range, which is less light transmission than everyday sunglasses usually allow (Butler and Chalfin, 2017). If side shields are not available, wiping mud or charcoal on the cheekbones under the eyes and to the side of the eyes can help reduce the reflection of light around the lenses. Protection is just as important on cloudy days, and snow blindness has occurred during snowstorms. Improvised protection can be made from pieces of cardboard with small slits in them.

Altitude-Related Problems

Occasionally SAR personnel are called upon to work at altitudes to which they are not accustomed. Some individuals may become ill if they travel to over 8,000 feet (2,438 meters) and ascend too quickly without taking time to acclimate. The reason this is a problem is that as you climb higher in altitude, the oxygen available in the air to breathe is reduced, which can lead to hypoxia (deficient oxygen reaching the tissues of the body). At 18,000 feet (5486 meters) elevation, there is approximately half the oxygen available than at sea level. Acute mountain sickness (AMS), high-altitude pulmonary edema (HAPE), and high-altitude cerebral edema (HACE) are three specific problems that can occur at high altitudes. SAR personnel must at least know of their existence and how to recognize them.

SEARCH AND RESCUE TIP

SAR personnel should be able to recognize the following altitude-related problems:

AMS: Acute mountain sickness
HAPE: High-altitude pulmonary edema
HACE: High-altitude cerebral edema

Mountain Sickness

Mountain sickness—also called **acute mountain sickness (AMS)** if sudden in onset—is not a disease, but a collection of symptoms that commonly occur to people who travel to over 8,000 feet (2,438 meters) in altitude without acclimating (taking time to become accustomed to the altitude). Generally, the symptoms begin with fatigue, loss of appetite, sleepiness, weakness, apathy, headache, and sometimes nausea and vomiting. Headache is by far the most common and most irritating symptom.

Headache may be blamed for it, but sleeplessness is another symptom of the syndrome. After a few days at altitude, the headache may be complicated by memory lapses, ringing in the ears, and difficulty walking. Severe indicators include difficulty walking, loss of consciousness, hallucinations, HAPE, HACE, and impaired judgment. If recognized immediately, treatment includes rest, fluid ingestion, pain medication for the headaches, and descent to a lower altitude. Sleeping aids may make the problem worse. If recovery is not quick, the patient must seek medical help at a lower elevation. Evacuation to a lower elevation is the best course of treatment. Never travel to higher elevations if a member of your team has AMS symptoms.

Prevention is accomplished by attaining higher elevations slowly. First, spend time resting at lower elevations, then progress higher at a slow rate. Descend at the first signs of illness. Some medications (e.g., acetazolamide and dexamethasone) may be helpful in preventing AMS when a physician familiar with high-altitude medicine administers them.

High-Altitude Pulmonary Edema

High-altitude pulmonary edema (HAPE) is fluid in the lungs brought on by ascending to an elevation exceeding 8,000 feet (2,438 meters) too rapidly. This can compromise a person's ability to breathe and, therefore, is considered dangerous and even lethal if not treated. Signs and symptoms include those of AMS plus coughing that produces white or red (bloody) mucus, weakness, shortness of breath, confusion, cyanosis (a bluish discoloration of the skin), loud breathing sounds, and rapid heart and breathing rates. The victim of such an illness will die if not evacuated to lower elevation (less than 5,000 feet [1,524 meters]) quickly.

Treatment includes evacuation to lower elevation immediately after the first signs and symptoms occur. Do not allow the patient to walk down, especially alone. Prevention is assured by never traveling above 8,000 feet (2,438 meters).

High-Altitude Cerebral Edema

High-altitude cerebral edema (HACE) is fluid on the brain that occurs from exposure to altitude without acclimating. HACE causes progressive neurological deterioration such as change in consciousness, inability to walk a straight line, impaired judgment, hallucinations, and coma. Treatment and prevention are the same as for HAPE.

Peripheral Edema

Swelling (edema) of the face, hands, and ankles is common at high altitude. This is often related to fluid retention and can be annoying, but by itself, it is usually not a serious problem. It usually resolves itself when physical exercise is halted and descent is started. If it is accompanied by breathing problems or neurological deterioration (e.g., change in consciousness, inability to walk a straight line, impaired judgment, hallucinations, and coma), evaluation for HACE and HAPE should be conducted, and, if discovered, the condition should be treated (Hackett et al., 2017).

Many high-quality alpine and mountain search and rescue training programs exist. However, rescuers should endeavor to take training that incorporates the relevant standards that address mountain search and rescue, including the latest versions of the following:

- ASTM F3027, *Standard Guide for Training of Personnel Operating in Mountainous Terrain (Mountain Endorsement)*
- ASTM F3028, *Standard Guide for Training of Search and Rescue Personnel Operating in the Alpine Environment (Alpine Endorsement)*
- ASTM F1773, *Standard Terminology Relating to Climbing, Mountaineering, Search and Rescue Equipment and Practices*
- ASTM F1655, *Standard Guide for Training First Responders Who Practice in Wilderness, Delayed, or Prolonged Transport Settings* (Section 6.1.5.1 deals with HAPE and HACE)

Water Deprivation

Dehydration is a condition that results from the excessive loss of body water. It is most often recognized by thirst, but thirst may be a late symptom. At elevation, thirst may be absent, and water consumption must be continuous because thirst is not always an accurate indicator of dehydration. At elevation, fatigue, weakness, and lightheadedness may be the first indicators. A person with severe dehydration will have a dry mouth and eyes, "loose" skin that stays pinched when pinched with the fingers (tenting), and may progress into unconsciousness and eventually death.

SAFETY TIP

Consume at least 4 liters of water per day in hot or extremely cold environments.

Treatment for dehydration is aimed at rest and consumption of liquids. If a person is unconscious, liquids cannot be consumed, and immediate evacuation is required. Preventing dehydration is one of the keys to health in the outdoors. Drink plenty of fluids, especially when working hard and sweating. Water needs increase at elevation and in both cold and hot climates. Push fluids at elevation and consume at least 4 liters of water per day in extremely cold or hot environments. Chapter 5, *Physiology and Fitness*, contains more information about hydration and health.

Blisters

Blisters are the bane of SAR personnel and the most common problem encountered in wilderness medicine (Lipman and Krabak, 2017). Blisters are fluid-filled pockets under the surface of the skin that are caused by friction against a particular part of the body (usually the feet) and are usually caused by ill-fitting footwear. They should be treated as soon as they are discovered, ideally before the blister has completely formed. The reddening of an area on the skin prior to becoming a full-blown blister is termed a *hot spot* and is simply red and irritated. In addition, the skin on a hot spot may feel like it moves easily over the underlying tissue.

Treatment of a hot spot involves applying a barrier over the area to minimize frictional forces. These barriers can include products such as moleskin, Elastikon® tape, Micropore® paper tape, kinesiology tape, Spenco® 2nd Skin® blister pads, Blist-O-Ban™ adhesive bandages, or even duct tape. Each of these barriers works best when applied preventatively before a blister forms. The barrier material should be adhesive so that it does not move across the skin when frictional forces are applied, and the application of a separate adhesive—such as tincture of benzoin or Tuf-Skin® Taping Base Spray—beneath the barrier may help. The shoes, boots, or other responsible garment should also be adjusted so that friction is minimized. If a fluid-filled blister has occurred, cut a hole in the moleskin, tape, or bandage the size of the blister ("donut hole") and apply enough layers to keep all pressure off the blister itself. Do not rupture the fluid-filled pocket unless travel is impossible otherwise. Where the fluid in a blister can leak out, bacteria can enter and cause an infection. If a rupture is necessary, then pierce the corner of the fluid-filled sack with a sterile (or as clean as possible) needle. The puncture may become infected, so apply a topical antibiotic or wash the area with soap and water to make certain it is clean, then cover it with a bandage or gauze.

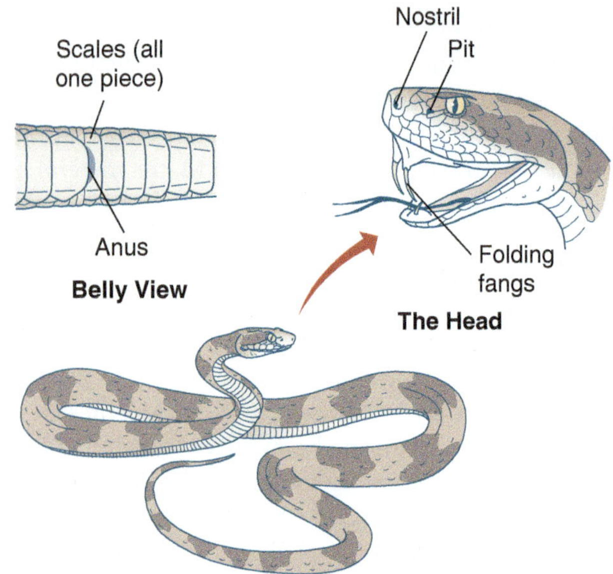

FIGURE 8-26 Positive identification of pit vipers (*Viperidae*), which includes rattlesnakes and copperheads.

Prevention of blisters is usually accomplished by acquiring and wearing properly fitted footgear. Some degree of success has been attained by always wearing two pairs of socks: a thin layer against the skin, and a second insulation layer with the thickness depending on the temperature. Applying a barrier in a spot likely to form a blister may work just as well. Massaging the feet at least daily promotes circulation and may decrease blisters. In addition, massaging may aid in the search for hot spots. Chapter 7 has more information about appropriate clothing.

Snakes

Snakes have long been the stuff of nightmares but are rarely a real problem for SAR personnel (**FIGURE 8-26**). Simply put, snakebites are quite rare. There are approximately 8,000 venomous snakebites in the United States each year (Norris et al., 2017). Approximately 20 to 25% of the most common types of venomous bites (pit vipers) will not have envenomation at all (dry bites), even when fang marks are present, and only 15% result in severe envenomation (Parrish et al., 1966). In the end, there are only about three deaths per year in the United States due to snakebite (Norris et al., 2017). To put it more plainly, one is far more likely in the United States to be injured or killed by a domestic animal such as a cat or dog than he or she is to be envenomated by a

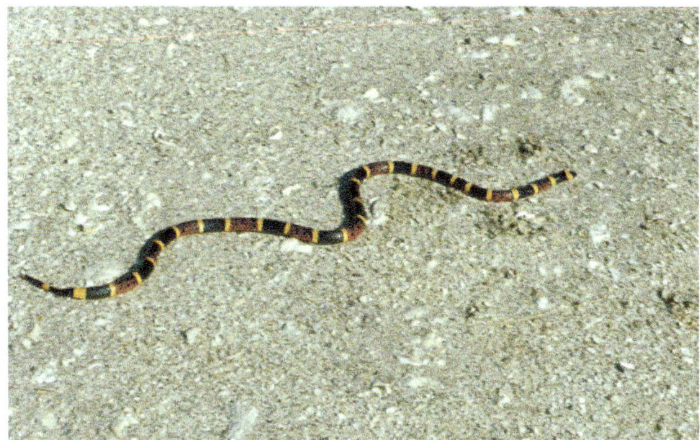

FIGURE 8-27 Identification of elapids (*Elapidae*), which includes coral snakes and sea snakes. Note that coral snakes can vary greatly in color. In the United States, however, consider any red-, black-, and yellow-banded snake a coral snake, especially if the red band touches the yellow (or white) band.

poisonous snake. In contrast, Mexico has more venomous snake species than any other country in the world and experiences as many as 150 deaths each year from snakebites (Gomez & Dart, 1995).

Following certain preventative measures substantially reduces the chances of having problems with snakes and their associated bites (**FIGURE 8-27**). Never stick your arm, hand, or finger in a hole; use a stick or branch. If a snake is sighted, stay clear of it and do not back it into a corner. Avoid contact with snakes or wild animals of any kind, especially if the exact type is unknown. Any snakebite where the snake type is unknown should be considered poisonous until proven otherwise.

If bitten by a snake, retreat and identify it before it gets away. If unable to identify it, take a photo of it, if possible, but do not try to kill it or transport it to the hospital with the patient. This wastes valuable time and leads to more bite injuries. See a physician after any snakebite. The measures that most reduce the chances of death or injury after a venomous snakebite are rapid transport, antivenin therapy, and intensive medical care. Certain attempts at field treatment should be avoided, including incising the wound(s), suction, tourniquets, electric shock, alcohol, and applying ice to the area (Norris et al., 2017).

If envenomation from a poisonous snake is suspected, the affected area should be cleaned and immobilized (splint extremities), and the patient should not be allowed to move around more than necessary. Suction of any kind—mechanical or oral—should not be applied to any snakebite, and the application of constricting bands above and below the bite is not recommended (Norris et al., 2017).

In summary, if a snakebite patient is simply transported directly to the nearest medical facility, no further prehospital treatment may be necessary.

SEARCH AND RESCUE TIP

Identification of coral snakes in the United States:
"Red touch yellow, kill a fellow; red touch black, venom lack."
Also, if every other band is yellow (or white), it's a coral snake.

Some safe practices and helpful tips when doing SAR work in snake country include the following:

- Do not place any part of your body in a position where it would be within striking range of a poisonous snake.
- Always watch where you put your feet. A walking stick may be used to probe areas where snakes may be hidden, such as under leaves or in rock crevices.
- Do not step over obstacles such as logs or large rocks. In snake country, the proper way to clear an obstacle is to step on top of it and then check below before moving forward.
- Use caution when walking, searching close to high banks, rock ledges, rock walls, and other high places where a snake may be resting.
- Try to select a clear space in which to land when jumping across streams, ditches, etc.
- Do not sit on stumps, logs, rocks, etc., without carefully looking over and around the spot.
- Wear gloves.
- Keep your eyes and ears open.
- If you see a snake, freeze and consider the situation. Walk around it—give it a wide berth—and try not to block its exit.

Insects

Stinging and biting insects can be a nuisance or even dangerous. SAR personnel would therefore do well to study the different insects in their area and follow some general guidelines regarding their management.

Insects most commonly confronted in field SAR situations include honeybees, wasps, ants, caterpillars, spiders, ticks, scorpions, and beetles. There are many different types of each of these insects, many of which have specific treatments unique to the particular insect. If insects are a serious problem in your area, further study may be required. For many insects, stinging and biting are most often a defensive action. When their home or life is threatened, they can be provoked to attack. Therefore, avoid such provocations, and you will likely avoid their potential result.

Generally, when a bite or sting is suspected (probably will be obvious), remove the patient from further exposure and apply cold to the area. If any debris is left on the skin, such as a stinger, scrape—do not pull—the object from the surface. Make sure all debris is removed completely. Wash the affected area with soap and water.

If a lethal bite or sting is suspected, or if severe symptoms occur, seek medical assistance immediately. If the patient is allergic to the sting or bite, or if symptoms consistent with an allergic reaction arise, medical assistance is needed immediately. This is a medical emergency. Serious symptoms include difficulty breathing, shortness of breath, severe hives and/or rash, swelling in the mouth or around the eyes, and unconsciousness. When these signs and symptoms occur, no time should be wasted. Seek medical assistance immediately. Apply the specific treatment to a particular sting or bite if it is known.

Prevention of bites and stings is directed at proper dress and the use of repellents. Keep the head and neck covered with clothing or netting in areas of high insect populations. The use of slippery materials (silk, nylon) is usually better than loose weave materials (cotton, wool), but any covering is better than nothing. Tie clothing at wrists and ankles or tuck in pant legs, and sleep under netting to prevent insect interactions. Use chemical repellents containing DEET (*N,N*-diethyl-3-methylbenzamide) as the active ingredient. Concentrations need not exceed 20–35% to be effective (Fradin and Day, 2002). A single application of DEET should be effective for about five hours. Some people are allergic to DEET, so watch for allergic reactions (e.g., reddening of the skin, skin irritation), and use it sparingly to avoid systemic absorption through the skin. Apply repellents in liquid form to the skin, spray the repellent on clothes, and keep both out of your eyes and away from mucous membranes. Compounds containing permethrin (synthetic chemical that acts like natural extracts from the chrysanthemum flower)—that kill insects rather than repel them—can also be applied to clothing, netting, and sleeping areas but not to the skin. Avoid using perfumes, colognes, and deodorant soaps before going into the field. Be aware that wearing brightly colored clothing may attract bees and wasps.

When chemical insect repellents do not seem to affect some types of fleas, black flies, horseflies, deerflies, chiggers, and gnats, the use of netting around the head, neck, and hands may be the only option available. Minimizing exposure in, or simply getting out of, highly infested areas is also prudent, when possible.

Ticks

A special word on ticks: they run a close second to mosquitoes as vectors of human disease. Tick-borne illnesses pose a potential threat to anyone who works or recreates in wilderness or in any outdoor areas. Tick-borne diseases in the United States include Lyme disease, Rocky Mountain spotted fever, Colorado tick fever, tick paralysis, relapsing fever, and tularemia. The Wilderness Medical Society suggests the following guidelines for preventing tick bites:

- Wear light-colored, protective clothing in tick-infested areas, especially long pants cinched at the ankles or tucked into boots or socks. Light-colored clothing makes ticks easier to spot.
- Spray the outside of clothes, netting, and around bedding with a permethrin-based spray, which is toxic to ticks and persists through several washings. It also works on mosquitoes, gnats, chiggers, and biting flies.
- Apply 20–35% DEET to exposed skin to repel ticks.
- Inspect all parts of the body at least twice daily for tick infestation.

To remove an embedded tick:

- Grasp the tick as close to the skin surface as possible with fine-tipped forceps (tweezers) but never fingers. Gradually pull straight out with steady pressure; do not crush or squeeze the tick's head or body.
- Ineffective removal methods that may increase the chances of disease transmission include applying kerosene, fingernail polish, isopropyl alcohol, a hot match head, a lit cigarette, or a heated piece of metal. These methods do not affect tick detachment and may induce the tick to push deeper into the skin, or to salivate or regurgitate into the wound, increasing chances of infection.
- Using the thin edge of a credit card or driver's license is NOT recommended for removing nymph and adult ticks from the skin (Cummings & Traub, 2017).
- After removal, wash and disinfect the site of the bite.
- After being in tick-infested areas, change clothes and place them in a plastic bag before entering your home. Laundering clothing in hot water and drying on high heat does not always kill ticks.

"Poisonous" Plants

Poison ivy, poison sumac, and poison oak are the most common cause of acute allergic contact dermatitis in the United States and can be found in every state (Freeman et al., 2017). Also referred to by their genus—*Toxicodendron*—they do not truly poison, but each can be extremely irritating to the skin.

Poison ivy is a climbing vine with three serrated-edged, pointed leaves. It grows east of the Rockies in the United States. In the northern and more western states, poison ivy grows as a nonclimbing shrub (**FIGURE 8-28**).

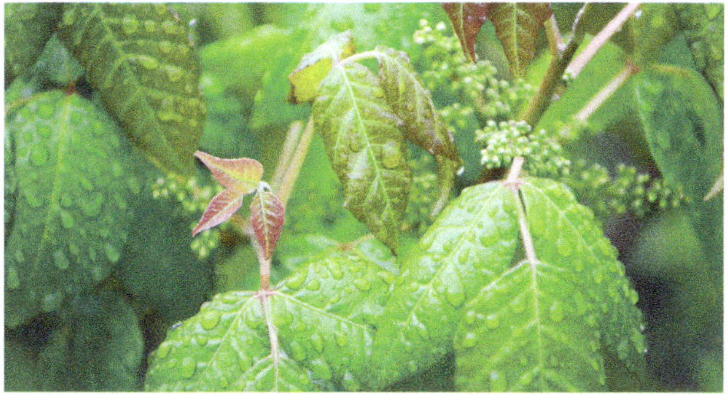

A

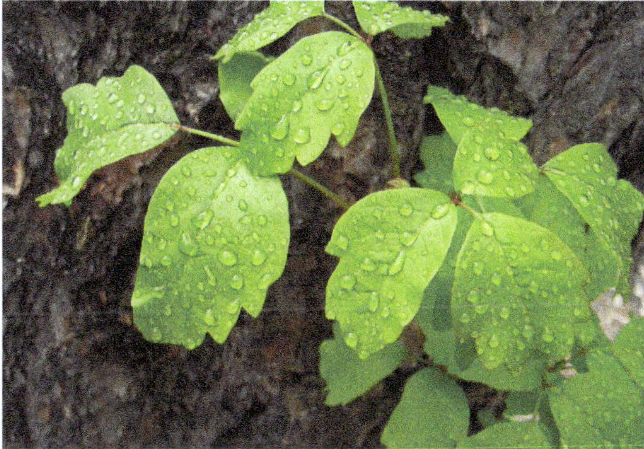

B

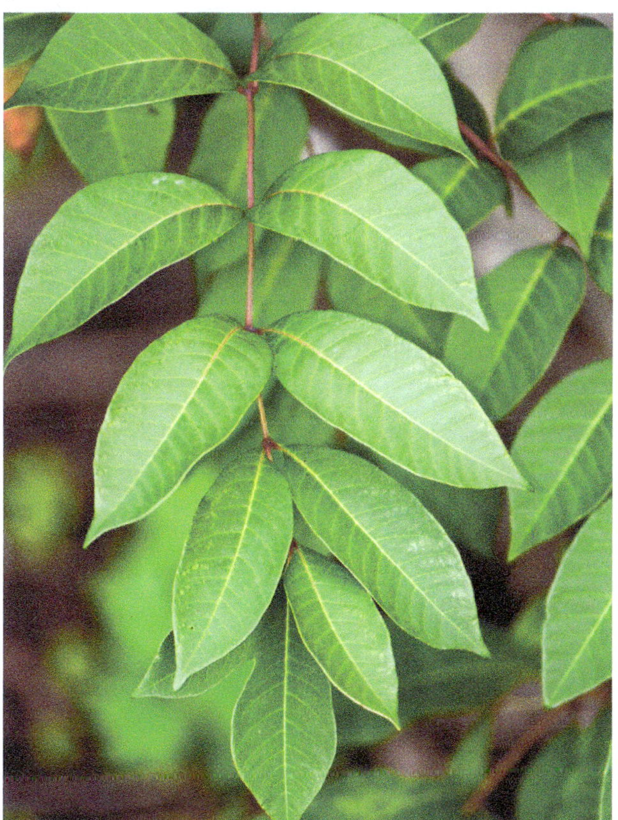

C

FIGURE 8-28 **A.** Poison ivy (*Toxicodendron radicans*). **B.** Poison oak (*Toxicodendron diversilobum*). **C.** Poison sumac (*Toxicodendron vernix*).

Poison oak also has three leaves. It grows in the sandy soil west of the Rockies as a small shrub. In the western United States, poison oak is a very large plant that grows as a standing shrub or climbing vine.

Poison sumac is a shrub or bush with two rows of 7 to 13 leaflets, and it is found most commonly in the peat bogs of the northern United States and in swampy southern regions of the country.

All parts of these plants contain urushiol, a clear, sticky, oily resin that causes rashes and itching of the skin. Urushiol resin remains stable, even in dead or dried plants and, therefore, is equally hazardous in the winter and summer. The resin can be carried by smoke that can be inhaled and affect the lungs if the plant is burned. Ingesting any part of the plant can cause a reaction in the oral cavity and gastrointestinal tract. Urushiol even stays stable in the necrotic blister, if it was not washed off completely, and can continue to irritate the skin and initiate new lesions (Freeman et al., 2017).

Different people react to the resin differently, but much success can be achieved by simply washing the suspected contact areas with soap and water as quickly as possible after exposure. The rash is not contagious after the resin has been washed from the skin, but if the resin has not been completely removed from the skin or clothing, submerging the affected area in a bath can spread it to other areas of the body.

It is estimated that 50–70% of the U.S. population is sensitive to urushiol, and that 10–15% are extremely sensitive to it and require emergency treatment should they come in contact with it (Freeman et al., 2017). Generally, the reaction ranges from mild to severe, and sensitivity can develop later in life. If you are allergic to poison ivy, you are also allergic to poison oak and poison sumac and may be allergic to cashew nut shell oil, mango fruit peels, and Japanese lacquer. A person is not as sensitive to urushiol the first time they touch it but can become severely allergic as the skin sensitizes to the resin.

Treatment for contact with urushiol includes drying (with lotions such as calamine) and itching control (by calamine, antihistamines, and oatmeal baths). Contaminated tools can be washed with a dilute mixture of bleach to inactivate the resin. The skin can be washed liberally with rubbing alcohol (isopropyl) to remove the resin, but contact time should be kept to a minimum to reduce the chances of alcohol absorption. A thorough rinsing with water must follow the use of rubbing alcohol to prevent spreading the oil on the skin. Contaminated clothing can be laundered with detergent and, even better, with bleach, which inactivates urushiol (Freeman et al., 2017).

Other plants commonly found that can cause skin irritations include buttercup, daisy, mustard, radish, crown-of-thorns, milk bush, daffodil, hyacinth, dogwood, barley, prickly pear, primrose, geranium, tulip, and some nettles (stinging). Some of these involve hair-like projections that get caught in the skin, so mere washing does not always help. Washing with a rough towel or specific treatments may work, though. Irritations that occur from the plants listed generally should be treated as an irritation from poison ivy.

In the field, contact with these plants is usually not suspected or even considered until symptoms arise. This is the time to wash the affected area thoroughly. Learn to recognize these plants and avoid contact if possible. Prevention is always better than treatment.

Handling a SAR Casualty

In SAR work, medical help may be miles away, and total medical ignorance can be dangerous or even fatal. When common sense is paired with basic knowledge of what to do and what not to do, an excellent outcome is possible.

Common sense is the most important component of necessary medical knowledge for SAR. Most problems arise from people not heeding warning signs or just ignoring the obvious. Heed the advice of those who know. Be prepared for the unexpected emergency. Be prepared physically, emotionally, and with the appropriate knowledge and equipment. Prepare for situations of risk by developing skills in less dangerous conditions. Do not tolerate horseplay in less-than-ideal conditions.

It is of utmost importance that the caregiver remains calm. If the rescuer panics, he or she can lose control of the situation. Acting calmly and purposefully establishes authority and reassures everyone. Do not further endanger yourself, the injured party, or others. Send for help (or more help) immediately, if necessary. You (the rescuer) are more important than your partners, your partners are more important than the victim, and the victim (injured party) is number three on the list of absolute priorities in SAR. Without you and your partners, there is no rescue, first aid, or search at all. The victim is not the last priority, just the third on a long list. The rescuer and his or her partners must have the skills, knowledge, and confidence that allow them to concentrate on the third priority: the patient. When these skills, knowledge, and confidence are lacking, the patient is not getting the care required.

SAFETY TIP

Absolute SAR priorities in order of importance:

1. You (the rescuer)
2. Your partners (other rescuers)
3. The victim or patient (the subject of your efforts)
4. Everything else

Never move a seriously injured person(s) unless he or she is in danger from the environment or needs to be moved for medical reasons. This is usually a moot point in SAR, because SAR work is rarely required where a person is not endangered by the environment or does not have medical problems. Do not allow a person to "walk it off" until lack of injury has been proven.

Never approach an injured subject from above. Approach from the side or below and travel to the subject from a safe position. Debris falling (this includes rescuers) on the patient can be detrimental to his or her health.

Re-evaluate the condition of the injured party at regular intervals. A change, for better or worse, can mean a change in approach to the incident and its urgency. Keep a written record, if possible, of everything that occurs regarding treatment rendered and medications given. This may serve to protect the interests of both the rescuer and the patient. This can also be valuable to the definitive healthcare personnel who will help the patient later.

If you must remove constricting clothing or jewelry to make the patient more comfortable, have a witness and place the objects in a safe place.

Always hope for the best but presume the worst. For example, a victim of trauma has a broken neck until proven otherwise. Consider the worst that a problem could possibly be and treat it correspondingly. Never administer medicines or perform procedures if you are unsure of, and untrained in, what you are doing. Never exceed your level of training. Know your limitations and do not overestimate your abilities. Follow the rule expressed in Latin as *primum non nocere*, which means "first, do no harm," and seek appropriate medical advice as soon as practical (**FIGURE 8-29**).

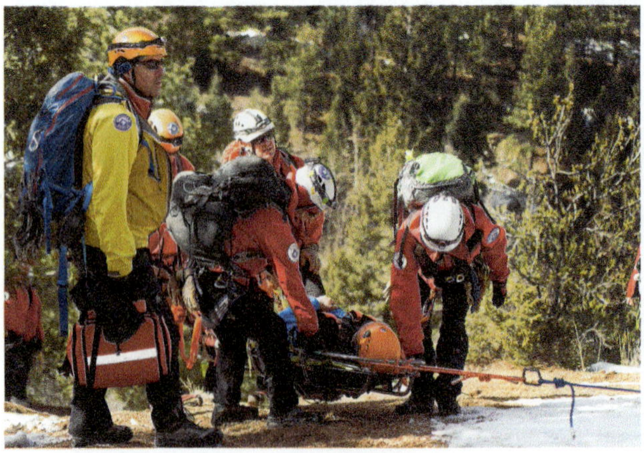

FIGURE 8-29 Know your limitations and do not overestimate your abilities. Follow the rule expressed in Latin as *primum non nocere*, which means "first, do no harm."

Wrap-Up

READY FOR REVIEW

- Hazards are generally caused by one of three things: nature, humans, or technology. In search and rescue (SAR) specifically, hazards may include environmental dangers, severe weather, difficult terrain, animals that may injure or harm, equipment failures and loss, injury, getting lost, and other threats to SAR personnel and operations.
- Specialized SAR environments bring on a diverse set of problems and potential complications for rendering aid to injured and/or stranded subjects. Each environment holds its own set of obstacles to increase the complexity and difficulty of a particular mission.
- Specialized SAR environments include vertical rock; caves and mines; water; cold, snow, and ice; and steep alpine terrain.
- The U.S. National Weather Service (NWS) suggests that when you see lightning or hear thunder you should immediately seek safe shelter in a building with electricity and/or plumbing or in a metal-topped vehicle with closed windows.
- Training in specialized, prehospital medical issues should be undertaken by all SAR personnel. Several organizations specializing in this type of training offer outstanding programs in wilderness medicine and first aid.
- Environmental challenges include hypothermia and cold injuries, heat-related problems, solar injuries, altitude-related problems, water deprivation, blisters, snakes, insects, and poisonous plants.
- Most problems arise from people not heeding warning signs or just ignoring the obvious. Heed the advice of those who know and be prepared for unexpected emergencies. Be prepared physically, emotionally, and with the appropriate knowledge, skills, and equipment.

SEARCH AND RESCUE TERMS

Acute mountain sickness (AMS) A collection of symptoms that commonly occur to people who travel to over 8,000 feet in altitude without acclimating (taking time to reach that altitude).

Avalanche path* A terrain feature where an avalanche occurs. Composed of a starting zone, track, and runout zone (American Avalanche Association, 2018).

Avalanche starting zones* The portions of an avalanche path where an avalanche releases (American Avalanche Association, 2018).

Avalanche track* The portion of an avalanche path between the starting zone and the runout zone (American Avalanche Association, 2018).

Bloodborne pathogens Microorganisms—such as viruses, bacteria, and similar microbes—that are present in human blood and can cause disease in humans (OSHA, 2017a).

Buoyancy The tendency of a body to float or sink in water or any other fluid (USCG, 2017).

Candle ice Ice that resembles many candles bundled together; commonly found in late winter or early spring.

Chilblains Itchy, reddish and purple, swollen lesions that occur primarily on the extremities due to longer exposure to temperatures just above freezing or sudden rewarming after exposure to cold.

Clear ice New ice formed by a long, hard freeze; considered to be the strongest ice.

Condition yellow A relaxed, heightened situational awareness where no threat exists but the individual is alert, observant, aware of his or her surroundings, and ready to respond to a problem or threat.

Dry suits Neoprene suits that trap air against the skin to provide both warmth and buoyancy while in the water.

Duty of care A requirement that a person act toward others with the watchfulness, attention, caution, and prudence that a reasonable person in the circumstances would use (Hill and Hill, 2017).

---

* Courtesy of Avalanche Encyclopedia, Avalanche.org, 2018.

Frazil ice The first type of ice to form; a thin, opaque film that floats to the surface.

Frazil slush Soft collections of frazil crystals that form in moving water where a current prevents a solid freeze.

Frostbite Partial or complete freezing of the skin and deeper tissues caused by exposure to the school.

Frost nip Early frostbite, characterized by numbness and pallor without significant tissue damage.

Granular convection A phenomenon where granular material subjected to vibration or shaking causes separation of the various sizes of the granules with larger ones rising to the surface.

Hazard Something that has the potential for harm.

Hazard mitigation Any sustained action taken to reduce or eliminate the long-term risk to people and property from hazards and their effects (Mitigation Planning, 2009).

Hazard controls Procedures adopted to minimize injury, reduce adverse health effects, and control damage to property (ANSI/ASSE, 2016; Safeopedia, 2017).

Heat cramps Muscle spasms that usually occur after vigorous exercise in hot weather and are generally relieved by rest and drinking water.

Heat exhaustion A form of shock that occurs when the body loses too much water and too many electrolytes through very heavy sweating after exposure to heat.

Heatstroke A condition of rapidly rising internal body temperature that occurs when the body's mechanisms for the release of heat are overwhelmed. Untreated, it can lead to death.

Hierarchy of hazard controls A system used to minimize or eliminate exposure to hazards (CDC/NIOSH, 2017).

High-altitude cerebral edema (HACE) An altitude illness in which there is a change in mental status and/or ataxia in a person with acute mountain sickness or the presence of mental status changes and ataxia in a person without acute mountain sickness.

High-altitude pulmonary edema (HAPE) An altitude illness characterized by at least two of the following: dyspnea at rest, cough, weakness or decreased exercise performance, or chest tightness or congestion. Also at least two of the following signs: central cyanosis, audible rales or wheezing in at least one lung field, tachypnea, or tachycardia.

Hypothermia A lowering of body temperature, which can endanger survival (USCG, 2017).

Hydraulic In river rescue, a backwash that traps and recirculates anything that floats (Chambers, 2016).

Inflatable Dependent on flexible air chambers that can be filled with air or other gas (usually carbon dioxide) for flotation (USCG, 2017).

Layered ice Ice formed from many layers of frozen and refrozen snow.

Low head dam A man-made structure, typically built to back up water in a reservoir (Chambers, 2016).

Normalcy bias The tendency of an individual to underestimate the possibility of something bad happening.

Personal flotation device (PFD) A device designed to maintain the wearer's head above water.

Risk An estimate of the probability of a hazard-related incident or exposure occurring.

Risk assessment A process to identify potential hazards and analyze what could happen if a hazard occurs (Ready.gov, 2017).

Rotten ice Old ice that is honeycombed with pockets of air bubbles; may crumble under the slightest pressure.

Runout zone* The portion of an avalanche path where the debris typically comes to rest (American Avalanche Association, 2018).

Safety Freedom from unreasonable risk.

Safety culture The attitude, beliefs, perceptions and values that people, usually in one industry or in one organization, share in relationship to safety.

Situational awareness Being aware of what is happening around you in terms of where you are, where you are supposed to be, and whether anyone or anything around you is a threat to your health and safety (Health and Safety Executive [HSE], 2018).

Snow blindness Essentially a sunburn of the eyes. Symptoms may not occur for many hours after the injury but include the sensation of a foreign body or sand in the eyes. Sensitivity to light (photophobia) is also common. Also called *photokeratitis*.

* Courtesy of Avalanche Encyclopedia, Avalanche.org, 2018.

Snow ice Opaque or milky-colored ice that is formed from the freezing of water-soaked snow; considered to be very weak.

Standard precautions Precautions applied to the care of patients in all healthcare settings, regardless of the suspected or confirmed presence of an infectious agent, for the purpose of preventing the transmission of infectious agents (CDC, 2017). Standard precautions include the use of personal protective equipment such as gloves, face masks, eye protection (goggles), and gowns (clothing covers). Formerly called *body substance isolation.*

Strainer In swift water, an obstacle that moving water can flow through, but that a swimmer or boat cannot. Some examples include trees, human-made obstacles, and debris. In swift water, strainers are life-threatening obstacles that should be avoided whenever possible.

Sunburn A first-degree burn (superficial, thermal burn) that causes reddening and pain of the skin after being exposed to sunlight. Swelling might accompany the reddening, and more prolonged exposure to sunlight might cause severe pain and blistering.

Sun protection factor (SPF) A measure of how well a sunscreen protects skin from UVB rays, which is radiation that causes sunburn, damages skin, and can contribute to skin cancer.

Swiftwater Water moving at greater than 1 nautical mile per hour (1.15 [statute] mile per hour) (NFPA, 2017a).

Trench foot A process similar to frostbite but caused by prolonged exposure to cool, wet conditions.

REFERENCES AND SUGGESTED READING

American Avalanche Association. 2018. Avalanche Encyclopedia. https://avalanche.org/avalanche-education/#avy-encyclopedia.

American Meteorological Association, Lightning Safety Group. 1999. Updated recommendations for lightning safety-1998. *Bulletin of the American Meteorological Society* 80, no. 10, 2035–2041.

American National Standard Institute/American Society of Safety Engineers. 2016. ANSI/ASSE Z590.3-2011 (R2016), *Prevention Through Design, Guidelines for Addressing Occupational Hazards and Risks in Design and Redesign Processes.* Park Ridge: IL. American Society of Safety Engineers.

American National Standard Institute/American Society of Safety Engineers. 2011a. ANSI/ASSE Z690.1-2011, *Vocabulary for Risk Management.* Park Ridge: IL. American Society of Safety Engineers.

American National Standard Institute/American Society of Safety Engineers. 2011b. ANSI/ASSE Z690.3-2011, *Risk Assessment Techniques* (National Adoption of: IEC/ISO 31010:2009). Park Ridge: IL. American Society of Safety Engineers.

ASTM, International. 2014a. Standard Practice for Single Person Cold Water Survival/Rescue Technique: HELP Position, F1729-96(2014). West Conshohocken, PA: ASTM, International.

ASTM, International. 2014b. Standard Practice for Multiple Persons Cold Water Survival/Rescue Technique: Huddle Position, F1728-96(2014). West Conshohocken, PA: ASTM, International.

ASTM, International. 2014c. Standard Guide for Ice Awls Self-Rescue Technique, F1766-97a(2014). West Conshohocken, PA: ASTM, International.

ASTM, International. 2014d. Standard Guide for Ice Staff Self-Rescue Technique, F1765-97a(2014). West Conshohocken, PA: ASTM, International.

ASTM, International. 2012a. Standard Guide for Hazard Awareness for Search and Rescue Personnel, F2890-12. West Conshohocken, PA: ASTM, International.

ASTM, International. 2012b. Standard Guide for Water Rescue Personal Flotation Device (PFD), F1823-97(2012). West Conshohocken, PA: ASTM, International.

Atkins, Dale. 2015. Ten years of avalanche rescues in the United States, 2003/04 - 2012/13. *Avalanche Rev.* 33, no. 3, 22–24.

Auerbach, Paul S., ed. 2017. *Wilderness Medicine*, 7th edition. St. Louis, MO: Elsevier, Inc.

Auerbach, Paul S. 2013. *Field Guide to Wilderness Medicine*, 4th edition. St. Louis, MO: Mosby, Inc.

Auerbach, Paul S. 2015. *Medicine for the Outdoors: The Essential Guide to First Aid and Medical Emergencies*, 6th edition. St. Louis, MO: Elsevier, Inc.

Backpacker.com. 2008. First aid: Hypothermia 101. http://www.backpacker.com/skills/hypothermia-101.

Ballard, Henry, Dale Atkins, and Lin Ballard. 2004. Probing for avalanche victims. Presented at the International Snow Science Workshop. Jackson, WY, September 19–24, 2004. http://training.scottishmountainrescue.org/files/2014/01/3HPS_ISSW_2004.pdf.

Boyd, Jeff, Pascal Haegeli, Riyad B. Abu-Laban, Michael Shuster, and John C. Butt. 2009. Patterns of death among avalanche fatalities: A 21-year review. *CMAJ,* 180, no. 5), 507–512.

Butler, Frank K. Jr., and Steven Chalfin. 2017. The eye in the wilderness. In *Wilderness Medicine*, 7th edition. Volume 1, edited by Paul S. Auerbach, pp. 1109–1127. St. Louis, MO: Elsevier, Inc.

Centers for Disease Control and Prevention. 2009. Infection control, standard precautions for all patient care. https://www.cdc.gov/infectioncontrol/basics/standard-precautions.html.

Centers for Disease Control and Prevention, The National Institute for Occupational Safety and Health. 2017. Hierarchy of controls. https://www.cdc.gov/niosh/topics/hierarchy/.

Chambers, Virgil. 2016. Low-head dams: A not-so clear and present danger. http://www.boatsafe.com/nauticalknowhow/lowhead.htm.

Cooper, Donald, ed. 2017. Event Safety Access Training [ESAT]. Slide deck developed for teaching safety fundamentals to the live event industry. Scottsdale, AZ: Event Safety Alliance.

Cooper, Dominic, and Lucas Finley. 2013. Strategic Safety Culture Roadmap. B-Safe Management Solutions Incorporated. http://www.behavioral-safety.com.

Cummings, Gregory A., and Stephen J. Traub. 2017. Tick-borne diseases. In *Wilderness Medicine*, 7th edition. Volume 1, edited by Paul S. Auerbach, pp. 968–993. St. Louis, MO: Elsevier, Inc.

Curtis, Rick. 2010. Outdoor action guide to hypothermia and cold weather injuries. Princeton, NJ: Princeton University. https://www.princeton.edu/~oa/safety/hypocold.shtml.

Danzl, Daniel F., and Martin R. Huecker 2017. Accidental Hypothermia. In *Wilderness Medicine*, 7th edition. Volume 1, edited by Paul S. Auerbach, pp. 135–162. St. Louis, MO: Elsevier, Inc.

Endsley, Mica R. 1995. Toward a theory of situation awareness in dynamic systems. *Human Factors*, 37, no. 1, 32–64. http://uwf.edu/skass/documents/HF.37.1995-Endsley-Theory_000.pdf.

Forgey, William W. 1989. *Hypothermia: Death by Exposure*. Pittsboro, IN: ICS Books.

Fradin, Mark S., and John F. Day. 2002. Comparative efficacy of insect repellents against mosquito bites. *New England Journal of Medicine* 347, no. 1,13–18.

Freeman, Esther E., Suchismita Paul, Joshua D. Shofner, and Alexa B. Kimball. 2017. Plant-induced dermatitis. In *Wilderness Medicine*, 7th edition. Volume 2, edited by Paul S. Auerbach, pp. 1414–1433. St. Louis, MO: Elsevier, Inc.

Freer, Luanne, Charles Handford, and Christopher H.E. Imray, 2017. Frostbite. In *Wilderness Medicine*, 7th edition. Volume 1, edited by Paul S. Auerbach, pp. 197–222. St. Louis, MO: Elsevier, Inc.

Linxweiler, Eric and Mike Maude, Editors. 2017. *Mountaineering: Freedom of the Hills*, 9th edition. New York: Mountaineers Books.

Giesbrecht, Gordon. 2011. Beyond cold water boot camp: 4 phases of cold water immersion. http://www.beyondcoldwaterbootcamp.com/en/4-phases-of-cold-water-immersion.

Giesbrecht, Gordon G., and Gerald K. Bristow. 1997. Recent advances in hypothermia research. *Annals of the New York Academy of Sciences* 813, no. 1, 663–675.

Gomez, H. F., and Richard C. Dart. 1995. Clinical toxicology of snakebite in North America. In *Handbook of Clinical Toxicology of Animal Venoms and Poisons,* edited by Jurg Meier and Julian White, pp. 619–644. Boca Raton, FL: CRC Press.

Gookin, John. 2010. Backcountry lightning risk management. 21st International Lightning Detection Conference, Wilderness Risk Management Conference. https://www.nols.edu/media/filer_public/fa/96/fa96d71d-df6b-487f-9e48-6b5a84de50b9/outdoor_lightning_risk_management-gookin.pdf.

Grissom, Colin K., Martin I. Radwin, Chris H. Harmston, Ellie L. Hirshberg, and Thomas J. Crowley. 2000. Respiration during snow burial using an artificial air pocket. *JAMA*. 283, no. 17, 2266–2271.

Grissom, Colin K., Martin I. Radwin, Scott McIntosh, and Dale Atkins. 2017. Avalanches. In *Wilderness Medicine*, 7th edition. Volume 1, edited by Paul S. Auerbach, pp. 40–71. St. Louis, MO: Elsevier, Inc.

Hackett, Peter, Andrew Luks, Justin Lawley, and Robert Roach. 2017. High-altitude medicine and pathophysiology. In *Wilderness Medicine*, 7th edition. Volume 1, edited by Paul S. Auerbach, pp. 8–29. St. Louis, MO: Elsevier, Inc.

Haegeli, Pascal, Markus Falk, Emily Procter, Benjamin Zweifel, Frédéric Jarry, Spencer Logan, Kalle Kronholm, Marek Biskupič, and Hermann Brugger. 2014. The effectiveness of avalanche airbags. *Resuscitation,* 85, no. 9, 1197–1203.

Health and Safety Executive. 2018. Leadership and Worker Involvement Toolkit: Knowing what is going on around you (situational awareness), Information sheet 6. http://www.hse.gov.uk/construction/lwit/assets/downloads/situational-awareness.pdf.

Hill, Gerald N., and Kathleen T. Hill. 2017. *The People's Law Dictionary: Taking the Mystery Out of Legal Language*. Fine Communications. http://dictionary.law.com/Default.aspx?selected=599.

Hilmo, Jonas, Torvind Naesheim, and Mads Gilbert. 2014. Nobody is dead until warm and dead: Prolonged resuscitation is warranted in arrested hypothermic victims also in remote areas—a retrospective study from northern Norway. *Resuscitation,* 85, no. 9, 1204–1211. doi: 10.1016/j.resuscitation.2014.04.029.

History.com. 2017. This Day in History: Avalanche kills thousands in Peru. A+E Networks. http://www.history.com/this-day-in-history/avalanche-kills-thousands-in-peru.

Hohlrieder, Matthias, Hermann Brugger, Heinrich M. Schubert, Marion Pavlic, John Ellerton, and Peter Mair. 2007. Pattern and severity of injury in avalanche victims. *High Altitude Medicine & Biology* 8, no. 1, 56–61.

Imray, Christopher, Charles Handford, Owen Thomas, and John Castellani. 2017. Nonfreezing cold-induced injuries. In *Wilderness Medicine*, 7th edition. Volume 1, edited by Paul S. Auerbach, pp. 222–234. St. Louis, MO: Elsevier, Inc.

Isaac, Jeffrey. 1998. *The Outward Bound Wilderness First-Aid Handbook: Revised Edition*. Guilford, CT: The Lyons Press.

Jensenius, Jr., John S. 2016. A detailed analysis of lightning deaths in the United States from 2006 through 2015. National Weather Service NOAA. http://www.lightningsafety.noaa.gov/fatalities/analysis06-15.pdf.

Johnson, G. Mark. 2003. *The Ultimate Desert Handbook: A Manual for Desert Hikers, Campers, and Travelers.* New York: Ragged Mountain Press/McGraw Hill.

Jordan, Ann T. 2003. *Business Anthropology.* Prospect Heights, IL: Waveland Press Inc.

Kithil, Richard. 1998. Lightning safety for campers and hikers. National Lightning Safety Institute. http://lightningsafety.com/nlsi_pls/ploutdoor.htm.

Kosinski, Sylweriusz, Tomasz Darocha, Jerzy Sadowski, and Rafał Drwila, eds. 2017. *Hypothermia: Clinical Aspects of Body Cooling, Analysis of Dangers, Directions of Modern Treatment. Warsaw, Poland.* Jagiellonian University Press.

Lipman, Grant S., and Brian J. Krabak. 2017. Foot problems and care. In *Wilderness Medicine*, 7th edition. Volume 1, edited by Paul S. Auerbach, pp. 533–549. St. Louis, MO: Elsevier, Inc.

Management of Health and Safety at Work Regulations. 1999. Risk assessment. 1999 No. 3242, Regulation 3. http://www.legislation.gov.uk/uksi/1999/3242/regulation/3/made.

Mapes, Lynda V. 2010. The Wellington Avalanche of March 1, 1910, near Stevens Pass is still the deadliest in U.S. history, with 96 lives lost. Seattle, WA: *The Seattle Times.* http://www.seattletimes.com/seattle-news/1910-stevens-pass-avalanche-still-deadliest-in-us-history/.

McIntosh, Scott E., Colin K. Grissom, Christopher R. Olivares, Han S. Kim, and Bruce Tremper. 2007. Cause of death in avalanche fatalities. *Wilderness & Environmental Medicine* 18, no. 4, 293–297.

McManners, Hugh. 2007. *The Complete Wilderness Training Book.* 2nd Revised Edition. New York: DK Publishing.

Mine Safety and Health Administration, U.S. Department of Labor. 2017. Mine Rescue Training. https://www.msha.gov/training-education/mine-rescue-training.

Mitigation Planning, 44 CFR §201.2 2009. Definitions. https://www.gpo.gov/fdsys/granule/CFR-2009-title44-vol1/CFR-2009-title44-vol1-sec201-2.

National Association for Cave Diving. 2016. Welcome to the official NACD website. http://www.nacdmembers.com/.

National Cave Rescue Commission, National Speleological Society. 2017. Resources. http://ncrc.info/Resources.

National Collegiate Athletic Association. 2014. 2014–2015 Sports Medicine Handbook. 25th edition. http://www.ncaapublications.com/productdownloads/MD15.pdf.

National Fire Protection Association. 2017a. NFPA 1670, *Standard on Operations and Training for Technical Search and Rescue Incidents.* Batterymarch, MA: NFPA.

National Fire Protection Association. 2017b. NFPA 1006, *Standard for Technical Rescue Personnel Professional Qualifications.* Batterymarch, MA: NFPA.

National Oceanic and Atmospheric Administration National Weather Service. 2017. Lightning safety tips and resources. http://www.lightningsafety.noaa.gov.

National Oceanic and Atmospheric Administration National Weather Service. 2014. NOAA knows. . .lightning. http://www.lightningsafety.noaa.gov/resources/lightning3_050714.pdf.

National Speleological Society Cave Diving Section. 2017. Training programs: Becoming a certified cave diver. https://nsscds.org/trainingprograms/.

Norris, Jr. Robert, Sean P. Bush, and Jennifer Cohen Smith. 2017. Bites by venomous reptiles in Canada, the United States, and Mexico. In *Wilderness Medicine*, 7th edition. Volume 1, edited by Paul S. Auerbach, pp. 729–760. St. Louis, MO: Elsevier, Inc.

Parrish, Henry M., John C. Goldner, and Stanley L. Silberg. 1966. Poisonous snakebites causing no venenation. *Postgraduate Medicine* 39, no. 3, 265.

Pavan-Langston, Deborah. 1996. *Manual of Ocular Diagnosis and Therapy.* 4th edition, Boston: Little, Brown.

Petzoldt, Paul. 1974. *The Wilderness Handbook.* New York: W.W. Norton & Company, Inc.

Radwin, Martin I., and Colin K. Grissom. 2002. Technological advances in avalanche survival. *Wilderness & Environmental Medicine* 13, no. 2,143–152.

Rawlins, Chip, and Colin Fletcher. 2002. *The Complete Walker IV*, revised edition. New York: Alfred A. Knopf, Inc.

Ready.gov. 2017. Risk assessment. https://www.ready.gov/risk-assessment.

Rosenberg, Joel. 2011. *The Carry Book: Minnesota Edition.* lulu.com.

Safeopedia.com. 2017. Hazard control: what does hazard control mean? https://www.safeopedia.com/definition/151/hazard-control.

Schein, E. & Schein, P. (2016). *Organizational Culture and Leadership, The Jossey-Bass Business & Management Series.* 5th edition. Hoboken, NJ: John Wiley & Sons. Reprinted with permission.

Skurka, Andrew. 2017. *The Ultimate Hiker's Gear Guide, Second Edition: Tools and Techniques to Hit the Trail.* 2nd edition. New York: National Geographic.

Stalsberg, Helge, Claus Albretsen, Mads Gilbert, Michael Kearney, Einar Moestue, Ivar Nordrum, Morten Rostrup, and Anne Ørbo. 1989. Mechanism of death in avalanche victims. *Virchows Archiv A Pathological Anatomy and Histopathology,* 414, no. 5, 415–422.

Survey & Cartography Section, National Speleological Society. 2017. SACS Home. http://caves.org/section/sacs/SACS/SACS_Home.html.

Tawrell, Paul. 2006. *Camping & Wilderness Survival: The Ultimate Outdoors Book.* 2nd edition. Lebanon, NH: Paul Tawrell.

U.S. Coast Guard. 2017. PFD selection, use, wear & care. https://www.dco.uscg.mil/CG-ENG-4/PFDSel/.

U.S. Department of Labor Occupational Safety and Health Administration. 2017a. Occupational Safety and Health standards, toxic and hazardous substances, bloodborne pathogens, 29 CFR 1910.1030(b). https://www.osha.gov/pls/oshaweb/owadisp.show_document?p_id=10051&p_table=STANDARDS.

U.S. Department of Labor Occupational Safety and Health Administration. 2017b. Occupational Safety and Health Administration. Shipyard employment eTool. https://www.osha.gov/SLTC/etools/shipyard/standard/ppe/general_ppe/lifesaving_equipment.html.

University of Minnesota. 2015. Minnesota sea grant, hypothermia prevention: Survival in cold water. http://www.seagrant.umn.edu/coastal_communities/hypothermia.

WebMD. 2017. Cosmetic procedures: Sun exposure and skin cancer. http://www.webmd.com/beauty/sun-exposure-skin-cancer#1.

Wilkerson, James A., ed., Ken Zafren, and Ernest E. Moore. 2010. *Medicine for Mountaineering*, 6th edition. Seattle, WA: Mountaineers Books.

Winkenwerder, William, and Michael N. Sawka. 2007. Disorders due to heat and cold. In *Cecil Textbook of Medicine*. 23rd edition., edited by Lee Goldman, Dennis Ausiello, William P. Arend, et al., pp. 763–767. Philadelphia, PA: Saunders, Elsevier Science.

World Health Organization. 2007. Standard precautions in health care: Aide-memoire. http://www.who.int/csr/resources/publications/EPR_AM2_E7.pdf.

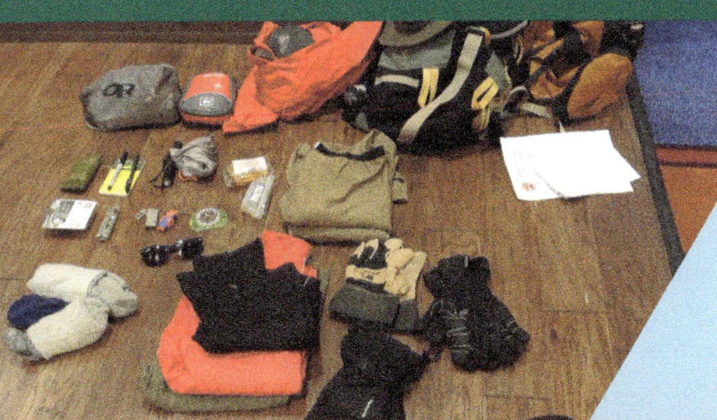

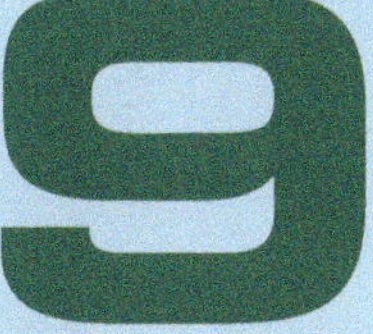

CHAPTER 9

The Ready Pack and Personal Equipment

OBJECTIVES

Upon completion of this chapter and the related course activities, the student will be able to meet the following objectives:

- List at least 10 of the 13 categories of equipment The National Association For Search And Rescue (NASAR) recommends be included in the 24-hour pack.
- For each of the 13 24-hour pack categories, identify items that could be included in that category.
- Discuss factors to consider when selecting the following equipment for use in SAR:
  - Head protection
  - Ground protection
  - Sleeping bag
  - Shelters
  - Nutrition
  - Hydration
  - Footwear
  - Illumination
  - Pack

Packing Right

The decision regarding what equipment should be included in a search and rescue (SAR) ready pack is mostly a personal one. Choosing the right basic equipment to bring into the field improves safety, speed, comfort, and durability (**FIGURE 9-1**).

Carrying the appropriate equipment is an essential part of SAR effectiveness and survival. SAR personnel must be intimately familiar with everything they carry so they know they have what they need to do their job. Being unprepared can quickly lead to becoming a casualty that distracts from the original SAR mission. Therefore, it is recommended that all SAR personnel construct their own SAR ready pack from scratch; it is more likely that unnecessary items will not be included and that all carried items are known and familiar to the person carrying them.

A **24-hour pack** is the suggested minimum that SAR personnel should carry during a mission (**FIGURE 9-2**). Its contents allow the person carrying it to be self-reliant and comfortable should a **bivouac** (temporary camp without tents or cover) become necessary while waiting for help or rescue. If the subject of a search is encountered, the contents of your pack can also be used to assist him or her until additional help arrives.

The 24-hour pack can be supplemented for longer missions. Correspondingly, the expanded packs are called "48-" and "72-hour" packs. In many regions where field SAR work can take personnel far from the safety and comfort of camps, 48- or 72-hour packs are minimum requirements. "Ready pack" is the generic term for any 24-, 48-, or 72-hour pack.

For efficiency, it is recommended that items selected for your 24-hour pack have multiple uses. For example, alcohol-based hand sanitizer can be used as a disinfectant

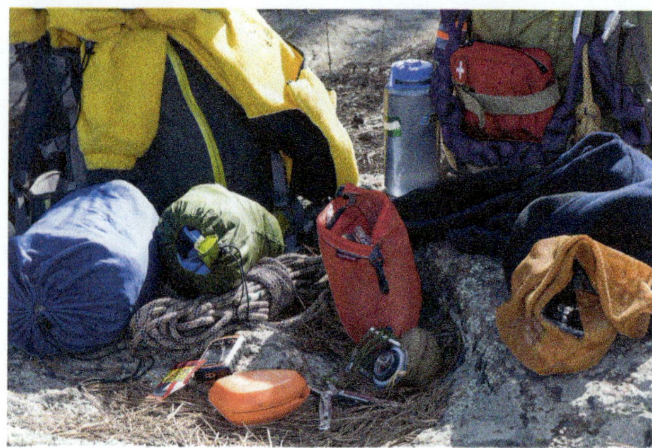

FIGURE 9-1 SAR personnel must be intimately familiar with everything they carry so they know they have what they need to do their job.
© 2016 Howard Paul, Photography for Communication and Commerce.

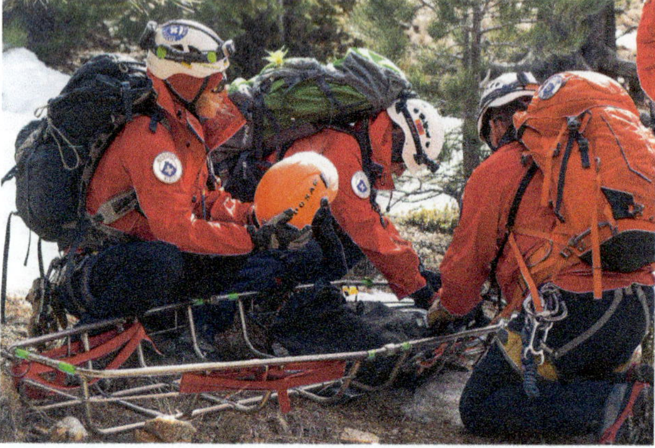

FIGURE 9-2 Carrying the appropriate equipment is an essential part of SAR effectiveness and survival.
© 2016 Howard Paul, Photography for Communication and Commerce.

or as a fire starter. Any item that has more than one use helps lighten and consolidate your pack. You can further conserve weight and improve efficiency by standardizing the batteries used by your communications, lighting, and navigation electronics. A lighter pack makes for a more effective searcher.

Setting up a 24-hour pack does not have to be overly expensive. You can save money by taking advantage of generous professional deals available to SAR personnel, your local team, and NASAR members (e.g., Experticity®). It is also important that you train with your 24-hour pack in conditions similar to those to which you will respond.

Ready Pack Contents

The contents of a ready pack can vary greatly from one region to another and from one user to another. Generally, however, certain components should be considered standard. NASAR recognizes this with their consolidated pack guide, which recommends that the categories of equipment carried in a 24-hour pack include the following (NASAR, 2016):

- *Survival/first aid/signaling.* A small, combination personal first aid survival kit should be part of any ready pack. Included should be small bandages, dressings, antihistamine capsules, and material for cleansing small wounds, as well as material that can be used to treat specific common wounds and illnesses, such as blisters, headaches, indigestion, and splinters. Attending to injuries and illnesses before they become bigger problems should be a goal. Survival and improvisational materials should be included, such as leaf bags, safety pins, wire, razor blade, para-cord/cordage, space blanket, water filter and purification capability (commercial filter/chemicals/UV), wire ties, duct tape, and fire-starting capability. Materials for signaling can include a whistle, signal mirror, smoke signal, strobe light, or improvised signal devices such as a chemical light stick twirled with para-cord ("buzz saw" signal). For consistency, members of a SAR team should carry the same model whistle so, should a whistle be blown, it can be quickly recognized as belonging to a team member rather than the subject. SAR team members may also wear the same color chemical or LED light on their pack at night so SAR members can identify each other in the field. Green chemical lights should be avoided when helicopter crews may be using night vision goggles (NVG) because the green light is difficult to see with NVGs.
- *Self-rescue.* A couple of carabiners; Prusik loops; a length of 1-inch, tubular webbing; and a multitool can be invaluable should self-rescue or self-belay be necessary. Rescue equipment carried to help the victim once he or she is located is considered specialized team gear that should be carried to where it is needed by the specially trained personnel who will use it.
- *Hygiene/personal items.* Goggles, tissues/toilet paper, feminine hygiene products, moist towelettes, sunglasses, prescription glasses (and spare pair), sunscreen, insect repellent, hand trowel/shovel, lip balm, and personal medications.
- *Navigation.* Navigation supplies should include a compass, map, pacing beads/counter, grid reader, protractor, map ruler, GPS, and altimeter.
- *Communications.* Communications supplies include a cell phone (with camera), radio, spare batteries, and charger, if applicable.
- *Light sources.* Light sources include hands-free (headlamp), secondary light source (light in weight),

chemical light stick(s), and common batteries for all lights.

- *Clothing and personal protective equipment (PPE).* Clothing and PPE would include a cap/hat, helmet, clothing appropriate for the environment, extra clothing, appropriate footwear, gloves (various types: surgical, leather, and/or insulated), eye protection (goggles, sunglasses), a high-visibility vest (ANSI/ISEA 201 compliant), extra socks, rainwear, trekking poles, gaiters, bandana, and dry bags for the contents (e.g., Ziploc®, Aloksak®, or equivalents). When deciding what is appropriate, consider that it WILL rain, it WILL snow, and it WILL be cold. Preparing for these potential problems can prevent an error in omission. In desert environments, do not think that it cannot get cold as well as hot. At the very least, extra socks, gloves, and a hat should always be carried.
- *Shelter.* Shelter components include a ground insulation/pad, shelter material (e.g., tarp, bivy), and multiple lead bags. Something that can be used to protect SAR personnel or the subject from the environment is useful as shelter. Tents can be adequate, but other material may be lighter, cheaper, and better suited for improvisation.
- *Food.* Although there are exceptions, generally, food should not be "meal" type; it should be of a type that can be eaten continuously to maintain strength and energy, rather than requiring special preparation and a "meal" period. Food should be nonperishable and nutritionally sound. Candy may taste good, but it does not supply needed nutrients and should be avoided. Foods that are high in salt or caffeine should also be avoided, and alcohol, tobacco, and recreational drugs should be prohibited. Carrying food in a pint- or quart-sized resealable, waterproof bag carries the advantage of being able to use that bag later to store any discarded food remnants or packaging, even after eating the food, without affecting the other contents of your pack. Carry out everything you carry in.
- *Hydration.* Hydration materials include a water bottle/canteen, hydration bladder, and sports drink mix powder. Always carry more water than you expect to need. For extended field encounters, variance may be required from standard practice. For instance, water filter/purification equipment may be necessary rather than carrying large quantities of water (water is very heavy to carry). Consumption of fluids is so important in SAR operations and during a survival situation that the additional weight and bother of carrying something that would make drinking water safe and enjoyable is justified. Lack of fluids (dehydration) has been implicated in so many deaths and injuries that anything that might promote fluid consumption is encouraged. Examples include powdered drink mixes, tea bags, instant coffee, and bouillon cubes. The user of these products, however, should realize the effects that the contents might have. For example, coffee and tea contain caffeine; sports drink mixes contain valuable electrolytes, but they also include plenty of sweeteners; and sweet drink mixes might have mostly sugar.
- *Load bearing/packs.* The pack should be an appropriate size for the contents and fitted to the wearer. Additional components are a waist/butt pack, radio chest harness, and pack (rain) cover.
- *Search equipment.* Search equipment includes photo identification, a pad (waterproof?) and pencil, binoculars/monocular, a tracking stick, flagging tape, and a measuring device (tape).
- *Resource-specific equipment.* This additional equipment is determined by the local authority.
- *Mission-specific equipment.* This additional equipment is determined by the mission.

The specific, recommended, minimum contents of a ready pack are included in NASAR's Consolidated Pack Guide, which can be found on its website (NASAR, 2016). These essential contents can be supplemented with items included to meet the desires and needs of the user. The content carried should be carefully chosen to supply the general needs of both the user and the mission. In NASAR's Guide, all contents have been chosen with improvisation in mind. All pieces can be improvised in at least two ways and most in many more.

Since the ready pack is meant to be carried at all times, weight is a serious consideration. This becomes especially relevant if additional items must be carried to support team efforts, to support advanced medical or technical skills, or to meet specialist needs such as a K9 handler carrying extra dog-related items. Many pieces of equipment that you might consider of marginal value (that is, questionable as to their value in such a pack) may be deleted to reduce weight. Improvisation is more thought-reliant than it is equipment-reliant, so even without certain gear, SAR personnel should have the ability to meet most challenges by thinking through them.

Expert Advice

The following advice from experienced outdoor and SAR instructors relates directly to carrying equipment in the field.

Keep the Pack with You

No matter what gear is collected and transported to the SAR mission site, it is all worthless if it is not where it is needed. Since there is not always warning before survival or improvisational skills are required, the ready pack needs to be with you all the time. Never set it down to go do something. Always have the pack with you. Do not respond to an incident without a ready pack (whether working in the field or not). Make it a habit to carry your ready pack with you everywhere.

Do Not Share

When you are in the field or at a mission site, your ready pack is your home, and your health, safety, and comfort depend on it. Do not offer ready pack contents to others unless they are in dire need. The same contents may be of value to you later.

Care for Your Ready Pack

Take care of your pack and its contents and give it the respect you would give any object that has the power to save or maintain your life. Just as food and water deserve proper storage and care, so does your ready pack. Just as you take care of rescue equipment, take care of your ready pack. Do not leave your ready pack unattended and its contents a target of pilfering. Review the contents often and maintain the contents required.

Hydration

Water often is carried more comfortably on a belt around the waist or in a hands-free hydration system with a bladder or reservoir secured in the pack and a watering tube extending outside the pack. These methods allow easy access so that water is consumed more often. Too often, SAR personnel pack away water and drink only at breaks. This can be dangerous, especially at altitude and in hot environments. Water needs to be consumed continuously during a mission, and if the water is packed away, the searcher is less likely to stay hydrated.

At nearly 8.5 pounds (3.9 kg) per gallon, with 1 imperial gallon taking up 231 cubic inches or 0.134 cubic feet (0.004 cubic meters), water is probably the heaviest material that will be carried. Carrying water properly—on the waist or tight against the back—more evenly distributes the weight, making it easier to carry.

Keep hydration systems and water bottles full. Water containers that are not full tend to slosh and shift in the pack, making travel more uncomfortable and difficult. However, water containers carried on the belt can shift and still be carried comfortably. If using hands-free hydration systems, always carry the bladder inside the pack, close to the searcher's back, aligned vertically with the spine to prevent spillage. An important consideration is the use of the cover to protect the water system. Bladders alone are not very durable and can rupture easily. This brings up another important point: always carry at least two different water containers in the unlikely event one ruptures.

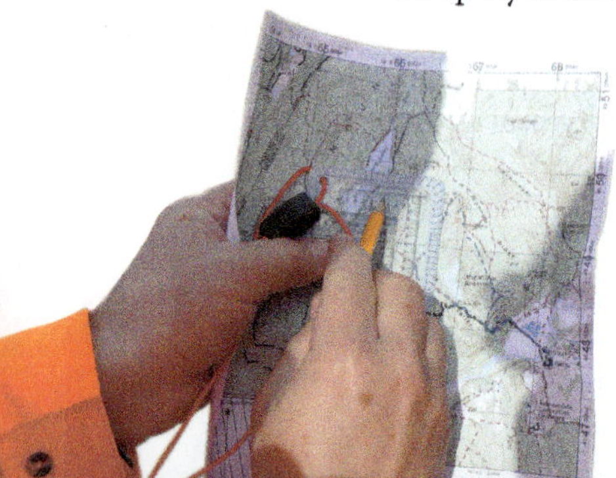

Equipment Accessibility

Several items included on the equipment list should be accessible to SAR personnel continuously without having to remove the pack. These items are termed "pocket items" and should be carried in an accessible pocket rather than in the pack itself. The decision to make a piece of equipment a pocket item is based on the item's frequency of use, size, and importance. Carrying some items in a pocket also allows more room in the pack or allows for a smaller pack.

Having something immediately available can also enhance safety. For example, keeping your whistle close at hand—say, attached to the front of your radio harness or pack chest strap—would make it quicker and easier to access should it be needed in an emergency. Many items qualify as potential pocket items, depending on the mission and the individual carrying them. They might include paper and pencil, a compass, a bandana or handkerchief, a whistle (on a lanyard attached to the pack or chest/radio harness), tissues, a watch (on the wrist), water (on a belt or with tube/straw access), and a personal first aid kit. Some items may be considered pocket items depending on the circumstances and situation. They include a flashlight (near dusk and at night), trail food (to munch on while traveling), sunglasses, sunscreen (where required), insect repellent (where required), a knife, a map, and similar items.

Research Contents

The decision of what to purchase for inclusion in your ready pack should not be made hastily. Research all equipment thoroughly before purchasing anything. Ask experienced SAR personnel their opinions and find out what has worked for others in different conditions. Get details on the equipment in which you are interested and compare them to similar equipment for quality, durability, and applicability to the SAR field. Equipment suitable for a specific type of outdoor environment may be entirely unsuitable for SAR work (e.g., a ski jacket may get torn to pieces in SAR work).

Equipment does not necessarily have to be expensive to be ideal for SAR work. In many cases, a military surplus garment or piece of equipment may be better than or just as effective as an expensive name-brand item. That said, consider purchases of SAR equipment as life-safety items. They are an investment, and they must protect and provide safety and comfort against the elements. Most name-brand technical gear has a lifetime warranty and has stood the test of time.

Take your time and find out what is best for you and your needs before spending a great deal of money. You might be surprised how inexpensive it can be to save someone's life.

Mission Readiness

Know what is in your ready pack and have it mission ready. Go through your pack and inventory the contents often. This keeps you familiar with the contents and helps identify problems before they make it into the field.

Keep your pack ready for the next mission by collecting and storing as much of the gear as possible together. Better yet, keep everything in the pack, ready to go, and simply check it often for completeness and serviceability. Food, water, and all perishables can be added at call-out. A separate bag can be added to the core equipment to supplement the clothing portion as necessary in different seasons and for different environments.

SEARCH AND RESCUE TIP

The bottom line is: Know what you have and always have it ready to go.

Personal Body Management and Protective Equipment

Several items may be required during SAR operations to minimize distractions and improve safety and comfort.

Insect Repellent

A nonchemical approach to repelling insects includes wearing clothing made of slippery material, such as silk and nylon, that covers exposed skin. Avoid loose-weave clothes that use materials such as cotton and wool when insects are a problem. Tying clothing at the wrists and ankles also aids in discouraging insects from sneaking inside. Netting may be required to repel some insects, such as gnats, fleas, black flies, horse flies, deer flies, and chiggers. Avoid the use of perfumes and deodorant soaps before going into the field.

Studies have shown that **DEET** (chemical name, *N,N-diethyl-meta-toluamide*) is still the most protective repellent, although it is not necessary to use products that contain more than 35% DEET (Fradin and Day, 2002). The U.S. government provides an informative fact sheet on DEET that describes how it can be used safely. This brief document should be reviewed by all personnel who intend to use DEET (CDC, 2017).

Sunscreen/Block

Creams and balms may be of value in preventing chapped body parts; however, consider how it might attract insects due to sweet smell before using too much.

Sunscreen/block can save much discomfort in terms of pain from sunburn. At altitude, the sun may not even feel hot, but its rays are burning your skin faster than at sea level. Sunscreen preparations are available that can block the harmful rays of the sun, but these must be reapplied frequently and may reduce the body's natural ability to regulate heat (sweating), which is why covering exposed skin with clothing is preferred. Look for products that provide a sun protection factor (SPF) of 30 or greater.

Eye Protection

When working in trees and brush (especially at night), it is advisable to wear protective glasses or goggles. These need not be heavy, and they should allow for ventilation around the eyes. Eye protection is also required any time members will be riding in, or working around, helicopters.

When traveling in hot, sunny areas or at elevation, sunglasses or tinted goggles should be worn to prevent eye injuries from overexposure to UV light (snow blindness, etc.). Sunglasses worn at altitude and in a reflective environment should block all UV radiation, have side shields, and limit the amount of visible light that is transmitted through them to the 5–10% range, which is less light transmission than everyday sunglasses usually allow (Butler and Chalfin, 2017).

Head Protection

Wearing a helmet is the best practice for head protection during field SAR work and is required any time members are riding in or working around helicopters, but there are many kinds of helmets, and not all of them are suitable for use in SAR. In cold weather, ventilation of the helmet may not be important, but it may be desirable in warm weather. Not all helmets can be worn on top of a winter hat or cap or maintain their integrity over time if paint, labels, or stickers are applied. Not all helmets are certified by their manufacturer to protect from side impacts or objects that fall from more than 3 feet (1 meter), both of which are likely in SAR environments. Only some manufacturers claim their helmets can be used in low temperatures, worn while climbing, stay on during a fall, or are even certified at all. Thus, serious consideration should be put into exactly which helmet you will need in a specific situation.

In the United States, the current standard required by OSHA for helmets worn on the job is ANSI Z89.1-2014 (OSHA, 2017). This standard provides performance and testing requirements for industrial helmets (i.e., hard hats). It establishes the types and classes of protective helmets, depending on the type of hazard encountered. It includes specifications for helmets designed to offer protection from top and lateral impact (Type II), or top-only impact (Type I), and a range of classifications for electrical conductivity (Class C = conductive; Class G = general, reduces exposure to low voltage conductors; Class E = nonconductive to 20,000 volts). Although a helmet that meets this standard may be suitable for some SAR work, it includes several requirements that may make a compliant helmet uncomfortable, at best, and unsafe, at worst, in many SAR environments.

The rough equivalent to ANSI Z89.1 in Europe is EN397, which sets out the performance and marking requirements for all PPE helmets. In this European standard, the protection provided to the wearer is against falling objects, which could cause brain or skull injury. It does not include side impact protection or significant helmet retention requirements, but it does allow for optional performance enhancements, claimed by the specific manufacturer, for use in low temperatures (even ultra-low temperatures), lateral deformation, and flame resistance (BSI, 2017a). Another European standard was developed for specialist mountaineering helmets: EN12492-2000. This standard includes requirements on helmet retention to ensure the helmet is not inadvertently removed and requirements that apply to wearers working at height. The International Climbing and Mountain Federation (UIAA™) also publishes a Mountaineering and Climbing Equipment standard regarding helmets: UIAA 106 (2013). The UIAA standard requires compliance with EN12492-2000 and adds specific labeling and testing requirements (UIAA, 2013). Helmets that meet these mountaineering standards are usually more appropriate for working in SAR environments, but many helmets are available that meet more than one of these standards. Thus, the following standards and capabilities are recommended for helmets that are used in a SAR environment:

- Meets the requirements of the EN12492 and EN397 standards for protection against impact
- Meets the requirements of UIAA 106
- Satisfies optional requirements of the EN397 standard concerning lateral deformation and use in cold temperatures
- Optional: Meets ANSI Z89.1-2014 Type II Class C
- Optional: Includes air vents
- Able to securely attach a headlamp

If you want to wear a winter hat or cap under the helmet, the helmet manufacturer must allow it in their certification of the helmet. If the helmet is not certified for this, wearing a hat may significantly reduce the protection the helmet provides. The same is true for painting the helmet and applying stickers. If the manufacturer does not specifically permit it in their certification of the helmet, it should not be done.

It is generally suggested that helmets should have an in-use life span of five years from date of first use or removal from storage. This length of time should be reduced if the helmet is used in an aggressive environment, incurs excessive wear and tear, or is stored in direct sunlight or a hot environment. If a helmet suffers an impact from a falling object, or is dropped from a height, the helmet should be replaced immediately. It may have been weakened by the incident, even if damage is not visible or apparent (PPE.org, 2017).

Sleeping Systems

Sleeping during a SAR mission may occasionally be required, so some information regarding what equipment might be necessary is provided. If a specific SAR mission does not warrant carrying all the equipment necessary to sleep comfortably in the field, as a minimum, members should carry something that can be used should an emergency bivouac be required (e.g., "space blanket," large garbage bag).

Ground Protection

A sleeping pad placed between your body and the ground while sleeping, sitting, or reclining can serve two purposes: it can insulate you from the cold ground and provide padding for a more comfortable resting position. For lengthy SAR operations, a sleeping pad is critical for comfort and warmth.

Ideally, insulating pads should be lightweight, soft, compact, waterproof, and efficient insulators. A thicker pad provides more insulation from the ground, but it is also heavier and bulkier. While sitting or lying on it, a pad should allow for insulating material to remain between you and the ground, even as your body compresses it. If it is too soft and compresses so much that you end up sitting or lying directly on the ground, the pad is not doing its job.

Open-cell foam is comfortable, lightweight, compressible, and provides good insulation when dry, but the open-cell structure absorbs water (like a sponge), so a waterproof cover for this type of pad is essential. The open-cell design is also not as durable and does not provide as much insulation as its closed-cell counterpart.

Closed-cell foam sleeping pads do not provide as much cushion as open-cell foam, but they are usually cheaper, far more durable, lighter, do not absorb water, and are more compact. A closed-cell foam pad can be strapped to the outside of a pack, endure rain and snow, and still perform perfectly as a sleeping pad. These types of pads can also be purchased in bright colors, which might be useful as a signal in an emergency. Because they are inexpensive, a closed cell foam pad can be cut up and used as a splint to pad an injury during transport, as a cervical spine brace during transport, or even as additional flotation. These are among the many reasons closed-cell sleeping pads are so popular with SAR personnel.

Although a traditional, single-chamber air mattress—inflated only by air—is not recommended as a sleeping pad used in SAR, variations on this theme have been developed that are much more appropriate for a sleeping pad. One includes two layered air chambers that are inflated separately with insulating, open-celled foam between the layers. The lower air chamber touches the ground and absorbs the unevenness of roots and rocks. It keeps the cold air in the chamber away from the user. The upper air chamber inflates separately and can be independently adjusted to a desired firmness while trapping air warmed by your body. The Sea to Summit® Comfort Plus Sleeping Pad is one example of this technology. Although it can be somewhat heavy and expensive when compared to other ultra-light alternatives, its comfort and warmth are excellent.

Self-inflating pads combine the comfort and warmth of open-cell foam with the compressibility of an air mattress. These sleeping pads enclose open-cell foam with an airtight chamber that includes a valve with which the internal air pressure can be controlled. The combination of foam and air cushions and thermally insulates users, keeping them warm and comfortable, but the air-filled device is susceptible to puncture. The tendency of open-cell foam to rebound allows the pads to self-inflate when the valve is opened, but blowing into the valve may be needed to hasten the inflation process. These pads are generally bulkier and weigh more than many of their closed-cell counterparts, and they often cost more than simpler options. However, their adjustability (letting more or less air in), warmth, and comfort are excellent.

A waterproof tarp on which your sleeping pad or tent can be placed provides an additional barrier between you and the ground. It protects your equipment and keeps it clean and dry while simultaneously reducing wear to the more expensive items. However, it does almost nothing to insulate you from the cold ground or lessen the impact from ground obstructions such as rocks and roots. A tarp can also be used to improvise a shelter, which is perhaps the most important reason to include it in your SAR ready pack.

Tree boughs, plastic trash bags filled with leaves, or just piles of leaves can be used as an improvised ground pad, but they should be considered only an improvisational replacement for the real thing—a lightweight, waterproof, comfortable, well-insulating ground pad.

Sleeping Bag

Full consideration must be given to the intended usage of a sleeping bag, as well as the needs of its user. When deciding how to choose a bag, consider these questions (**FIGURE 9-3**):

- In what temperatures will the bag be used (temperature rating)?
- What type of insulation do you desire or need (insulation type)?
- How much room do you need in the bag, and how important is the bag's weight?
- What features do you require (zipper location and types, draft collars, hood, stash pockets, pad loops, foot area shape, extra insulation, etc.)?

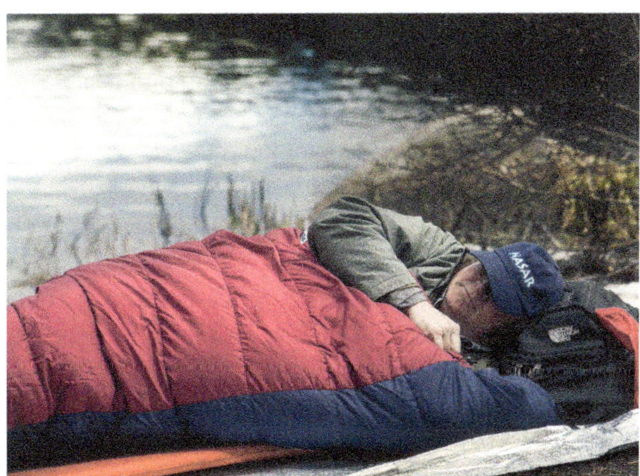

FIGURE 9-3 Full consideration must be given to the intended usage of a sleeping bag, as well as the needs of its user, when deciding how to choose a sleeping bag. Note the use of a ground pad, for comfort and insulation, and tarp, to protect the bag and pad.

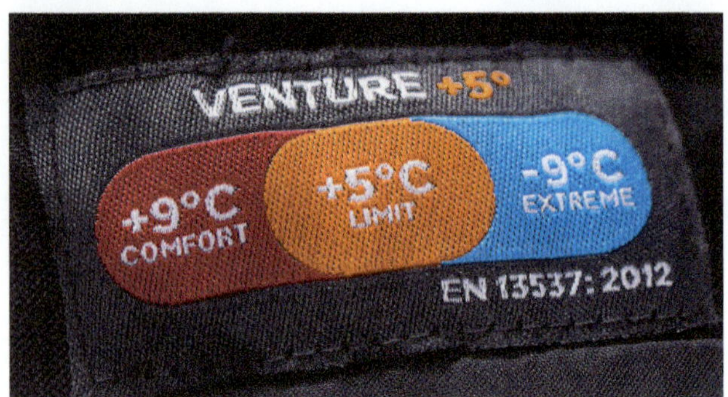

FIGURE 9-4 Label in Zajo Venture (UK) sleeping bag showing temperature ratings according to the EN 13537:2012 European standard, which was recently replaced with EN ISO 23537-1:2016. There is no current U.S. equivalent to this standard. The "limit" value is a good measure to use for comparisons between bags.
Courtesy of Donald Cooper.

A European Norm (EN) standard exists for temperature ratings of sleeping bags: EN ISO 23537-1:2016, which recently replaced EN 13537 (**FIGURE 9-4**). Although this is a European standard, it is recognized and used in many parts of the world. The standard requires that all sleeping bags claiming to meet the standard be tested and labeled with the following temperature ratings (BSI, 2017b):

- *Comfort.* The temperature at which a standard female can expect to sleep comfortably in a relaxed position.
- *Lower limit.* The temperature at which a standard male can sleep for eight hours in a curled position without waking.
- *Extreme.* The minimum temperature at which a standard female can remain for six hours without risk of death from hypothermia.

Note that these ratings assume that the subject is using a sleeping pad and tent and is wearing one base layer of thermal underwear. A "standard male" is assumed to be 25 years old, with a height of 5 feet 8 inches (1.73 meters) and a weight of 161 pounds (73 kilograms); a "standard female" is assumed to be 25 years old, with a height of 5 feet 3 inches (1.60 meters) and a weight of 132 pounds (60 kilograms). Since everyone's body, whether one sleeps cold or hot, and what qualifies as comfort is different, the best use of EN ISO 23537 may be in comparing sleeping bags with each other. When comparing, the "comfort" and "lower limit" temperature values—found on the labels of bags that meet the standard—are the best to use.

Insulating Material

The insulating material affects the cost, warmth, weight, and construction method. Selected specific materials are discussed in depth in Chapter 7, *Search and Rescue Clothing*, in the section on clothing.

Down. Down is the fine, insulating, fluffy feathers found under the stiffer feathers of ducks and geese. Its natural function as an insulator has made it the standard insulating material for lightweight sleeping bags. The primary reasons for its popularity are its light weight and compressibility for a given amount of insulation. Down is also soft, nontoxic, breathable, resilient, and should be stored uncompressed. On the negative side, down is expensive and loses its insulation when wet, which is why the down in most sleeping bags today is treated with a water-resistant chemical. In addition, down bags require special care in use and cleaning.

Polyester. Polyesters are synthetic fibers that are washable, durable, nonallergenic, and softer than other synthetic fabrics, giving it a softer, more comfortable feel. Polyester fibers can be manufactured in almost any thickness and design, can be molded with a hollow core for added insulation, and are hydrophobic (repels water). Polyester has less loft, is heavier, and is bulkier than down, but its fibers retain insulative properties when wet and are relatively inexpensive. Many modified polyester fibers are on the market today, including Polartec®, PolarGuard™ (Delta), Primaloft®, Thinsulate™ (mixture of polypropylene and polyethylene terephthalate [PET], thinner than polyester fibers), and Climashield® (Apex).

Hybrid. Sleeping bags are now available that combine down and synthetic fills. These combinations can allow the benefits of each material to offset the disadvantages of the other. The two materials may be blended throughout the bag, or the synthetic may be placed on the bottom with the lofty down filling the top.

Construction

Sleeping bags are compared generally by their quality of construction, their loft, and their effective temperature range.

Quality of construction is determined primarily by the reputation of the manufacturer. A reputable manufacturer stands behind its products, offering repair or replacement of damaged items.

Loft is generally used to specify the total thickness of a sleeping bag after it has had time to fluff up to its full thickness. Some manufacturers use it to specify the thickness of one wall. The criteria for determining loft should be determined for each product before a comparison is made so that the thickness of the actual insulating layer can be determined and compared.

In constructing a sleeping bag, one fundamental goal is to create a uniform loft throughout the bag to eliminate thin or cold spots.

- Fiberfill is produced in battings and is sewn into sleeping bags in sheets, with some variations.
- Down and some synthetic materials are subject to matting and shifting, so a method of baffling is necessary to control the filling to create a uniform loft.
- The channel block (side-block baffle) is a longitudinal baffle in bags that extends the length of the bag on the side opposite the zipper to prevent down from shifting around the circumference of the bag.
- The zipper baffle (draft tube) is an insulation-filled tube that extends the length of the bag on the inside of the zipper. Its purpose is to prevent heat loss through the zipper.
- The use of heavy-duty nylon or noncorrosive synthetic zippers has eliminated much of the problems encountered with earlier metal zippers: snagging, breakage, freezing, and the danger of skin-to-metal contact in extreme cold. The full-length zipper is most popular and versatile, especially if it has a double tab to allow it to be opened from either end for ventilation. When buying a bag, the main zipper can be ordered to open on the right or the left, depending on the desire of the buyer.
- The shells of nearly all sleeping bags are now made of nylon. It is strong, breathable, wind resistant, and lightweight. Specifically:
  - Taffeta nylon is a flat-weave fabric with a softer, more comfortable texture and a higher thread count than ripstop nylon.
  - Ripstop nylon has the same strength as taffeta but has extra heavy threads every 3/16 inch to 1/4 inch that prevent tears from running, making ripstop more durable than taffeta.
  - Cotton shells are still used in some rectangular bags where weight and water considerations are not as important. These are not recommended for anything outside of a child's slumber party.

Shapes and Sizes

The rectangular bag is the roomiest and the least expensive shape, but it is usually heavy, and its roominess creates superfluous air space to heat. The additional material can make this style of bag too heavy, but the extra room usually makes it more comfortable. A semi-rectangular design is a compromise between a rectangular and mummy bag and has qualities of both.

The mummy bag is contoured to the body shape: wider at the shoulders and hips and narrower though the legs and feet. It is the lightest, warmest, and most efficient design, but it allows very little room for moving around inside. Most mummy bags have a hood closure to cover the head and neck, drawcords to close openings, and an enlarged foot area (footbox) for comfort and additional insulation. Mummy bags specifically designed for women are available and are usually shorter, narrower at the shoulders, and wider at the hips. These may also include extra insulation in the upper body and footbox.

Short and extra-long bag sizes are also available. A bag too long may cause cold feet, and a bag too short may cause great discomfort. Choosing the right length is important.

Care of Sleeping Bags

Clean the bag when it gets dirty, but make sure to follow the manufacturer's instructions when doing so. Generally, do not wash sleeping bags in top-loading washing machines with central agitators, use detergents, or roughly handle a water-soaked bag. Generally, sleeping bags should be stored unstuffed, but again, it is important to follow the manufacturer's instructions for storage.

Sleeping Warmer Inside a Sleeping Bag

There are several ways in which a rescuer can sleep warmer inside a sleeping bag:

- Sleep inside a shelter or tent (~10°F [5.5°C] warmer).
- If you do not have a tent, improvise a windbreak.
- Do not set up camp in a ravine or valley bottom; it is warmer downwind just below peaks at higher elevations.
- Sleep in one layer of dry clothing in a good bag; synthetic long underwear is preferred.
- Protect the head, neck, and shoulders, and wear a wool stocking hat in cold weather.
- Huddle with others for warmth, or press sleeping bags together.
- If your feet are cold, put on socks or booties or reduce constriction of socks.
- Improve ground insulation; add insulation beneath the sleeping pad, add a second pad, or buy and use a better pad.
- Add a sleeping bag liner, or sleep on extra clothes placed inside the bag.
- Keep your sleeping bag dry.
- Use a vapor barrier in extreme cold (waterproof barrier over or around the sleeping bag); watch for condensation, which can wet the bag and clothing.
- Eat a high-calorie or high-fat food or drink just before getting into the bag.

SEARCH AND RESCUE TIP

Your shelter is your multipurpose tool for protection against many discomforts: insects, wind, rain, cold, heat, and sun.

Shelters

Tarps are lightweight, inexpensive, and versatile. Those made from coated nylon or poly fabrics with several grommets allow a variety of ways to rig a shelter. Pitched properly, tarps can provide considerable water and wind protection (**FIGURE 9-5**). The flexibility and versatility of a tarp, as well as its multiple improvisational uses, is why it should be part of the SAR ready pack.

A bivouac sack, or bivy sack, is essentially an overbag that provides shelter and protection from the elements for one person in a sleeping bag. It provides added warmth and weather protection in a small, lightweight package, and works well as an emergency shelter. A bivy sack is a good option for one- or two-night outings when you want a bit more than an improvised tarp shelter and where minimum bulk and weight is necessary.

Tents are generally heavier and more expensive than tarps or bivy sacks, but they provide the maximum security and protection. While not normally part of a SAR ready pack, there are SAR operations that require the use of a tent.

In most applications, warmth is a secondary consideration. However, where it is important, such as in winter use, tent warmth is a function of size, fabric, and design. Given the same design, a smaller tent is warmer than a large one. A double-walled tent is warmer because of the insulation value of the air space enclosed between the walls.

A double-wall tent uses two layers of fabric: an inner layer that is breathable but not waterproof and an outer layer (rainfly) that is waterproof but not breathable. A single-wall tent uses one layer of fabric to provide both breathability and waterproofness, but it generally does neither as well as the double-wall tent. A double-wall tent is heavier, protects better from the wind, and relies more on the placement of stakes and guy lines to adjust and readjust the rainfly. A single-wall tent is simpler and quicker to set up, can be self-standing, and requires fewer tie downs. Single-wall tents produce more condensation, which can leave gear inside the tent wet. Double-wall tents are better ventilated and usually have more doors and vestibules for more flexibility in how the space is used. Single-wall tents usually work best in alpine environments where it's typically dry and cold. Double-wall models are best when it is raining and humid and where extra gear storage is necessary.

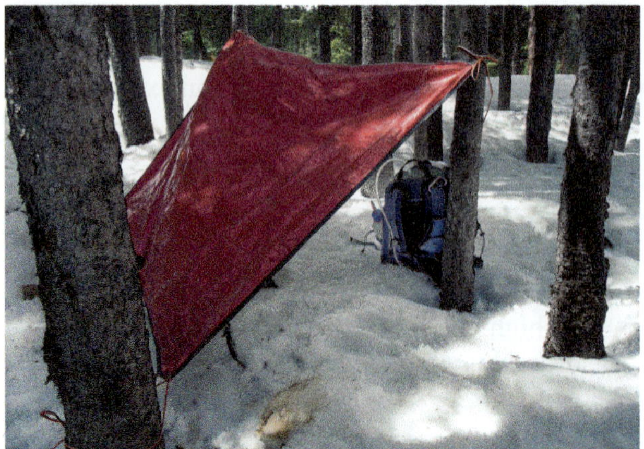

FIGURE 9-5 Pitched properly, tarps can provide considerable water and wind protection.

Three-season tents are designed for use in the summer, spring, and fall, and four-season tents are intended for use in all seasons, including winter. Three-season tents are designed to withstand all but winter conditions and thus are good at handling wind, rain, and severe weather. Four-season tents are usually designed with more poles to withstand snow loads better, and a lower profile to minimize the effects of wind. Summer (one-season) tents are also available, but these are mostly just all-mesh insect shelters with one or two solid fabric panels to provide shade.

Weight is a function of tent fabric, size, pole number, and pole design. A significant part of a tent's weight can be concentrated in the pole system. Total weight must consider the main tent, rainfly, poles, pegs, guy lines, and carrying sack. Generally, a two-person tent is heavier than a one-person tent, a four-season tent is heavier than a three-season tent, and a double-wall tent is heavier than a single-wall tent.

Size is usually determined by personal preference, based on the intended use of the tent (i.e., one, two, or more people). One-person backpacking tents are frequently tapered in both length and height to maximize the size of the limited space and have a simple pole system, all to reduce weight. Increased tent capacity is associated with a heavier tent.

An important function of a properly pitched tent is insect protection. Most tents use mesh panels to cover the inside of each tent opening. This provides insect protection while allowing for ventilation. This is less important in cold environments but most important in humid, warm climates. Summer tents may be made of nearly all mesh, whereas four-season tents, designed for mountain and winter use, make minimal use of mesh panels.

Considerations for tent fabrics include water repellency, breathability, wear resistance, weight, and wind resistance. Nylon is the most common tent fabric and is made in many weaves and thicknesses. For the breathable portions, most tents use thin-strand, ripstop nylon, which is lightweight and resists tears, or taffeta, which is a very soft and light nylon. Rainflies are made from nylon coated on one side with urethane or a similar treatment.

The most complex tent design uses a system of exterior poles to which the tent is attached. However, the more complex the system, the more dependent the system is on each piece of the frame; the loss of one piece can render the whole frame useless.

Tent poles are usually made of aluminum alloy, fiberglass, or carbon fiber. Aluminum poles are the most popular, are very strong, and are adequate for almost all SAR uses. Tubular aluminum poles are usually corded together to make setup fast and easy. Easton aluminum is a more expensive and stronger type of aluminum and is often used with high-end tents. Carbon fiber offers slightly more strength and durability than even the highest-grade aluminum, which may still crack under severe cold conditions. Carbon fiber tent poles are lighter, do not corrode, can be found in the highest-end tents and tent equipment, and are used most often in professional mountaineering where state-of-the-art equipment is required.

Food and Water

Because of the almost infinite variety of foods available, it can be very frustrating to plan a menu for SAR operations when you must pack meals into the field. Your choices vary from simple ready-to-eat items or add-hot-water meals to gourmet cooking, but these two facts remain: (1) you do not need much food during SAR operations, and it may be provided for you, and (2) most novices carry much more food than they need or will eat. While it may be impossible to starve over the three or four days of a SAR incident, food may be necessary to maintain comfort and energy for demanding operations. If food is required, consider the weight and space the food will take before packing.

Carrying what it takes to cook a meal is usually not preferred during SAR operations. It is better to carry ready-to-eat food that meets your nutritional needs and involves minimal packaging. **Trail mix** is a frequent alternative to carrying a full meal.

If you choose to carry what it takes to cook a meal, as a minimum you will need a pot in which to cook, one or more utensils with which to eat, a stove (preferred over building a fire), and nutritional food items to cook, ideally in one pot.

TABLE 9-1 shows a meal preparation strategy used by experienced outdoors people and SAR personnel. Realizing that large meals are not encouraged during daily operations in the field and that light snacks are generally used during SAR activities, dinner may be the only substantial meal of the day. One-pot meals are a quick and easy method of preparing a well-balanced dinner meal for the day. One-pot meals should be designed to consist of carbohydrates, protein, and seasonings/sauce. Carbohydrates and fats are important for quick and lasting energy. The process is simple and easy to prepare and helps ensure a more balanced meal.

Stoves

Although not essential for SAR work, a stove may be a good option if extended time is spent in the backcountry. A good mountaineering/backcountry stove should have a low profile with a wide base for added stability. The top of the stove should be wide enough to provide a good base for whatever you carry to put on it (e.g., cooking pot, steel cup). The main danger in stove operation is in overheating the fuel. For maximum safety, follow the manufacturer's operating instructions, and make sure to get a proper safety and operating briefing from the dealer before using it.

Types of Stoves

A chemical fire (Sterno, Heat Tabs, Canned Heat, solid fuel tablets) has a restricted heat output and is heavy for the amount of heat produced. Stoves that use alcohol directly for combustion have similar characteristics, but they also are simple to operate, lightweight, and easy starting. They are adequate for heating a cup of tea or soup or melting snow for drinking water, but they are usually inadequate for cooking a meal or boiling a larger pot of water.

Other liquid-fuel stoves usually burn white gasoline or kerosene, and some burn both. They have a high and controllable heat output but require priming (using a small amount of easily ignitable fuel to heat the burner) to start and special precautions in handling.

White gasoline (a purified form of gasoline) is widely used and generally available but is extremely volatile (Class IB flammable liquid). It is especially dangerous when fuel fumes can collect in an enclosed space, for example, when refueling a stove in a tent.

Coleman® fuel, or similar liquid fuels, can be used in stoves that burn white gasoline. It is slightly less volatile and tends to burn cleaner, and there is less stove

TABLE 9-1 One-Pot Meals*

Carbohydrates	Proteins	Seasonings/Sauces
Minute rice	Sealed/packaged tuna, shrimp, or meat	Tomato flakes/add water-type of powdered sauces
Instant potatoes	Chicken, salmon	Salt, pepper
Macaroni	Spam, corned beef	Onion or garlic salt
Spaghetti/pasta	Sealed/packaged roast beef in gravy	Cloves or cinnamon
Noodles	Cheese	Gravy mixes
Top Ramen™	Meat or bacon bar	Cheese sauce mix
Kraft™ dinners	Bacon bits	Parsley flakes
Lipton™ dinners	Beef stick, pepperoni	Bouillon cubes
Tuna Helper®	Salami, summer sausage	Sour cream sauce
Rice-a-Roni™	Freeze-dried meats	Vegetable flakes
Cup-a-Noodles®	Margarine, butter	Powdered milk
Dehydrated soups	Tuna casserole	Dried parsley, onion, and/or green pepper

* A "one-pot meal" is prepared by choosing one item from each of the three columns and combining/cooking them together.

clogging. In addition, Coleman® fuel is more widely available than white gasoline.

Kerosene is much less volatile (Class II combustible liquid) than other liquid fuels; however, it requires a separate, more easily ignited priming fuel (usually alcohol), has a distinctive and bothersome odor, and burns with a dirty, sooty residue, especially if the stove is not in top condition.

In extreme cold, precautions must be taken to avoid spilling any liquid fuel on the skin. Most types of liquid fuel do not freeze but remain liquid down to very low temperatures. This extreme cold combined with the evaporative cooling effect can cause instant frostbite if it comes into contact with the skin.

Gas cartridge stoves use liquefied gases (such as butane or propane) under pressure in sealed canisters (**FIGURE 9-6**). As the canister's pressure is released, the enclosed liquid boils, releasing the flammable gas. Since butane boils at 10°F (−12°C) and propane boils at −45°F (−43°C), the ability of these canisters to produce flammable gases can be substantially reduced in cold temperatures. If the contents are released at or just below its boiling point, very little or no flammable gas is produced. Thus, to operate properly, the canisters

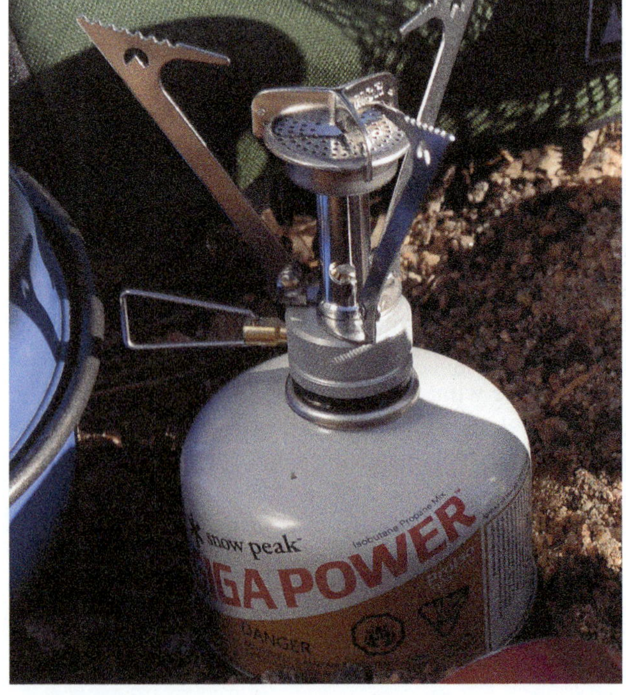

FIGURE 9-6 Gas cartridge stoves use liquefied gases (such as butane or propane) under pressure in sealed canisters.

must be kept warm, which is why many keep them in their coat or sleeping bag. Propane is more efficient as a fuel because it works at lower temperatures. However, it also takes more pressure to liquefy because of its lower boiling point, so the canisters in which it is contained must be stronger and, therefore, heavier—a distinct disadvantage when the canister must be carried.

In comparison to other commercially available camp stove fuels, these liquefied gas cartridges are the most expensive per unit of heat. However, they do offer extreme convenience and simple and reliable stove valve operation, and they require no priming. In many parts of the world, gas cartridge stoves are replacing white gas stoves as the backcountry standard (Hovey, 2017).

A modern camping stove, like any other mechanical device, can malfunction. Often this happens at a very inconvenient time. The stove's chief enemies are the wind and the operator's impatience. When problems arise, take your time to identify possible causes before pouring on more fuel to preheat the generator.

A relatively new and unique stove technology is now on the market that burns only wood and uses heat from the fire and a thermoelectric generator to generate up to 3 watts of (peak) power. The power charges an electronic device connected to its 2-amp USB port with any excess power saved to its internal battery. The BioLite® CampStove 2 includes a wood combustion chamber that uses an internal fan to inject air back into the burn chamber to increase the intensity of the fire. Although it may take a bit longer to heat up than other stoves, the manufacturer claims this high heat creates a hotter, more efficient burn that consumes smoke, creating a smokeless fire. Weighing in at just over 2 pounds (0.9 kg) and about the size of a football, the stove can be purchased with a number of accessories, including a flex light that connects to, and is powered by, the USB port (BioLite, 2017). The cost is a bit more than some other camp stoves but not all of them. This is an example of how technology continues to improve how field SAR work is done.

If you carry a stove, regardless of the type, always carry the recommended tools and repair kit for your particular model. Generally, your preventative maintenance and use of the proper fuels helps reduce camp stove frustrations.

Water Bottles and Hydration Systems

Water containers come in many sizes and shapes, but the best have certain characteristics in common. They are light, durable, strong, and have a wide mouth.

Water bottles can be made of stainless steel, aluminum, high-density polyethylene (HDPE), low-density polyethylene (LDPE), copolyester, or polypropylene; the main difference between them being the flexibility of the material. Stainless steel bottles made of culinary (food grade) stainless are excellent choices, but some people find they impart a metal taste to the water. Some polycarbonate and aluminum water bottles incorporate or are lined with material that contains bisphenol A (BPA), an unhealthy additive that should be avoided (Hovey, 2017). Look for "BPA Free" on the label of a new bottle (**FIGURE 9-7**).

Weight is always a factor, but keep in mind that the container must be able to withstand the rigors of SAR work. This means that it must be able to take a beating and not become ruptured, bent, or punctured. Plastic usually supplies this best, especially if it is a type of plastic that can withstand the contents freezing without breaking. Ask about this when purchasing one.

Vinyl hydration bladders (hydration systems) can be carried in one's backpack or on one's back like a rucksack (**FIGURE 9-8**). These allow the wearer to drink from the bladder without having to get into the backpack or open a bottle. They generally come in sizes that hold up to 0.8 gallons (3 liters) of water. A tube attaches to the bottom of the bladder and wraps over the shoulder of the wearer to a mouthpiece that can be operated hands-free with a special bite valve on the end. The system can be integrated into varying sizes of packs, or it can be worn alone. Either way, the easy access to water while moving is well suited for SAR field operations. Note that because the tube is exposed to the environment, it may require special attention in very cold weather to prevent it from freezing. Also, always carry at least two methods of storing and carrying water.

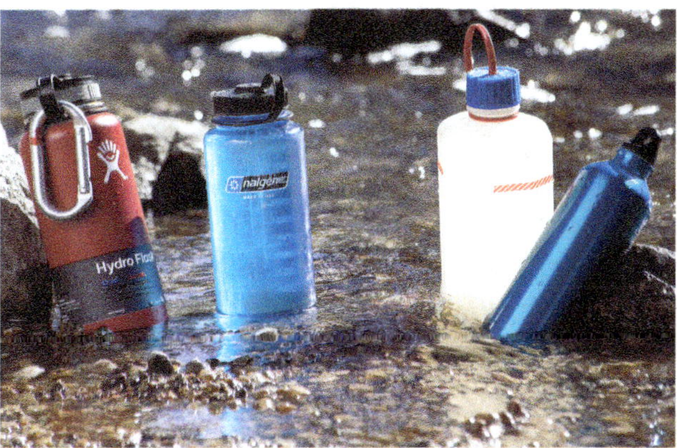

FIGURE 9-7 Water bottles, from left to right: stainless steel, wide-mouth Hydro Flask®; BPA-free, wide-mouth Nalgene®; old, small-mouth water bottle made with BPA; and aluminum bottle potentially lined with BPA resin.

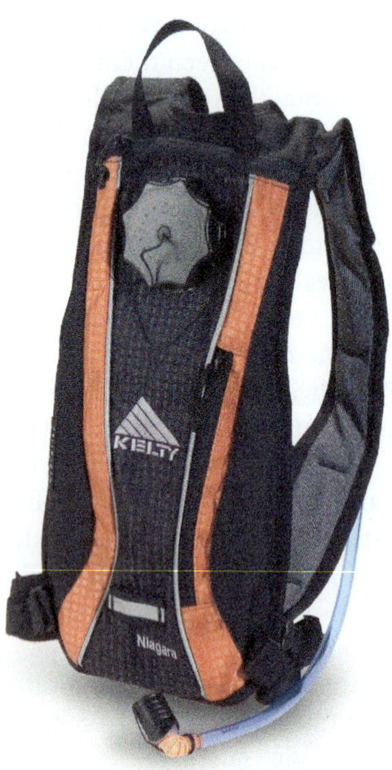

FIGURE 9-8 A hydration system can be integrated into varying sizes of packs, or it can be worn alone. Either way, the easy access to water while moving is well suited for SAR field work.
Courtesy of CMC Rescue, Inc.

Water is too important for your only water container to be damaged or lost.

In freezing weather, wrap water bottles in insulated sleeves, which can be improvised with neoprene or foam and duct tape, and carry them inside your coat or close to your back in your pack. Hydration bladders should be treated similarly. In hot environments, water bottles may be frozen, or hydration bladders may be filled with ice cubes and topped off with water. Not only is the cold water refreshing, but carrying cold water containers close to the body may help cool the body and reduce heat stress.

Do not wash your water bottles in a dishwasher, including stainless steel and aluminum ones, unless the manufacturer has explicitly stated they are dishwasher safe. After use, wash all water containers thoroughly with hot, soapy water. Before storing them, disinfect them with a solution of chlorinated water (1 teaspoon bleach in 1 liter [0.25 gallon] of water) to minimize mold and bacterial growth (Hovey, 2017).

Boots

Tennis shoes and thin, leather-soled footgear are extremely hard on the feet in hilly and mountainous terrain, which is why they are not recommended in SAR work. Boots that protect the ankle and the feet are the preferred footwear for SAR operations.

Boots should be adequate for their intended usage. They should provide good ankle support and have nonslip soles. The manufacturer's recommendations should be followed on methods and materials for waterproofing and cleaning.

Working in cliffs and high-angle terrain requires tight-fitting, stiff-soled boots. Hiking requires a lighter, more flexible boot.

Generally, avoid boots that reach much higher than the ankle because ventilation to the feet may be hindered and ankle movement restricted. The use of a good pair of gaiters with lower cut boots may be better than high-topped boots. Also, avoid boots with tight-fitting scree collars because they can ultimately cause a degree of **tendinitis**. Boots with backs that slope forward above the heel can also cause this injury.

Boots must fit correctly. Boots that fit loosely are better ventilated, keep your feet drier and warmer, and cause fewer hot spots and blisters than snug-fitting boots. However, many still feel the need to wear boots too snug. To ensure a proper fit, Paul Petzoldt, one of America's most accomplished mountaineers and creator of the National Outdoor Leadership School (NOLS), recommended the following in his book *The Wilderness Handbook* (Petzoldt, 1974, p. 48). This advice remains germane to this day.

> . . . take off all socks, place the bare foot in the boot without lacing it, and push the foot as far forward as possible. Stand with full weight on the feet, with toes touching the end of the boot, and bend knees forward. There should be enough room between the heel and the back of the boot to insert a finger without pressure. People who wear larger sizes should allow slightly more space . . . from 5/8 inch for size seven to one inch for size 12.

Now put on the socks that you will wear in the field, lace the boot comfortably, and stand. If there is pressure that stretches the boot outward, the boot is too tight, and you need a larger width. Kick the toe of the boot against a solid surface. If your toes touch the end of the boot, you need a larger size.

See Chapter 7 for more information on boots and foot care.

Tools and Equipment

During SAR operations, a few tools can be invaluable when attempting to repair essential equipment, improvise, or just make yourself more comfortable. A map, compass, and knife are essential in SAR work.

Map and Compass

The specifics of what to look for, how to use a map and compass, and definitions of map and compass terms are covered in Chapter 10, *Maps and Navigation*.

Knife

Criteria for a knife are simple but rarely followed. A knife for use in field SAR work should have two folding blades of different sizes (a fixed blade is not recommended), neither of which is over 3 inches long. One blade should be very sharp, and one should be small and pointier. Multitools that include pliers and multiple integrated instruments such as scissors, screwdrivers, wire cutters, a saw, and a serrated knife blade are ideal but much heavier (up to 0.5 pounds [0.23 kilograms]) than a simple, well-made, two-bladed knife. Gerber®, Leatherman®, and SOG®, among others, make high quality multitools that are excellent for SAR work (**FIGURE 9-9**).

Paramedic or trauma shears are stout scissors specially designed for quickly and safely cutting clothing away from a patient when using a knife blade might be difficult or dangerous. Their rugged design and longer lever arm enable them to cut through many materials that might be difficult for a knife blade (e.g., seat belts, leather, wire, sheet metal, and thick plastic). Including a pair of these shears in your SAR ready pack is recommended (**FIGURE 9-10**).

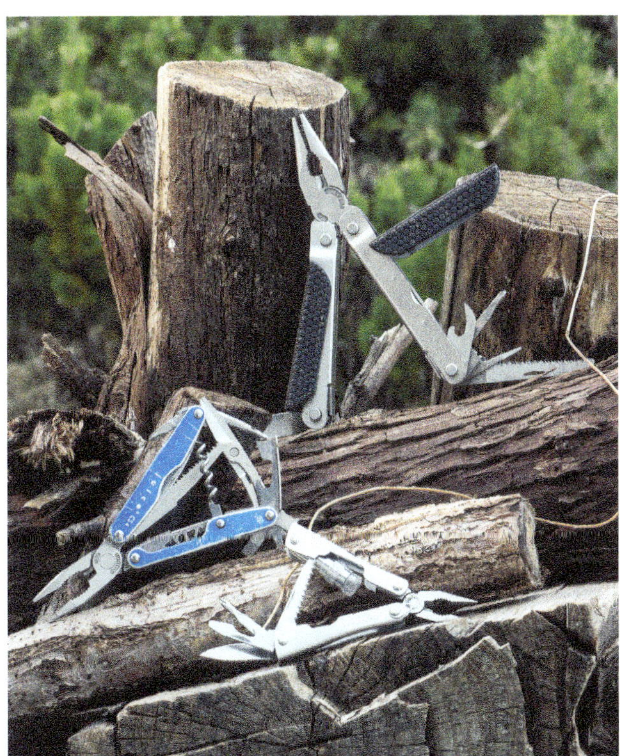

FIGURE 9-9 Three examples of multitools.

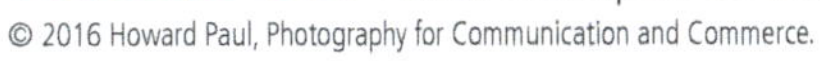

© 2016 Howard Paul, Photography for Communication and Commerce.

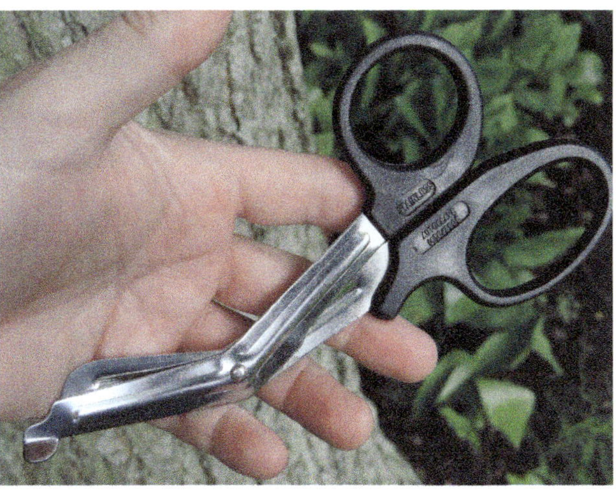

FIGURE 9-10 An example of multipurpose trauma shears.

Courtesy of Donald Cooper.

Trekking Poles

Trekking poles or a walking stick can be helpful when carrying a heavy pack over a long distance or when walking in steep terrain. They can help hold you up as well as offer assistance in probing those holes where snakes may lurk. They can also double as a tracking stick (see Chapter 13, *Tracking*), a shelter pole, or an expedient field splint. Weight is a factor, and so is bulk, so avoid logs that could as easily serve as a telephone pole, and use one or two that are easily packed but can support your body weight.

Headlamp/Flashlight

A headlamp can be invaluable in SAR work, especially but not exclusively at night (**FIGURE 9-11**). SAR fieldwork usually demands a medium-brightness beam that is longer burning than it is bright. In most field situations, a little light for several hours is better than a bright light for a few minutes.

Light-emitting diode (LED) bulbs have mostly replaced traditional, incandescent (tungsten) light bulbs in headlamps intended for outdoor use. LEDs are more efficient, allowing for improved battery life, and do not burn as hot. Headlamps that use xenon and halogen bulbs are also available. They produce a very bright, white light but burn very hot and consume power at a much higher rate. Hybrid lights are also available that include a xenon or halogen bulb alongside an array of (usually three) LED bulbs. This provides the flexibility to switch between the bright, white light of the high power-consuming bulb and the dimmer but lower power

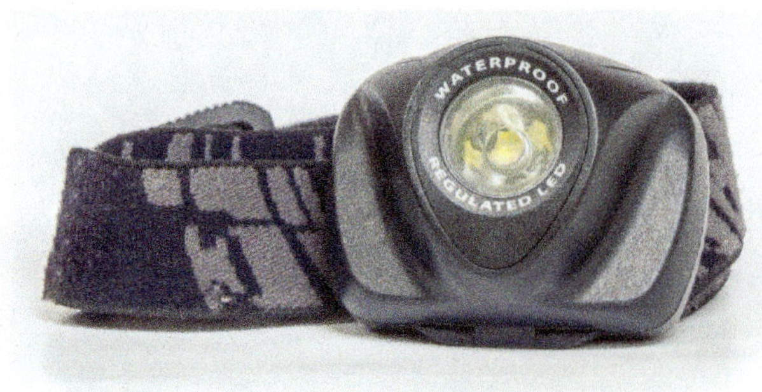

FIGURE 9-11 A reliable headlamp is a convenient light source for SAR work.
© t00n_in/Shutterstock.

LED bulbs. Modern headlamps usually offer a number of other features such as a flashing mode for signaling, an adjustable beam (wide and narrow), a red light option to preserve night vision (highly recommended), and a power off lock to prevent the device from being accidentally powered on while being carried in a pack. Headlamps should be durable, waterproof, and compatible with your helmet.

Do not become dependent on a light when working in the field. If you let your eyes adjust to the darkness, enough ambient light often exists to allow you to work quite safely. Save the headlamp for finding the toilet paper and other important uses. Do not waste it when you do not need it.

Always carry extra batteries and bulbs, and if working at night, carry at least one additional complete light source. When carrying more than one headlamp, the parts should be interchangeable between devices, and, ideally, the batteries should be interchangeable with your other electronic devices. Many different sizes and types of flashlights may be useful in certain situations, but avoid large heavy car battery or law enforcement type lights. They are heavy, use many batteries, are bulky to carry, and are not recommended.

Hand lanterns/flashlights are fine for many outdoor activities, such as searching from or near a vehicle, but a headlamp is the preferred light source for field SAR work. It keeps your hands free to perform other tasks, and it always points where you are looking.

SAFETY TIP

NEVER shine a flashlight/headlamp into someone's eyes in the field. Not only is it impolite, it ruins their night vision for several minutes and can be hazardous.

Repair/Sewing Kit

A repair kit consisting of wire, pliers (multitool), needle, thread, etc., is handy for minor repairs such as torn clothing and broken pack parts, but its potential weight and bulk could make it unsuitable for light 24-hour ready packs.

General "Hell Bag"

This is simply a small bag of possible items. These include anything that might come in handy for comfort, repairs, and emergencies. Tape, screwdriver, screws, wire, pliers, clevis pins, stove parts, flashlight/headlamp parts, string, cord, horseshoe nails, etc., are all possibilities. The lighter you want to pack, the smaller the bag. A small nylon bag or, better yet, a sealable plastic bag, can be carried in a pocket (if small enough) or crammed into a small spot in your pack.

Equipment Purchasing

Since most people involved in SAR are volunteers and have limited funds, finding economical ways to purchase the necessary equipment is always desirable. Here are two suggestions that you can likely extrapolate into other seasons.

The best time to purchase winter gear is at the end of winter. Thermal underwear, winter coats, insulated gloves, hats, and waterproof outerwear are all discounted at the end of the winter season to make room for new inventory. Similarly, the best time to purchase summer gear is at the end of summer. Sunblock, sunglasses, lightweight clothing, daypacks, water bottles, and other summer items are on sale to make room for the next season. Take advantage of it.

Equipping your SAR pack need not be expensive, but do not hesitate to spend the appropriate amount on the most important items: boots, jacket, and pack. Investing in quality in these items is a wise investment that you will benefit from for years.

Toiletries

Personal hygiene is important in the backcountry, and toiletries can help achieve and maintain it. Most consider certain toiletry items necessities; however, many of these can be done without or improvised from other pack contents. Typical toiletries include the following:

- Toilet paper
- Toothbrush and toothpaste
- Dental floss
- Biodegradable, all-purpose camp soap (used on skin and dishes)
- Feminine hygiene products
- Shaving equipment (razor, blades, small mirror, soap/shave cream)

- Hairbrush/comb
- Towel (microfiber travel towel works well)

Decide for yourself which items are actually a necessity and which are merely a comfort, and pack accordingly.

Some hygiene items are more important than others. For instance, toilet paper is so light and useful that no one should be without it in the backcountry. Anyone who has ever had to do without it knows how important it is. Packing it in a sealable plastic bag keeps the paper dry.

We are taught that both toothpaste and toothbrush are important for oral hygiene, but what is really the priority is getting the mouth clean on a regular basis. Simply rinsing the mouth frequently with clean water and scrubbing the teeth with a towel, on occasion, can serve the purpose.

Packs

Selection and use of a pack is a function of the following variables:

- Your intended use and needs.
- The individual characteristics of the various types of packs.
- Your body structure.
- The combined weight and space (cubic inches/centimeters) of all the items that you intend to put inside.
- The type of SAR mission—equipment needs depend on the mission and the operating environment.

To help decide how big a pack you need, make a pile of the equipment that you intend to carry. Separate the items into different piles: items that will go into the pack itself, items that will be attached to the outside of the pack, and items for your pockets. Use this pile as an estimate of the size you will need. For comparison, the average paper grocery bag holds about 1400 cubic inches (23 liters).

Types of Packs

The vast quantity and types of packs on the market, and the speed at which they all change, requires that fitting any pack for type, size, body shape, and specific use be done by a professional. Do not underestimate the importance of getting qualified assistance when choosing and fitting a pack, especially a large one. There are too many variables to discuss here, so only general guidance is provided.

Lumbar Packs

Belt, waist, and lumbar packs are small bags designed to wear as a belt around the waist. They work well in good weather when carrying only a relatively small amount of equipment is needed.

- Capacity: 100 to 800 cubic inches (1.6 to 4.9 liters), 3 to 20 pounds (1.4 to 9 kilograms)
- Uses: Carrying lunches, the essentials, cameras, and personal gear. Lumbar packs are well suited for non-wilderness/urban searches where members may need to carry search equipment but are not required to carry a great deal of overnight and survival gear.

Day Packs

Day packs or rucksacks are small, usually frameless packs designed for shorter excursions, which is one reason they include only minimal padding in the shoulder straps and belt.

- Capacity: 700 to 1000 cubic inches (11.5 to 16.4 liters), 20 to 25 pounds (9 to 11.3 kilograms)
- Uses: Carrying general day-hiking equipment such as a spare jacket, hat, gloves, food, water bottle, and emergency gear.
- Options include:
  - A waistband, usually with less padding than other types, helps prevent the pack from shifting on the back.
  - Vertical or horizontal partitions provide more efficient loading and access.

Backpacks

Backpacks are larger packs designed to hold more weight and then allow that weight to be carried comfortably over long distances. There are two major types of backpacks: external frame and internal frame. External-frame packs use aluminum tubes to form a stiff frame on the outside of the pack, and the nylon pack and waist belt are attached to the frame. An external-frame pack allows air to circulate beneath its suspension system, which keeps the back cooler and more comfortable. External-frame packs carry and distribute heavy loads more comfortably, but they are bulkier and make it hard to pass through confined spaces or thick woodlands, which is why they are not usually the best option for those working in SAR.

To add support, internal-frame packs incorporate adjustable plastic or aluminum stays into sewn vertical pockets in the pack, and because these packs hug the body, they are warmer. Internal-frame packs are narrower and more flexible than external frame packs, thus they make it easier to balance and maneuver in tight spaces, while climbing, and through densely wooded areas. Internal-frame packs are usually the best choice for SAR.

Internal-frame packs are better suited for activities requiring good balance and freedom of movement (**FIGURE 9-12**). They fit close to the back, provide for a lower center of gravity, and are flexible. Rigid (external) pack frames with fitted bags provide the most comfortable and convenient method of carrying large loads on extended trips.

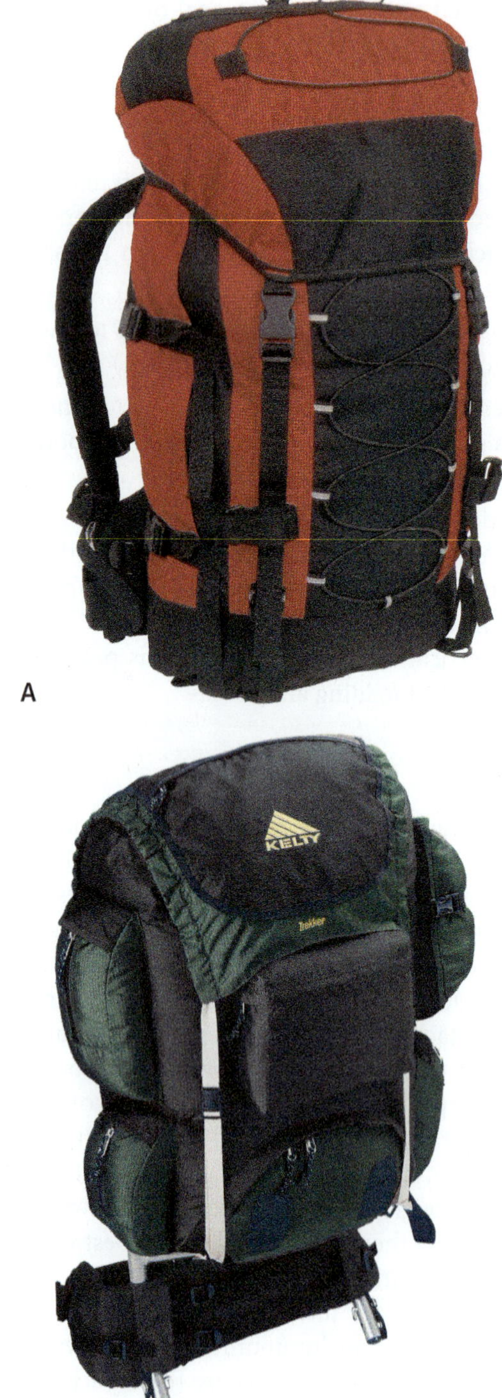

FIGURE 9-12 **A.** An example of a large internal-frame pack. **B.** An example of a large external-frame pack.

A: © jonpic/E+/Getty; B: Courtesy of Kelty.

- Capacity: Up to 6000 cubic inches (100 liters), up to 80 pounds (36 kilograms), weight limited only by user's strength
- Uses: Extended trips of several days, heavy or bulky loads
- Options:
  - Waist or hip suspension systems help distribute weight between the hips and the shoulders.
  - Most packs have multiple outside pockets that provide convenience in organizing and finding equipment easily.
  - Packs may be a single compartment or may be divided into various arrays of zippered compartments.
  - Top-loading packs have one large compartment that opens at the top and closes with a drawstring and a covering flap. Panel-loading packs have a large zipper that opens at the front to allow access to the entire contents of the pack.

Pack softer items in a soft bag placed near your back inside the pack. Avoid overloading either by weight or bulk. Pack the contents with heavy items high and near the back, least needed items at the bottom, and frequently used items in the outside pockets. Waterproof all items individually in plastic bags. Although most pack fabrics are water resistant, water can enter the pack through leaky seams or when it is opened. Blowing sand or snow can be forced right through zippers and open compartments, so be careful choosing when and where to open your pack.

How to pack your pack can be just as important as what to pack. On smooth, flat ground, heavy items are kept high in the pack so that much of the weight comes straight down and is balanced. On rough ground, or if you are going cross-country over steep inclines, heavier gear should be lower down near the center of the pack. If you are bouldering or traveling through deep snow, the weight should be placed on the bottom to form a lower center of gravity that helps maintain balance. No matter where the weight is placed, the heavier items should be as close to your back as possible. This conserves energy and aids with balance.

Stuff sacks made of nylon and net bags can be used to compartmentalize items in your pack. Use compression bags for bulky items such as sleeping bags and extra clothing. Resealable freezer bags can be used to store small items. Carry a few extra for protecting electronic devices and other items affected by moisture. Minimize what you hang on the outside of the pack. Most backpacks are treated to be water resistant, but line the pack with a thick, durable garbage bag to keep the contents dry, and carry a pack cover for severe weather. If an extremely wet environment is expected, consider the use of various sizes of dry bags, like paddlers use.

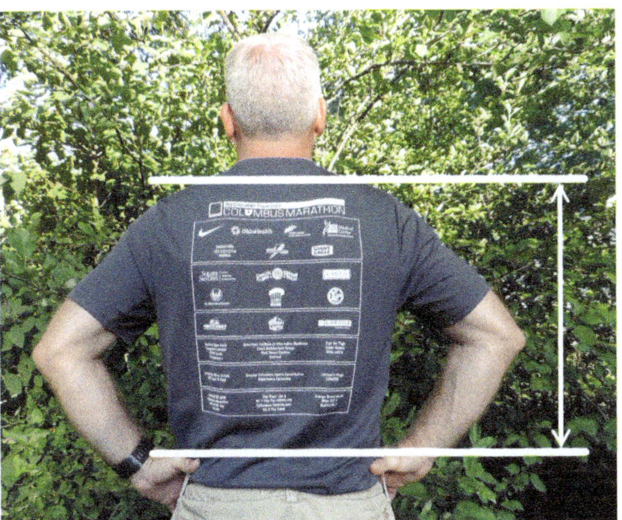

FIGURE 9-13 Your torso length is measured on your back as the distance between an imaginary horizontal line drawn across the top of your shoulders and an imaginary horizontal line drawn across the top of your pelvis.
Courtesy of Donald Cooper.

Making It Fit

To be comfortable, a pack must fit properly. Most packs made today are available in various sizes and with adjustable suspension systems. Pack manufacturers often publish tables that detail which size pack would fit you best. The two most important measurements are your torso length and your hip measurement. These two measurements suggest the general range of sizes that may work for you. Your torso length is measured on your back as the distance between an imaginary horizontal line drawn across the top of your shoulders (superior lateral aspect of the clavicles) and an imaginary horizontal line drawn across the top of your pelvis (superior iliac crests) (**FIGURE 9-13**). Your hip measurement is measured with a tape measure around the top of your hips (superior iliac crests). To ensure that your pack is a good fit, get it sized by a professional at a reputable outdoor shop.

With the pack loaded to capacity and the hip belt placed where you want it (make sure it is snug), the shoulder straps should be high enough that you can drop a shoulder down without the strap falling off that side. The straps should be aligned perpendicular to the shoulders with only a small portion of the weight of the pack resting on the shoulders.

Many packs today are designed with a variety of adjustable suspension features to assure a good personal fit. Do not let the variety of buckles, straps, sliders, and pins overwhelm you. Load the adjustable pack to maximum weight, put the pack on, and adjust the shoulder and lift straps until the weight moves off your shoulders and onto your hips. Most of the weight should be on your hips while the pack is pulled snugly against the body. Adjustments should be made while wearing the pack, so at least for the first time wearing it, you may need assistance from another person. A woman should wear a pack made for her anatomy. Larger packs should have more padding in the waist belt and shoulder straps and should be able to be adjusted while being worn.

Packs without hip belts contain few, if any, adjustments. You will be carrying all the weight on your shoulders. For SAR work, except in the most accommodating situations, get a pack with a hip belt that has multiple adjustments or fits you perfectly.

Donning a Backpack

Donning a heavy backpack can be challenging and even dangerous. It can be accomplished alone or with assistance, which is by far the safer approach. Backpackers have forever hoisted their packs over one shoulder, much like putting on a coat, followed by fishing the other arm through the remaining strap. Some approach the pack while it is on the ground, face down and, in a single move, toss it over their heads and onto their backs. Both are acceptable practices when done correctly, but both have the potential to cause back injuries. During SAR operations, personnel become fatigued, emotional, and adrenaline charged, which is when the risk of mistakes and preventable injuries increases. Since SAR personnel should never be alone and without a partner in the field, the buddy system can be used to mitigate this risk.

When donning a pack, the owner should grasp the pack from the suspension side, using his or her legs and a straight back, and rise to a standing position while lifting the pack. The owner can then pass the pack to a partner who has assumed a stable stance, ready to accept the load. As the partner accepts the load, the partner announces "mine" to indicate the owner can release the load. This is the owner's signal that the partner has control of the load, and it is safe to let go. As the owner lets go, he or she would respond, "yours." The owner would then release the grip on the load, turn around, and begin to don the pack, including adjusting shoulder and waist straps to a comfortable fit. Once the owner feels ready to assume the load, he or she announces, "mine," to which the partner responds "yours" and releases the pack. The two can now switch roles, and the one wearing the pack can assist the other with donning theirs. If done correctly, neither person has to endure an injury-causing lifting or twisting motion while carrying a heavy load. With the assistance of a partner, the same process in reverse can be used to remove your pack.

Wrap-Up

READY FOR REVIEW

- Carrying the appropriate equipment is an essential part of SAR effectiveness and survival.
- Personal body protection items may include insect repellant, sunscreen, eye protection, and head protection.
- Sleeping systems for SAR missions depend on the environment and the likelihood of need but usually include ground protection and a sleeping bag.
- In terms of shelter, tarps are lightweight, inexpensive, and versatile. Tents are heavier but offer more protection from the elements.
- When determining the food to pack, consider that (1) you do not need much food during SAR operations, and it may be provided for you, and (2) most novices carry much more food than they need or will eat.
- Water containers come in many sizes and shapes, but the best have certain characteristics in common. They are light, durable, strong, and have a wide mouth.
- Boots should be adequate for their intended usage. They should provide good ankle support and have nonslip soles. Follow the manufacturer's recommendations on methods and materials for waterproofing and cleaning.
- During SAR operations, a few tools can be invaluable when attempting to repair essential equipment, improvise, or just make yourself more comfortable. Three items have been recognized as essential in SAR work: a map and compass, a knife, and a repair/sewing kit.
- Decide for yourself which toiletries are a necessity and which are merely a comfort, and pack accordingly. Remember that many items can be improvised.
- To help decide how big a pack you need, make a pile of the equipment that you intend to carry. Separate the items into different piles: items that will go into the pack itself, items that will be attached to the outside of the pack, and items for your pockets. Use this pile as an estimate of the size you need.

SEARCH AND RESCUE TERMS

24-hour pack Also called a *ready pack*, the suggested minimum equipment and pack that SAR personnel should carry at all times during a mission. It allows the person carrying it to be self-reliant and comfortable should a bivouac become necessary while waiting for help or rescue.

Bivouac Temporary camp without a tent or cover.

DEET Abbreviation for chemical name, N,N-diethyl-meta-toluamide, a potent insect repellant.

Tendinitis An inflammation of the sheath of the Achilles tendon, or soreness above the heel, caused by continuous pressure over long periods of time.

Trail mix A type of snack mix, specifically a combination of granola, dried fruit, nuts, and sometimes chocolate, developed as a food to be taken along on hikes; also called *gorp*.

REFERENCES AND SUGGESTED READING

Auerbach, Paul S. 2013. *Field Guide to Wilderness Medicine*, 4th edition. St. Louis, MO: Mosby, Inc.

Auerbach, Paul S. 2016. *Medicine for the Outdoors: The Essential Guide to First Aid and Medical Emergencies*, 6th edition. Philadelphia, PA: Elsevier.

Auerbach, Paul S., ed. 2017. *Wilderness Medicine*, 7th edition. St. Louis, MO: Elsevier, Inc.

BioLiteEnergy.com. 2017. CampStove 2: Fire gets an upgrade. https://www.bioliteenergy.com/products/campstove-2?gclid=CJivg56-49MCFYi2wAod3SABwA.

BSI. 2017a. BS EN 397:2012+A1:2012, Industrial safety helmets. http://shop.bsigroup.com/ProductDetail?pid=000000000030269397.

BSI. 2017b. BS EN ISO 23537-1:2016. Requirements for sleeping bags, Part 1: Thermal and dimensional requirements. Brussels, CEN.

Butler, Jr., Frank K., and Steven Chalfin. 2017. The eye in the wilderness. In *Wilderness Medicine*, 7th edition. Volume 1, edited by Paul S. Auerbach, pp. 1109–1127. St. Louis, MO: Elsevier, Inc.

Fradin, Mark S., and John F. Day. 2002. Comparative efficacy of insect repellents against mosquito bites. *New England Journal of Medicine* 347, no. 1,13–18.

Getchell, Annie, and Dave Getchell. 2000. *The Essential Outdoor Gear Manual: Equipment Care, Repair, and Selection*, 2nd edition. New York: International Marine/Ragged Mountain Press.

Gilpatrick, Gil. 2012. *Building Outdoor Gear: Easy to Make Projects for Camping, Fishing, Hunting, and Canoeing*, revised 2nd edition. East Petersburg, PA: Fox Chapel Publishing.

Hostetter, Kristin. 2012. *Backpacker Magazine's Complete Guide to Outdoor Gear Maintenance and Repair: Step-By-Step Techniques to Maximize Performance and Save Money*. Guilford, CT: Falcon Guides.

Hovey, John R. 2017. Nonmedical backcountry equipment for wilderness professionals. In *Wilderness Medicine*, 7th edition. Volume 2, edited by Paul S. Auerbach, pp. 2409–2428. St. Louis, MO: Elsevier, Inc.

International Climbing and Mountain Federation. 2013. Mountaineering and climbing equipment: Helmets, UIAA 106. http://theuiaa.org/documents/safety-standards/UIAA_106_Helmets_March_2013.pdf.

Johnson, G. Mark. 2003. *The Ultimate Desert Handbook: A Manual for Desert Hikers, Campers, and Travelers*. New York: Ragged Mountain Press/McGraw Hill.

Linxweiler, Eric and Mike Maude, Editors. The Mountaineers. 2017. *Mountaineering: Freedom of the Hills*, 9th edition. New York: Mountaineers Books.

Manning, Harvey, and Bob Cram. 1986. *Backpacking: One Step at a Time*, 4th edition. New York: Vintage Books.

McManners, Hugh. 2007. *The Complete Wilderness Training Manual*, 2nd revised edition. New York: DK Publishing.

National Association for Search and Rescue. 2016. Consolidated pack guide: A pack guideline for NASAR education and certification programs. http://www.nasar.org/consolidate_pack_guide_announcement.

Occupational Safety and Health Administration. 2017. Occupational Safety and Health standard: Personal protective equipment, head protection, 1910.135. https://www.osha.gov/pls/oshaweb/owadisp.show_document?p_table=STANDARDS&p_id=9785.

Petzoldt, Paul. 1974. *The Wilderness Handbook*. New York: W.W. Norton & Company, Inc.

PPE.org. 2017. Social media for the safety industry: PPE certification for head protection. https://www.ppe.org/ppe-certification-head-protection/.

Rawlins, Chip, and Colin Fletcher. 2002. *The Complete Walker IV*, revised edition. New York: Alfred A. Knopf, Inc.

U.S. Centers for Disease Control and Prevention. 2017. Fact sheet for the general public: Fight the bite for protection from malaria: Guidelines for DEET insect repellant use. https://www.cdc.gov/malaria/toolkit/DEET.pdf.

CHAPTER 10

Maps and Navigation

OBJECTIVES

Upon completion of this chapter and the related course activities, the student will be able to meet the following objectives:

- Define the following terms:
  - Contour lines
  - True north
  - Magnetic north
  - Grid north
  - Azimuth
- Demonstrate the use of the Universal Transverse Mercator (UTM) grid system to determine the coordinates for a given point.
- Identify the key features of the orienteering compass.
- Describe how to take a bearing in the field and transfer it correctly to the map.
- Describe how to obtain a bearing on the map and transfer it correctly to the field.
- Explain the process of navigating around an obstacle.
- Explain the four methods to adjust for magnetic declination.
- Describe one method for estimating distance traveled in the field.
- List three advantages and three limitations of global positioning system (GPS) units as employed during search operations.

Navigation in Search and Rescue

Search and rescue (SAR) is an inherently **spatial** problem. Whether SAR personnel are searching for a lost skier or rescuing a hiker with a broken ankle at a known location, the ability to safely and efficiently navigate through the wilderness using a map, compass, and/or GPS is vital. To do this, personnel must have a working knowledge of basic geographic concepts, including coordinate systems, maps, compasses, and the **global positioning system (GPS)**.

Georeferencing Methods and Coordinate Systems

There are numerous ways to describe the location of a **feature**. Perhaps the most basic way is to use specific place names, such as "Swan Lake," or "Kelly's Diner." References can also be relative to such known points (e.g., 1 mile south of Swan Lake). These references can be measured in travel distances (e.g., 4 miles west of Swan Lake) or in map distances (e.g., 1 inch east of Kelly's Diner on a specific map). Another way to describe a location is by referencing an addressing system, (e.g., 123 Main Street). If everyone using these systems understands the reference, the system works. Maps may not even be necessary if everyone is familiar with the area and specific **landmark** names.

Although these types of **georeferencing** systems require little or no training and are easily learned, they may not be suitable in SAR situations. They are often too ambiguous, not precise enough to be used in most environments, and may be difficult to transmit via radio. Therefore, this basic approach may work best as a backup to other more sophisticated mapping systems.

Geographic Coordinate System: Latitude and Longitude

One way to identify points on the curved surface of the Earth is with a system of reference lines called **parallels** of **latitude** (horizontal) and **meridians** of **longitude** (vertical). On some maps, the meridians and the parallels appear as straight lines. On most modern maps, however, the meridians and the parallels appear as curved lines. These differences are due to the mathematical treatment required to portray a curved surface on a flat surface so that components of the map (such as distance) are shown with minimum distortion. The system used to portray a part of the round Earth on a flat surface is called a map projection. The most important thing for you to know as a responder is that map projections must be clearly transcribed in verbal, written, and digital communication.

To simplify the use of maps and to avoid the inconvenience of pinpointing locations on curved reference lines, map makers superimpose on the map a rectangular grid consisting of two sets of straight, parallel lines, uniformly spaced, each set perpendicular to the other. This grid is designed so that any point on the map can be designated so by its latitude and longitude or by its grid **coordinates** (see UTM below), and a reference in one system can be converted into a reference in another system. Such grids are usually identified by the name of the particular projection for which they are designed. Each search and rescue team should have trained staff and access to software tools that can convert between different **coordinate systems**.

SEARCH AND RESCUE TIP

Distance hint for all USGS maps: One minute (1′) of latitude, regardless of the scale of the map, or globe, equals 1 nautical mile (1.15 statute miles, or 1.18 kilometers). Therefore, 1 degree (1°) of latitude equals 60 nautical miles (about 69 statute miles, or 111 kilometers).

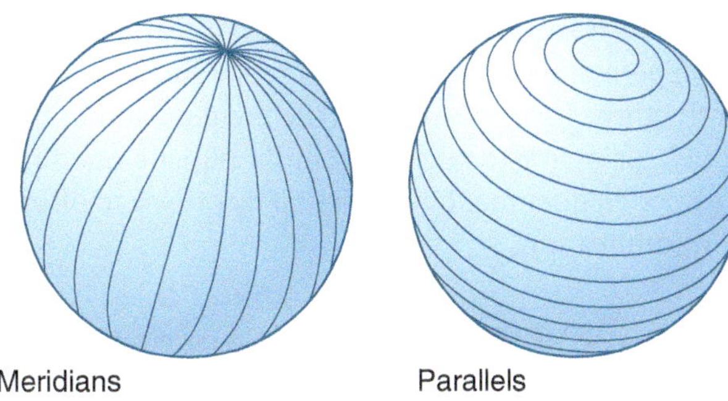

FIGURE 10-1 Examples of meridians (longitude) and parallels (latitude).
Courtesy of the United States Geological Survey.

The **geographic coordinate system** (latitude and longitude) uses a grid system that covers the entire globe and uses lines of longitude (meridians), which run north-south, and latitude lines (parallels), which run east-west (**FIGURE 10-1**). Quite a bit of skill is required to accurately describe a point in the field with this system, but it gets much easier with practice. This system is not nearly as effective for ground personnel as it is for those who do not require as much accuracy (e.g., on aircraft or boats), but works fairly well for all-around, general use, especially when coordinate information must be exchanged between air and ground forces or between international units.

Latitude starts at the equator, considered zero, with a big circle that encompasses the entire globe midway between both poles. The angular distance of any point on Earth north or south of the equator is measured in degrees, with 90 being the maximum at each pole. Lines of latitude are parallel to the equator and are referred to as parallels.

Longitude lines run vertically, connecting the North Pole to the South Pole, with the starting point (0 degrees longitude) at the prime meridian, which runs through the British Royal Observatory in Greenwich, England. From this point there are 180 degrees going west and 180 degrees going east, converging at the International Date Line on the opposite side of the globe from the prime meridian. Longitude locations are given as x degrees east, or x degrees west, of the prime meridian.

One degree of either latitude or longitude equals 60 minutes, and 1 minute equals 60 seconds. Plotting a point to within one navigational second is accurate to within approximately 1000 square feet. This is very accurate as mapping methods go, but it is very difficult to define 1 second (1.3 mm) on a 7.5-minute map; 15-second accuracy is much more realistic.

Latitude and longitude can be written in three different formats:

- Degrees, minutes, seconds (DD° MM' SS")
- Degrees, minutes, decimal minutes (DD° MM.mm')
- Degrees, decimal degrees (DD.DDDD°)

While it is common for ground, maritime, and aviation personnel to have different preferences for which of the three formats are used, the incident action plan (IAP) for major incidents should designate one form for written documentation, digital records, and official communication.

Universal Transverse Mercator System

In 1947, the U.S. Army adopted a special grid for military use throughout the world called the **Universal Transverse Mercator (UTM)** grid (Snyder, 1987). This system is used by ground search and rescue teams because it can be easily taught, uses distance-based coordinates (meters), and works well at the local level. In this grid, the world between 84° N and 80° S latitude is divided into 60 north-south zones, each covering a strip 6 degrees wide in longitude. These zones are numbered consecutively beginning with Zone 1, located between 180° W and 174° W longitude, and progressing eastward to Zone 60, between 174° E and 180° E longitude. Thus, the conterminous 48 United States are covered by 10 zones, from Zone 10 on the West Coast through Zone 19 in New England (**FIGURE 10-2**). In each zone, coordinates are measured north and east in meters (where 1 meter equals 39.37 inches, or slightly more than 1 yard). The **northing** values are measured continuously from zero at the equator, in a northerly **direction**. To avoid negative numbers for locations south of the equator, the designing cartographers assigned the equator an arbitrary false northing value of 10,000,000 meters. A central meridian through the middle of each 6-degree zone is assigned an **easting** value of 500,000 meters. Grid values to the west of this central meridian are less than 500,000, and to the east, more than 500,000 meters.

The UTM grid is shown on all quadrangle maps prepared by the U.S. Geological Survey (USGS). On 7.5-minute quadrangle maps (1:24,000 and 1:25,000 scale) and 15-minute quadrangle maps (1:50,000, 1:62,500, and standard-edition 1:63,360 scales), the UTM grid lines are indicated at intervals of 1000 meters, either by blue ticks in the margins of the map or with full grid lines. The 1,000-meter value of the ticks is shown for every tick or grid line. In addition, the actual meter value is shown for ticks nearest the southeast and northwest corners of the map. If the map does not already have the grid lines marked, the lines can be hand-drawn by connecting the blue tick marks.

On the 7.5-minute map, each tick is represented by four numbers. The first two numbers are in superscript (e.g., $^{49}98$). The numerals in superscript represent the 1,000,000- and 100,000-meter grids. The last two numerals represent the 10,000- and 1,000-meter grids. Thus, using the northing (that is, the left and right margins), $^{49}98$ represents 4,998,000 meters north of the equator. Computer programs exist that can convert these figures into latitude and longitude, and most GPS units can easily switch between UTM and latitude/longitude.

To use the UTM grid, you can place a transparent grid overlay (interpolator or grid reader, **FIGURE 10-3**) on the map to subdivide the grid, or you can draw lines on the map connecting corresponding ticks on opposite edges (**FIGURE 10-4**). The distances can be measured in meters at the **map scale** between any map point and the nearest grid lines to the south and west. The northing of the point is the value of

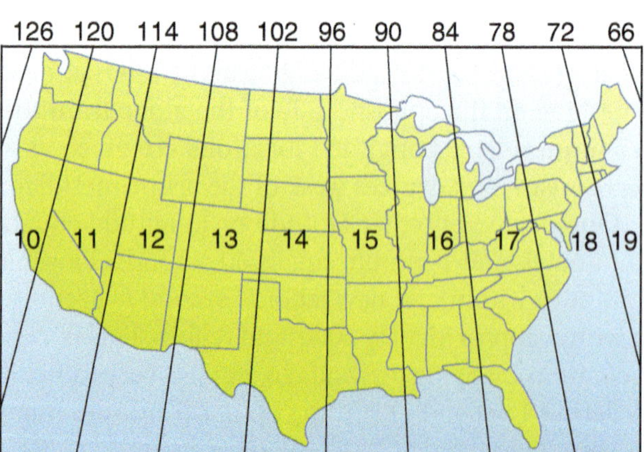

FIGURE 10-2 The Universal Transverse Mercator (UTM) grid that covers the conterminous 48 United States comprises 10 zones, from Zone 10 on the West Coast through Zone 19 in New England. Degrees of longitude are indicated across the top of the map.
Courtesy of the United States Geological Survey.

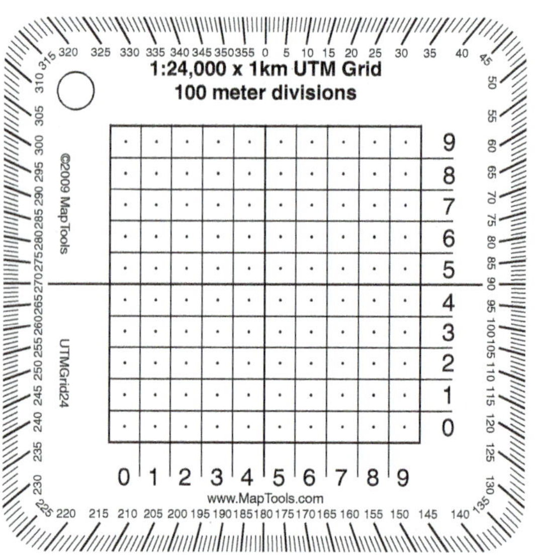

FIGURE 10-3 Map grid reader for interpolating points on a map.
Courtesy of maptools.com.

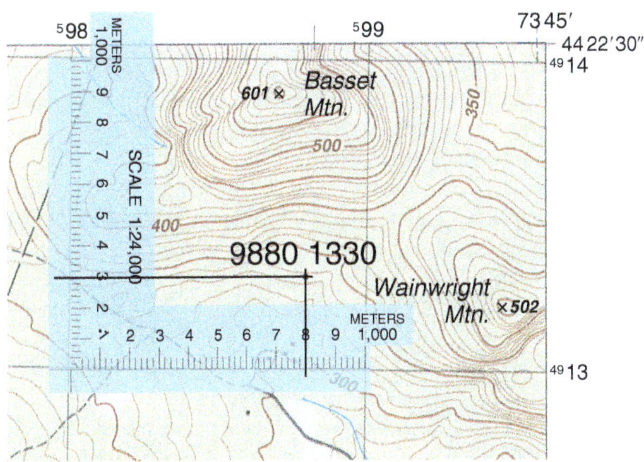

FIGURE 10-4 Finding a UTM point using an interpolator. To plot a point at coordinates of 9880/1330, the easting (9880) is first located by finding the blue tick marked with the upper case 98 on the bottom or top margin of the map then measuring an additional eight-tenths of the way (800 meters) to the tick line at 99. The northing is located by finding the blue tick marked with the upper case 13 on the right or left margin of the map then measuring an additional 300 meters north (approximately one-third of the way to the tick line at upper case 14).

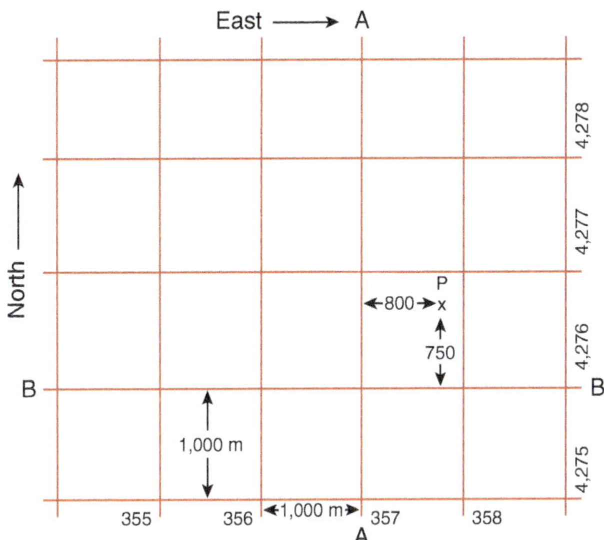

FIGURE 10-5 In Zone 19, the grid value of line A-A is 357,000 meters east. The grid value of line B-B is 4,276,000 meters north. Point P is 800 meters east and 750 meters north of the grid lines. Therefore, the grid coordinates of point P are east 357,800 and north 4,276,750. Ignoring the superscript numerals, the UTM point would be read, "Zone 19, 57800 76750," and is theoretically within 1 square meter accuracy.

the nearest grid line south of it plus its distance north of that line; its easting is the value of the nearest grid line west of it plus its distance east of that line (**FIGURE 10-5**).

In use, the numerals in superscript are most often ignored when describing points on a UTM grid. Thus, a point falling midway between ^{3}61 and ^{3}62 (easting) and ^{49}97 and ^{49}98 (northing) would be described as 61,500/97,500. The use of all 10 digits to describe a UTM point describes a point to within 1 meter and is called "10-digit accuracy." In actual use, the right-most (fifth) digits in the description of the easting and northing are infrequently used because describing a point to within 100 square meters (10 × 10 m) is usually sufficient for land navigation. This level of accuracy requires the use of only eight digits. So, the same point may more realistically be described as 6150/9750 (eight-digit accuracy). Measurements in this system are always made from the left margin to the point, then from the bottom margin to the point (Read-Right-Up).

United States National Grid

The **United States National Grid (USNG)** is an unambiguous, nationally consistent alpha-numeric georeferencing system that can be easily implemented using both printed maps and USNG-enabled GPS devices. It can be used for area gridding, as well as pinpoint locations, and it is the primary georeferencing source used by state, local fire/rescue, and Federal Emergency Management Agency (FEMA) Urban Search and Rescue (US&R) teams. In addition, the georeferencing matrix included in the U.S. Land SAR Addendum provides guidance on which georeferencing system each SAR responder should be using. It recommends that the USNG be used as the primary method of georeferencing for land search and rescue operations (NSARC, 2011, p. 4-51) (**FIGURE 10-6**).

The USNG standards were first proposed in 2000 and adopted by the Federal Geographic Data Committee (FGDC) for National Spatial Data Infrastructure (NSDI) applications in 2002. The USNG was implemented to alleviate problems associated with other georeferencing systems. For example, when multiple agencies representing different jurisdictions responded to an incident, each agency often used a different coordinate reference system. This reduced interoperability created communication problems between the agencies and presented a situation where it was difficult for people to efficiently convert from one system to another. Also, when latitude and longitude were used, it could be difficult for field personnel to accurately determine the location of a place on a paper map. In addition, during large-scale disasters, street signs and other landmarks may be destroyed, and the USNG can be used without this infrastructure.

Georeference System User	United States National Grid (USNG)	Latitude/Longitude DD-MM.mm[1]	GARS[2]
Land SAR Responder[3]	Primary	Secondary	N/A
Aeronautical SAR Responders[4]	Secondary	Primary	As Needed
Air Space Deconfliction[5]	N/A	Primary	N/A
Land SAR Responder/ Aeronautical SAR Responder Interface.[6]	Primary	Secondary	N/A
Incident Command:			
Air SAR Coordination	Secondary	Primary	N/A
Land SAR Coordination	Primary	Secondary	N/A
Area organization and accountability[7]	Secondary	Tertiary	Primary

[1] During SAR operations (and to avoid confusion) Latitude and Longitude should be in one standard format: DD-MM.mm. If required, use up to 2 digits to the right of the decimal. If required, allow 3 digits in the degrees field for longitude (i.e., DDD-MM.mm). Do not use leading zeros to the left of the decimal for degrees or minutes that require fewer than the maximum number of possible digits to express their value. The minimum number of digits is always one, even if it is a zero. (Example: Recommended: 9-0.3N 4-2.45W; Not Recommended: 09-00.300N 004-02.45W).

[2] GARS: Global Area Reference System.

[3] Land SAR responders use U.S. National Grid; however, a good familiarity with latitude and longitude is necessary to ensure effective interface between Land and Aeronautical SAR responders (Note: Land SAR includes SAR on flooded terrain).

[4] Aeronautical SAR responders will use latitude and longitude for SAR response. However, aeronautical SAR responders that work directly with Land SAR responders should understand the U.S. National Grid system for effective Land SAR/Aeronautical SAR interface.

[5] Air space deconfliction will only be implemented and managed using latitude and longitude.

[6] Aeronautical SAR responders working with Land SAR responders have the primary responsibility of coordinating SAR using USNG. However both groups must become familiar with both georeference systems.

[7] Describes the requirement for providing situational awareness of SAR operations geographically to Federal, military, state, local and tribal leadership. Provides for quick reference to send SAR resources closest to incident.

FIGURE 10-6 National SAR Committee's Georeferencing Matrix (NSARC, 2011). This matrix indicates what type of georeferencing system should be used in various types of SAR situations.

Data from from National Search and Rescue Committee [NSARC]. (November, 2011). Land SAR Addendum to the National Search and Rescue Supplement to the International Aeronautical and Maritime Search and Rescue Manual, Version 1.0. Table 4-7-1: National SAR Committee's Geo-referencing Matrix, p. 4-51. Retrieved from https://www.hsdl.org/?abstract&did=715465.

The USNG is functionally equivalent to the Military Grid Reference System (MGRS), and the basic coordinate values and numbering are identical to UTM coordinate values over areas of the United States. The USNG is simple to use and utilizes a grid zone designation, a 100,000-meter square identification, and grid coordinates. For example, the USNG coordinates for the Washington Monument in Washington, DC, are 18S UJ 23483 06479.

The U.S. geographic area is divided into 6-degree longitudinal zones designated by a number (as is the UTM system) and 8-degree latitudinal bands designated by a letter (FGDC, Standards Group, 2001). Therefore, each area is denoted by this unique alphanumeric Grid Zone Designator (GZD). In **FIGURE 10-7**, "18S" identifies a specific GZD.

Each 6-by-8-degree GZD is then covered by a specific scheme of 100,000-meter squares where a two-letter pair identifies each square. In Figure 10-7, "18S UJ" identifies a specific 100,000-meter square in the specified GZD.

A point within the 100,000-meter square can further be defined using the UTM grid coordinates. An even number of digits is always used. The first half defines the easting, and the second half defines the northing. The number of digits specifies the precision (**TABLE 10-1**). The grid coordinates are always read "right, then up."

Township and Range: U.S. Public Land Survey System

The U.S. Public Land Survey (USPLS) was a survey method devised to subdivide and describe land parcels. Although it is not a primary system for planning and navigating during a SAR, it is still referenced by some people, especially in very rural areas, so it is beneficial for SAR personnel to have a basic understanding of it. The Public Land Survey System, as it was known, began in 1785 in the territories northwest of the Ohio River. In each area that was to be mapped, a starting

Reading US National Grid (USNG) Coordinates: *"Read right, then up."*

Information Sheet 1 in this series. FGDC-STD-011-2001 From www.fgdc.gov/usng

The example below locates the Jefferson Pier at USNG: 18S UJ 23371 06519.

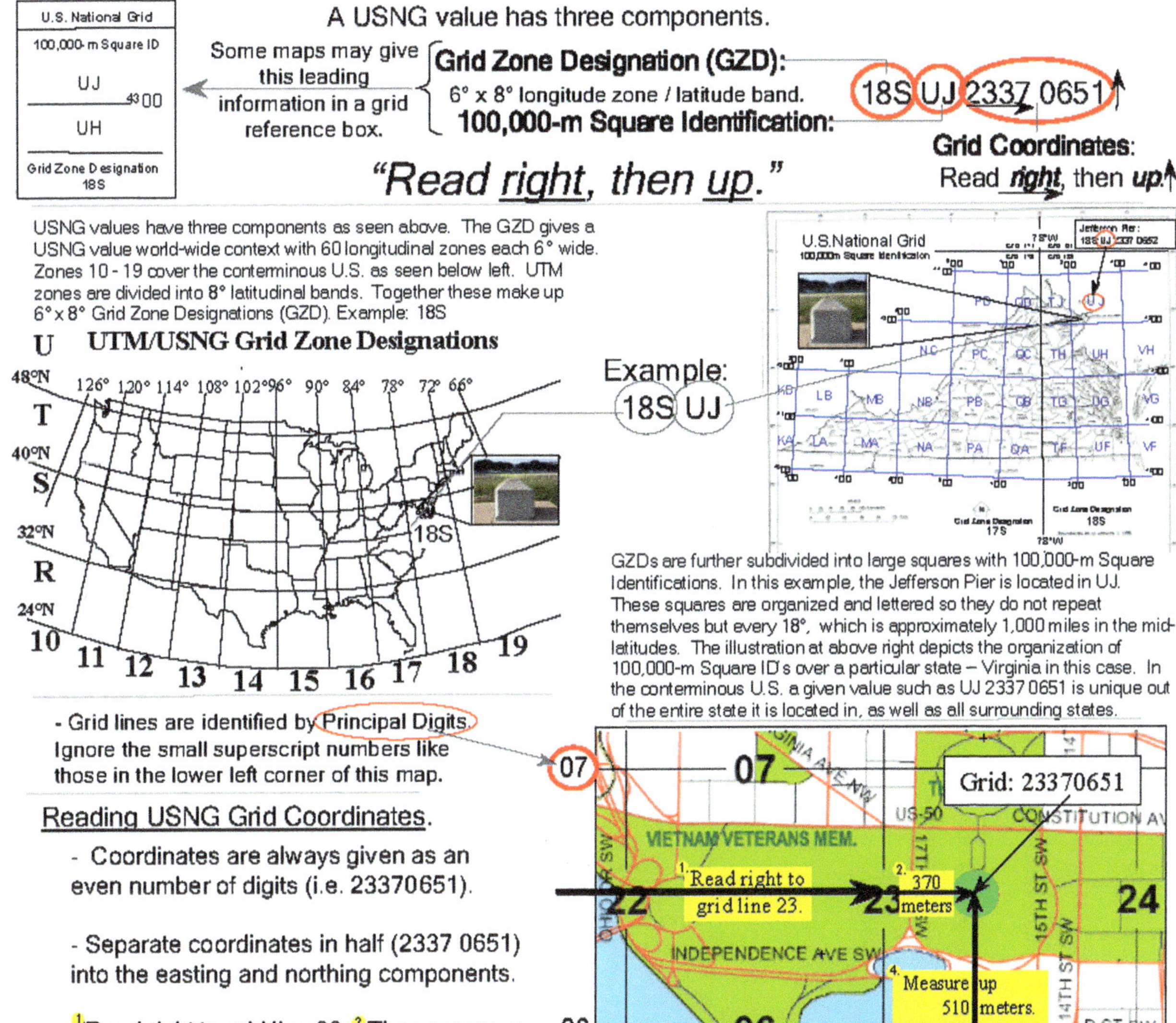

- [1] Read right to grid line 23. [2] Then measure right another 370 meters. (Think 23.37)

- [3] Read up to grid line 06. [4] Then measure up another 510 meters. (Think 06.51)

***A complete reference is*: 18S UJ 2337 0651**

Grid:	Point of Interest:
228 058	FDR Memorial:
231 054	George Mason Memorial:
2338 0710	Zero Milestone:
2275 0628	DC War Memorial:
222 065	Lincoln Memorial:

Grid: 2306 — TIDAL BASIN — JEFFERSON MEM. — Potomac River — [3] Read up to grid line 06. — 05 — 4305000mN — 322000mE — UTM format. — USNG: 18S UJ 23 — Datum: NAD 83 — 24 — 0 — 1,000-m

Ignore the small UTM superscript numbers that are provided for reference purposes. UTM numerical values are best suited for determining direction and distance as in surveying. USNG alpha-numeric values are best suited for position referencing because they can be given as only grid coordinates in a local area and with only the precision required for a particular task.

FIGURE 10-7 Instructions for using USNG.

Reproduced from Federal Geographic Data Committee. (2008). US National Grid Executive Summary and Information Paper. p. 3. Retrieved from https://www.fgdc.gov/usng.

point was established, and all points in the area were referenced relative to that point. The reference point for the Washington–Oregon survey, for example, was established near Portland, Oregon, in 1851 and is called the Willamette Stone. A true north-south line runs through the stone and is called the Willamette Meridian. An east-west line runs through the stone and is called the Willamette Baseline. These are also referred to as the principal meridian and principal base line, respectively.

From this starting point, townships, which are parcels of land that are 6 miles by 6 miles, were surveyed on a grid to the north, south, east, and west. These townships were then further subdivided into 36 numbered sections of 1 square mile (640 acres) each (**FIGURE 10-8**).

A specific point on the map is described by first identifying the township in which it falls. The township number is described as either north or south of the principal baseline and east or west of the principal meridian. For example, the township shown as shaded in Figure 10-8A is two townships (tiers) south of the principal baseline and three ranges (columns) from the principal meridian. Thus, the township is described as "Township 2 South, Range 3 West" or "T 2 S, R 3 W."

A point in a township could be further described by its section number. Sections are numbered consecutively, starting at the northeast corner and ending in the southeast corner of the township. Section 31 is at the lower left of the township, and section 6 is at the upper left in Figure 10-8B. Indicating the section in which a point is located plots it to 1 square mile accuracy. A point can be

TABLE 10-1 Precision Using U.S. National Grid Georeferencing System

USNG Grid Reference	Precision
18SUJ20	Locates a point with a precision of 10 kilometers
18SUJ2306	Locates a point with a precision of 1 kilometer
18SUJ234064	Locates a point with a precision of 100 meters
18SUJ2348306479	Locates a point with a precision of 1 meter

SEARCH AND RESCUE TIP

Throughout the years, there have been many unique mapping systems implemented at the local level. Two of these systems are the Uniform Mapping System (UMS) and the San Diego Mountain Rescue Team System (SDMRT). The UMS was devised in Washington state in the mid-1960s and used letters and numbers to describe points. It was tied into Sectional Aeronautical Charts (1:500,000) that were broken down into a grid and used by the Civil Air Patrol and the U.S. Air Force. UMS was also keyed into 15-minute topographical (topo) maps (15° latitude by 15° longitude; 1:62,500 scale).

The SDMRT used a simple system to describe a point on a map by identifying the map scale and quadrant and then indicating the distance, in inches, from the left map margin as well as the distance from the bottom margin (Read Right Up). For example, point A is 12-1/2 inches from the left and 4-3/8 inches from the bottom of the 7.5-minute series, Northampton Quadrangle topo map. Although this was simple, fast, and easy to learn, it was useless without a map and cannot be strictly considered a method of absolute navigation.

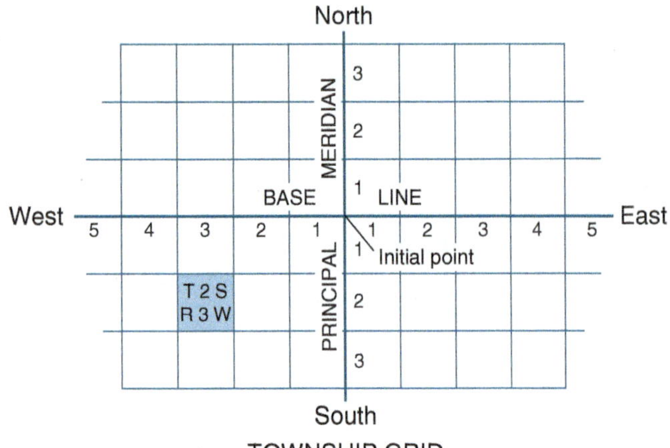

6	5	4	3	2	1
7	8	9	10	11	12
18	17	16	15	Section 14	13
19	20	21	22	23	24
30	29	28	27	26	25
31	32	33	34	35	36

TOWNSHIP 2 SOUTH, RANGE 3 WEST

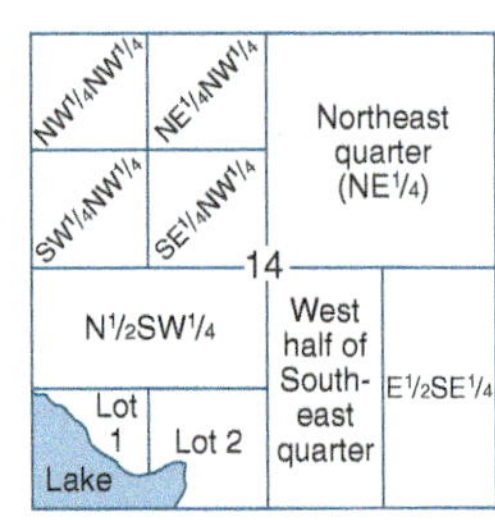

FIGURE 10-8 General diagram of the U.S. rectangular system of surveys.

Courtesy of the United States Geological Survey.

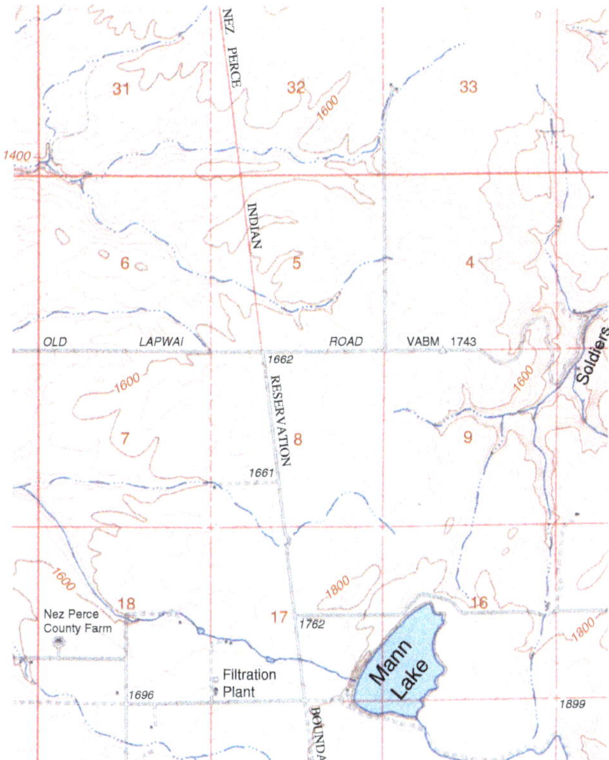

FIGURE 10-9 Examples of red township and range boundaries on a map.

Courtesy of the United States Geological Survey. Lewiston Orchards Quadrangle: Idaho–Washington: 15 Minute Series. Retrieved from https://store.usgs.gov/product/289566.

more accurately described by indicating that corner (1/4) of the section where the point is located. Describing a point as being within the NW corner of a section describes a point within 160 acres of accuracy. Describing a point as being in the SW corner of the NW corner of a section describes a point within about 40 acres of accuracy. A description of a point within 40 acres of accuracy would look like: SE 1/4, NW 1/4, Section 14, T 2 S, R 3 W.

Most of the western United States is surveyed using this system; however, the survey was never completed and, therefore, is not applicable in some parts of the country (particularly in the East and Texas). For this reason, not all USGS maps have township and range lines on them as does the map in **FIGURE 10-9**. It is also important for SAR personnel to recognize that while these red lines are found on many maps, they should not be used for navigation since the lines do not always run true north-south or true east-west as originally intended. It should also be noted that this system is rarely used in SAR, but it is still occasionally referenced in certain parts of the country.

Maps

A map is a pictorial representation of the Earth's surface. In SAR, reading a map allows SAR personnel to associate the graphic details appearing on the map with the physical features in the field, and vice versa.

As a minimum, maps for land navigation should provide the following information:

- An accurate depiction of terrain in a scale that is appropriate to the mode of transportation (e.g., walking, flying, boating). "Scale" is the ratio of the area represented by the map to the same area in the terrain (e.g., 1 to 24,000).
- The major terrain features such as hills, valleys, and ridges.
- Human-made features such as buildings, trails, and roads.
- An accurate depiction of measurable relief, elevation, and contour (lay of the land).
- The location of water and water courses (important information for SAR personnel and search planning).

Topographical Maps

Topographical (topo) maps portray the shape and elevation of the terrain while showing a graphic representation of selected human-made and natural features on a part of the Earth's surface plotted to a definite scale. These are probably the most commonly used maps for SAR operations and are a familiar source of geographic knowledge. There are pros and cons to using a topographical map, and they should not be used as the only source of geographic information when planning SAR missions. Updated geographic layers, institutional knowledge, and verification from the field should be used to supplement these maps.

The USGS publishes topo maps in a variety of scales; the most popular for land SAR is the 1:24,000 or 7.5-minute map (**FIGURE 10-10**). These maps have quadrangle dimensions of 7.5 minutes in latitude and longitude, the bounding parallels and meridians being integral multiples of 7.5 minutes. The series includes the few maps whose boundary lines are offset or extended to cover islands, irregular coastal features, or areas needed to complete mapping to political boundaries.

USGS topo maps are supposed to be updated every five to 10 years, but in reality, it is often longer, and some maps are over 30 years old. Because of this, they accurately depict terrain and relief (elevation and slope), but the human-made features in the terrain may occasionally differ from what the map depicts due to the extended length of time between map updates (**FIGURE 10-11**). The 7.5-minute series maps are the most commonly used maps in ground SAR work because of the appropriateness of scale and wide availability. They are also available as downloadable digital files from the USGS Locator and Downloader (USGS, 2015a).

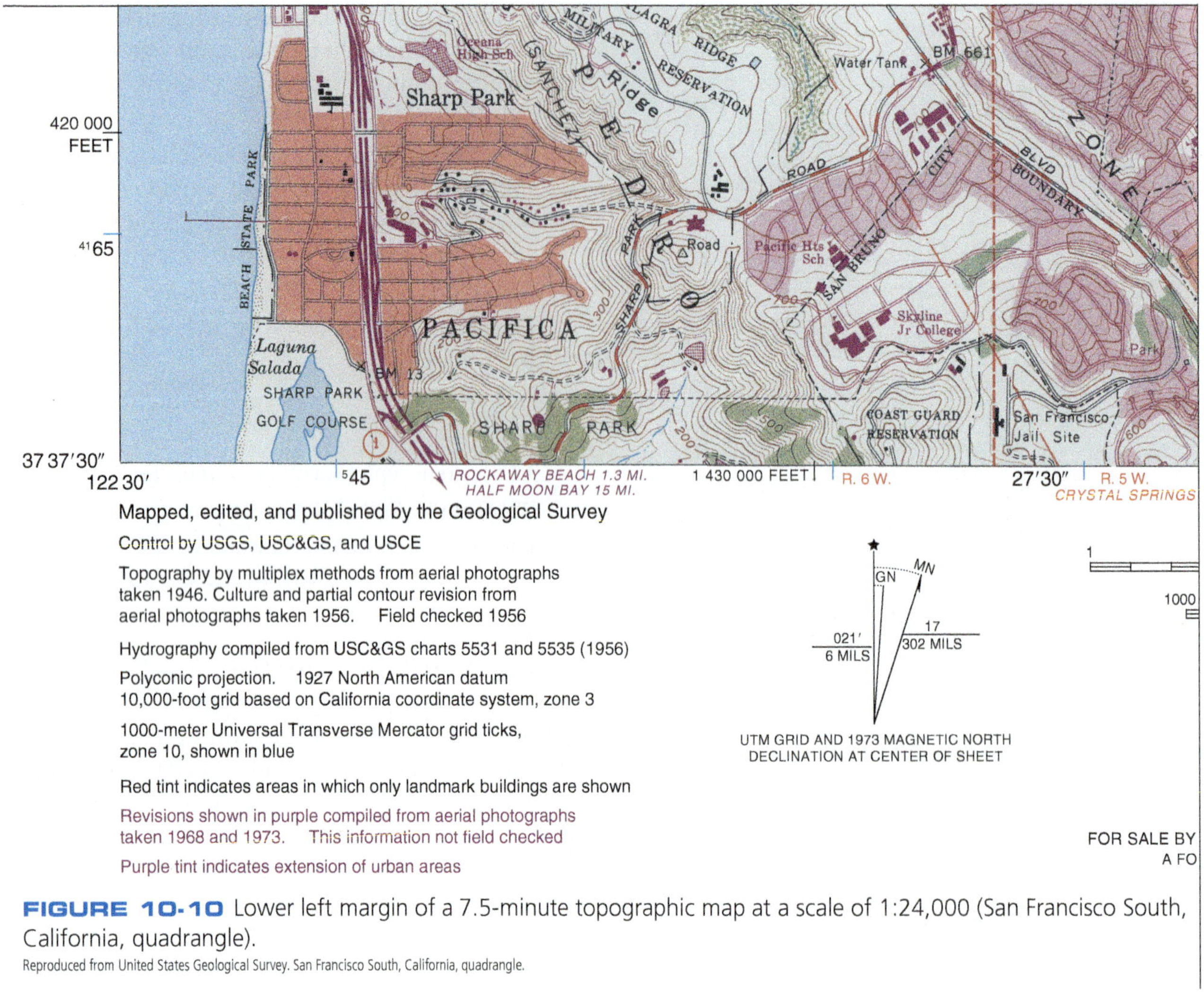

420 000
FEET
4165
37 37′30″
122 30′
545
ROCKAWAY BEACH 1.3 MI.
HALF MOON BAY 15 MI.
1 430 000 FEET
R. 6 W.
27′30″
R. 5 W.
CRYSTAL SPRINGS
Sharp Park
PACIFICA
Laguna
Salada
SHARP PARK
GOLF COURSE
SHARP PARK
BEACH STATE PARK
Water Tank
BM 661
BM 13
Pacific Hts
Sch
Skyline
Jr College
COAST GUARD
RESERVATION
San Francisco
Jail Site
Park
Mapped, edited, and published by the Geological Survey
Control by USGS, USC&GS, and USCE
Topography by multiplex methods from aerial photographs
taken 1946. Culture and partial contour revision from
aerial photographs taken 1956. Field checked 1956
Hydrography compiled from USC&GS charts 5531 and 5535 (1956)
Polyconic projection. 1927 North American datum
10,000-foot grid based on California coordinate system, zone 3
1000-meter Universal Transverse Mercator grid ticks,
zone 10, shown in blue
Red tint indicates areas in which only landmark buildings are shown
Revisions shown in purple compiled from aerial photographs
taken 1968 and 1973. This information not field checked
Purple tint indicates extension of urban areas
GN
MN
021′
6 MILS
17
302 MILS
UTM GRID AND 1973 MAGNETIC NORTH
DECLINATION AT CENTER OF SHEET
1
1000
FOR SALE BY
A FO

FIGURE 10-10 Lower left margin of a 7.5-minute topographic map at a scale of 1:24,000 (San Francisco South, California, quadrangle).

Reproduced from United States Geological Survey. San Francisco South, California, quadrangle.

260
275 ×
200
20
100

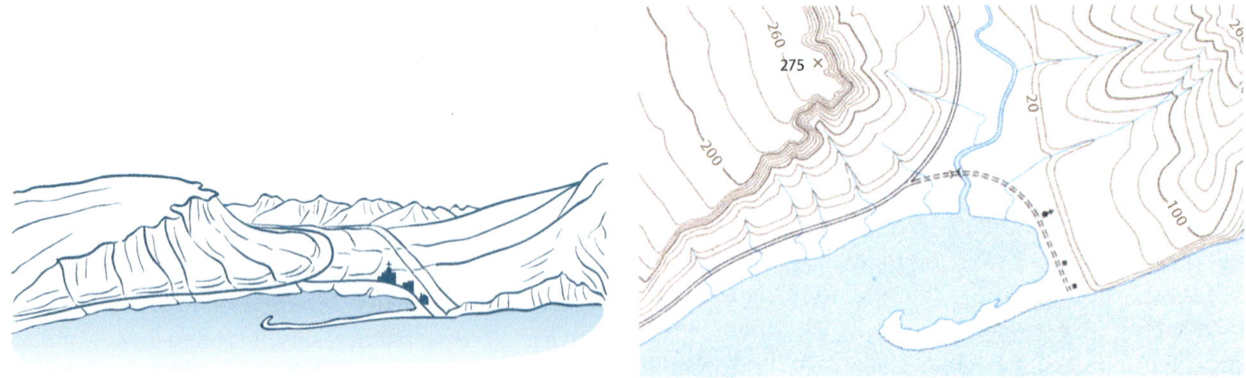

FIGURE 10-11 The terrain on the left (**A**) is depicted by the topographical map on the right (**B**).

Courtesy of the United States Geological Survey.

The top of a USGS topo map is always true (geographic) north. Thus, the vertical lines of longitude on the map point north and south, and the horizontal lines of latitude point east and west.

The space outside the margin line (called the *margin*) on USGS topographical maps identifies and explains the map. The marginal information corresponds somewhat to the table of contents and the introduction of a book;

it tells briefly how the map was made, where the quadrangle is located, which organizations are responsible for the contents, and gives other information to make the map more useful.

Each map is identified in the upper right margin by its quadrangle name, state or states in which it is located, series, and type (**FIGURE 10-12**). It is usually named after a prominent, immovable place or landmark within the mapped area. If the quadrangle includes areas of more than one state, the state names are shown in the title in the order of decreasing area. The "series" refers to the area mapped in terms of minutes or degrees; "type" is either topographic or planimetric (no topographic features). If a new 7.5-minute map covers a part of a published 15-minute quadrangle, a note is added giving the position of the 7.5-minute quadrangle.

The title block in the lower right margin shows the quadrangle name, state name, and the geographic

PENINSULA QUADRANGLE
OHIO—SUMMIT CO.
7.5 MINUTE SERIES (TOPOGRAPHIC)

FIGURE 10-12 Quadrangle name found in the upper right margin of a USGS topographical map.
Courtesy of the United States Geological Survey.

index number (**FIGURE 10-13**). For a 7.5-minute map, the margin also gives the position in relation to the 15-minute map, if applicable, and the year the map was published. The geographic index number is the geographic position of the corner of the map nearest the Greenwich meridian and the equator, followed by the series, such as "7.5-minute." Just to the left of the title block is a diagram of the location of the quadrangle within the state. If there have been any major physical changes to the terrain since the map was published, these changes are often indicated on the map in purple, and the map may have another date in the margin, also in purple, next to the words "photo revised" or "photo inspected."

Adjoining quadrangle names are shown so that map users may know that topographic data are available for these adjacent areas (**FIGURE 10-14**).

Geographic coordinates are shown at all four map margin corners and along the margin lines at 2.5-minute intervals for 7.5-minute maps (**FIGURE 10-15**). Coordinates for both the state (each state has its own zone grid based on various projections) and UTM grid systems are shown near the map margin corners.

The credit legend is located in the lower left margin (see Figure 10-10). Because of the almost infinite number of possible combinations of data, credit legends cannot be rigid. However, they usually include the

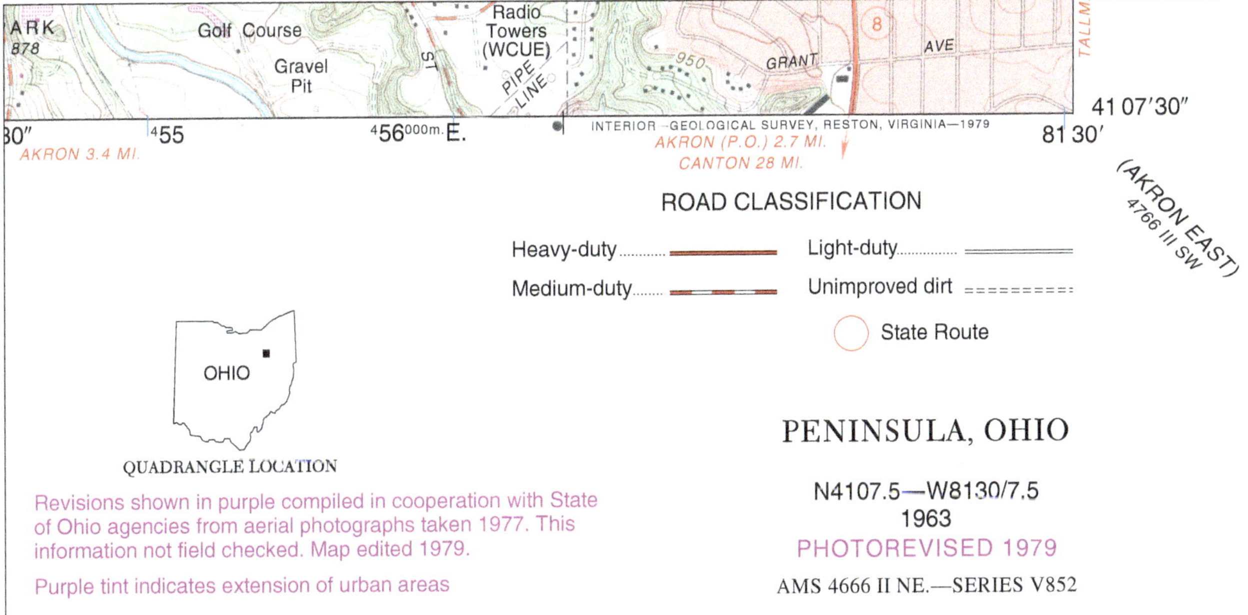

FIGURE 10-13 Lower right margin of a USGS topographical map.
Courtesy of the United States Geological Survey.

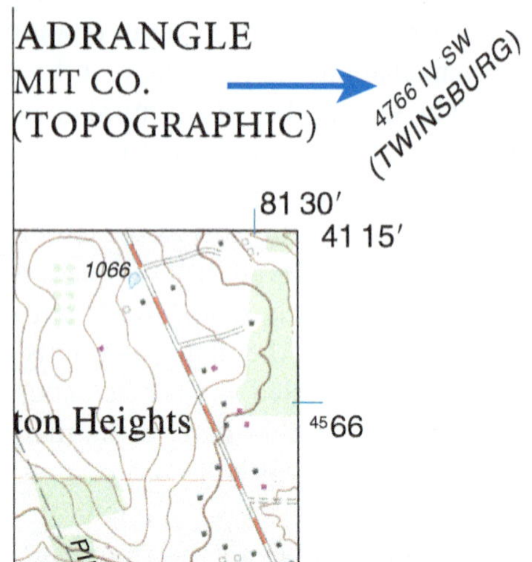

FIGURE 10-14 Adjoining quadrangle name indicated by blue arrow. This example shows the upper right map margin.
Courtesy of the United States Geological Survey.

name of the mapping agency, the name of the editing and publishing agency, the name of the agency that furnished the geodetic (the science that deals with the measurement and mathematical description of the size and shape of the Earth) control, the method by which the mapping was performed, a credit note for hydrographic (the science that deals with measurement and description of the physical features of the Earth's oceans, seas, and other waterways) information, and informative and explanatory notes.

The **magnetic declination** for the year of field survey or revision is determined to the nearest 0.5 degree from the latest isogonic chart. It is shown by a diagram centered between the credit legend and bar scale (**FIGURE 10-16**). The **declination** diagram indicates the angular relationship among **true north**, **grid north**, and **magnetic north**. If the map is over 10 years old, it is a good idea to check and confirm the declination information included on the map.

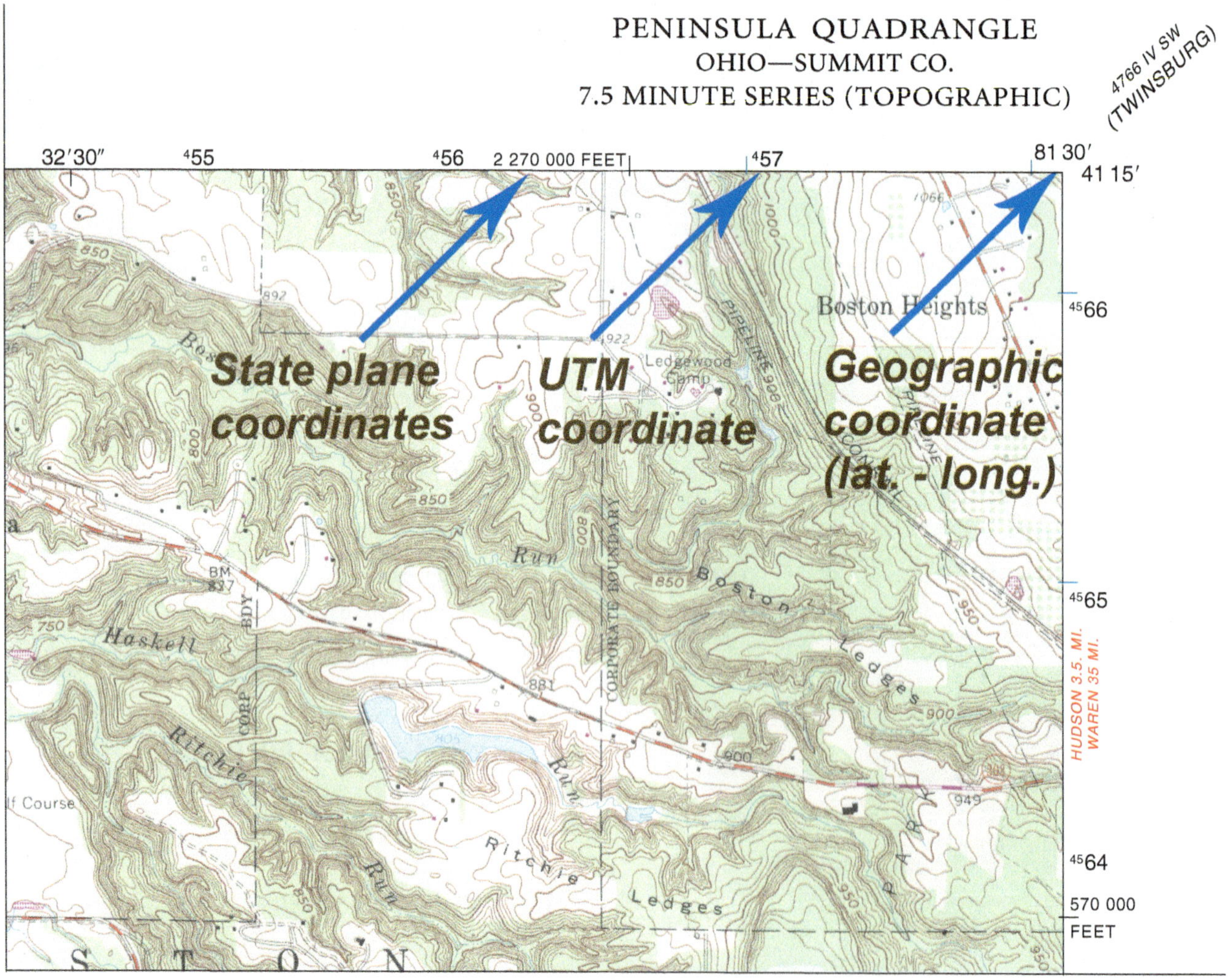

FIGURE 10-15 UTM coordinates, state plane coordinates, and geographic coordinates (latitude and longitude) at the map margin corners of a 7.5-minute topographical map.
Courtesy of the United States Geological Survey.

The center of the lower margin contains the following information, arranged in the order indicated:

1. Publication scales expressed as a ratio.
2. Bar scales in metric and imperial units.
3. Contour–interval statement. If the map contains supplementary contours, a statement to that effect is added. When the maximum elevation on the quadrangle is less than the specified contour interval, a note stating, "entire area below 5 feet" is used in place of the standard contour interval.
4. Vertical **datum**. The statement, "Datum is mean sea level" is on standard survey topographical maps printed prior to 1975. On maps published since, the statement is "National Geodetic Vertical Datum of 1929."
5. Depth-curve sounding statement, where applicable.
6. Shoreline and tide-range statements, shown on maps that include tidal shoreline.
7. Map accuracy statements. The standard statement is, "This map complies with national map accuracy standards."

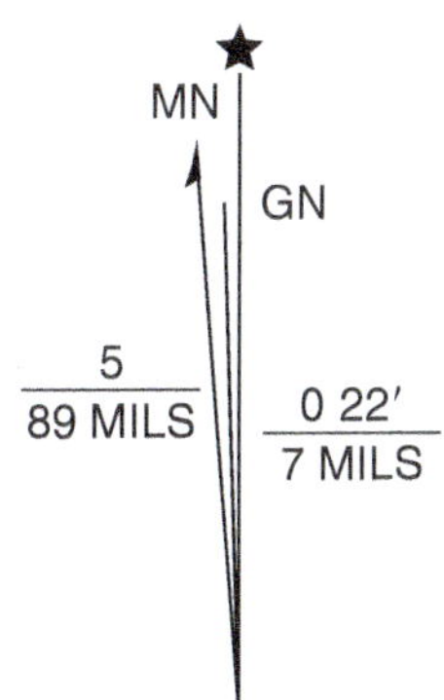

FIGURE 10-16 Magnetic declination diagram on a USGS topo map, found in the bottom margin of the map.
Courtesy of the United States Geological Survey.

The bar scales (distance determination) are located at the bottom center margin of the map (**FIGURE 10-17**). Distance can be determined by measuring the distance on the map with a piece of paper, a piece of string, or a ruler, then comparing the measured distance to the bar scale, which is in meters, miles, and feet. The metric system (meters) is the measurement of choice for SAR.

A legend explaining the various road symbols that are shown on the map is placed in the lower right margin (**FIGURE 10-18**). This legend is tailored for each map to include only the classes of roads and route markers that are shown in the body of the map. Trails are not included in the legend unless there are no roads on the map.

The year of the data shown on the map is printed beneath and as part of the title in the lower right margin (see Figure 10-13). The latest date of field completion or revision is used. It remains unchanged in future reprintings but is changed when the map is revised. If minor cartographic corrections are made for a reprint, a note in small type is added under the year (e.g., "1957, Minor Revision 1973").

Road destinations are shown in the map margin for convenience in determining the distance to the next town or important road junction beyond the map border and to facilitate **orientation** of the map with respect to well-known features.

The USGS has a free pamphlet that has every map symbol found on a topo map (USGS, 2015b) (**FIGURE 10-19**). These free pamphlets should

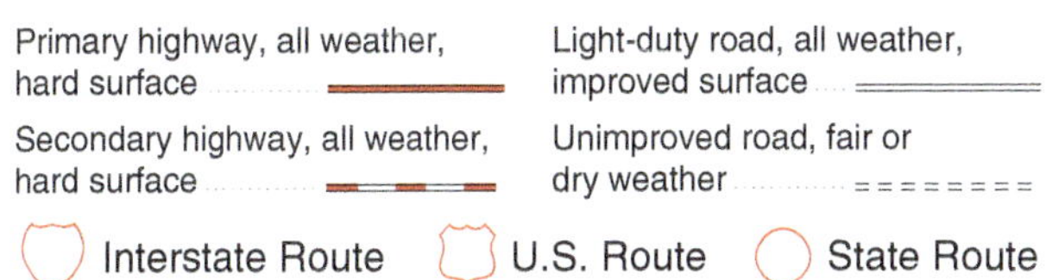

FIGURE 10-18 Legend showing various road symbols.
Courtesy of the United States Geological Survey.

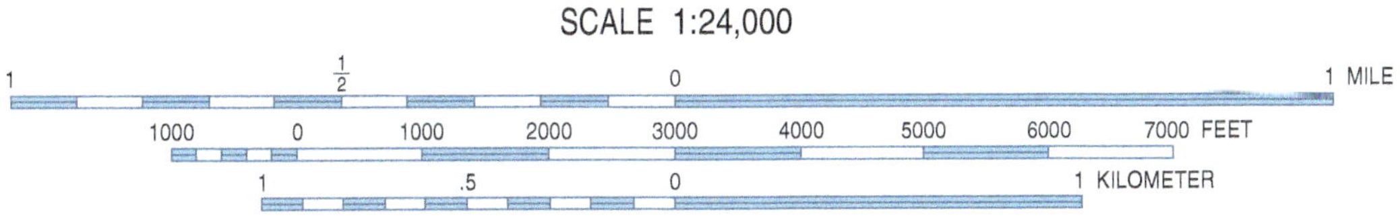

FIGURE 10-17 The scale and contour interval in the bottom margin of a USGS topographical map.
Courtesy of the United States Geological Survey.

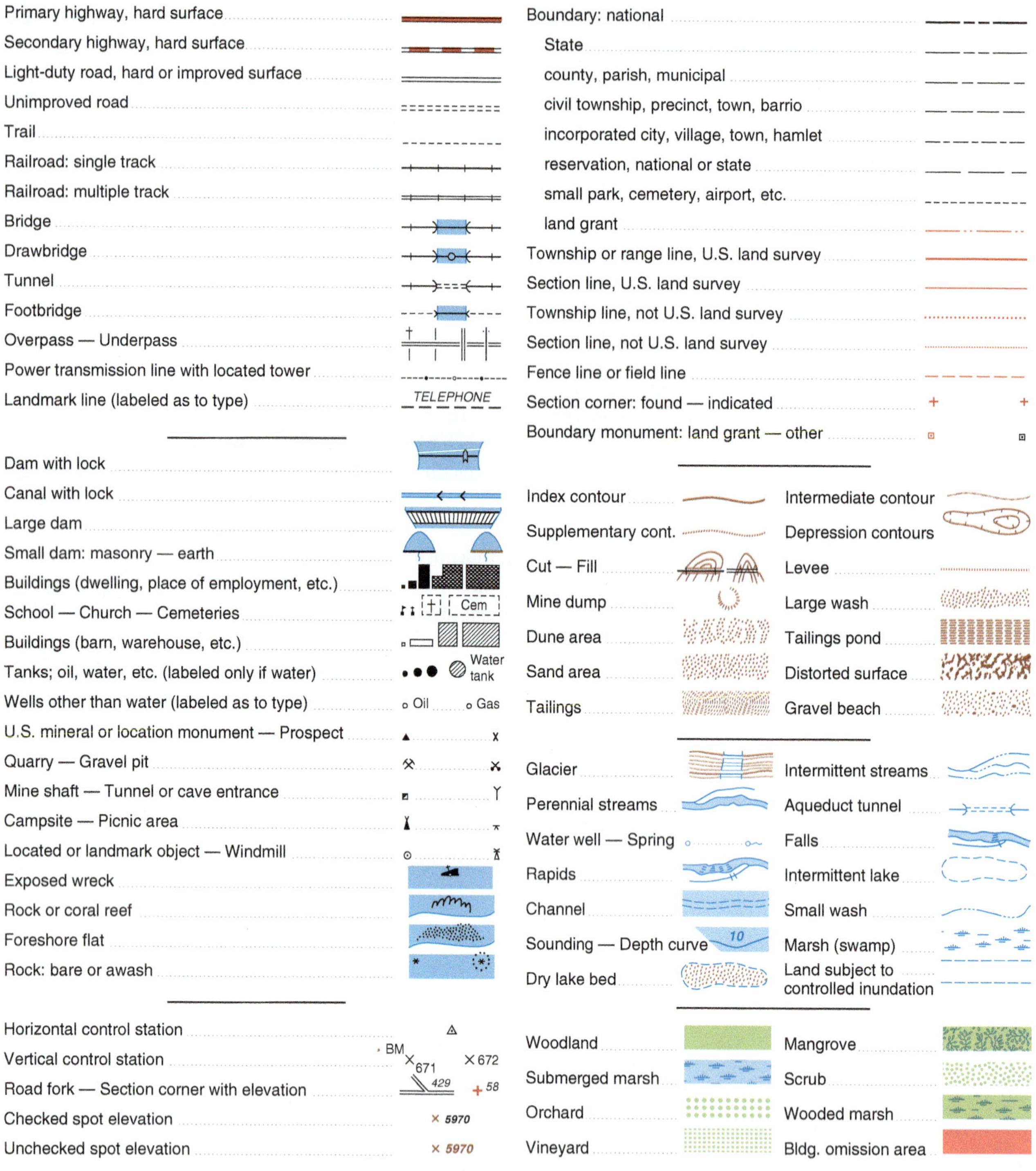

Primary highway, hard surface
Secondary highway, hard surface
Light-duty road, hard or improved surface
Unimproved road
Trail
Railroad: single track
Railroad: multiple track
Bridge
Drawbridge
Tunnel
Footbridge
Overpass — Underpass
Power transmission line with located tower
Landmark line (labeled as to type) TELEPHONE

Dam with lock
Canal with lock
Large dam
Small dam: masonry — earth
Buildings (dwelling, place of employment, etc.)
School — Church — Cemeteries Cem
Buildings (barn, warehouse, etc.)
Tanks; oil, water, etc. (labeled only if water) Water tank
Wells other than water (labeled as to type) Oil Gas
U.S. mineral or location monument — Prospect
Quarry — Gravel pit
Mine shaft — Tunnel or cave entrance
Campsite — Picnic area
Located or landmark object — Windmill
Exposed wreck
Rock or coral reef
Foreshore flat
Rock: bare or awash

Horizontal control station
Vertical control station BM 671 672
Road fork — Section corner with elevation 429 58
Checked spot elevation 5970
Unchecked spot elevation 5970

Boundary: national
State
county, parish, municipal
civil township, precinct, town, barrio
incorporated city, village, town, hamlet
reservation, national or state
small park, cemetery, airport, etc.
land grant
Township or range line, U.S. land survey
Section line, U.S. land survey
Township line, not U.S. land survey
Section line, not U.S. land survey
Fence line or field line
Section corner: found — indicated
Boundary monument: land grant — other

Index contour
Intermediate contour
Supplementary cont.
Depression contours
Cut — Fill
Levee
Mine dump
Large wash
Dune area
Tailings pond
Sand area
Distorted surface
Tailings
Gravel beach

Glacier
Intermittent streams
Perennial streams
Aqueduct tunnel
Water well — Spring
Falls
Rapids
Intermittent lake
Channel
Small wash
Sounding — Depth curve 10
Marsh (swamp)
Dry lake bed
Land subject to controlled inundation

Woodland
Mangrove
Submerged marsh
Scrub
Orchard
Wooded marsh
Vineyard
Bldg. omission area

FIGURE 10-19 Topographical map legend available from USGS (USGS, 2015b).
Data from United States Geological Survey. Topographic Map Symbols. Retrieved from https://pubs.usgs.gov/gip/TopographicMapSymbols/topomapsymbols.pdf.

be available where topo maps are sold, or are free from the USGS by writing, calling, or by visiting their website.

Colors on the Map

Generally, there are six colors on the map (**FIGURE 10-20**). Brown denotes **contour lines**, green is for vegetation, blue for water, black for human-made objects, red for human-made features such as roads and built-up areas, and purple for new changes or updates on the map. When contour lines are showing elevation on glaciers or snow-capped mountains, these lines are blue.

Contour lines represent relative elevation (**FIGURE 10-21**). Each contour line on the map connects all points at the same elevation above sea level. There are three types of contour lines: index, intermediate, and supplementary. Every fifth line is darker and has a number superimposed on it, indicating the elevation along that particular line. This darker contour is an “index” contour line. The

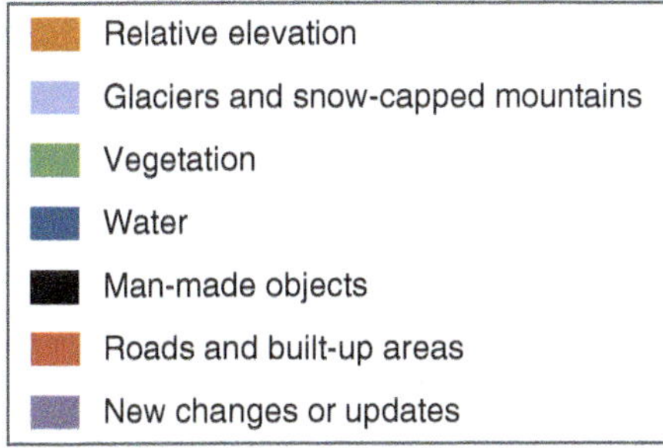

FIGURE 10-20 Map colors.

Courtesy of Donald Cooper.

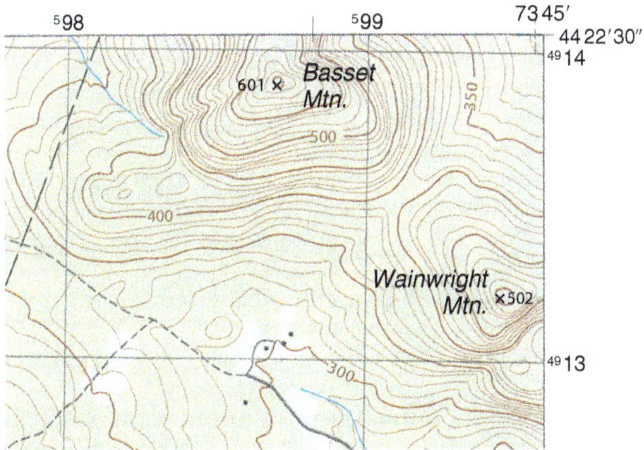

FIGURE 10-21 Brown contour lines on a USGS topographical map.

Reproduced from United States Geological Survey. (1979). Lake Placid, New York. 7.5x15 Minute Series (Topographic). 4473-231-T25. Retrieved from https://store.usgs.gov/product/288394.

lighter brown contour lines are called "intermediate" contour lines, and they fall between index lines and are not numbered. Supplementary contour lines are dashed lines that may be used when the terrain is very flat and there are large distances between adjacent contour lines. A supplementary contour line shows a difference in elevation that is half of the elevation of the contour lines between which it falls. The contour interval can be found in the bottom margin of the map, usually near the distance scale. When successive contour lines are close together, the terrain is steep. Contour lines that touch indicate a cliff, but contour lines do not cross. Widely spaced contour lines indicate a gently sloping or flat terrain.

Terrain Features

All terrain features evolve from a complex landmass known as a *ridgeline* (**FIGURE 10-22**). This ridgeline should not be confused with, and is not a synonym for, a ridge, which is an individual terrain feature. A ridgeline is a line of high ground, usually with variations in elevation along its top and low ground on all sides, which is the source of many terrain features. A ridge is simply one of the terrain features that may arise from a ridgeline.

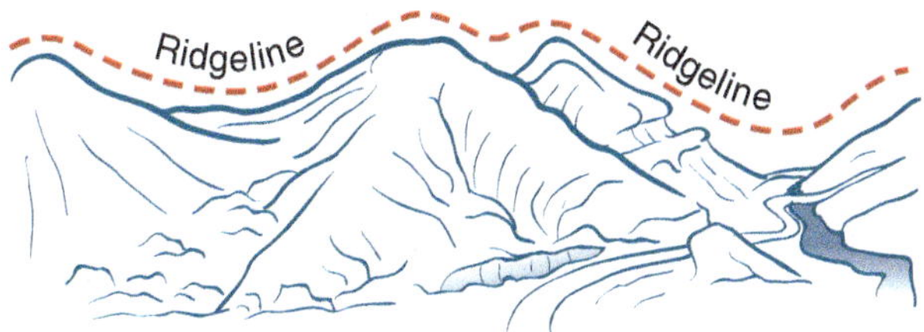

FIGURE 10-22 A ridgeline, not to be confused with a ridge, is the source from which all terrain features evolve.

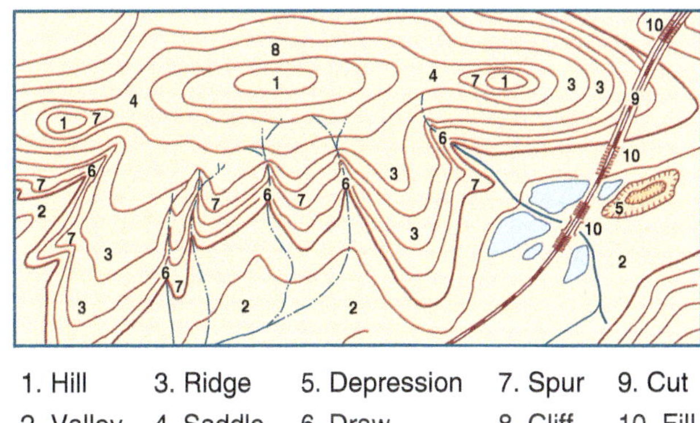

FIGURE 10-23 Examples of major (1–5) and minor (6–10) features.

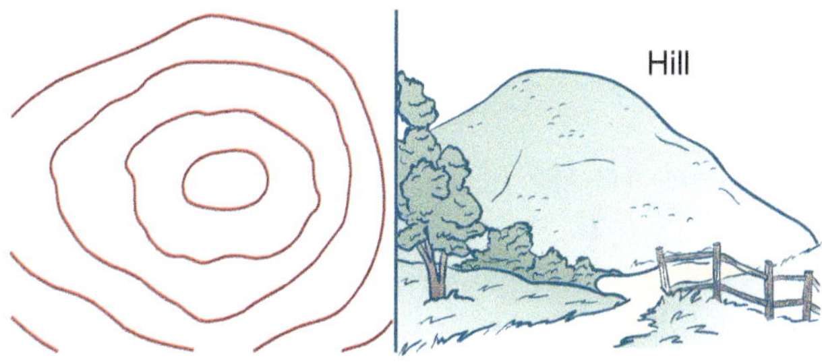

FIGURE 10-24 Hill.

A total of 10 natural or human-made terrain features may arise from a ridgeline, each with unique and notable characteristics. These features fall into two categories: major and minor (**FIGURE 10-23**).

Major Terrain Features. Major terrain features include the following:

- *Hill.* A hill is an area of high ground. From a hilltop, the ground slopes down in all directions. A hill is shown on the map by contour lines forming concentric circles (**FIGURE 10-24**). The inside of the smallest closed circle is the hilltop. It is important to note that it is rare to have a completely flat hilltop. It is very possible that the hill rises slightly in elevation beyond the very top contour line, but the elevation is less than the contour interval.
- *Saddle.* A saddle is a dip or low point between two areas of higher ground (**FIGURE 10-25**).

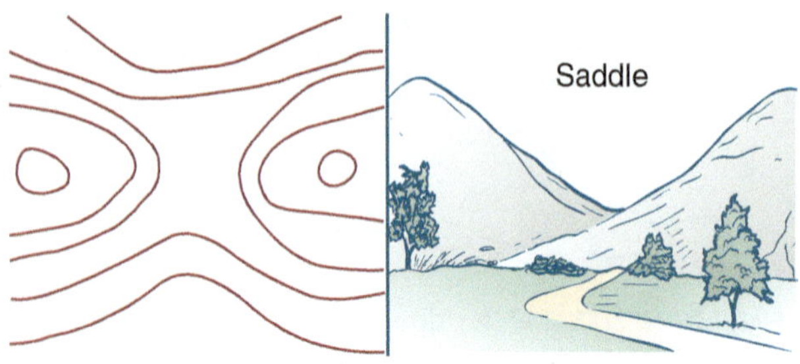

FIGURE 10-25 Saddle.

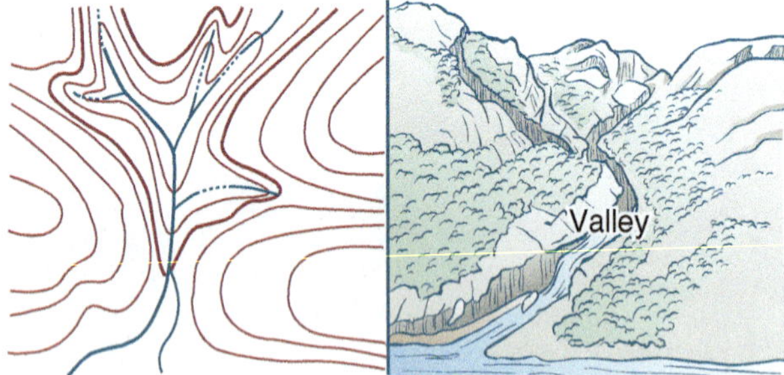

FIGURE 10-26 Valley.

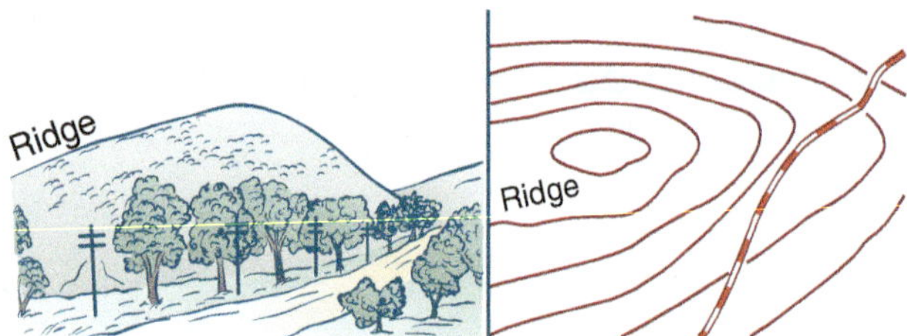

FIGURE 10-27 Ridge.

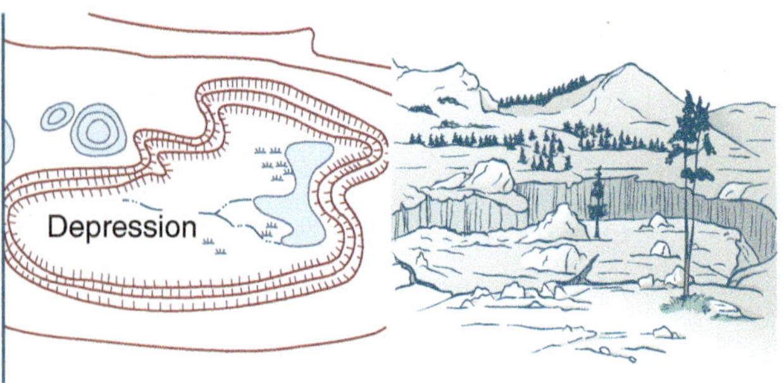

FIGURE 10-28 Depression.

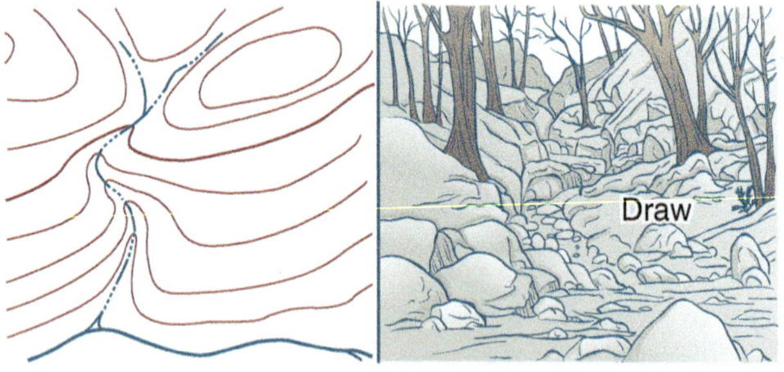

FIGURE 10-29 Draw.

A saddle is not necessarily the lower ground between two hilltops; it may be simply a dip or break along a level ridge crest. If you are in a saddle, there is high ground in two opposite directions and lower ground in the other two directions.

- *Valley*. A valley is a stretched-out groove in the land, usually formed by streams or rivers (**FIGURE 10-26**). A valley begins with high ground on three sides, and it usually has a course of running water through it. If standing in a valley, there is high ground in two opposite directions and a gradual incline in at least one other direction. Depending on its size and where a person is standing, it may not be obvious that there is high ground in the third direction, but water flows from higher to lower ground. Contour lines forming a valley are either U-shaped or V-shaped. To determine the direction water is flowing, look at the contour lines. The closed end of a contour line (U or V) always points upstream or toward high ground.
- *Ridge*. A ridge is a sloping line of high ground (**FIGURE 10-27**). If you are standing on the centerline of a ridge, you normally have low ground in three directions and high ground in one direction with varying degrees of slope. If you cross a ridge at right angles, you may climb steeply to the crest and then descend steeply to the base. When you move along the path of the ridge, depending on the geographic location, there may be either an almost unnoticeable slope or a very obvious incline. Contour lines forming a ridge tend to be U-shaped or V-shaped. The closed end of the contour line points away from high ground.
- *Depression*. A depression is a low point in the ground (**FIGURE 10-28**). It could be described as an area of low ground surrounded by higher ground in all directions, or simply a hole in the ground. Usually only depressions that are equal to or greater than the contour interval are shown. On maps, depressions are represented by closed contour lines that have tick marks pointing toward low ground. Examples of a depression include inside the cone of a volcano and a pit that serves as the opening to a cave.

Minor Terrain Features. Minor terrain features include the following:

- *Draw*. A draw is a less developed water course than a valley (**FIGURE 10-29**). In a draw, there is essentially no level ground and, therefore, little or no maneuver room within its confines. If you are standing in a draw, the ground slopes upward in three directions and downward in the other direction. A draw could be considered the initial formation of a valley. The contour lines depicting

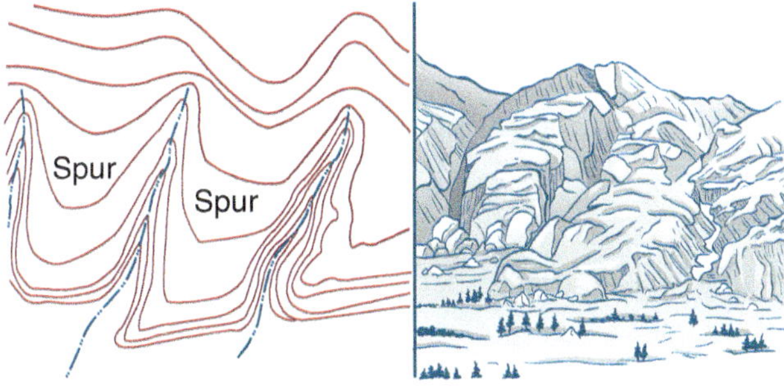

FIGURE 10-30 Spur.

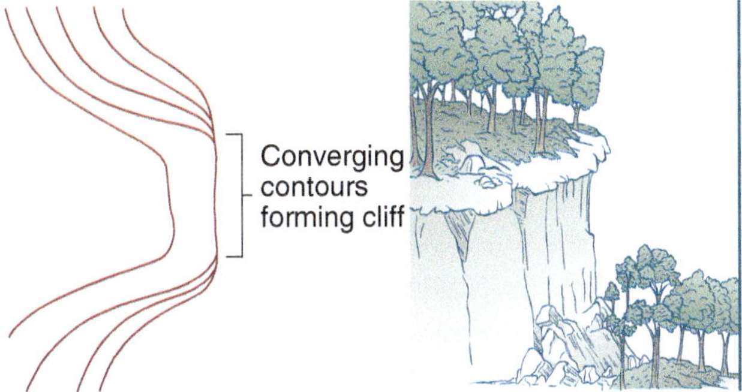

FIGURE 10-31 Cliff.

a draw are U-shaped and V-shaped, both pointing toward high ground.

- *Spur.* A spur is a short, continuous sloping line of higher ground, normally jutting out from the side of a ridge (**FIGURE 10-30**). A spur is often formed by two roughly parallel streams cutting draws down the side of a ridge. The ground slopes down in three directions and up in one. Contour lines on a map depict a spur with the U or V pointing away from high ground.
- *Cliff.* A cliff is a vertical or near vertical feature; it is an abrupt change of elevation. When a slope is so steep that the contour lines converge into one "carrying" contour or contours, this last contour line has tick marks pointing toward low ground (**FIGURE 10-31**). Cliffs are also shown by contour lines very close together and, in some instances, touching each other.
- *Cut/fill.* A cut is a human-made feature resulting from cutting through raised ground, usually to form a level bed for a road or railroad track. Cuts are shown on a map when they are at least 10 feet high, and they are drawn with a contour line along the cut line. This contour line extends the length of the cut and has tick marks that extend from the cut line to the roadbed, if the map scale permits this level of detail (**FIGURE 10-32**). A fill is a human-made feature resulting from filling a low area, usually to form a level bed for a railroad track. Fills are shown on a map when they are at least 10 feet high, and they are drawn with a contour line along the fill line. This contour line extends the length of the filled area and has tick marks that point toward lower ground. If the map scale permits, the length of the fill tick marks are drawn to scale and extend from the base line of the fill symbol.

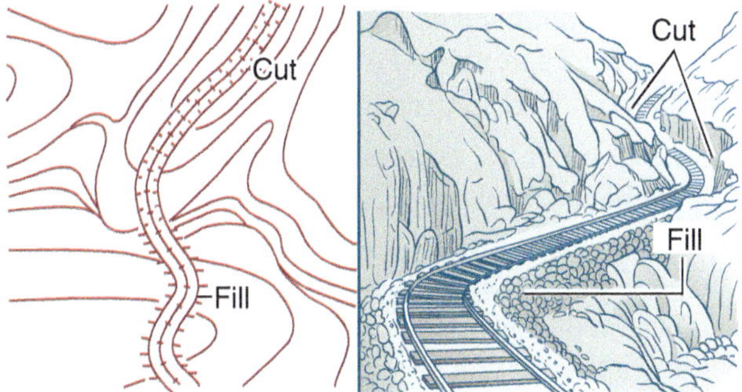

FIGURE 10-32 Cut/fill.

Incident Specific Maps

Easy-to-use mapping software and fully functional geographic information systems (GIS) (discussed further in Chapter 11) have made it possible to create custom maps for specific incidents, which can then be printed for SAR personnel or viewed on mobile electronic devices or tablets. These maps can incorporate not only **topography** lines but aerial imagery as well. This can enhance rescuers' situational awareness, but it should be stressed that imagery alone is not a map. More importantly, GIS allows for the inclusion of updated and information-rich layers to aid in SAR operations and planning. Two important concepts regarding layers are *base data* and *incident data* (National Wildfire Coordinating Group [NWCG], 2014).

Base data are layers that exist before the incident and are used to provide the base features for mapping (e.g., roads, land ownership, DRGs). These data are not edited during the incident and should be readily accessible as minimum essential data sets for every SAR team. Minimum essential data sets are the layers needed to meet the business needs of maps and analyses during search operations for a given region. Incident data are layers created or edited in support of the incident. For missing person search operations, these might include the initial planning point (IPP), clues, search assignments, incident command assets, and more. For more information on this topic, refer to Durkee and Glynn-Linaris (2012) in the Reference section.

There are numerous map products that can be created on an incident, including IAP maps, briefing maps, and assignment maps, all of which might be useful in operations and by incident management teams (NWCG, 2014). Regardless of the type of map created, they should each include the following cartographic (map) elements as defined by the acronym STANDL (Scale, Title, Author, North arrow, Date of preparation, Legend):

- *Scale.* A graphical expression of a fixed distance (i.e., scale bar) is preferred. A textual description, such as 1:24,000 or 1inch = 1 mile is useful only if the map is printed at the desired output size. If a map is scanned or printed at different dimensions, only the graphical scale bar will work.
- *Title.* The basic description of the map, including items such as incident name, incident identifier, and map type. The title may also include the operation date for which the map was prepared and the operational period.
- *Author.* The person or group that prepared the map.
- *North arrow.* The graphical display used to orient the map correctly. This element could also include additional direction indicators for magnetic declination or grid angle.
- *Date of preparation.* The date appears near the author's name on the map. Software tools allow the automatic insertion of this element onto the map with minimal effort.
- *Legend.* The key that describes the meaning of the symbols found on the map.

Other elements that may need to be included are a source statement(s), a **graticule**, and the datum, especially if the map is intended to be used for navigational purposes. If it is believed the base map or base data may not represent current conditions in the field (e.g., new roads, changes in trail path, hazards), it should be explicitly stated on the map.

Compass

There are generally two different styles of compass: an **orienteering compass** (clear base plate) and a **lensatic compass** (military). The environment and the local team standards determine which compass will work best for a response. Regardless of the style, all compasses have similar basic features (**FIGURE 10-33**). Knowing the proper names for the parts of a compass is important when learning how to use it and when purchasing a compass for SAR.

A quality compass for use in SAR includes the following:

- *Base plate or base.* Clear, rectangular, and with various measurement markings and UMT scales. It is also beneficial to have a small magnifying glass in the base plate.
- *Bezel, dial, ring, or compass housing.* Marked clockwise in 360 degrees, in 2-degree increments.

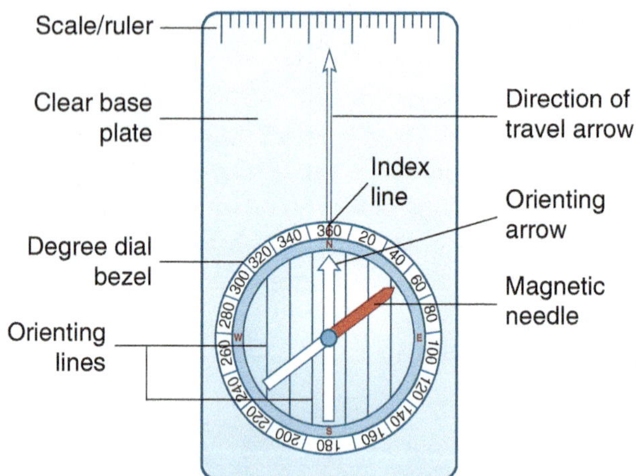

FIGURE 10-33 Knowing the proper names for the parts of a compass is important when learning how to use it.

- *Bearing/orienting lines.* Parallel lines within the bottom, center of the dial. These orienting lines are used with the map to obtain headings. Most compasses also have an outline of a compass needle, called an orienting arrow, also within the dial, or possibly two marks near the north end of the capsule. These items are used to align the magnetic needle with the orienting arrow so that an **azimuth** (**bearing**) can be followed.
- *Magnetic needle.* For most compasses, the red or colored end points toward magnetic north. The magnetic end of the needle may be indicated by a small luminous dot at the point of the needle. In a quality compass, the magnetic needle usually pivots on a jeweled bearing for smooth action. To help the needle move smoothly and settle quickly, the dial is filled with a non-freezing liquid.
- *Direction-of-travel arrow.* On most compasses, this is an arrow inscribed in the base plate of the compass, the base of which forms the index or lubber line. In higher quality compasses, this direction-of-travel arrow might be something as small as a small luminous mark near the front end of the compass. The direction-of-travel arrow must be pointing in the desired direction of travel while navigating.
- *Index line or lubber line.* Location where the degree reading (azimuth) is read, usually at the bottom of the direction-of-travel arrow. The index line is also called the *index mark.*
- *Sighting mirror.* A mirror, usually on the hinged cover of the compass, that has a fine line that runs from the top (near a rifle-like sight) to its bottom within the center of the mirror. This center line can also be an extension of the direction-of-travel arrow. Not all compasses have a sighting mirror. However, a higher quality compass with a sighting mirror is

recommended for SAR. This feature on your compass helps make more accurate sightings, plus the mirror might also be used for signaling during an emergency.

- *Grid lines in the base plate.* Quality compasses are available with 1:24,000 UTM and 1:62,500 UTM grids embedded in the base plate. This can be a very useful feature for SAR navigation.

The other category of compass is the lensatic compass. This is a good quality compass that is mostly used by the military. The lensatic compass is useful to those who already know how to use it; however, it may be difficult to use accurately, especially for a beginner.

There are many other kinds of compasses on the market, including some electronic varieties. These compasses have no moving parts, but the electronic units rely completely on batteries to function properly—a significant shortcoming. SAR personnel must first learn to use an orienteering-type compass before learning other navigational devices such as GPS and other types of compasses.

SEARCH AND RESCUE TIP

The environment and the local team standards determine which compass will work best for a response.

Navigating with a Compass

When first learning how to use a compass, it is important to remember good compass posture. To hold the compass for use, stand still with your arms comfortably at your sides, elbows bent so that both hands can hold the compass directly in front of your body. For most people, this position will have the compass at either chest-level or belt-level. The next step is to ensure that the direction-of-travel arrow is pointing in the same direction as your toes. To get where you want to go, your toes must always be pointing in the same direction as the direction-of-travel arrow on the compass. Hereafter, when you move the compass to a specific **heading**, move your entire body as a solid extension of the compass. Make sure that you hold the compass level so that the needle may move freely to settle on a direction.

For practice, try facing in the direction of 160 degrees. This is a three-step process:

1. Turn your compass bezel (dial ring) so that 160 degrees is on the index line.
2. Use good compass posture. Hold the compass level with the direction-of-travel arrow pointing in the same direction as your toes.
3. Turn your entire body and compass (as one unit) until the magnetic end of the floating needle is directly aligned over the pointed end of the orienteering arrow painted on the bottom, center of the bezel.

The magnetic needle will still point to magnetic north, but you will now be facing a magnetic heading of 160 degrees.

To determine the bearing of a distant object (e.g., radio tower, mountain peak) from you, do the following:

1. Use good compass posture. Hold the compass level with the direction-of-travel arrow pointing the same direction as your toes and turn your body until you are facing the distant object.
2. Turn your compass dial until the pointed end of the orienting arrow in the bottom center of the bezel is perfectly aligned under the pointed end of the magnetic needle.
3. Read the heading (number on the dial ring) at the index line at the base of the direction-of-travel arrow.

Be sure to check for anything near you, or on you, that might be metallic. Depending on how close you are to metallic items, the magnetic needle could be affected by the metal object(s). Keep these items away from your compass when it is in use: belt buckles, watches, jewelry, brass-colored objects (many have steel in them), eyeglasses, automobiles, frame packs, utensils, ink pens, whistles, radios, vehicles, mobile phones, and anything else metallic or magnetic. Note that power and telephone lines (anything conducting or producing electric current) can also cause deviation. Also, be aware that there are certain areas of the United States that have a high mineral content in the ground that can affect your compass. One such area located in Arkansas is appropriately named Magnet Cove.

When using a compass with a sighting mirror, use the same procedures, but the compass may have to be brought up to eye level to view distant objects using the sight. In doing so, it is still best to use both hands and keep the compass level. Most sighting mirrors have a fine line down the center that helps you align with the distant object. The mirror casing also has a "gun site" at the top of the mirror casing, which makes it easier to sight the distant object. When the sight, direction-of-travel arrow, your toes, and the image of the index line are all aligned, any object viewed through the sight is directly on the heading set on the compass.

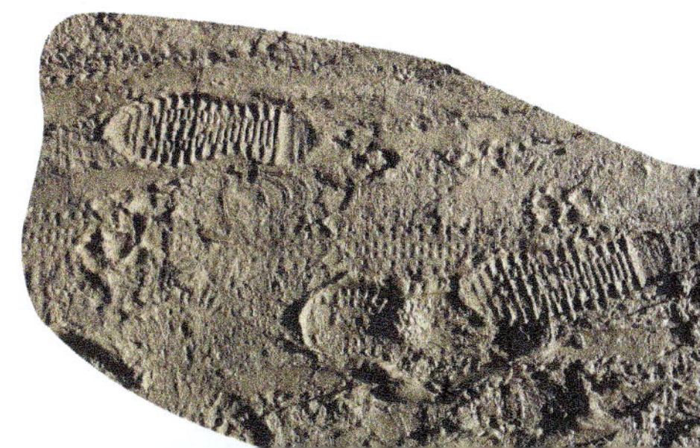

SEARCH AND RESCUE TIP

Remember that the magnetic needle of a compass is influenced by metallic objects such as belt buckles, watches, whistles, and radios. It can also be affected by anything producing an electric current, as well as ground containing a high mineral content.

Cardinal directions are those directions that correspond to bearings that are multiples of 90 degrees. North is either "0" or 360 degrees, east is 90 degrees, south is 180 degrees, and west is 270 degrees. **Intercardinal directions** fall between cardinal directions (i.e., northwest falls between north and west, southeast falls between south and east, etc.). If you are familiar with the cardinal directions in relationship to your position, it is easier to estimate direction of travel.

Occasionally, the term **back azimuth** is used to describe a direction that is 180 degrees from one's azimuth, bearing, or heading. This is simply another way of indicating the direction opposite one's direction of travel.

When in the field, SAR personnel should always know where north is located, with or without a compass. This provides a constant awareness of one's direction of travel and may come in handy should improvisational navigation be required.

Following a Heading

Following a lengthy compass heading through rough terrain can be challenging and requires practice. To follow a heading over some distance, do the following:

1. Once you have selected a heading, with the direction-of-travel arrow and your toes facing the direction that you wish to travel, sight an object in the distance. The object, such as a distinctive tree, rock, or other unique feature, must be something that is attainable, immovable, and visible.
2. Once you have confirmed your object in the distance, close your eyes for just a few seconds. Then, open your eyes to reconfirm that you can easily find your object again.
3. Reconfirm your heading to that object and lower your compass. Now, simply walk to the object. The route you take to the object is irrelevant. You can meander as much as you like as long as you can always see your target object. Once you arrive at your object, repeat the process with another distant object. Continue to repeat the process until you reach your destination. Generally, the farther away the sighted object is, the more accurate the heading will be over a long distance. The closer the sighted object is, the less accurate the heading will be over a long distance.

Traveling a long distance on a compass bearing can be challenging but gets easier with practice. The real challenge is searching well while moving between objects and navigating around obstacles and over rough terrain. Thus, in SAR, competent navigation becomes a critical and necessary secondary skill without which your primary purpose (searching) could not be accomplished. Navigation with a map and compass must become so easy and natural to SAR personnel that they can safely focus on other issues—such as finding the lost subject.

Using Map and Compass Together

When using an orienteering compass with a map, the compass is used primarily as a **protractor** and ruler. The 360-degree dial—in association with the orienting lines in the base of the bezel—serves as the protractor, and the straight sides of the rectangular base plate serve as a straight edge. When using the compass as a protractor, the magnetic needle can be completely ignored. A map grid reader, such as is shown in Figure 10-2A, can also be used as a protractor.

To determine the heading from one point to another on the map, place the compass on the map so that one edge of the base plate touches both the starting point and the destination, with the **direction-of-travel arrow** pointing in the direction of the destination. Then, turn the dial ring until the orienting arrow, with the arrow pointing north, is parallel to the nearest north-south meridian. The heading from the starting point to the destination is now indicated on the dial ring at the index line. Remember not to use the red township and range lines on a topographic map for navigation, as they are not true north/south or true east/west lines.

The scales on the bottom margin of the map can be used to measure distance on the map. On a 1:24,000 scale map, 1 inch on the map equals 24,000 inches (or 2,000 feet) in the terrain. To get the distance in feet in the terrain, measure the inches on the map and multiply by 2000. The bar scale can also be used directly by marking on the edge of a piece of paper the distance between two points on the map. Then, measure it against the bar scale in the bottom margin of the map (**FIGURE 10-34** and **FIGURE 10-35**). The base plate on the compass or the compass lanyard, in lieu of the paper, also works well.

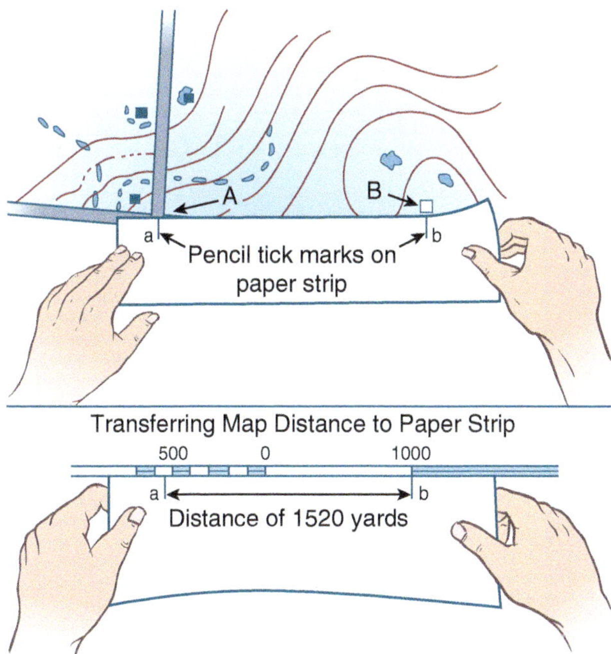

FIGURE 10-34 Measuring straight line map distances. Use a ruler, a piece of paper, a lanyard, or a ruler edge of a compass to indicate distance, then compare it to the map scale.

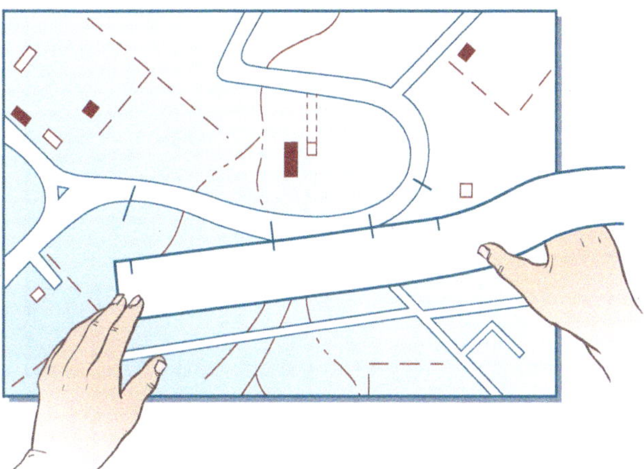

FIGURE 10-35 Measuring curved line distances.

Adjusting for Magnetic Declination

The geographic North Pole and the magnetic North Pole are not at the same location. The geographic North Pole is the northernmost point on the Earth, geodetic latitude 90 degrees north, where all lines of longitude converge, and the basis for "true" north. In contrast, the magnetic North Pole is in the northern hemisphere where the Earth's magnetic field points vertically downwards. Unlike the geographic North Pole that remains stationary and does not move, the magnetic North Pole moves over time due to magnetic changes in the Earth's core. The angle between the direction the magnetic needle points (magnetic north) and true north is called *declination*. Due to the geology of the Earth, the magnetic needle on a compass points to the North Pole (true north) only when the compass is along a line in the United States that (as of 2004) generally runs from just east of New Orleans, through the middle of Alabama and the eastern tip of Arkansas, through eastern Iowa and eastern Missouri, through eastern Minnesota and western Wisconsin, and up to the magnetic north pole just north of Hudson Bay. This line along which a compass needle points to both true north and magnetic north is called the *agonic* line (**FIGURE 10-36**). East of this line, a compass needle points west of true north (west or negative declination); west of this line, a compass needle points east of true north (east or positive declination). In the United States, declination varies from 20° west in Maine to 30° east in parts of Alaska. The declination diagram in the bottom margin of a topo map indicates the declination in the center of the map at the time the map was printed (**FIGURE 10-37**).

If you know the magnetic declination of the area in which you will be navigating, you have four options:

1. Ignore it.
2. Adjust for it on the compass.
3. Adjust for it by drawing magnetic meridians (north-south lines) on the map.
4. Adjust for it mathematically.

Ignore It

In some situations, magnetic declination can be ignored altogether. When using a compass without a map, all references should be made to magnetic north, so declination is irrelevant. If you are operating on the agonic line (see previous section) where the angle between magnetic declination and true north is zero, magnetic declination can be ignored even when using a map and a compass together.

The same philosophy may be applied when the compass being used has 2-degree increments on the dial ring and you are operating in an area with a declination of less than 1 degree. The level of accuracy at which you are navigating makes adjusting for small declinations unnecessary. The inverse is also true: If your compass is extremely accurate and has 0.5-degree increments on the dial, and you are using the compass with a map, corrections should be made for even the smallest magnetic declination.

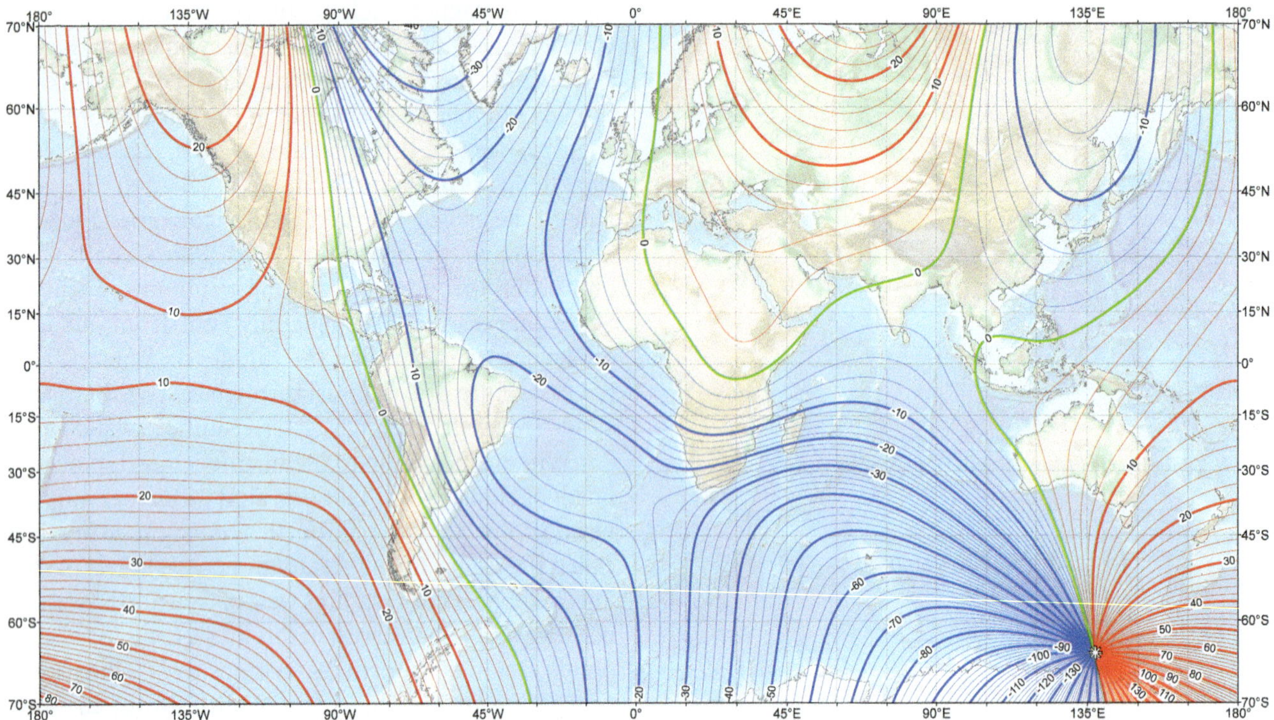

FIGURE 10-36 Approximate magnetic declination around the Earth in 2010. The green lines are agonic lines on which declination is zero.

Courtesy of the National Centers for Environmental Information, formerly the National Geophysical Data Center.

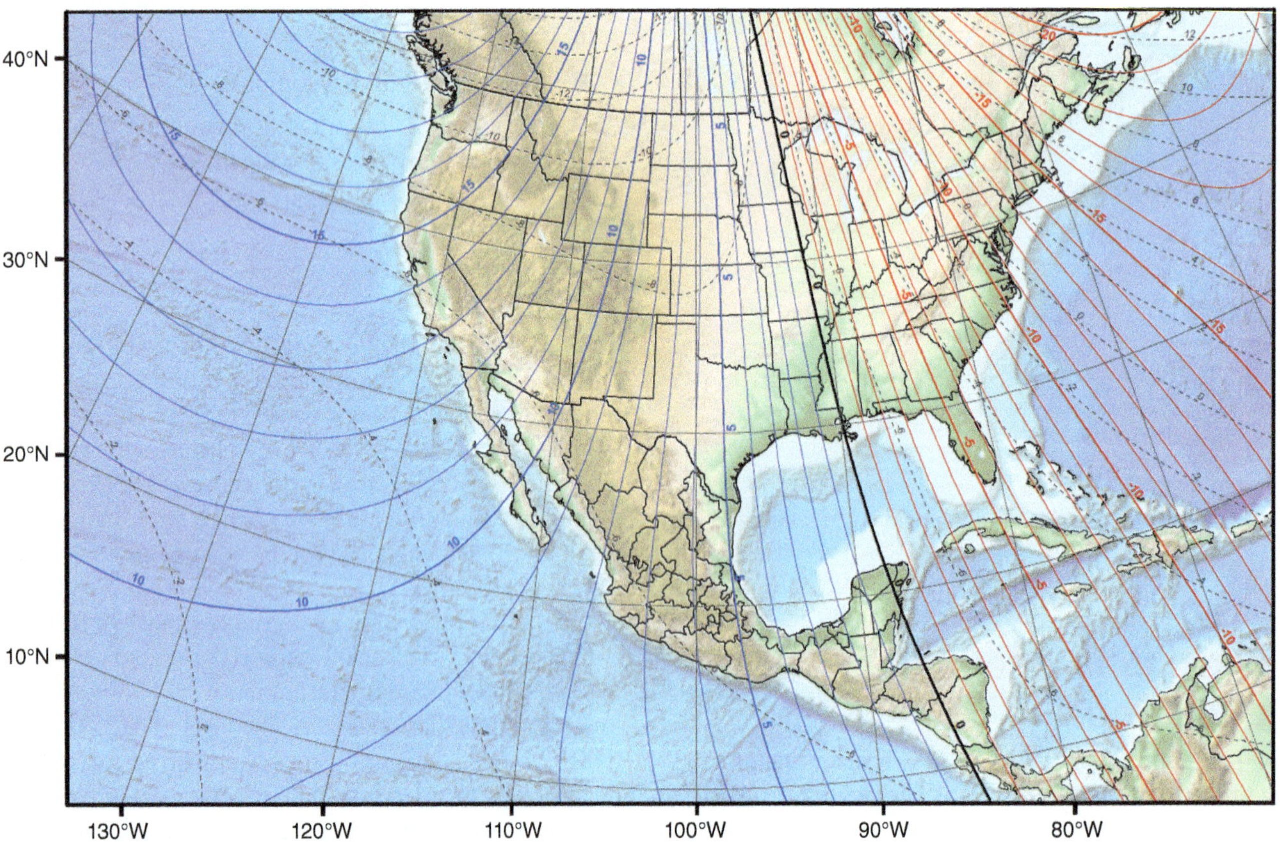

FIGURE 10-37 Approximate magnetic declination in North America in 2010. The dark black line that passes through Minnesota, Iowa, Missouri, Arkansas, and Mississippi is the agonic line on which declination is zero.

Courtesy of the National Geophysical Data Center, produced from the World Magnetic Model (WMM), 2010.

TABLE 10-2 Correcting for Magnetic Declination

	East Declination	West Declination
Map to Compass	Subtract declination	Add declination
Compass to Map	Add declination	Subtract declination

Adjust the Compass

Some compasses have a small screw on them that allow the user to adjust the compass for declination. This is a simple and easy method of adjusting for declination that is often used in SAR. What adjusting the compass does is offset the orienting arrow and the index line in the base of the bezel just enough to compensate for declination when the compass is used as a protractor with a map. Once adjusted, the orienting arrow in the bezel is no longer parallel to the orienting lines. A scale marked in the bezel allows the index line to be offset in relation to the orienting lines for the precise amount and direction of magnetic declination.

Make sure to check the adjustment on the compass each time it is used with a map and every time you travel to another area that might have a different declination.

Draw Magnetic Meridians on the Map

Another way to account for magnetic declination is to prepare the map by adding magnetic north lines to it. If magnetic north-south lines are drawn on the map, the magnetic needle on a compass will point to the north end of the lines drawn on the map. Adding these lines requires a protractor, a long straight edge, and the angle of declination. On computer-generated topo maps, the lines can be added with a click of the mouse. Because of the difficulty in accomplishing this manually, especially with multiple maps, this method is not recommended for SAR. In addition, since the map probably has UTM grid lines on it, adding the magnetic lines could make the map difficult to use because of too many lines.

If this method is used, the actual angle in the magnetic declination diagram in the bottom margin of the map must not be used as the basis for the magnetic meridians. The USGS, which produces the topo maps, specifically warns against this method. They claim that the angle of the declination diagram is meant to show only relative directions of true, grid, and magnetic north, not the actual angles. In addition, magnetic declination varies over time, and the declination diagram may be obsolete.

Mathematical Correction

Mathematically adjusting a bearing to compensate for magnetic declination is another option. To use this method, you must first know if the declination is east or west. Determine this by inspecting the declination diagram in the bottom margin of your map. If the "MN" is to the left of the star in the diagram, the declination is west. If the "MN" is to the right of the star in the diagram, the declination is east. Next, you must determine if you are going from the map to the compass (e.g., plotting a bearing based on the true north lines on the map, then using the bearing to navigate with a compass) or going from the compass to the map (e.g., taking a bearing with a compass then plotting it on the map). This combination gives you four options for mathematically correcting for magnetic declination, and each of the four options has a rule for correcting for declination (**TABLE 10-2**). Since most SAR personnel are unlikely to use both easterly and westerly declinations—they mostly stay on one side of the agonic line or the other—the rules necessary to mathematically correct for declination are usually reduced to two.

The simplicity of the rules makes remembering them easy, but the similarity between the options also makes it likely that they may be confused with each other. Worse, using the wrong set of rules (adding when you should have subtracted) doubles the error of declination. It is recommended that a small note be added to one's map case or compass that includes the two rules most likely to be used, or just copy Table 10-2, reduce it in size, cut it out, and attach it to your map case or compass. This precludes the need to remember the various rules and reduce the chances of error.

Declination Correction Examples. Here are two examples of using the magnetic declination adjustment rules to correct the magnetic declination:

> *Example 1:* You are in the western United States. In the bottom margin of your map, you note that the declination diagram indicates that the magnetic declination is 4 degrees east. You plot a **course** on the map from point A to point B using true north and determine that the bearing is 100 degrees (true). What is the bearing you would follow in the field to travel from point A to point B? Using the magnetic declination adjustment rules found in Table 10-2, you determine that the declination is east, and you are going from

the map to the compass, so the rule that applies is to "subtract declination." Since the map course was 100 degrees, and the declination is 4 degrees east, the magnetic course to follow in the field is a bearing of 96 degrees (100 – 4 = 96).

Example 2: You are in the eastern United States. The declination diagram indicates that the magnetic declination is 9 degrees west. You follow a compass heading of 355 degrees (magnetic) to travel from a church to a distant peak. Arriving at the peak, you note that there are many similar peaks in the area, and you want to determine which one on the map you are on. You want to draw a line on the map that indicates the route you just traveled. Using the magnetic declination adjustment rules found in Table 10-2, you determine that the declination is west, and you are going from the compass to the map, so the rule that applies is to "subtract declination." The corrected bearing for the map would be 346 degrees (355 – 9 = 346). Using your compass as a protractor, enter 346 degrees at the index line of the compass. With the direction-of-travel arrow pointing from the church to the peak on the map and the edge of the compass base plate next to the church, turn the entire compass (base plate and all) until the orienting lines in the compass bezel are aligned with the true north lines on the map. Draw a line from the church along the edge of the compass base plate. The peak on which you stand is on that line.

When adjusting for declination, it is very important that it be compensated for properly (according to one of the accepted methods described above) and only ONCE. Accounting for declination twice is just as bad as accounting for it improperly. Be very careful and practice often.

SEARCH AND RESCUE TIP

Orient your map by turning it so that north on the map points to north in the landscape.

Using the Map and Compass in the Field

An important step in using a map as a guide in the field is to orient it. Orienting the map means turning it so that north on the map points to north in the landscape. Once this is done, the terrain and human-made features on the map should align with the same features in the field. To do this, inspect the map and the surrounding landscape and, using a compass to help determine when you are facing north, turn your body while holding the map until the compass, map, and landscape all match. This can also be done while turning the map and compass on the ground (**FIGURE 10-38**).

It also may be useful to determine your exact location on the map. Either of two approaches should work to determine your location, depending on your situation: observation and resection (triangulation).

In the observation or inspection method, simply visually identify features or landmarks in the landscape by looking around. Then, slowly turn the map around until the features on the map match the features within sight of where you are standing (**FIGURE 10-39**).

In the resection method, a compass is required but the method starts the same way: Look around and identify features or landmarks in the landscape around you. Then, determine the bearing from your location to the feature/landmark you see (**FIGURE 10-40**).

Map Orientation With Compass

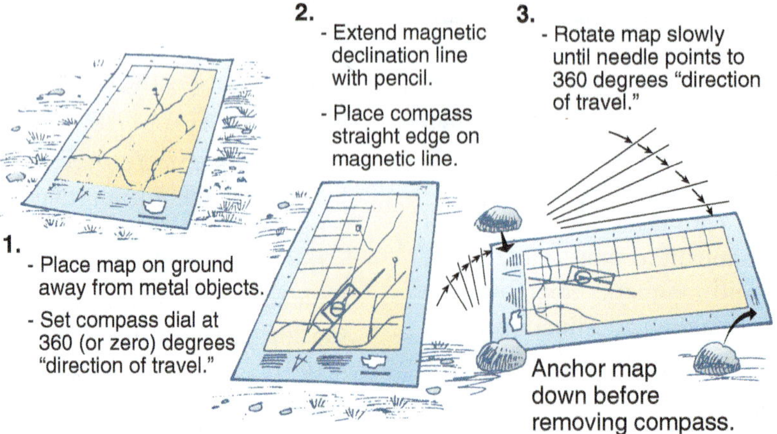

FIGURE 10-38 Orienting the map to the surrounding landscape using a compass.

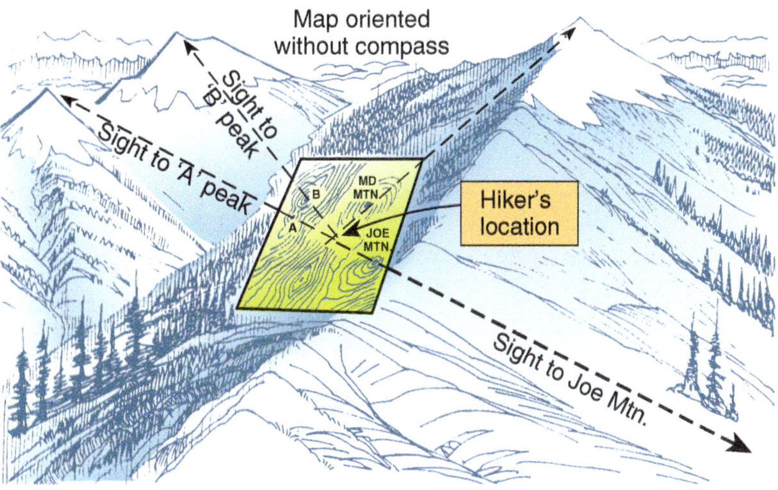

FIGURE 10-39 Determining your position on the map without a compass, through observation of prominent features or landmarks in the terrain.

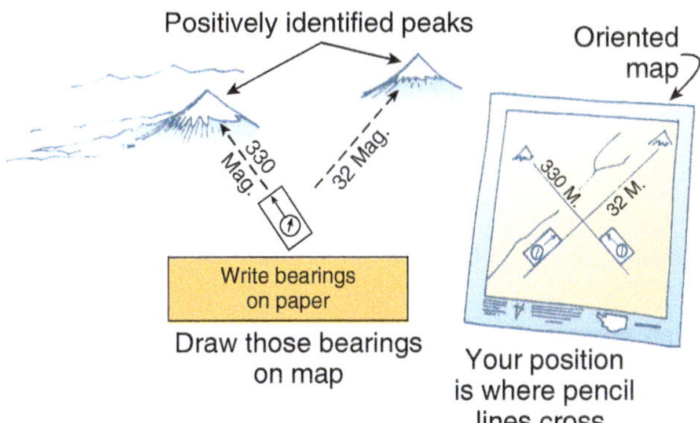

FIGURE 10-40 Determining your position using a compass and map together (resection). Using three prominent points can add accuracy to the position.

Let us assume that the bearing is 70 degrees (magnetic) to a radio tower on a nearby mountain peak and try an example.

Leave the heading of 70 degrees on your compass and place the compass (now used as a protractor and ignoring the magnetic needle) on the map with the edge of the base plate immediately next to the distant object (tower on mountain). While keeping the edge of the base plate on the map next to the tower, pivot the edge of the compass around the tower until the orienteering lines in the bottom of the bezel are aligned with the north-south grid lines on the map. When using this method, the orienting arrow on the compass should always be pointing to the top (north) of the map. Once everything is aligned, draw a line with the edge of the compass through the distant object (the tower in this example). Your location is somewhere on this line. To narrow down your location on this line, select another distant object that is approximately 90 degrees from the first object you chose. For our example, let us assume you also see a water tower at a bearing of 160 degrees. Follow the same procedure as you did with the first distant object and draw a second line on the map. The intersection of the two lines is very close to your location on the map. For greater accuracy, take bearings to three objects or landmarks.

Other Compass Skills

Traveling at night with a compass presents many of the same problems as traveling through dense underbrush. Using a flashlight properly with a compass at night can simplify things substantially, and using a flashlight improperly at night can hinder the most skilled navigator. A dim, wide-beamed light can be held underneath the base of the compass, pointed primarily in the direction of travel, to allow some light for reading the compass at night. However, care must be taken not to shine the light in anyone's eyes. When the needle is aligned with the orienteering arrow, the light can be directed in the direction of travel where an object can be sighted. Some compasses also have a small light integrated into the compass. The light is small and just the right size to easily see the heading while not disturbing night vision.

Traveling around obstacles is often necessary in the field when using a compass for navigation. The easiest way to travel around an obstacle, such as a lake, pond, cliff, or other hazard, is to sight an object beyond the

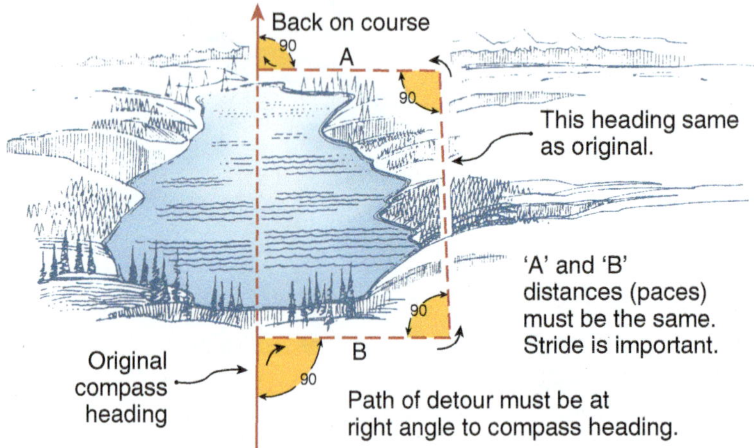

FIGURE 10-41 Navigating accurately around obstacles. Take a 90° turn right or left of the obstacle. Count paces until you are clear of the obstacle (B). Resume the original bearing until you are past the obstacle. Take a 90° turn opposite of the first turn and walk the exact same distance you did to clear the obstacle (A). Continue on the original bearing.

obstacle and then travel to that object by the easiest route possible. This approach, however, is limited to those obstacles that can be seen over or through. When obstacles cannot be seen over or through, a completely new course may be required, or a method similar to the one in **FIGURE 10-41** can be used.

Measuring Distance by Stride: Tally

A method of estimating distance in the field may be required for some situations in SAR. Distance can be estimated by knowing the length of one's stride and multiplying it by the number of strides walked.

Being able to estimate distance traveled in the field can be of value in several situations that often arise in SAR. For instance, estimating distance can be of value when a mapped object or area is a known distance from a starting point (measured from a map) and searchers want to know when, in their travels, to start looking for the object or area. Also, being able to estimate how far a clue was found from the start of a search might be valuable during debriefing.

The English term *mile* is derived from a Roman term meaning "1000 Roman Paces" or double steps. The Romans considered the pace to be five times the length of a Roman legionnaire's foot and, thus, the Roman mile was 5,000 feet. It wasn't until much later that the English mile was redefined as 5,280 feet.

One step is the distance one walks when measured from one foot to the other. A stride, on the other hand, is equivalent to two steps, or the distance between where one foot strikes the ground and where the same foot strikes the ground again. The Roman stride was nearly 6 feet, but the average stride today is usually considered 5 feet on level, unencumbered ground. Stride varies depending on many variables such as leg length, terrain, weather, darkness, fitness, and many others.

Measuring your stride is sometimes referred to as *finding your tally*. To find your tally, you need to set up a course in your local terrain and practice. Use a long piece of string and measuring tape to set up a meandering route in the woods of some easily remembered distance such as 50 meters or 100 feet. It is important not to use a straight-line course because your stride needs to naturally adjust for low branches, thick underbrush, and other natural obstacles. Walk the string route several times over several days, and keep track of the number of strides it takes to cover the course. Walk the route with your 24-hour pack in the morning while you are still energetic, and then also walk the route with your pack in the late afternoon after several hours of hiking or other physical exercise. Once you have completed the course several times, under several conditions, take the number of strides for each trial and obtain an average (add up the total strides and divide the sum by the number of trials. This is your personal tally for determining distances in your terrain. If your course was 100 feet long and it took an average of 20 strides to cover the course, your tally is 20 strides for 100 feet, or 5 feet per stride.

Strides can vary substantially from one individual to another, so it is important for individuals to know their own personal stride length. Once one's stride has been determined, a method of counting strides over long distances becomes necessary. To do this, some have tied knots in string every 100 strides to keep all counting less than 100. Moving pebbles from one hand or pocket to another every 100 strides, moving beads on a string, and other similar techniques have also been used. In SAR, especially when accurate count is important, a good method is to carry a small hand counter (also known as an inventory counter) and use it to count strides, or every 10 strides, or every 100, etc.

Applying counted strides from the field to a map is not always as simple as it seems. A person's stride changes in different terrain. Tall grass, uphill, downhill, sand, rocks, and other types of terrain affect one's stride. A topo map shows only a two-dimensional view of an area. In steep areas, horizontal distances on a map may not equal traveling distances in the field.

These and many other problems are significant considerations when estimating distance, but, unfortunately, no easy answer exists. Many rules of thumb have been proposed, but it is probably better if all SAR workers simply keep records of their traveling, estimate their personal differences, and make their own conversions for field work.

One appointed tally person per team can constantly keep track of distance traveled from a starting point. This can be valuable when estimating where in a search segment a clue is found, for example, or anytime a rough estimate of distance traveled is desired. Because of how much concentration it takes to constantly count strides during a search, it may not be prudent to ask only one person to keep the tally, operate the radio, and navigate simultaneously.

Global Positioning System

The global positioning system (GPS) is a space-based radio-navigation system consisting of a constellation of satellites and a network of ground stations used for monitoring and control. SAR team members often use a handheld GPS receiver to display their coordinates and the route they have taken on a handheld device. However, GPS is a complex system capable of providing great benefit to SAR operations if used correctly. If GPS is used incorrectly, especially in conjunction with the communication of coordinate based locations, it can create an unsafe condition for rescuers and be detrimental to SAR operations. It is also important to recognize that this is a technology that is always evolving, especially with introduction of complementary technology such as GPS receivers embedded in mobile devices (e.g., smartphones and tablets) and wireless communication infrastructure that provide location-based services. Here we present the basics of how GPS works and how it is commonly used in SAR operations.

A minimum of 24 GPS satellites orbit the Earth, providing users with accurate information on position, velocity, and time anywhere in the world and in all weather conditions. GPS is operated and maintained by the U.S. Department of Defense (DoD).

GPS has three parts: the space segment, the user segment, and the control segment. The space segment consists of at least 24 satellites, each in its own orbit altitude of approximately 12,550 miles above the Earth. Each of the GPS satellites takes 12 hours to orbit the Earth. The user segment consists of receivers, which you can hold in your hand or mount in your vehicle. The control segment consists of one master control station, an alternate master control station, 12 command and control antennas, and 16 monitoring sites. This array of control stations tracks the GPS satellites and confirms that they are in proper working order.

The principle behind GPS is the measurement of distance (or range) between the receiver and the satellites. The satellites also specify exactly where they are in their orbits above the Earth. If the exact distance from a satellite in space is known, then we are somewhere on the surface of an imaginary sphere with radius equal to the distance to the satellite radius. If the exact distance from two satellites is known, then we are located somewhere on the line where the two spheres intersect, but when there is a third measurement from a satellite, there are only two possible points where we could be located. One of these is usually impossible, and the GPS receivers have mathematical methods of eliminating the impossible location.

The GPS satellites are positioned in orbit so that signals from six of them should be received nearly 100% of the time at any point on Earth. Signals from six satellites are required to get the very best position information. GPS satellites are equipped with very precise clocks that keep accurate time to within 3 nanoseconds, which is three billionths of a second. This precision timing is important because the receiver must determine exactly how long it takes for signals to travel from each GPS satellite to calculate its position. To measure precise latitude, longitude, and altitude, the receiver measures the time it took for the signals from a minimum of four separate satellites to get to the receiver.

For the system to accurately establish position, altitude, and velocity, the receiver must "acquire" four satellites. The acquisition of signals from three satellites can convey one's position on the Earth's surface, but a fourth signal is required for altitude information. "Acquire" means that the unobstructed signals from four satellites need to be received by the receiver. For

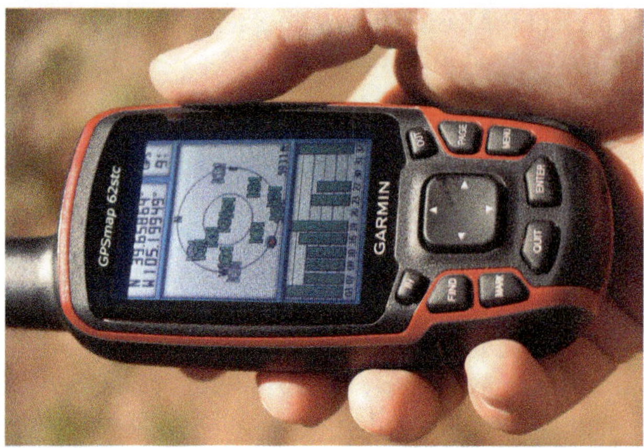

FIGURE 10-42 Example of GPS unit used in SAR (Garmin GPSmap 62stc) showing its satellite page.
Courtesy of Jarod Doke.

this to happen, there must be four satellites above the horizon above the receiver; the system is designed to achieve this everywhere on Earth. Because the GPS signal is in the 1 GHz (gigahertz, or 1000 megahertz) range, terrain (e.g., trees, hills, buildings), the metal from a vehicle (e.g., car roof, airplane fuselage, boat cabin), and even the human body can block the signal and make acquisition difficult or impossible. Clear, line-of-sight access between the receiver's antenna and the satellites is necessary for best results. Keep this in mind if you are trying to obtain GPS signals from a deep ravine or in a forest with heavy tree cover.

The GPS system can tell you your location anywhere on or above the Earth to within about 300 feet. Even greater accuracy, usually within less than 3 feet, can be obtained with corrections calculated by a GPS receiver at a known fixed location.

GPS receivers can be hand carried or installed on aircraft, ships, tanks, submarines, cars, and trucks. These receivers detect, decode, and process GPS satellite signals. The typical handheld receiver is about the size of an old cellular telephone, but the newer models are even smaller (**FIGURE 10-42**).

Handheld GPS units are used by outdoor enthusiasts as well as SAR teams. However, it is critical to note the applications and limitations of such units before purchasing or using one in the field. The many challenges involved in the use of GPS by untrained personnel include the following:

- The device requires line-of-sight to the satellites and does not work in all terrains (e.g., deep canyons, heavy tree canopy, urban environment with tall buildings).
- GPS should not be used as the sole navigation device; it should complement other conventional approaches to navigation.
- The less than perfect accuracy is not always acceptable, especially for altitude.
- Human error (input error) is always a possibility.
- The position display can easily be misread, and the display can give the impression of far greater accuracy than the device is capable of producing.
- Especially considering today's GPS technology, which requires great current consumption, batteries can fail at any time. Typical battery life of most GPS units is between four and six hours.
- Many GPS units are not waterproof and require special protection during bad weather. The GPS units also need additional protection if crossing streams or near other water sources.

It is important to note that the GPS receiver is simply another tool in the land navigation skill tool box, and it should never be considered a substitute for map and/or compass knowledge. In the hands of a skilled navigator, a GPS unit can provide significant benefits in the areas of expediency, precision, documentation, and reference. GPS is dependent on multiple variables, many of which are beyond the control of the user; these include power supply (batteries), satellite integrity, and signal strength. If one of these elements were to fail or be substantially weakened, the operator would be required to rely completely on alternate navigational skills. Regardless of the GPS equipment used and available, SAR personnel must be well versed in map and compass skills prior to use of a GPS unit.

SAFETY TIP

A GPS unit is a very precise and beneficial tool but has limitations outside the control of the user. Therefore, a GPS unit should never be considered a substitute for map and compass skills.

The information contained herein is of a general nature and pertains to no specific model or type of GPS unit. The intention is to provide general information that is pertinent to most available models. It is highly recommended that SAR personnel attend a hands-on GPS training program and practice with GPS units in an outdoor setting before using the unit in a real-world SAR operation.

Common Components and Nomenclature

Although there are a variety of GPS units made by various companies, they all possess common components that are integral to their function.

Battery

Most GPS units take either two or four AA batteries that are housed in a plastic casing located in the base or back of the unit. GPS unit instruction manuals may state that the unit is "water resistant" or "waterproof." Read the specifications to determine the limits of each unit. While any appropriately sized batteries will work in the GPS unit, alkaline batteries generally produce the best results. Ni-cad and NiMH batteries are convenient because they are rechargeable; however, the rechargeable type of batteries usually do not have the full power of the alkaline batteries, plus the rechargeable batteries require the use of a charger. The more expensive lithium batteries may provide the best performance in cold-weather operations.

Always keep batteries stored at room temperature when not in use. It is also a good idea to carry at least one extra set of batteries as a backup. When outdoors, store the unit and spare batteries near the body within layers of clothing to avoid exposure to extreme cold or heat. In the event the batteries become very cold, re-warm them before use to avoid reduction in battery life. This can be done by holding the batteries in the palm of your hand for several minutes prior to use. Some GPS units may have an internal memory battery to retain information while the normal batteries are removed. These backup batteries recharge automatically when the regular batteries are replaced. This process takes approximately 24 hours if the backup battery is completely drained. Memory batteries usually have a lifespan of about three months; after this time, all user information and the almanac will be lost until the unit has reacquired a satellite signal and the information is renewed. Most of the newest generation GPS units do not require a backup battery because the data are stored in nonvolatile memory.

To limit the number and weight of the batteries, it would be wise to choose a GPS unit that uses the same battery as your light sources.

Keypad

On many of the older style GPS units the keypad is placed on the face, whereas some of the newer models have placed many of the keys or buttons along the sides. Most of the keys are adorned with a short label or some type of icon to signify its function, and many of the keys are also multifunctional. This means that a specific number of keystrokes can control a specific function or depressing a key for a specified period of time can access another function. For example, pressing a key one time may display a certain menu, whereas pressing the same key two times in succession displays another. The interface keys are so diverse from one unit to the next that it is best to refer to the instruction manual to determine the functions associated with each key. If possible, try to find a unit that has a safety on the "on" button to help keep the GPS unit from being turned on by accident while in your pack.

Some of the newer GPS models use a touch screen interface; however, these units may be difficult to operate in the cold or while wearing thick winter gloves.

Antenna

Almost all handheld GPS units house an internal antenna and provide the option of a plug-in external antenna. The antenna receives information called **ephemeris** from satellites in the form of a two-spread spectrum radio frequency signal (~1575 MHz). The antenna is often housed in the top of the GPS unit. Any obstruction between the antenna and the satellite may degrade the signal quality and hinder accuracy or proper functioning. This kind of signal degradation is often referred to as antenna masking. Reception is best at high elevations with 360 degrees of visibility; however, this does not mean that your GPS does not work while in densely forested areas. It is important to note that foliage does degrade signal quality and hence may lengthen acquisition time, possibly increase the estimated position error (EPE), and slow down ephemeris updates. Also note that if you are trying to use your GPS in a steep canyon or an area of heavy foliage, it is more than likely that the antenna cannot receive appropriate signals from satellites for a correct display.

Satellite Characteristics

It is not necessary to know everything about the satellites to use a GPS unit properly, but some basic information may be useful, especially as it relates to terms that are frequently used to describe the GPS system.

Selective Availability

Before May 2000, all civilian GPS units received satellite information that contained built-in errors that limited accuracy. This error was designed for security reasons and was referred to as selective availability (SA). The use of SA has now been discontinued, so theoretically all GPS units can now achieve an accuracy of approximately 12 to 15 meters horizontal and vertical.

Differential GPS

Differential GPS (DGPS) is a method of improving the accuracy of a GPS receiver by adding a local reference station to augment the information available from the satellites. It also improves the integrity of the entire GPS system by identifying certain errors. The estimated accuracy while using DGPS is approximately 3 to 5 meters horizontal and vertical. In DGPS operation, a station, often called a beacon, transmits correction data in real time that is received by a separate box, called a beacon receiver, which in turn sends the correction information to the GPS receiver.

Wide Area Augmentation System

The Wide Area Augmentation System (WAAS) is the latest method of providing improved accuracy from the GPS system. It is similar in principle to the DGPS capability that is built into most of the recent GPS units, except that a second receiver is not required. Instead of a beacon receiver, the correction data are sent via a geostationary satellite and are decoded by one of the regular channels already present in the GPS receiver. Thus, up to two of the 12 channels can be designated to decode regular GPS signals or can be used to decode the WAAS data. This works using a set of ground stations all over the United States that collect correction data relative to the area of the country where they are located. All data are then packaged together, analyzed, converted to a digital correction format by a master station, and then uploaded to the geostationary satellite, which in turn transmits the data down to the GPS receiver. The GPS receiver then figures out which data are applicable to its current location and then applies the appropriate corrections to the receiver.

The WAAS system is still being set up and will be improved with more satellites in the future (possibly dozens worldwide). Because of the type of satellites used, a clear view of the southern sky is required to benefit from WAAS from the northern hemisphere. This means WAAS units are very useful on an airplane or perhaps a boat, but they may be less useful to someone on the ground with a limited view of the horizon.

Global Navigation Satellite System

An alternative to the familiar GPS is the global navigation satellite system (GLONASS), a space-based satellite navigation system operated by the Russian military (Federal Space Agency, Information-Analytical Centre, 2015). It also has global coverage and comparable precision. At the time of this writing, this system had at least 24 satellites, which may add an additional ability to acquire coverage in areas with obstruction (e.g., buildings, tall trees, canyons). Be sure to read the specifications for your GPS receiver to see if it can take advantage of both GPS and GLONASS.

GPS Unit Screen Pages

Most GPS units display information in the form of screen "pages." Although various manufacturers display their pages slightly differently, they all have certain characteristics in common.

Satellite Page

The satellite page is usually the first functional screen or page to be displayed by the GPS unit (see Figure 10-42). Although the satellite page varies from unit to unit, most GPS satellite screens are similar. Some of the newer GPS units display more information, and a select few display less. The purpose of the satellite screen is to convey the current status of the connection between the GPS receiver and the GPS satellites.

Receiver Status. The receiver status is the current type of satellite lock or mode. There are several messages that could be displayed to give the user a better idea of the current status of their GPS unit. These messages include:

- *Searching*. Unit is currently searching the sky for satellites.
- *AutoLocate*. Unit is collecting new almanac data.
- *Acquiring*. Unit is collecting data prior to its first lock.
- *2D Nav*. Unit has a lock on horizontal position and is looking for a three-dimensional lock.
- *3D Nav*. Unit has a lock on both the horizontal and vertical positions and is tracking normally.
- *2D Diff*. Unit has the two-dimensional lock using DGPS data.
- *3D Diff*. Unit has the three-dimensional lock using DGPS data.
- *Not Usable*. Unit was not able to compute a solution.
- *Poor Coverage*. Unit is attempting to compute a position but is having difficulty.
- *Enter Altitude*. Unit is requesting the user to input the approximate altitude to aid in acquiring a signal.
- *Simulator*. Unit is in simulator mode.

Battery Life. There is a graphic representation of the battery life based on alkaline batteries, with the exception of a select few GPS units that allow the user to define the battery type. Some units do not display the battery life if connected to an external power source, while others may display a full battery. Many newer units have placed this feature on a different page.

Satellite Signal Strength. A bar graph represents the signal quality between particular satellites and the GPS receiver. The numbers on the bottom of the graph represent the individual satellites. The bars above each satellite number correspond to the signal strength of that satellite. If no bars are displayed, then no connection has been established. If a hollow bar is displayed, the receiver has found the satellite and is collecting data from it. When a solid bar is displayed, the receiver has collected data (ephemeris) from the satellite. Some GPS units have slight variations in their display. For example, a select few units use solid bars to identify when the receiver has acquired the satellite and a hollow bar to signify that it has collected the ephemeris. For almost all 12-channel GPS units, 12 openings are displayed in the bar graph. The receiver attempts to acquire all 12 satellites but chooses the best four satellites from which to collect information. If the receiver is WAAS enabled, it may leave two openings strictly for WAAS satellites. Currently, WAAS satellites are distinguishable by a number designation above 32.

Satellite Position. This diagram depicts the relative location of each satellite within range. When a GPS unit is first turned on, these satellites are arranged in accordance to the receiver's location and built-in almanac (stored data). The almanac is fairly accurate if the receiver has acquired near the location before. This is often referred to as a warm start. If the user has traveled more than 300 to 500 miles with the unit off, then the almanac may have significant errors, and the receiver may take longer to acquire. In many cases, the GPS unit prompts the user to redefine the general location to aid in acquisition (a cold start). The unit's satellite almanac updates once the GPS has collected ephemeris. Each satellite in the diagram is represented by its respective number and corresponds with the number shown in the satellite signal strength bar graph. The concentric circles represent the relative position of the satellites in the sky. The top of the screen typically represents north, so satellites represented at the bottom of the screen would be south of the receiver's current position. Some models allow control over where north is represented. The center of the diagram represents directly overhead, the first circle beyond the center denotes 45 degrees above the horizon, and the final circle corresponds to the horizon itself. In the sample page, above satellite 09 would be on the southeast horizon.

Estimated Position Error. Sometimes labeled as "accuracy," the estimated position error (EPE) is the way the receivers attempt to give the user an idea of the approximate position discrepancy between what is given by the GPS unit and its true position. This number can be represented in either feet or meters depending on the unit display properties found in the menu options. It is important to note that this number is a rough estimation and, in many cases, cannot be trusted. It is best to double the EPE number displayed to provide a safe margin of error.

Position Page

In many of the newer GPS units, the position information has been integrated with other pages and is sometimes called the trip computer page (**FIGURE 10-43**). The purpose of this screen is to provide the user with pertinent information concerning his or her position. This page displays several optional fields, meaning some may be modified to show different information. In this section, the most widely used and pertinent of these fields are discussed. Depending on the unit used, these terms may be labeled differently (with or without acronyms), or not be available.

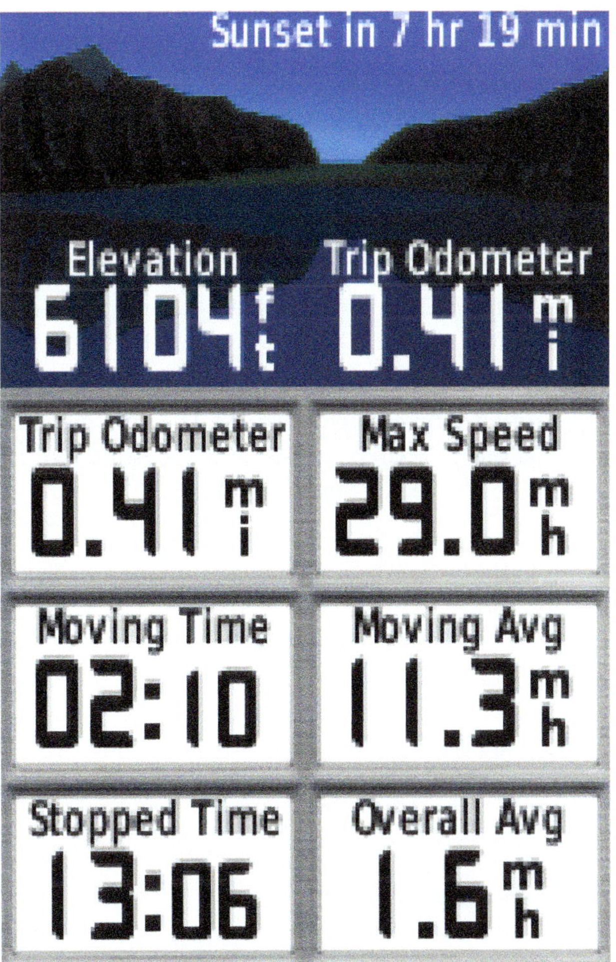

FIGURE 10-43 Trip computer page on a Garmin GPSmap 62stc.

Optional Field Terminology. The following terms may be used in the field as well:

- *Position.* The current position of the receiver displayed in the position format and datum designated by the user in the menu options.
- *Time.* The current time displayed in the format designated by the user in the menu options.
- *Speed (SPD).* The current speed the unit is traveling displayed in the format designated by the user in the menu options (sometimes called *speed over ground [SOG]*).
- *Bearing (BRG).* The direction from the current location to the destination. In many new GPS models, this is displayed in cardinal direction, degrees, or mils. For use in land navigation, it is best to set this for degrees. It is also important to note that the value may vary depending on the north reference setting. If using a GPS unit with a compass, the north reference should be set at magnetic north.
- *Course over ground (COG).* Direction of the line connecting your previous position with your next position. This value is dependent on your definition of north, which could be true north, magnetic north, grid north, etc., depending on the GPS setting (sometimes called *course*, *track* [TRK], or *heading* [HDG]).
- *Distance (DST).* The distance between the receiver's current position and the desired destination displayed in the format designated by the user in the menu options.
- *Altitude (ALT).* The current altitude of the receiver displayed in the format designated by the user in the menu options.
- *Estimated time of arrival (ETA).* The estimated time that the user will reach the desired destination, calculated by velocity made good.
- *Estimated time en route (ETE).* The estimated time required to travel to the desired destination, calculated by velocity made good (sometimes called *time to go* [TTG], or *time to*).
- *Turn (TRN).* The angle difference, in degrees, between the bearing to the destination and the current course of the user. "L" represents turn left, and "R" means turn right (sometimes called *course to steer* [CTS]).
- *Velocity made good (VMG).* The speed at which the user closes in on a destination along a desired course (sometimes called *vector velocity*).
- *Cross track error (XTE).* The distance off the desired course in either direction (sometimes called *off course* or *course error*).
- *Odometer.* A running tally of the distance traveled by the user.

Compass/Highway Page

The screen in **FIGURE 10-44** shows an example of the compass page (sometimes called the *pointer page*) on the top and the highway page on the bottom. Both pages are used as a reference page when navigating to a **waypoint**. Once again, it is important to note that this screen varies somewhat depending upon the model of GPS.

Compass Page. This page is labeled the compass page because of the compass-like diagram depicted. Although this diagram looks like a compass, it is not and should never be used as such. Some GPS models have an electronic compass built into them, and although they can be used as a compass, they do not

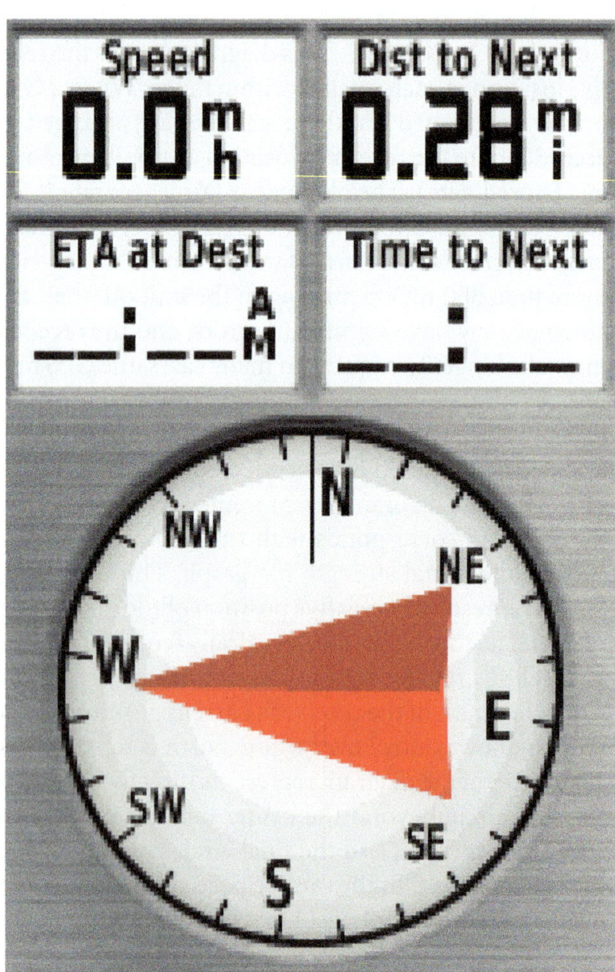

FIGURE 10-44 The compass page of a Garmin GPSmap 62stc.

rival the accuracy or functionality of a traditional compass. The electronic compass needs to be selected within this page and calibrated before it can be used, otherwise the diagram of the compass may give the current track (TRK, see course over ground [COG]) like the models that do not have a built-in electronic compass. This feature does not work correctly if the receiver is not in motion. This happens because all the GPS is doing is displaying what direction the user has traveled from when it last updated its ephemeris. Most receivers have an update rate of once per second, but it is important to understand that TRK displayed is only as accurate as the position information. Within the compass diagram is the bearing indicator arrow. This arrow depicts the bearing and the direction that the user must travel in order to reach the currently selected waypoint. Along with the compass diagram and direction indicator, several optional fields are displayed, as well as the name of the destination or waypoint. (See the Position Page section for a description of these optional fields.)

Highway Page. This page looks similar to the compass page, with the exception that the highway diagram is in the place of the compass diagram. The highway diagram consists of a three-dimensional perspective road, with the receiver's position at the base of the road and the desired destination at the other end. If the user is heading directly toward the destination, the road appears straight, and if the user drifts off course, the road veers left or right to inform the user to compensate for the course deviation. As with the compass page, various optional fields are present, as well as the name of the destination or waypoint (see the Position Page section).

Map Page

This page contains a graphical representation of the unit's current position, nearby waypoints, possibly the user's track log, and a map of the area if loaded into the GPS unit. Each GPS manufacturer uses its own map software. This software is under constant development and is progressively expanding to meet the various needs and desires of the community. The layout of this page can vary significantly from model to model; however, nearly all models have a pan feature (ability to go side to side), the ability to zoom in and out, and some type of scale. Some models also have optional fields displayed, such as the example in **FIGURE 10-45**. Review the owner's manual for specific instructions in using this page.

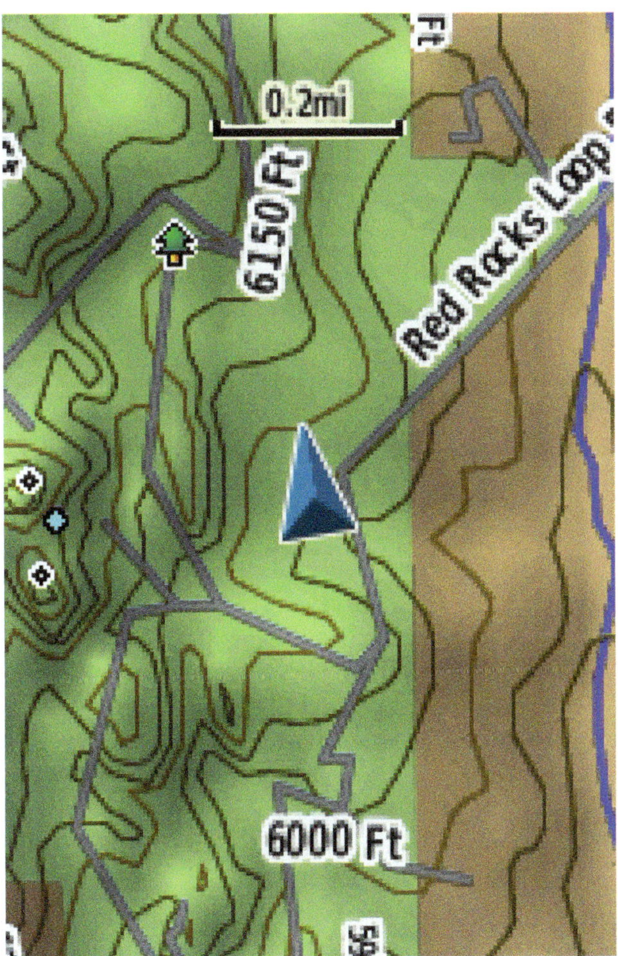

FIGURE 10-45 Map page of a Garmin GPSmap 62stc.

Menu Page

Most menu pages are accessed by simply scrolling through the different screens; however, some GPS units use an actual menu button to display this page. Within the menu, the user may find a slew of various options for customizing the receiver and interfacing with other features. The submenus found within the main menu vary from unit model to unit model. It is important to note which submenus are needed to customize the receiver to function properly when used during navigation.

Customizing GPS Settings

Using a GPS for land navigation requires several skills, including the ability to alter GPS unit settings and input waypoints and routes.

The purpose of altering the unit's settings is not only to personalize the user's preferences but also to set up the GPS to work in conjunction with a map and compass. If the settings of the receiver do not correspond to the grid format or datum of the available maps, the position information cannot be translated from the GPS unit to the map. If the magnetic declination is not set to work with a compass, the discrepancy found when using both could confuse the user and lead to faulty navigation. The following information addresses where and when to alter the GPS unit's settings during land navigation. With all the different manufacturers and models of GPS units, it would not be practical to give the exact button configurations for every type. It is best left for the user to consult the receiver's user manual to learn the exact location and button configuration for the specific unit. Most of these settings can be found in the main menu.

Units

This setting determines what types of units are displayed by the GPS. The typical unit settings include statute (i.e., miles, feet, inches), metric (i.e., kilometers, meters, millimeters), and nautical miles (marine-based units). Most models default to the statute system. For some models, there is one field to alter the unit settings, and the settings are established throughout the entire receiver. Many of the newer GPS units allow the user to customize variable information fields to display different unit settings. For example, the distance may be given in meters (metric system), while the altitude is displayed in feet (statute system).

Datum

A datum is a mathematical model of the Earth's shape and dimensions that is used in conjunction with a grid projection to create a coordinate system used for plotting a position on the Earth's surface. Different maps often have a different datum that affects the projection format. If the corresponding map datum is not selected within the GPS unit, the coordinates given by the receiver could be inaccurate up to 900 meters depending upon the datum selected. The map datum is normally given in the marginal information of a USGS topographical map listed under horizontal datum. Most GPS units default to WGS84.

Position Format

The position format is the grid projection used to designate a coordinate system for plotting a position on the Earth's surface. When using a GPS in conjunction with a map, the user needs to select the position format that corresponds to the one to be used with the map. Maps typically have several grid systems on them. The most common within the United States include latitude/longitude (hddd.ddddd°, hddd°.mm.mmm′, and hddd°.mm′ss.s″), and Universal Transverse Mercator (UTM) grids. Most GPS units default to latitude/longitude.

Time/Universal Time Coordinate (UTC)

The GPS receiver automatically determines your local time from UTC once it has collected these data from the satellites. A select few receivers require the correct time deviation of the area's local time from the UTC to be inputted. If an incorrect time deviation is input, the position information may be inaccurate. Some GPSs can adjust the UTC offset, and it is always a good idea to check and ensure the correct data are entered. It is also important to remember to compensate for daylight savings time during this operation. Many units automatically do this, and some have the option of being set to automatic update or user specified.

Magnetic Declination

Magnetic declination (also known as *variation*) is the angular difference between true north and magnetic north. This variation comes into play when using a compass with a map during navigation. When using a GPS device in conjunction with a compass, it is important to ensure that the correct declination is loaded into the receiver; otherwise the GPS may give a faulty bearing. Typically, this setting is referred to as the north reference. Most GPS units have an auto feature in that the proper declination is set as soon as the unit has acquired. The most common options in the receiver for the north reference are that of true north, mag north, grid north, and user. True north uses the north value without compensating for magnetic variation. This is fine to use as long as the user is not using the GPS information in conjunction with a compass (unless the user compensates for the magnetic variation in some manner). Mag north automatically calculates the proper declination once the GPS has acquired, and then the unit bearing information is ready to be used with a compass. The grid north option references north, based on the grid projection of the area. In most cases, this option should not be used. The user option allows the user to select a north point. If "user" is selected, it is important that the declination be adjusted when operating the receiver in a different area or with a different map.

Waypoints

Waypoints are position coordinates that the GPS unit stores in its memory. Different models have a different limit on the number of waypoints that can be stored. Most units can store a minimum of 250 waypoints, while the newer units usually have a capacity for up to 1000. Different models also have different means for marking a waypoint; the user manual should be referenced to see how this is done. When marking a waypoint with the GPS, you may have the option of designating a name or symbol for ease of reference in the future. Most models default the name with a number identification from 001 to 999 depending on available openings. For example, if the user inputs a waypoint at 001, then the next default waypoint name automatically goes to 002. Once the name and the symbol are designated, the waypoint is stored in the unit's database for future use. Most units store only the horizontal data, but a select few also can store the elevation. To aid in accuracy, some receivers also have an averaging feature that allows the unit to assign the waypoint to a more accurate position. Once the unit has done this, it assigns a figure of merit (FOM) to indicate the probable accuracy of the position information.

The user can also input coordinates of a position without having to travel there. For most units, this is done by accessing the main menu and selecting the waypoints or landmarks submenu. It is best to refer to the receiver's user manual to see how this is done. Before this is done, the user needs to ensure that the position format and datum are set to the map from which the coordinates are derived. The user is then given several data fields to input, including waypoint name, possibly symbol (if supported), position coordinates, and user comments (if supported). Once the user has input the proper information and saved it, the waypoint is stored in the receiver's memory for future reference.

Yet another means to plot a waypoint is to use an existing waypoint as a reference point, and then input the distance and bearing from this reference point. This information is normally gleaned from a map and compass. This method of plotting a waypoint is often referred to as projecting a waypoint, and it is less reliable than the methods described earlier.

Tracks

A track is essentially an electronic bread crumb that can be used to retrace a user's steps or document where they have been. This "track log" is a series of points with detailed information of the path taken, including location, time, and elevation. The interval for tracks can be set by the user to distance, time, or, on some models, "auto." *Distance* creates track points after the user moves a specified distance, such as every 50 meters. *Time* records track points after a specified time has lapsed, such as every 30 seconds. *Auto* allows the user to select one of five intervals ranging from "least often" to "most often." These selections allow the GPS itself to decide when to drop a point. This usually occurs when the user changes speed dramatically or when they turn more than 25 meters from a straight-line projection from their last point. Field crews participating in SAR should typically set this option to "time." This provides information on how long a person searched in a particular place. If the setting was set to "distance," then a person could spend hours searching a small area, and it may only record a few number of points. However, with "time" selected, the same searcher could spend the exact same amount of time in the same area, but it could later be determined where exactly in that area the searcher was.

Tracks can be invaluable during SAR operations. Teams with GPS units can be sent into the field to search for a missing subject with their track logs turned on. Once they return to the command post, those tracks can be downloaded and displayed on a map. This information can then be used to determine probability of detection and whether any part of the assigned search segment was missed.

Routes

A route is a collection of waypoints strung together to reach a final destination. Many users find this option unnecessary because the final destination can simply be input into the receiver as a waypoint. Routes can come in handy if a direct approach to the final point is not possible or if the distance to the final point is significant. To circumnavigate around an obstacle, simply input waypoints that head toward the final point but take a course around the obstacle. Once the user has reached the first waypoint, the GPS unit directs the user to the next waypoint and so on until the final point is reached. The number of waypoints is dependent on the type and the size of the obstacle to be avoided. Waypoints should be determined by using a map to plot the best possible route. Once this is done, the user should input a waypoint for each section of travel that requires a direction change. If traveling a large distance, it is a good idea to break the line of travel into several waypoints to aid in the accuracy of the travel information displayed by the receiver, namely the ETE and ETA. Routes also can be used to designate rest stops with a line of travel. To create a route with the GPS unit, the user must input all applicable waypoints and group them together. How this is done is dependent upon the particular receiver model and can be found in the user manual.

SAR personnel who are expected to use GPS equipment—like any specialized equipment—must be trained in its use, practice with it often, and possess a full appreciation of its limitations.

Wrap-Up

READY FOR REVIEW

- Whether SAR personnel are searching for a lost skier or rescuing a hiker with a broken ankle at a known location, the ability to navigate through the wilderness safely and efficiently using a map, compass, and/or GPS is vital.
- Reading a map allows SAR personnel to associate the graphic details appearing on the map with the physical features in the field, and vice versa.
- There are generally two different styles of compasses: an orienteering compass (clear base plate) and a lensatic compass (military). The environment and local team standards determine which compass will work best for a response.
- When using an orienteering compass with a map, the compass is used primarily as a protractor and ruler. The 360-degree dial—in association with the orienting lines in the base of the bezel—serves as the protractor, and the straight sides of the rectangular base plate serve as a straight edge.
- A method of estimating distance in the field may be required for some situations in SAR. Distance can be estimated by knowing the length of one's stride and multiplying it by the number of strides walked.
- SAR team members often use a handheld GPS receiver to display their coordinates and the route they have taken on a handheld device.

SEARCH AND RESCUE TERMS

Azimuth See *bearing.*

Back azimuth 180 degrees opposite from one's azimuth, bearing, or heading.

Bearing The direction of an object measured in degrees from north. Azimuth, bearing, and heading are often used interchangeably.

Cardinal directions The four principal points of the compass: north, south, east, and west.

Contour lines On a map, contour lines represent relative elevation and connect all points at the same elevation above sea level. On a USGS topographical map, it is brown and may be either darker brown and include elevation numbers (called an index contour line) or a lighter brown that is not numbered and falls between the index contour lines (called an intermediate contour line).

Coordinates A set of values represented by the letters x, y, and optionally z or m (measure) that define a position within a spatial reference. Coordinates are used to represent locations in space relative to other locations.

Coordinate system A reference system consisting of a set of points, lines, and surfaces, and a set of rules, used to define the positions of points in space in either two or three dimensions.

Course Plan of travel using a compass, map, or both.

Datum The reference specifications of a measurement system, usually a system of coordinate positions on a surface (a horizontal datum) or heights above or below a surface (a vertical datum).

Declination The horizontal angle between geographic north and magnetic north from the point of observation.

Direction The relative location of one terrain feature to another; similar to bearing, azimuth, and heading but usually described in terms of points of the compass rather than degrees.

Direction-of-travel arrow The arrow or line on the base plate of an orienteering compass that points in the direction of travel when the compass is oriented.

Easting A figure or a line representing eastward distance on a map (expressed by convention as the first part of a grid reference, before northing).

Ephemeris A table giving the coordinates of GPS satellites at several specific times during a given period.

Feature (1) an object in a landscape or on a map, or (2) a shape in a spatial data layer, such as a point, line, or polygon, that represents a geographic object.

Geographic coordinate system Navigating using a system of reference lines called parallels of latitude and meridians of longitude.

Georeferencing Defining and establishing the location of an object in physical space.

Global positioning system (GPS) A space-based radio navigation system consisting of a constellation of satellites and a network of ground stations used for monitoring and control.

Graticule A network of longitude and latitude lines on a map or chart that relates points on a map to their true locations on the Earth.

Grid north The north established by the vertical UTM grid lines on the map. In the declination diagram of a USGS topographical map, grid north is usually indicated by the letters "GN," and the grid north line has no arrow on it.

Heading See *bearing*.

Intercardinal directions The four points of the compass between the four cardinal points: northeast, southeast, northwest, and southwest.

Landmark A feature in the landscape that can be readily recognized—anything from a prominent tree or rock to a building or lake.

Latitude The angular distance along a meridian north or south of the equator, usually measured in degrees. Lines of latitude are called *parallels*.

Lensatic compass A (formerly) typical military, field, magnetic compass having a magnifying lens for reading the compass scale.

Longitude The angular distance, expressed in degrees, minutes, and seconds, of a point of the Earth's surface east or west of a prime meridian (usually the Greenwich meridian). All lines of longitude are great circles that intersect the equator and pass through the north and south poles. Lines of longitude are called *meridians*.

Magnetic declination (or just declination) See *declination*.

Magnetic north The direction to which the compass points. In the declination diagram of a USGS topographical map, magnetic north is usually indicated by the letters "MN," and the magnetic north line has an arrow on it.

Map scale The ratio or relation between distance or area on a map and the corresponding distance or area on the ground.

Meridians Lines of longitude.

Northing A figure or line representing northward distance on a map (expressed by convention as the second part of a grid reference, after easting).

Orientation The process of determining one's location in the field with the help of landscape features, map, or compass, or with all three combined.

Orienteering compass A compass especially designed to simplify the process of finding one's way with map and compass. It usually has a compass housing mounted on a rectangular base plate in such a way that it can be turned easily.

Parallels Lines of latitude.

Protractor Instrument for measuring angles, usually in degrees.

Spatial Of or relating to space.

Topography The shape or configuration of the land, represented on a map by contour lines, hypsometric tints, and/or relief shading.

Topographical (topo) maps Type of map that portrays the shape and the elevation of the terrain with lines, while showing a graphic representation of selected man-made and natural features on a part of the Earth's surface plotted to a definite scale.

True north A line from any position on the Earth's surface to the North Pole. All lines of longitude are true north lines. In the declination diagram of a USGS topographical map, true north is usually indicated by a star.

Universal Transverse Mercator (UTM) Navigation grid system used worldwide.

United States National Grid (USNG) An unambiguous, nationally consistent, alpha-numeric georeferencing system that can be easily implemented using both printed maps and USNG-enabled GPS devices.

Waypoint Set of coordinates that identifies a point in physical space.

REFERENCES AND SUGGESTED READING

ASTM International. 2014. *ASTM F3071-14, Standard Guide for Basic Wilderness GPS/GNSS Use (GPS/GNSS-IW) Endorsement*. West Conshohocken, PA: ASTM International.

ASTM International. 2014. *ASTM F3072-14, Standard Guide for Intermediate Wilderness GPS/GNSS Use (GPS/GNSS-IIW) Endorsement*. West Conshohocken, PA: ASTM International.

Bowditch, Nathaniel. 2017. *The American Practical Navigator*. Springfield, VA: National Geospatial-Intelligence Agency. https://msi.nga.mil/NGAPortal/MSI.portal?_nfpb=true&_pageLabel=msi_portal_page_62&pubCode=0002.

Burns, Bob, Mike Burns, and Paul Hughes. 2004. *Wilderness Navigation: Finding Your Way Using Map, Compass, Altimeter, & GPS*, 2nd edition. New York: Mountaineers Books.

Durkee, George and Vanessa Glynn-Linaris. 2012. Using GIS for wildland search and rescue. Redlands, CA: ESRI. http://www.mapsar.net/files/gis-for-wildland-search-and-rescue-ebook.pdf.

El-Rabbany, Ahmed. 2002. *Introduction to GPS: The Global Positioning System*. Norwood, MA: Artech House.

Federal Geographic Data Committee. 2015. How to read a United States National Grid (USNG) spatial address. Reston, VA: Federal Geographic Data Committee. https://www.fgdc.gov/usng/how-to-read-usng/index_html.

Federal Geographic Data Committee. 2015. *United States National Grid*. Reston, VA: Federal Geographic Data Committee. https://www.fgdc.gov/usng.

Federal Geographic Data Committee, Standards Working Group. 2001. *United States National Grid*. Reston, VA: Federal Geographic Data Committee. http://www.fgdc.gov/usng/fgdc_std_011_2001_usng.pdf.

Federal Space Agency, Information-Analytical Centre, Russia. 2015. GLONASS. https://www.glonass-iac.ru/en/.

Gatty, Harold. 1999. *Finding Your Way Without Map and Compass*. Mineola, NY: Dover Publications.

Jacobson, Cliff. 2007. *Basic Essentials Map & Compass*, 3rd edition. Guilford, CT: Falcon Guides.

Johnson, G. Mark. 2003. *The Ultimate Desert Handbook: A Manual for Desert Hikers, Campers, and Travelers*. New York: Ragged Mountain Press/McGraw Hill.

Kals, W. S. 2005. *Land Navigation Handbook: Sierra Club Guide to Map, Compass and GPS*. Sierra Club Outdoor Adventure Guide, Second edition. Berkeley, CA: Counterpoint Press.

Kjellström, Bjorn, and Carina Kjellström Elgin. 2009. *Be Expert with Map and Compass*, 3rd edition. Somerset, NJ: John Wiley & Sons.

Linxweiler, Eric, and Mike Maude, Eds. 2017. *Mountaineering: Freedom of the Hills*, 9th edition. New York: The Mountaineers Books.

Manning, Harvey, and Bob Cram. 1986. *Backpacking: One Step at a Time*, 4th edition. New York: Vintage Books.

McManners, Hugh. 1998. *The Complete Wilderness Training Book*. New York: DK Publishing.

National Search and Rescue Committee. 2011. Land SAR Addendum to the National Search and Rescue Supplement to the International Aeronautical and Maritime Search and Rescue Manual, Version 1.0. https://www.hsdl.org/?abstract&did=715465

National Wildfire Coordinating Group. 2014. GIS standard operating procedures on incidents [GSTOP], PMS 936. Boise, ID: National Wildfire Coordinating Group.

Petzoldt, Paul. 1974. *The Wilderness Handbook*. New York: W.W. Norton & Company, Inc.

Rawlins, Chip, and Colin Fletcher. 2002. *The Complete Walker IV*, revised edition. New York: Alfred A. Knopf, Inc.

Snyder, John Parr. 1987. *Map projections: A working manual, U.S. Geological Survey Professional Paper 1395*. U.S. Department of the Interior, U.S. Government Printing Office, Washington, DC. http://pubs.er.usgs.gov/djvu/PP/PP_1395.pdf.

U.S. Geological Survey. 2015a. Map locator & downloader. http://store.usgs.gov/b2c_usgs/usgs/maplocator/(ctype=areaDetails&xcm=r3standardpitrex_prd&carea=$ROOT&layout=6_1_61_48&uiarea=2)/.do.

U.S. Geological Survey. 2015b. Topographic map symbols. http://pubs.usgs.gov/gip/TopographicMapSymbols/topomapsymbols.pdf.

CHAPTER 11

Resources and Technology

OBJECTIVES

Upon completion of this chapter and the related course activities, the student will be able to meet the following objectives:

- Describe and provide an example of each of the three categories of search and rescue (SAR) resources.
- Describe at least two ways that human resources can be used to search an area.
- List at least three functions that human resources can perform to support a SAR mission.
- Describe the advantages that the two primary animal resources can provide to a SAR mission.
- Describe an example of an informational resource.
- List at least two types of search sensor technology.
- Identify at least three different examples of equipment and technology resources and describe their value to a SAR mission.

Resources

A resource, in regard to search and rescue, refers to a person, group, or piece of equipment that has the ability to contribute to an operation or organization. A resource is simply an asset that lies ready for use or can be drawn upon for aid. A single person is termed an *individual resource*, whereas a collection of individuals and their equipment may be called a *group resource*. A canine team is a resource, and so may be a fisherman with a fish-finder. Anyone or anything that could serve as an asset in a search and rescue (SAR) event may be considered a resource.

At its most fundamental level, SAR requires participants to be proficient in a wide variety of skills and information. However, operational effectiveness in SAR occasionally requires the use of individuals and/or groups that have special knowledge. Here, some common and some not-so-common areas of specialization are discussed. Although this text does not go into detail describing each particular search and rescue resource, the following information is intended to offer a general description of the various specialties and equipment that may be called upon to help resolve a SAR problem.

There are many ways to categorize SAR resources, but common methods most often depend on the type of specialization of the particular resource. In the end, categorizing resources boils down to three basic subdivisions:

- Human and animal
- Informational
- Equipment and technology

It is a combination of these three subdivisions that provides SAR personnel with the potential resource base to solve operational problems. Rarely does a single resource offer only one option or application to a task. Rather, it is a thorough understanding of resource capability and complementary applications that gets the job done. The intent here is to familiarize SAR personnel with what is available and the potential application of these resources.

It is impossible to identify all the potential information sources that are available to individual SAR teams. This chapter is intended only as a primer to provide an overview of the vast array of options available regarding what might be useful in SAR incidents and to expose SAR personnel to some of the resources with which they might become involved. In this age of information technology, nearly all data imaginable exist somewhere. It is up to the individuals and teams who need these data to determine exactly how to get it.

Human and Animal Resources

The emphasis under this category is on the capability of the resource. Equipment or an unusual environment may be involved, but it is usually only incidental to the application of some specialized, required skill or capability.

Ground Searchers

Three types of human search resources (**ground searchers**) are discussed: rapid (hasty) search teams, area searchers, and human trackers. Each has its own uses, benefits, and limitations.

Rapid (Hasty) Search Teams

Rapid (hasty) search teams are small (usually three members), well-trained, highly mobile, self-sufficient, clue-conscious teams that provide the backbone for state-of-the-art search efforts. They use rapid action search tactics in locations most likely to produce clues or, better yet, the subject(s), quickly. The efficiency and usefulness of hasty teams are based on how quickly they can respond and the accuracy of the initial information.

Rapid (hasty) search teams quickly deploy to a specific location where the subject is likely to be and search it thoroughly (e.g., point of interest, house, barn, parking lot, or campsite). This type of search can also be conducted along a linear feature such as the intended or estimated route of travel of the subject or a travel aid such as a trail or drainage. Rapid (hasty) search teams look not only for the subject but also clues that suggest other areas to search, which is referred to as reconnaissance.

Ideally, these teams should include two or three individuals who are:

- Track and sign aware
- Clue oriented
- Familiar with the local terrain and dangers
- Completely self-sufficient
- Able to skillfully interview witnesses
- In possession of pinpoint navigational skills, including the ability to record their tracks using a GPS-enabled device
- Capable of traveling quickly into the field (mobile)
- At least advanced first aid trained

Rapid (hasty) teams usually operate under standard operating procedures so that they do not have to wait for specific instructions, and they carry all the equipment they might need to help themselves and the subject for at least 24 hours. Rapid (hasty) search teams may be activated so quickly that they do not have a map or much information to work with. They are good for reconnaissance and bringing back information early in a search, and they should be deployed immediately, without delay.

Sources of rapid (hasty) teams usually include organized SAR teams and some emergency response agencies.

Area Searchers

Using a more systematic approach to searching, area search teams may include up to seven members but usually not more. They operate in a very coordinated fashion, often using some type of line search, with a goal of searching a bounded segment in a relatively thorough manner. An area search requires segment boundaries that are readily identifiable both on a map and in the field. Often, these boundaries are also likely routes the missing subject may have traveled, such as natural topographical features (e.g., ridges, streams, drainages, field edges) or manmade features (e.g., roads, trails, fences, power or utility transmission line clearings). Because the boundaries are often likely routes of travel, all boundaries of a segment are considered part of the segment as it is searched. The specific tactics used depend on the type of resource available and the terrain in the segment.

Route (Area) Search. A route search is a systematic, direct search tactic that is guided by a natural or manmade feature. For a parallel route search, two or three searchers spread out on, and perpendicular to, a trail, road, stream, or other linear feature on which a subject may have traveled or may be found. They follow and guide on the linear feature, and their **search lanes** are parallel, thus this technique's name. On a serial route search, searchers line up one after the other on the linear feature and travel on it for their search. For more information on route searches, see Chapter 15, *Search Operations*.

Grid (Area) Search. A **grid search** is a high-**coverage (coverage factor)**, very thorough, systematic search, usually reserved for looking for clues and evidence

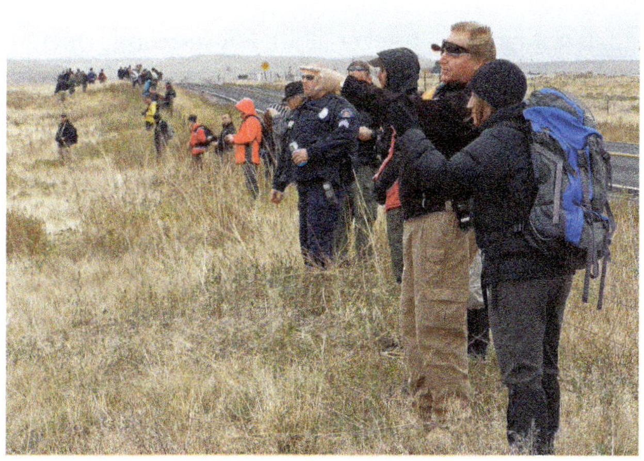

FIGURE 11-1 Grid searching is resource-intensive and tends to be very damaging to evidence.

(**FIGURE 11-1**). The objective of grid (area) search is to search a segment to a measurable, often high, level probability of detection (POD). In the field, this would require that searchers have the ability to record their search track accurately, such as with a GPS-enabled device. The classic approach to grid searching involves several individuals (almost always too many) standing in a line and then walking together through an area in search of either evidence or subjects. However, such resource-intensive approaches to searching are generally less preferred to those that utilize fewer personnel in a more efficient manner (e.g., rapid [hasty] teams, tracking, dogs, aircraft). Although grid searches can be invaluable in the right situation, they are usually so damaging to the search area and evidence that they are used only as a last resort.

When looking for human subjects, the preference is usually for smaller, more efficient search teams to be used, such as rapid (hasty) teams, to search quickly through trails, linear features, and locations likely to contain the subject. Grid (area) search teams require many searchers, up to seven per team, often making such teams difficult to coordinate and manage. Unlike many other resources, grid teams may consist of a mixture of trained and untrained searchers and, thus, may have severe limitations in terms of when and where they can be used. As a minimum, at least half of any grid team should be trained in navigation, search techniques, team organization, communication, and other skills that can allow the safe supplementary use of untrained personnel. It is also important to note that when grid teams are used in a segment, any clues not discovered in the area may well be destroyed forever.

Grid search teams can also attempt to cover large segments, which usually translates to a relatively low coverage and a less thorough search. In practice, searchers can space themselves widely apart while searching, even out of visual sight of each other, to cover a larger area in less time, resulting in a lower coverage. Thus, these teams must have more skilled members who can travel and act somewhat independently. This relative independence requires that members of this type of team be skilled at navigation, communication, self-sufficiency, survival, and general search techniques. The often large distances between searchers allows fewer people per team, so it is easier to administrate and coordinate with other resources. These types of teams often mix sound (yelling, whistle-blowing) into their visual searches, but some use sound techniques as a primary tactic. For more information on grid (area) searches, see Chapter 15.

Sound Sweep. Although yelling the subject's name has long been part of ground search operations, sound sweep is a specific method of searching a relatively large area quickly. It requires that the subject be responsive to sound and is based on the idea that sounds can often be heard even when the subject cannot be seen. In practice, it requires a carefully coordinated approach that has searchers with radio communications perform a widely spaced grid search pause at predetermined intervals during their search and blow their whistles, ideally simultaneously, then listen for a response. For more information on sound sweeps, see Chapter 15.

Expanding Circle Search. When there is evidence that a missing subject was at a specific geographic location (i.e., last known position [LKP] or point last seen [PLS]), a tactic that has been effective involves an experienced, track-aware search team (usually three members) spiraling outward from where the evidence was discovered, looking for sign of the subject's passing. They usually look for tracks from which to track the subject. Searchers conducting an expanding circle search can easily destroy clues they do not see as they walk over them, so this tactic is best suited to highly skilled, track-aware searchers or trained trackers. This type of search can also be useful following the contour of a hilltop working downward.

Human Trackers

Trackers use primarily their visual senses to search for evidence left by a person's passing (**FIGURE 11-2**). They "cut" or look for **sign** (discoverable evidence) by examining the area where the subject would likely have passed. This process of looking for the first piece of evidence from which to track is called **sign cutting**. Following the subsequent chain or chronology of sign is called *tracking*. In SAR, most trackers use a stride-based approach called the "Step-by-Step" Method. This method

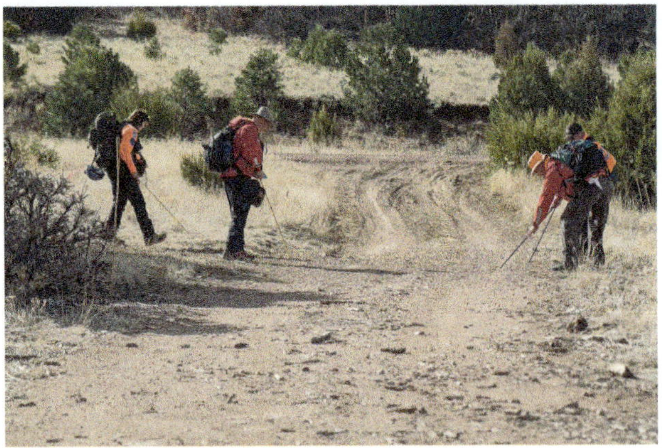

A

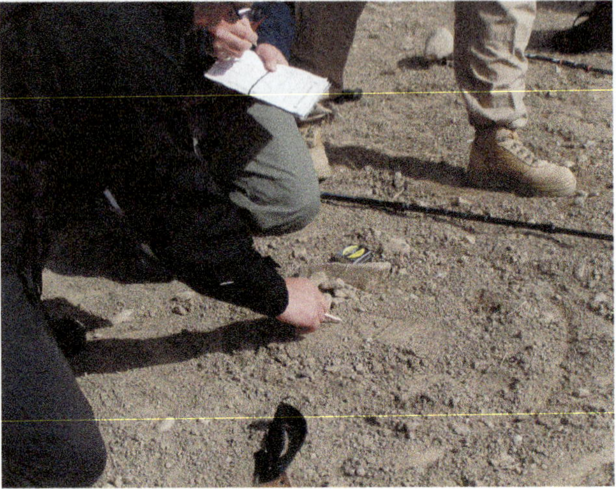

B

FIGURE 11-2 A. Human trackers use primarily vision to search for evidence left by a person's passing. **B.** Trackers examine subtle clues to piece together what happened.

A: © 2016 Howard Paul, Photography for Communication and Commerce; B: Courtesy of Donald Cooper.

is simple, methodical, and emphasizes finding every piece of possible evidence left by a subject.

Tracking is a very visual skill and requires a great deal of practice and experience to achieve even a limited level of effectiveness. However, all searchers should be trained to a minimum level, referred to by many as "track aware." This entry level allows all searchers to at least be aware that tracks and related evidence exist. First, searchers must know to look for this type of evidence. Second, they must learn how to find it. In the end, the most important role for tracking is undoubtedly its ability to determine the direction of travel of the subject quickly and thus limit the search area.

Organized SAR groups are a good source of trackers, as are the U.S. Border Patrol and some other law enforcement and military agencies. However, care should be taken to assess the individual's unsubstantiated tracking ability. In most SAR situations, depending on someone who claims to be able to track but cannot do it is far worse than not having a tracker at all. For more information on tracking, see Chapter 13, *Tracking*.

Technical Rope Rescuers

As used here, the word *technical* precedes components of search and rescue where very specialized techniques are applied to the study of a science, art, or craft. Technical rope rescue applies to those specific rescue techniques that involve rope and its related equipment.

Rope rescue is required in many different environments and is often what novices envision when thinking about rescue in general. In reality, rope rescue is a complex tool used in the rescue function to achieve a goal that cannot otherwise be achieved. Rope rescue is a very specialized discipline that involves equipment such as ascenders, pulleys, friction devices, and carabiners; it includes skills such as tying knots, rigging a mechanical advantage system, and rappelling.

When rope rescue is required, there is almost always an elevation differential necessitating the use of rope rescue equipment to either raise or lower both rescuers and subjects. Because it does not take much of a fall to seriously injure a person, rope rescue is considered both hazardous and exciting.

Organized SAR teams are a good source of rope rescue resources in terms of both equipment and personnel. However, fire service, law enforcement, park services, and often emergency medical agencies have substantial rope rescue capabilities that should not be overlooked.

More information on rope rescue and evacuation can be found in Chapter 16, *Rescue*.

SEARCH AND RESCUE TIP

Sign cutting is the process of looking for the first piece of evidence from which to track.

Management

Management resources are often among the most important to the success of an incident, especially when extended operations and planning are required. Several specific types of management resources are often keys to effective command and control.

Search Planning and Management

The specific functions required to plan and manage a search effectively, especially an extended, complex, or large one, often require many uniquely qualified individuals. Chapter 3, *Incident Management*, describes

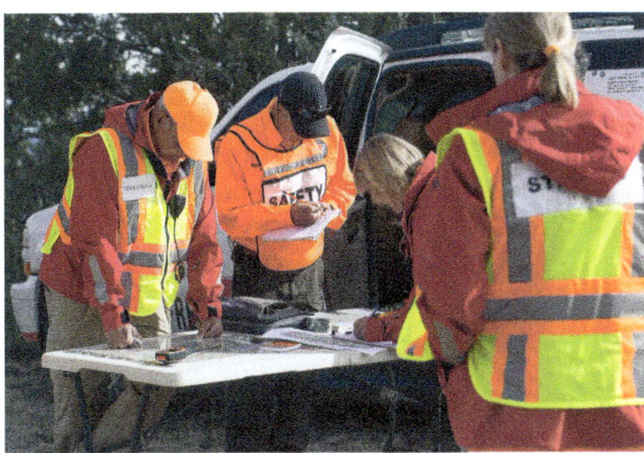

FIGURE 11-3 Management resources are among the most important to the success of any incident and should not be taken for granted.

the fundamentals of the incident command system and the functions required in the management of any incident. Certain functions are particularly important in a search, such as investigation, communications, and search planning. Excellent, position-specific training is available for each of these areas, and individuals with these skills can be invaluable during a SAR event (**FIGURE 11-3**). However, do not overlook individuals who may not be formally trained in SAR but still possess the necessary skills to manage the incident and those working to address it.

Organized SAR and incident management teams are good sources of these specially trained individuals, and access to them should be pre-planned because they are not always available within the immediate area or jurisdiction.

Logistical Support

Food, shelter, and other logistical concerns are often difficult obstacles during a SAR event. Using specially skilled personnel in this support function can often make a substantial difference in the comfort and safety of all human resources.

Sources of these specialists are often numerous and can be provided by civic organizations, the Red Cross, the Salvation Army, faith-based groups, auxiliaries of emergency services agencies (e.g., fire department auxiliary), military bases, and private vendors.

Investigators/Interviewers

Investigation is a skill that is required in every SAR event. Getting the information required to institute an effective search takes a great deal of practice and skill. In the end, a properly conducted investigation often means the difference between success and failure. One crucial skill involved in investigation is extracting information from people through asking questions or interviewing. A novice may ask extraneous questions, sometimes not ever getting to the right ones, and usually takes far too long to extract the pertinent information. The most skilled interviewers know exactly what questions to ask, how to ask them, and whom to ask. A properly conducted interview often abbreviates the entire investigation process and produces both planning information (where should we look?) and searching information (what should we look for?).

Law enforcement agencies are typically the source for the best interviewers because interviewing is an integral part of their job. However, search and rescue organizations, social workers, counselors, and other similar specialists can also be effective.

GIS Specialist

Maps are a critical component for planning and operations in search incidents. Geographic information systems (GIS) are the integrated collection of computer software and data used to view and manage information about geographic places, analyze spatial (relating to space) relationships, and model spatial processes. If possible, GIS specialists should be involved from the very beginning of a search incident to make sure that all location-based information is accurately recorded, visualized, and analyzed. A GIS specialist is typically placed under the planning section in a search incident, but the paper and digital map products they use may be used by anyone involved on the incident. They may work closely with Plans and Investigations to record clues and plan search assignments. The operations section will want to assign someone to download GPS data from ground and air resources to show search progress. As GIS technology advances and becomes more "real-time," the GIS specialist becomes even more critical, and their role may expand well beyond the production of paper maps (Durkee and Glynn-Linaris, 2012). For more information, see Chapter 10, *Maps and Navigation*.

Communications Support

In addition to the internal communications systems of responsible organizations and support agencies, specialized communication support, such as portable radios, cell phones, radio operators, and even Internet access, is often available from:

- REACT units
- CB clubs
- HAM operators

In many areas, one phone call to the right person can get all the necessary communication resources supplied at an incident.

Facilities

An important component of the incident command system, especially when the command structure grows large, is predesignated incident facilities. When many people must be fed, housed, rested, and given a place to work, the physical requirements can be both numerous and extraordinary. Some thought should be given to accommodating the following resources during the planning stages of larger incidents.

- Administrative and support personnel
- Extra telephones and lines
- Computer and fax equipment
- Photocopy equipment
- Transportation (trucks, buses, aircraft)
- Sanitation facilities (dumpsters and portable toilets)
- Temporary shelter (tents, canopies, mobile homes)
- Portable heaters or air conditioners

The incident command system describes six primary facilities: incident command post, staging area, incident base, camp, helibase, and helispot. Not all incidents require the use of all these facilities. However, an incident command post and a staging area will likely be established on all but the smallest incidents. In incidents where greater numbers of responders are required, a **mobilization center** may be established. Ideally, all facilities should be located outside the search area and remote from the PLS and LKP.

As the size of an incident grows, so do the requirements of the physical facilities. Resources that improve the comfort and usability of these facilities can be invaluable as the incident increases in size and complexity. For more information on predesignated facilities, see Chapter 3.

Critical Incident Stress Management Teams

There are hundreds of critical incident stress management (CISM) teams in the United States and many more in other parts of the world. CISM teams comprise mental health professionals, trained emergency services personnel (peers), and clergy who provide an organized means by which individuals who have experienced a critical incident can be helped. A critical incident is an event faced by emergency workers that creates unusual or acute emotional reactions that interfere with their ability to function.

Environment-Specific Personnel

The harsher the environment, the more difficult it is to meet SAR operational objectives. Harsher and more hazardous environments also require personnel to be able to overcome both environmental and operational challenges simultaneously. Thus, specialized groups have evolved to address those special situations.

Many standards are available that address SAR operations in and around the various environments. NFPA 1670, *Standard on Operations and Training for Technical Search and Rescue Incidents*, NFPA1006, *Standard for Technical Rescue Personnel Professional Qualifications*, and multiple ASTM standards address aquatic-specific operations, and more may be available by the time you read this. Reviewing and becoming familiar with these standards is highly recommended for SAR personnel who may operate in or around these environments (NFPA 2017a, NFPA 2017b, ASTM 2017).

More information on the specific hazards of the various environments, as well as how to travel through them, may be found in Chapter 8, *Safety in SAR Environments*, and Chapter 12, *Foot Travel for SAR Personnel.*

Mountaineers

Mountainous or alpine environments often involve both technical terrain (steep slopes, scree slopes, rock cliffs, etc.) and inclement weather in addition to their relative remoteness. The combination of dangerous terrain; diverse, severe weather; and extreme isolation makes this environment one of the most dangerous on the planet for SAR.

SAR personnel working in this environment are required to be prepared for just about anything. It may be warm, it may snow, or it may rain. It may be calm, or wind may make it difficult to stand. Simple hiking may be suitable for most travel, but rock and ice climbing, snowshoeing, and belaying may also be required. The catch phrase is, "be prepared for anything," including unusual medical conditions (**FIGURE 11-4**). For example, acute mountain sickness, also known as altitude illness, is a condition related to working at high altitudes that can be fatal if not recognized and treated properly.

SAR units that specialize in the skills and equipment required to effectively and safely operate in remote alpine environments can be found throughout the United States but are mostly located in the Rocky and Coastal Mountain areas of the west. Many of these units are affiliated with the Mountain Rescue Association (MRA), a nonprofit organization dedicated to the research, development, and distribution of search, rescue, communications, and medical information, primarily as it relates to the alpine environment (MRA, 2017).

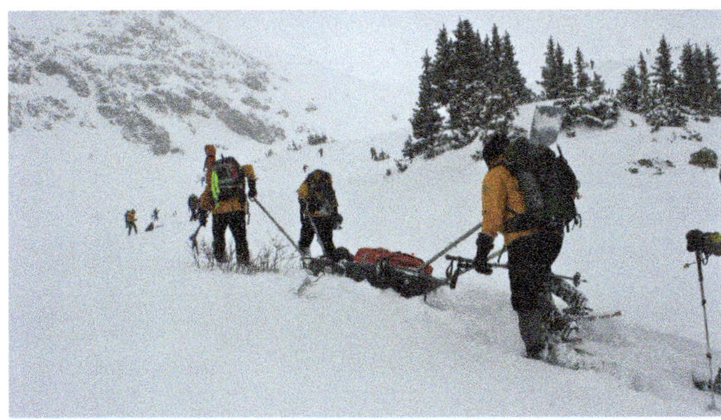

FIGURE 11-4 SAR personnel working in the mountain/alpine environment are required to be prepared for just about anything.
Courtesy of Dale Atkins.

SAFETY TIP

Be prepared for anything in mountainous environments, as weather is unpredictable, terrain is dangerous, and extreme isolation is common.

Ice, Snow, and Cold

Just about every SAR unit must deal with a cold environment at one time or another, but some have the additional challenge of dealing frequently with extreme cold, ice, and snow. Alpine and arctic units must often travel through cold environments, over ice and snow, to meet their objectives. For these units, and others working in similar environments, technique and equipment measures beyond those taken by most units may be required. Avalanche shovels, transceivers, and probes are the tools of the SAR trade in snow-covered alpine terrain. Crampons, snowshoes, Nordic skis, and arctic clothing are also frequently required by members of units operating in cold, snow, and ice-covered environments. Hypothermia and frostbite are a common concern, and cold weather emergency service units must be adept at recognizing and treating them.

The National Ski Patrol is an educational organization dedicated to serving the public and the ski industry by promoting ski safety and providing educational services so the membership can deliver emergency care. Ski patrollers often become involved in SAR in the cold and snow environment and, much like the MRA, serve as a good place to turn for information regarding training (NSP, 2017).

Subterranean (Cavers)

The underground environment is special in that nowhere else can a person experience such absolute darkness, the distinctive odor of wet rock and mud, constant cool temperatures, and perfect silence. Perhaps this is what has drawn people into caves for thousands of years, thus requiring someone to go in after individuals who have become lost or injured.

Caves and mines are common in today's society. Construction projects, mining, and spelunking (caving) are daily occurrences requiring individuals to exist and travel safely underground. SAR in these areas is particularly specialized because the environment necessitates equipment and skills that are considered only conveniences in other places. The absolute darkness requires multiple sources of reliable light, the dampness and cool temperatures require addressing the extreme potential for hypothermia, and the confined nature of the environment requires safety equipment to prevent injury. Many of the skills and equipment from other SAR disciplines are used in the subterranean environment (ropes, rescue hardware, etc.), but modification of techniques and equipment are also required to maintain safety and effectiveness.

Today, confined space and cave rescue units are well equipped to deal with lost or injured people in the underground environment. Teams that specialize in confined space rescue usually limit themselves to the urban setting and specific environments such as tanks, basements, and the like. However, cave rescuers specialize in the natural underground environment and are likely the resource of choice in a caving incident. Not only are local cavers familiar with the general environment, but they may also likely know the layout of the particular cavern involved.

In 1941, the National Speleological Society (NSS) was formed. From their association with others with similar interests, local cavers formed chapters (grottos), and from there, potential rescuers found a place to exchange ideas. The first people called to rescue a lost or injured caver were other cavers, so local grottos often formed their own formal or informal cave rescue groups. Over the years, regional networks and eventually a national network evolved (NSS, 2017).

In 1979, the National Cave Rescue Commission (NCRC) received its charter from the NSS and continues to be affiliated with the Cave Rescue Section of the NSS. The NCRC is not a response organization but rather a communications network, operated by volunteers, developed to coordinate cave rescue resources throughout the United States. In addition, the NCRC also serves as an equipment cache for specialized cave rescue equipment, a clearinghouse for cave rescue information (training, equipment, personnel, etc.), and a sponsor of training seminars (NCRC, 2017).

The Mine Safety and Health Administration (MSHA) is a federal agency charged with establishing and enforcing standards for the health and safety of mine workers in the United States. They are a good source of information regarding equipment and safety in the subterranean environment. Additional resources that might be helpful in supplying equipment are mining equipment stores and outdoor recreational equipment retailers (MSHA, 2017).

Aquatic (Water SAR)

Aquatic environments include everything from surf to rivers and lakes. Each specific type of aquatic environment has its unique characteristics and hazards, including those shared with other environments (e.g., hazardous materials, confined space, caves).

All responders to the aquatic environment must be trained and equipped for the specific types of situations in their area. For instance, coastal teams must be able to negotiate heavy surf and possibly strong currents; teams in the mountains or near fast-flowing rivers/irrigation canals must train in swiftwater rescue techniques with the possible use of rope systems. U.S. Air Force pararescue personnel are equipped to drop mid-ocean to assist distressed boats or downed aircraft; the Navy trains surface swimmers to rescue pilots who have either ditched or ejected over water.

The most common surface operations for aquatic rescuers will likely be of the swiftwater variety (**FIGURE 11-5**). This usually consists of rigging a rope system; equipping the rescuer with wet suit, helmet, knife, gloves, harness, boogie board, and fins; preparing a standby rescuer (or diver) similarly equipped; rigging safety ropes downstream; and then trying to reach and retrieve the victim.

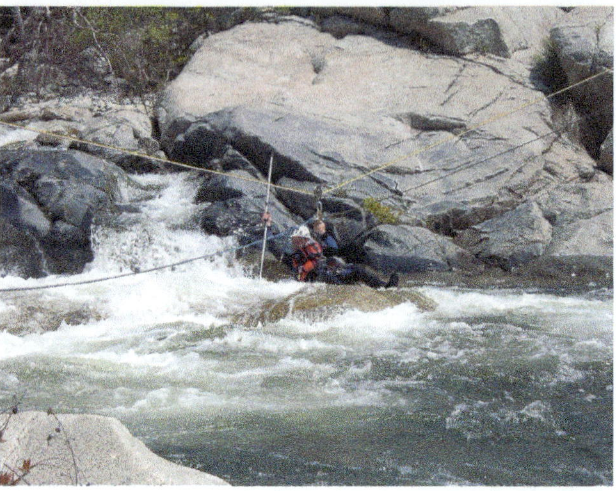

A

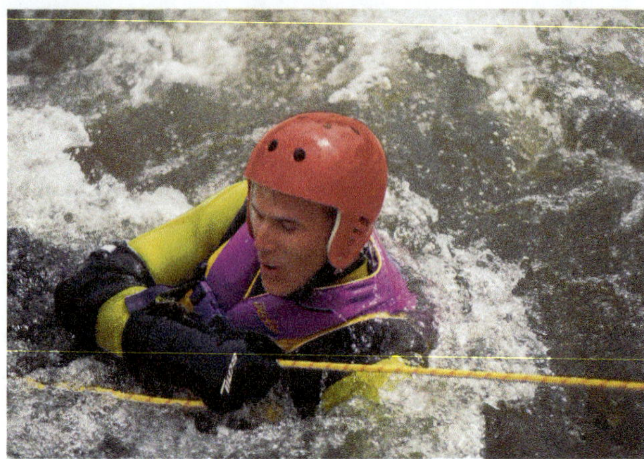

B

FIGURE 11-5 **A.** The most common surface operations for aquatic rescuers will likely be of the swiftwater variety. **B.** Personal protective equipment used in fast-moving water is unique and designed specifically for this environment.

A: Courtesy of Jorene Downs/NASAR; B: © 2016 Howard Paul, Photography for Communication and Commerce.

Water rescue, particularly swiftwater, is one of the most dangerous areas of technical rescue. Although advances in technology have made water rescue safer, rescuers still need to receive special training before undertaking rescue in this environment. There are numerous cases where rescuers have drowned trying to save a victim because improper equipment and techniques were used or because of inadequate training (IAFC/NFPA, 2011). Rescuers must learn how to recognize hidden hazards associated with water, such as current, water level, low-head dams, backwashes, hydraulics, and any hazard not apparent on the surface. In addition, moving water has the capability of pinning individuals against rocks, submerging them in turbulence, or impaling them on rocks, branches, and debris. All water rescuers should be trained in self-rescue techniques and should be familiar with local water (and ice) conditions.

Where the victim submerges below the surface of the water, similar rigging, techniques, and equipment need to be applied by divers. Diving is many times more dangerous to rescuers than surface operations and should, therefore, be approached much more cautiously and only by those completely familiar with its unique hazards and techniques.

Aquatic rescue expertise can usually be procured from local water rescue units or specially trained individuals, public safety dive-rescue units, or organized dive organizations (e.g., Divers Alert Network, NAUI, PADI, SDI/TDI, SCUBA Clubs).

Hazardous Materials

Hazardous materials, often called *hazmat*, refers to any substance or chemical that may be harmful or dangerous to humans (OSHA, 2017a). The realm of hazardous materials touches so many aspects of emergency response that the federal government has enacted legislation (Superfund Amendment and Reauthorization Act [SARA], Title III) and regulations (Code of Federal Regulations [CFR] 1910.120), that require all responders who have a possibility of encountering hazardous materials to have at least basic and recurrent recognition training. For personnel who mitigate and manage a hazardous material incident, additional training is required (OSHA, 2017b).

Although all rescuers (in an ideal world) should have hazardous materials recognition training, hazmat technicians with considerable training and skill are needed to handle anything more than the most minor spill or leak. In the United States, this type of resource is usually available through the fire service.

At the most practical level, SAR personnel confronted by a hazmat situation should stay well away from the location of any hazardous materials and move uphill and upwind before calling hazmat trained responders to address the situation.

Confined Space

According to the National Fire Protection Association (NFPA), a confined space is a space that has all the following characteristics:

- Is large enough and so configured that a person can enter and perform assigned work
- Has limited or restricted means for entry or exit
- Is not designed for continuous human occupancy

Examples of confined spaces include tanks, vessels, silos, storage bins, hoppers, vaults, wells, trenches, cisterns, and pits.

To perform a rescue in a confined space requires very specialized equipment and skill. In addition, federal legislation and regulations apply to operations in most types of confined spaces. Why does the federal government care so much about this particular environment? Because this environment has claimed disproportionately more workers' and rescuers' lives than other environments and has earned the respect and attention of both rescue personnel and regulatory agencies (IAFC/NFPA, 2011).

If rescue operations in a confined space are necessary or anticipated, qualified confined space rescue personnel must be procured, and the local fire department is a good place to start. Industrial complexes and utility companies may also have resources available.

Animals

Although many animals may have some use in a SAR operation, two stand out as being used regularly around the world in search and rescue: dogs and horses.

Generally, animal resources should be staged uphill and upwind from fuel stores, generators, vehicle exhaust, port-a-potties, and other sources of fumes and gases that might be toxic to the animals or impair their value as a SAR resource. They should also be provided shade when staged in direct sunlight and protected from both extremes of temperature and severe weather when possible. In short, animals used in SAR generally need the same support as their human counterparts.

Just like all SAR personnel, dog handlers and horse riders who plan to participate in SAR operations must be trained, equipped, and conditioned to operate as a member of a SAR team, even without their animal. Being expert in working with dogs and horses has a place in SAR operations, but animal-specific expertise alone it is not enough to keep you and your colleagues safe during SAR operations. Build and possess competence and confidence in basic SAR skills before bringing specialized expertise to bear in a SAR incident.

Canines

A canine team comprises one or more dogs (usually only one) and a human handler. There are two types of dogs that are commonly used in SAR: tracking/trailing dogs and air scenting (searching) dogs. Each type differs in its approach to searching, and its value depends on varying factors. Considerations such as when in the search the animals are used (early or late), weather, and skill of the handler all enter into determining the type and effectiveness of the team.

Humans give off a constant stream of scent, like an invisible smoke, which is mostly made up of skin cells that are constantly being shed at an estimated rate of 40,000 per hour (Grabianowski, 2017). These cells, their associated bacteria, and body secretions are detectable by a dog as they either float through the air or come to rest in the environment. Air scenting dogs detect the scent as it floats through the air, while tracking/trailing dogs detect the scent (along with crushed vegetation) as it comes to rest on the ground (snow, rubble, or water). Tracking/trailing dogs frequently work on a lead, require a scent article to establish the scent, and follow very closely on the trail of where a person traveled, regardless of the wind. Air scenting dogs, on the other hand, work off lead to follow a subject's scent to its source and do not require a scent article. Specifically bred and trained air scenting dogs can even discriminate between individual humans (Syrotuck, 2000; Judah, 2014).

The most skilled dog handlers train for years with the same animal to assure that it is an eager worker with an agreeable temperament, has good manners, and learns to communicate with its handler. The communication flow is two-way, however. The dog learns what is desired and expected of it, and the handler learns to read what the dog is sensing. The ability of a handler to know when the dog is on the trail or has "alerted" to scent is acquired through many hours, and often years, of practice (**FIGURE 11-6**). It is this ability, and the degree to which it is honed, that differentiates a trained SAR dog handler from a dog owner.

As with most specialized resources, dog teams are only as good as their training and experience. It is not unreasonable for a SAR manager to ask about a dog team's experience and training, and they should have no problems describing it. However, there are few universally set standards or qualifications for dogs and their handlers. Although some qualifications have been set by various organizations (e.g., NASAR, American Rescue Dog Association, FEMA), and some performance standards exist (ASTM F1879, F3070, and F3144), strict adherence is often not required. It is also important to note that the best dog teams have handlers who are skilled at far more than just dog handling. Just like with other resources, cross training in navigation, communication, and other SAR skills are important.

Dog teams are a highly efficient resource and are often quite effective as first responders or as part of a rapid (hasty) team. They can search large areas in a fraction of the time it would take human, visual searchers to do the same. Dogs work well at night when visual searching is difficult and usually require very little support beyond transportation. They work well in most environments and have been used successfully to locate subjects and clues buried in snow, rubble, and even under water (the scent floats to the surface). Generally, dog units are available through organized SAR units, law enforcement agencies, and specialized SAR dog organizations

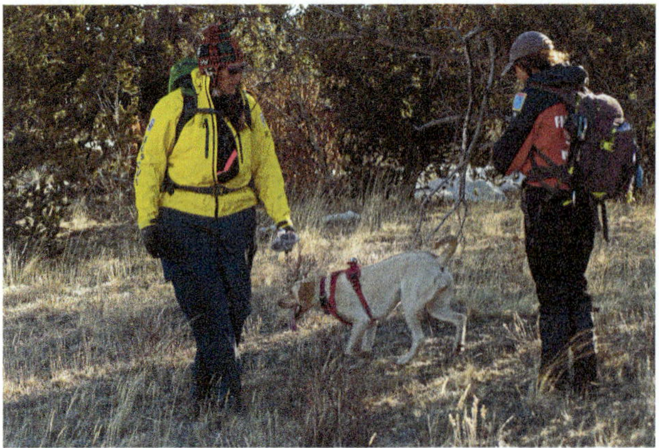

FIGURE 11-6 The most skilled dog handlers train for years with the same animal to assure that it is an eager worker with an agreeable temperament, has good manners, and learns to communicate with its handler.

SEARCH AND RESCUE TIP

A SAR dog handler must have the ability to know when the dog is on the trail or has "alerted" to scent—an ability that is acquired through many hours, and often years, of practice.

Equine

Horses and mules act primarily as a means of transportation for equipment and at least one rider who may be a searcher. Unlike many other vehicle-resource combinations, horses and skilled riders can travel far with very little support in difficult terrain. Horses can be valuable for transporting supplies and equipment as well as for searching remote or rough terrain. A horse and rider can cover far more terrain in a shorter period of time than a person on foot, and a horse, with its highly developed senses of hearing, sight, and smell, is often able to locate a subject before human, visual searchers are able to do so. The problem is that a horse can be quite damaging to the terrain and certain evidence, and it may be difficult to search for small or subtle bits of evidence from horseback. If their limitations are understood, horses can be a valuable asset, especially in the right circumstances.

Law enforcement agencies, local riding stables, and horseback guide services are all good sources of horses and experienced riders. An increasing number of regions also have organized equestrian units (mounted search and rescue) that specialize in the use of horses and their unique traits for SAR.

Informational Resources

Informational resources are those databases and technical information sources that can be accessed when research is necessary for both planning and operational decision making. Information sources such as technical manuals, the Internet, poison control centers, U.S. Weather Service (NOAA), state and local SAR databases, lost subject behavior studies, geographic base layers, and accident statistics from the National Safety Council all provide a rich source of data for complex problem solving in SAR.

As an example, weather information can be difficult to acquire without specialized training like that offered to pilots or by private weather service providers. Federal Aviation Administration (FAA) resources such as Flight Service Stations (FSS) and Air Route Traffic Control Centers (ARTCC) are usually available around the clock with current weather and predictions. However, radio and TV news organizations, specialized cable weather channels, the U.S. Department of Commerce's NOAA, and military bases can all provide accurate current and forecast weather information. There are few sources that are better for weather information in the United States than an experienced, current pilot who can access the federal aviation system's (FAA, FSS, ARTCC) weather information. Usually, all he or she might need is a telephone (800-WX-BRIEF in the United States). Contacting the National Weather Service is also an option, especially if the call is made by a public safety official during an emergency, but one option that may be better—albeit more costly—is access to a commercial weather service provider such as those listed on the National Weather Service website (NOAA NWS, 2017).

Accurate and up-to-date geographic base layers should be used during operations. Consider contacting the local GIS office at the county or state level for minimum essential datasets for your maps. Many of these datasets are now available online to those who know how to use them. See Chapter 10 for more information on this topic.

Equipment and Technology

In SAR, equipment and technology can combine to deliver operational and support capabilities that as little as 10 years ago were not even possible. Specialized transportation such as aircraft and specialty vehicles, electronic devices, and extraordinarily capable communications equipment are just a few examples of this constantly expanding realm of resources being applied to meet SAR objectives.

Aircraft

Aircraft can serve the same purpose as grid searchers, only from a greater distance, at a greater speed, over a larger area, and usually with a lower level of coverage (thoroughness).

Within a search effort, aircraft can serve both as a tactical tool to look for clues and as transportation for personnel and equipment. Both fixed-wing and rotor-wing aircraft have their place in SAR and, like other resources, have their advantages and limitations. Among the most obvious limitations are the expense and complex use requirements of aircraft. Aircraft not only take very specialized personnel and cost a great deal to operate, they also have very strict weather and environmental restrictions. For instance, it would be difficult to search from—or even fly—an aircraft in a snowstorm, and terrain (heavy timber, thick tree crowns, heavy underbrush, etc.) may prevent searching the ground from the air. However, most of these difficulties can be adequately addressed and minimized in a well-developed preplan.

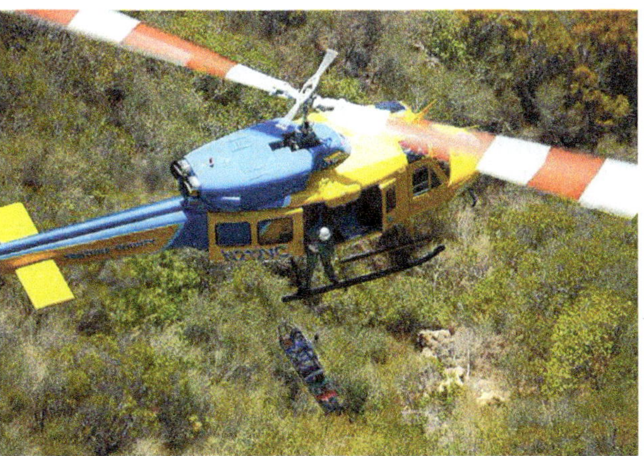

FIGURE 11-7 Helicopters are useful for the movement of supplies and equipment, search area evaluation (planning), and as a search platform.
Courtesy of CMC Rescue, Inc.

Helicopters are useful for the movement of supplies and equipment, search area evaluation (planning), and as a search platform (**FIGURE 11-7**). The military is a common source for this type of resource, usually through a local base or the rescue coordination center (RCC), but many private and/or volunteer providers also offer services.

The MAST (Military Assistance to Safety and Traffic) program was created in November 1973. Under this law, the U.S. Army and Air Force have identified certain units to assist local governments in maintaining an effective emergency service. The MAST program is a temporary measure to fill local needs in areas where civilian assets are insufficient or nonexistent, and units are authorized to provide direct support in coordination with local governments, medical facilities, and law enforcement agencies. After approval for mobilization, MAST units are directed to conduct specific missions.

In those areas where there is adequate private helicopter assistance, the MAST units may not be active. Private ambulance services, often hospital based, are available in most parts of the country.

Fixed-wing aircraft are useful for search area evaluation and for actual searching under certain terrain and vegetation conditions. Affixing a radio repeater to an orbiting fixed-wing aircraft can increase the range and connectivity of radios operating in rough terrain that otherwise limits line-of-sight communications.

Sources of aircraft for SAR include:

- Military: Primarily through the RCC or a local military base
- Civil Air Patrol (CAP): Through the RCC or a local CAP unit

- Government contract
- Private and volunteer clubs and groups

Unmanned Aircraft Systems

An unmanned aircraft system (UAS), sometimes called an unmanned aerial vehicle (UAV) or drone, is an aircraft without a human pilot onboard—instead, the UAS is controlled from an operator on the ground. In the United States, it is most important to understand the law and regulations regarding the use of UAS before considering their use for a SAR mission. The devices are now regulated in the United States by Title 14 of the Code of Federal Regulation (14 CFR) Part 107 (FAA, 2018). In addition, there is a wide variety of sizes and propulsion mechanisms, and the technology is rapidly evolving. Initially UAS were used primarily by military and civil protection agencies, but recreational and commercial use is now widespread. More research is needed on how to process the data they collect, but early experiments (Goodrich et al., 2007; Silvagni et al., 2016; Waharte and Trigoni, 2010) and use-cases show great promise for increasing the mobility and effectiveness of search efforts using photo and video sensors.

Specialized Vehicles

This type of resource includes local units or individuals with vehicles capable of responding in special terrain/environmental conditions, such as:

- Over-snow vehicles
- Four-wheel-drive vehicles
- All-terrain vehicles
- Mountain bikes

Sensor Technologies

Locating equipment has many different applications. Their uses range from determining where a subject lies within a collapsed building to locating a rescuer who needs assistance. Locating technology is useful for coordinating searches over vast areas because it can help determine which areas have been searched and provide a geographic reference to base operations.

The newest and most sophisticated locating equipment employs advanced computers, listening devices, cameras, and satellites to assist with locating a subject or tracking a rescuer. The capabilities and applications of recently developed advanced locating and tracking equipment have made rescue operations much more efficient. However, there are still many rescue needs that have not been satisfied with the existing technology. Many of the systems presented here have been developed for military or scientific purposes and then adapted to SAR applications. This section describes some advances, capabilities, and limitations of locating technology.

Thermal Imaging (Infrared)

Thermal imaging devices were developed for the military and are now used by police to track criminal activity in the dark. Thermal imaging devices use infrared technology to sense heat. Typically, infrared equipment displays a monochrome or color image highlighting as little as 0.1°F difference between an object and its background. This allows a human body to be seen in complete darkness or in a smoke-obscured environment. The more intense the heat source, the brighter the image appears in the display. The display produces a silhouette-type image of a person but does not show detailed features.

Fire fighters have adapted thermal imaging cameras to look for victims through smoke at a fire. This application incorporates infrared viewing technology into either a fire fighter's helmet or a handheld device. These devices are primarily designed for structural firefighting but may be adapted for technical rescue. Thermal imaging devices are now available that weigh less than 1 pound.

The operating principle of this type of device is the same as the forward-looking infrared (FLIR) units described in the following section. All objects radiate a certain amount of heat, which travels outward as detectable energy. Because of differences in the amount of heat being radiated, the viewer detects each difference as more intense or less intense. Thermal-imaging devices can be used in daylight or darkness and can be extremely useful because of their ability to see through smoke, dust, heavy rain, falling snow, fog, camouflage, and light vegetation.

Thermal imaging equipment has multiple applications, but it is expensive and may have significant limitations (**FIGURE 11-8**). Infrared radiation cannot be detected through concrete, rock, brick, wood, or even thick drywall. Thus, infrared locating technology has limited value at structural collapse sites.

The handheld devices are ruggedly designed for limited exposure to areas near a fire or water. They can usually be used for one to two hours before the batteries die. Some units must be turned off hourly to cool down, since their airtight design does not allow for easy cooling of internal components.

Forward-Looking Infrared

Thermal, infrared imaging, and forward-looking infrared (FLIR) units are used to scan wide areas, most often from aircraft, and have numerous applications for SAR. In water rescue operations, they can be used during the day or night to scan the surface for a subject. They are

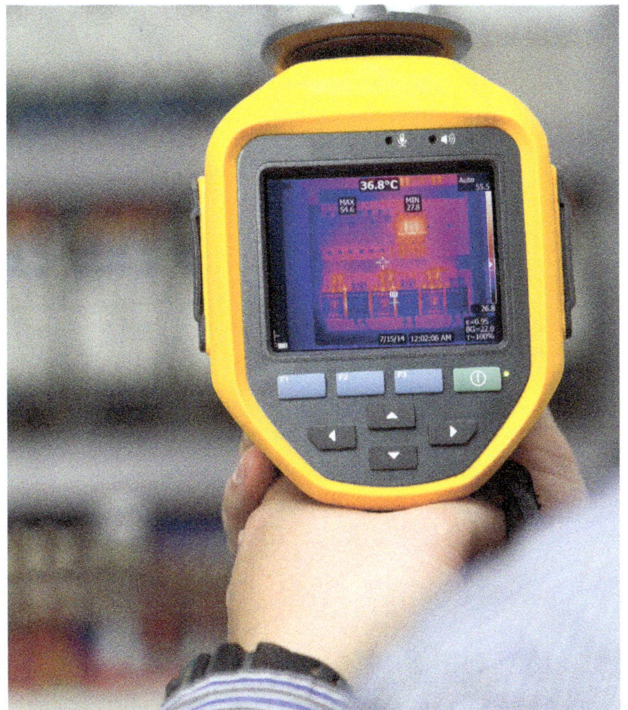

A

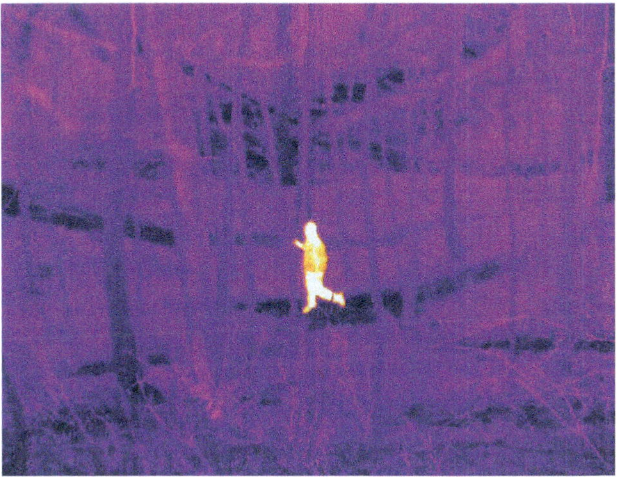

B

FIGURE 11-8 Thermal imaging equipment has multiple applications, but it is expensive and may have operationally relevant limitations.
A: © poneak/Shutterstock; B: © Edward Kinsman/Science Source/Getty.

useful on wide rivers, lakes, or other large bodies of water where it may be difficult to pinpoint the location of a subject. Handheld thermal imaging cameras, similar to TV cameras, can also be used by rescuers in helicopters or on the ground. The more powerful FLIR units, used mostly by aircraft, are very expensive.

FLIR was first used in law enforcement in 1984 and uses a thermographic camera that senses infrared radiation in a wide application of search environments. The technology involves registering temperature differences of houses, trees, cars, and people (so slight as to be almost nonexistent) and projecting these temperature differences onto a computer monitor. The system has now become a widely accepted law enforcement resource.

The units themselves (a tough polymer/plastics "cyclops"-looking ball or cylinder) can be easily adapted to the mount on a normal helicopter's searchlight or spotlight bracket. Installation takes minimal time, and it can be affixed to nearly any helicopter. The detector moves up and down, and left to right, and is controlled by a handheld (computer linked) joystick that has various buttons and toggles to control field of view switching (wide or narrow), optimal signal presentation, and travel sweep. For many units, the best operating altitude is between 600 and 800 feet (180 and 250 meters) where a 300- to 450-foot (100- to 150-meter) wide ground swath can be observed.

On the imaging screen (if white is selected as warm), the eerie, almost photonegative-type image shows tree branches on a cold winter's night as warmer (almost white) with tree trunks (which lose less heat) being darker. Houses show up distinctively radiating white through glass windows, while cars and trucks show a distinctive glow over their engine compartments.

Tests and actual searches tend to be more successful at night when ambient temperatures are most uniform and no artifacts of localized heating by sunlight distort findings. Forested areas can be penetrated well, although dense leaf growth or evergreen cover requires greater operator skill to detect visual differences. The units have been tested and used under actual conditions of fog, rain, snow, and extreme cold with excellent results. Images of people, dogs, and various forms of wildlife are clearly visible, as are tracks in the snow (less than 15 minutes old). In field tests, ground team members have been asked to quickly identify themselves by showing a portion of their skin. Individuals wrapped in sleeping bags that were difficult to detect were immediately visible when they showed their faces or put a hand or arm out.

Trees, roads, fields, shacks, or buildings all have marginally different temperatures that the monitor translates into a very clear picture. These can be recorded on videotape and replayed later. Even the smallest heat sources, such as the place where a vehicle has stopped and started again, and even where individuals have stopped and then continued, can be detected.

Subjects who cannot verbally communicate their location, such as unconscious individuals, may be spotted using infrared devices. Some thermal imaging units can see several feet below the surface of the water. This capability could assist with locating a submerged victim, a victim in very shallow water, or even a body, since it may still emit enough heat to activate these units for hours after death.

Helicopter-mounted FLIR units can sense heat variations as far as 10 miles or more but may cost over $100,000. The handheld models, which use a less powerful lens, cost in the range of $16,000. More expensive models can see up to 500 yards.

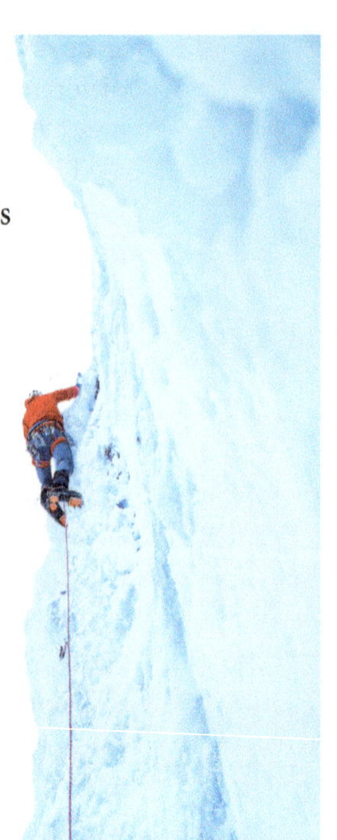

Light Amplification (Night Vision)

Another technology for nighttime searching is light amplification devices. Unlike the infrared technology that can "see" humans in complete darkness, night vision units require some ambient light, whether it be residual light at dusk, light from street lamps, or, in some cases, infrared light. For example, light amplification devices can be used to search a river at night if there is some light projected onto the search area from the shore. The newest units, however, can work on overcast nights because they are very sensitive to infrared light that penetrates clouds.

These devices do not project detectable energy. They amplify the existing or ambient light at night to project an image on the scope or viewer. Ambient light may come from moonlight, starlight, or the glow from cities and towns. Light from flares, searchlights, and laser illumination improves the viewing capability but should not be viewed directly by the device. Image-intensification devices are adversely affected by fog, smoke, heavy rain, and falling snow.

Night vision technology was originally designed to help helicopter pilots see the ground during the night. For SAR applications, it allows rescuers to distinguish objects at distances as far as 200 yards (183 meters). The units provide viewers with an electronically enhanced video image that enables them to see people, buildings, vehicles, and the landscape. Some night vision units magnify images one to two times while amplifying the light up to 100,000 times. These units, however, cannot see through foliage, dense smoke, or fog as the infrared units can. Night vision units come in binocular, monocular, scope, and goggle styles. Low-end models cost approximately $500.

The standard military models of NVGs are normally equipped with an infrared light source and a positive control switch that permits close-in viewing from 10 inches to infinity. This allows a person wearing the device under low light conditions to do everything from read a map to drive a vehicle. The units weigh about 1.5 pounds (0.68 kilograms) and are capable of continuous operation over a 15-hour period before battery replacement is required. Some also have a high light cutoff feature that shuts power down to the goggles when they are exposed to bright light. Therefore, it is important to note that during night helicopter operations where NVGs are in use by the aircraft crew, it is essential that ground personnel do not shine or flash lights directly at the aircraft. Rather, the appropriate method of signaling such an aircraft is to shine a light, or lights, toward the ground.

Cost of the units can vary from $1000 to $4000, but despite this substantial price tag, the technology has found a place with numerous police and government agencies and has proven quite useful in SAR.

Videography, Photography, and Photo Interpretation

Of course, videographic and/or photographic evidence indicating the whereabouts of a search subject would be outstanding, but acquiring it takes a great deal of planning, equipment, and skill. For instance, trail- or road-blocks could be replaced with remote video cameras, but the setup and monitoring of such equipment could be more trouble than it's worth. Aerial photographs could show evidence such as human-made signals, tracks, discarded evidence, or wreckage, but acquiring such photographs would take a great deal of resources (aircraft, pilot, photographer, photographic equipment, etc.) and an enormously skilled interpreter (to analyze the photographs), so the argument becomes, "Is it worth the trouble" rather than "Can we do it?"

Additional problems arise for SAR managers with these types of resources. For instance, how is the location of evidence on an aerial photograph transferred to a map that can be used by field search crews? What is the scale on a particular aerial photo? Questions like these are not insurmountable but require a great deal of forethought and planning to address.

Real-time video has had widespread acceptance in certain settings such as building collapse and confined space rescue. Small, maneuverable cameras can be slipped into small spaces to visually examine a void where victims may be trapped or where rescuers may soon enter. Also, rescuers now can have a video camera built into their helmets to broadcast a constant visual image to supervisors who view the hazardous environment from relative safety. Such use of video technology not only enhances the safety of rescuers, it also allows viewing of areas that otherwise may never have been viewed. The application for field SAR units has yet to be exploited.

Sonar

Sonar (sound amplification and ranging) technology can be useful in some underwater searches. Only a few SAR teams use this technology at present, partly because of the expense of the equipment and partly because of the challenge of deploying it quickly by trained operators. Sonar is often used by boaters to determine the depth of water or locate fish ("fish-finder"), but similar technology specific for use in SAR is available (**FIGURE 11-9**). It plots objects detected underwater on a display monitor located in the rescue boat. With proper training, rescuers can learn how to differentiate the profile of a human body from fish, debris, and other objects in the water. A body on the bottom—a likely location—can be very difficult to locate using sonar because of the very slight differential created by the width of the body as compared with other objects on the bottom. Improvements in technology, however, have improved this capability significantly.

Sound and Vibration Detection

Sound and vibration detection devices occasionally available in SAR situations include equipment able to detect sound over great distances (such as powerful unidirectional, low-level microphones), from remote locations (wired or wireless microphones), through various media (concrete, collapsed structures), and in low sound situations. Like any unusual resource, their limitations and use should be thoroughly investigated so that, should the need arise, SAR personnel are prepared to benefit fully from the technology. Everyone should always be on the lookout for not only applications for new technology but also new applications for old technology. Sound detection devices are a good example of the latter.

The requirements of the urban SAR (US&R) environment give rise to a great opportunity to reevaluate current technology to meet new needs. For instance, vibration and sound detection devices are being used in collapsed structures to listen for the cries, movement, and even the breathing and heartbeats of trapped victims. This type of application of technology, of course, is expensive, but when such resources are required, nothing else will suffice.

FINDER, which stands for Finding Individuals for Disaster and Emergency Response, is a good example of this. FINDER is a collaboration between NASA's Jet Propulsion Laboratory and the Department of Homeland Security's Science and Technology Directorate. The device, about the size of a small suitcase and used with a laptop computer, sends a very low-powered microwave signal through rubble before analyzing the reflections of those signals coming back from tiny motions caused by victims' breathing and heartbeats. In tests, FINDER detected heartbeats through 30 feet (9.1 meters) of rubble or 20 feet (6 meters) of solid concrete. In addition to finding victims buried in the wreckage of a collapsed building, NASA believes the device could also be used to find subjects lost in wilderness settings, entombed in avalanches, and trapped in a burning building (Landau, 2015).

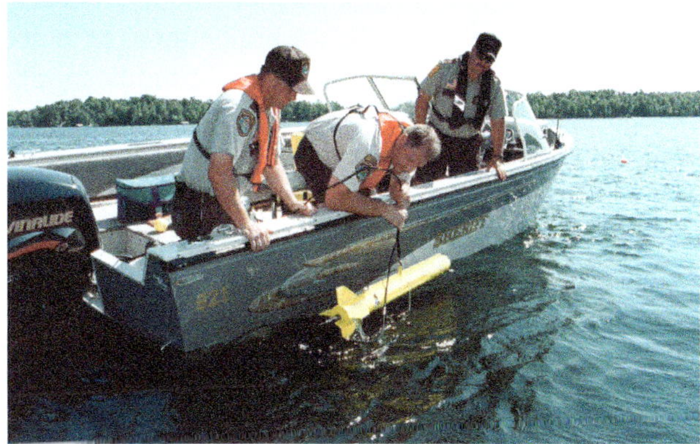

FIGURE 11-9 Side-scan sonar has been used very effectively in SAR work in the underwater environment. Pictured is the "tow fish" that is towed in the water by the search boat.

Avalanche Beacons/Transceivers

In the early 1970s, avalanche rescue beacons, or transceivers, were introduced in the United States. Since then, these devices have become the most-used personal rescue devices in the world. The reason is that, when used properly, there is no faster, more efficient, or more effective way of locating buried avalanche victims; numerous documented cases of lives being saved have been attributed to their use.

Costing anywhere from $50 to $200, these devices are available from most outdoor and winter equipment shops. Their use is simple. Avalanche beacons emit a signal on one or two frequencies when they are set on "transmit" (457 kHz is now the international standard). If the wearer of one of these devices were to become buried in an avalanche, rescuers could turn their beacons on "receive" to pick up and home in on the signal from the buried unit. Various search patterns combined with evaluation of the strength of the signal are then used to narrow down the location of the buried beacon. The signal carries about 100–150 feet (30–46 meters), but frequent practice and well-maintained and properly used beacons are necessary to make the system work. Although skilled practitioners can usually find a subject in less than five minutes after picking up the signal, the use of these devices is not straightforward. Effective use takes frequent practice and thorough knowledge of the devices and their limitations. More information on avalanche beacons can be found in Chapter 8.

Communications Equipment

An abundance of highly advanced communications equipment is available to rescuers today. Communications equipment provides a vital link between rescuers, especially if they are separated visually. It allows them to communicate needs, findings, distress calls, and even images of the incident to other rescue personnel or to a remote location. A functional communications system is essential to maintaining organization and safety at any rescue scene.

Communications equipment is particularly important to rescuers entering dangerous environments. The lack of proper communications has been an issue in cases involving injuries and death to rescuers. Often, rescuers who enter a confined space, for example, are out of visual and audible contact with nonentry personnel. During such incidents, if the entry rescuers were to experience a life-threatening situation and need assistance, communications technology might be the only means of requesting help.

Communications technology can transmit a signal over a radio frequency or hard wire cable. Radio signals can be blocked by walls and metal and are limited by distance or other barriers. Communications systems that use radio frequency transmission are considered at most 95% reliable. Hard wire communications are the only media considered nearly 100% reliable, but they are limited by practical considerations, such as the length of the communications cable.

The type of communications system used should be dictated by the needs of rescuers and the types of situations they anticipate. For instance, rescuers who are entering a confined space or cave containing walls and other barriers that may inhibit radio frequency transmission should use hard-wired systems if they are available. This section discusses communications equipment designed and used for a variety of different rescue systems.

Radio Frequency Systems

The standard handheld and mobile communications radios used by most emergency services and rescuers transmit over radio frequencies (RF). The frequency of different systems varies from 25 MHz to the 800-MHz band. RF systems have strengths and weaknesses that make them more applicable in certain rescue situations than in others.

RF-based communications systems generally can transmit over a large area. Given a constant transmission power, the lower frequency signals travel farther than the higher frequency signals, but they do not penetrate barriers as well as a higher frequency signal. For example, a 40-MHz (VHF) signal from a standard mobile radio can travel 50 or more miles without a signal repeater, but it is very unlikely that an 800-MHz (UHF) signal with the same power could match this without ideal atmospheric conditions. Conversely, it is much harder for a 40-MHz unit to transmit through an area surrounded by concrete than it is for an 800-MHz unit. Well-designed RF systems with repeaters can transmit hundreds of miles. Also, RF systems generally allow the user to choose between several channels or talk groups (**FIGURE 11-10**).

There are many limitations associated with RF systems. Higher frequency RF units depend on signals bouncing around to reach the person on the other end. Obstructions such as concrete, metal, tunnels, and atmospheric conditions (e.g., an electric storm) can prevent a transmission from reaching other users. Static interference can make transmissions unintelligible. Outside interference may also leak in from others using similar frequencies.

RF is the best method of communication in incidents where rescuers are geographically scattered over an area or for surface-level communications at a small-scale incident. It is one of the best methods of communications for rescuers involved in wilderness search, urban search, trench rescue, water rescue (surface communications only), or any other surface-level operations environment. It is generally not as reliable for operations involving subsurface communications (i.e., confined space such as a sewer system or subway), underwater communications, or communications deep within a building heavily partitioned with walls and floors. In these situations, the RF signal may have trouble getting outside to a repeater or other rescuers. However, some technology discussed in the following section can help to conduct or carry an RF signal out of a confined area.

Terrestrial Trunked Radio Systems

Trunking technology is designed to accommodate many users on a small amount of radio spectrum (frequencies). Conventional radio systems are limited in the number of channels available to emergency personnel and match

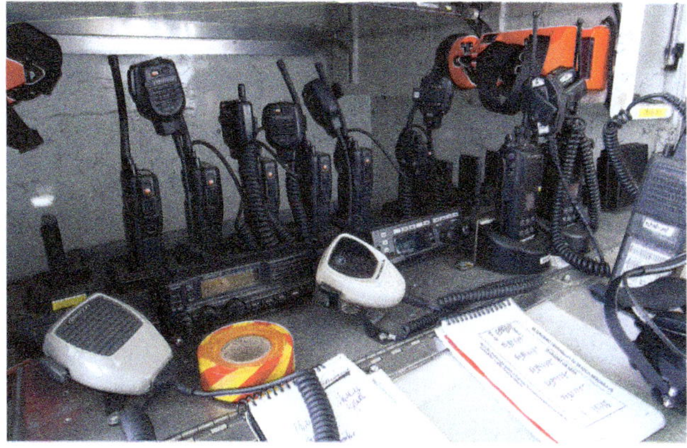

A

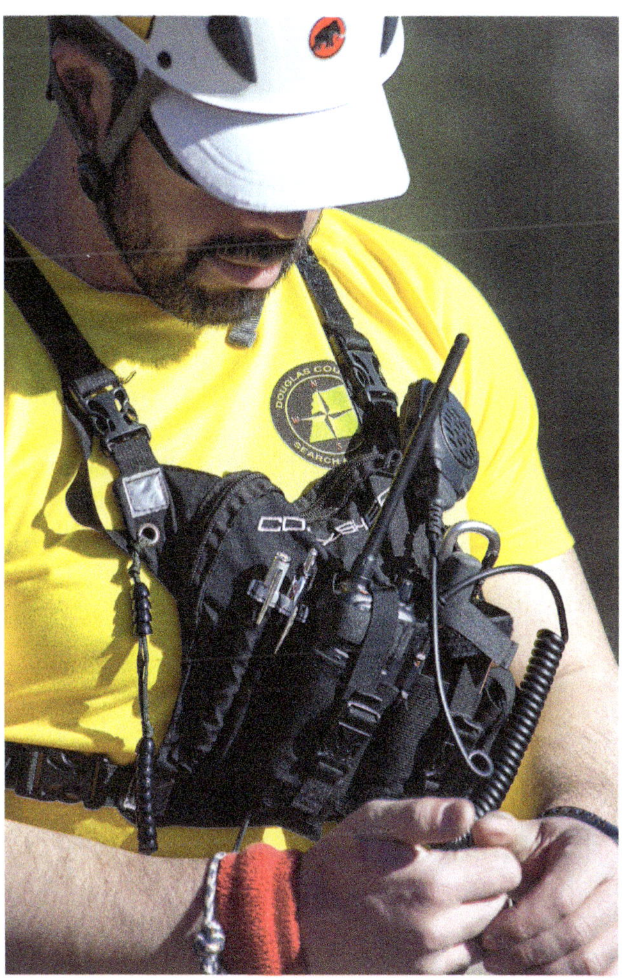

B

FIGURE 11-10 **A.** A variety of handheld (portable) and mobile radio frequency (RF) devices. **B.** A radio harness is commonly used to safely carry a portable radio in a convenient position in the field.

one radio channel per frequency. For example, a jurisdiction that is allocated four emergency frequencies by the Federal Communications Commission (FCC) would have four emergency channels.

In a trunked system, channels are allocated by a centralized computer controller, so a few radio frequencies can be used by multiple users. Trunked systems can offer hundreds of talk groups, even though the system may use only a small number of discrete frequencies. The heart of a trunked system is a computer that assigns a user an open frequency. However, the computer selection process is invisible to the user. The multiple talk group capability of trunked radio systems offers many advantages at small- and large-scale SAR incidents.

SEARCH AND RESCUE TIP

Trunked radio systems can allocate many "talk groups" to just a few frequencies, offering many advantages over conventional radio systems that match one channel per frequency.

A trunked system can be designed to allow communications among multiple agencies. This allows fire, police, public works, and other agencies to communicate with one another and facilitate communications during a disaster. The technology also allows other jurisdictions responding for mutual aid to be connected to the radio system so that no patching of frequencies is necessary. One limitation with the trunked system is that if the signal does not reach the central trunked system receiver, the transmission does not reach other radios that are connected to the system. Also, if the computer goes down, most of the system becomes inoperative, but most handheld units are programmed so that, should they not be able to reach the trunked system, they are able to talk to each other on the same frequency when they are in line-of-sight.

Also available and in use today are patching devices (intelligent audio communication gateways) that can connect different radio systems. These devices can allow communications between very different radio systems such as VHF, UHF, HF, P25, military radios, and even cellular and landline phones. However, when more individuals are using the same channels and talk groups, chaos can follow. Interconnecting radio systems must be done carefully by experts in the technology and its use.

Wireless Communications

Following major disasters, terrestrial telephone systems may be totally disabled or severely limited. Communications cables may be down, incoming and outgoing calls may jam circuits, and switching stations may be destroyed. Many rescue teams have begun to use alternative telephone systems such as cellular and satellite phones to work around the potential telephone problems.

When hard-wired systems are out of service, wireless, cellular phones are a viable alternative, if the cellular receiving sites are not destroyed or overtaxed. However, with the increasing number of cellular phones in use by the public, cells may also become jammed and prevent rescuers' calls from getting through. Cellular transmissions may also not get through if the user is in an area where signals cannot reach a receiving cell tower.

A cell phone carried by missing persons can be a valuable tool when used by trained investigators and cell phone analysis technology. Cellular service providers, when requested by law enforcement, offer some of the following services to assist in locating the origin of cellular calls (NSARC, 2011):

- *Call trace/cellular tower locator*. If there is a connection, the carrier can determine which cell tower is receiving the call and, if power and antenna height are available, an approximate arc of distance from the cell tower.
- *Call trace modified*. After the call is initiated and the technician is notified, the caller can be instructed to call back at a specified time, and the technician can determine through the use of signal strength at several cell sites a more accurate probable position of the caller.
- *Cell traffic recording*. A carrier can determine the cell location of the last call placed by the subscriber given the cellular phone number.
- *Tap*. This function provides notification when a call is made from the user's phone. It is beneficial in overdue cases.

Cell phones can also be useful for the communication of geographic information. For instance, in environments where network coverage is available, there are platforms for live tracking searchers in the field. Where network coverage is not reliable, there are mobile applications that allow for the download of GPS tracks and waypoints.

Using a smart phone with Internet access and Apple FaceTime, Google Hangouts, Skype, or other real-time video chat service can allow SAR managers to use the phone's camera to see the location of the subject's phone to help the user orient himself or herself in an attempt at self-rescue. When available, this technology can allow those remote from the subject to visually examine injuries, enhance situational awareness, and assess the scene in a way that verbal description cannot match.

Since cell phones have limitations, SAR personnel should quickly try to get at least the following information from a lost subject who is using a cell phone (NSARC, 2011):

- Ask the caller for the following details:
  - Complete cellular telephone number (including area code)
  - Type of cell phone.
  - Cellular service provider or carrier
  - Availability of other means of communications
  - Remaining battery strength in cell phone
- Establish a communications schedule or require the caller to call back at a scheduled time, if possible.
- Ensure the user understands that the cell phone, if there is sufficient battery strength, must not be turned off, so that further communications can be established.
- Ask if the user has an alternate power source available.
- Ask if the user can send and receive text messages to conserve battery life.
- Obtain a good alternative point of contact.

One particularly ingenious, yet elegantly simple, smart phone app that has been developed in the U.K is called SARLOC (developed by Russ Hore of the Ogwen Valley Mountain Rescue Team in North Wales). If a lost subject has a smart phone with its geolocation feature enabled and access to the Internet, the subject is sent a text with a link to a web page. Opening this link opens a page in the phone's browser, which queries the phone to identify its location as a Lat/Long coordinate, which is then displayed to the user and automatically sent to the SAR team. On many occasions, this simple app has saved lives and precluded the need for large search operations.

A satellite telephone or "sat phone" is a type of wireless mobile phone that connects to geosynchronous or low Earth-orbiting (LEO) satellites instead of terrestrial cell sites (**FIGURE 11-11**). They provide similar functionality to conventional mobile telephones but bypass the entire local cellular telephone system altogether. Satellite telephones can bypass the jammed circuitry of a disaster scene. These more expensive units are particularly useful for rescuers in remote areas where neither land line nor cellular systems are available.

Hard-Wired Systems

Hard-wired systems are the most reliable communication systems available because users are directly connected. Some systems use a console to interconnect several users. This allows for duplex communications, where two or more of the rescuers can talk simultaneously and everyone hears them (similar to a conference telephone call). The systems generally use headsets, sometimes with throat microphones, which are attached to the wire that runs to a central console. The headsets and microphones are very compact, and the transmit button can be placed in a rescuer's palm or the system can be voice activated. These features facilitate movement within a confined space or inside a protective suit.

Hard-wired systems can be used effectively at incidents where RF signals cannot penetrate, such as

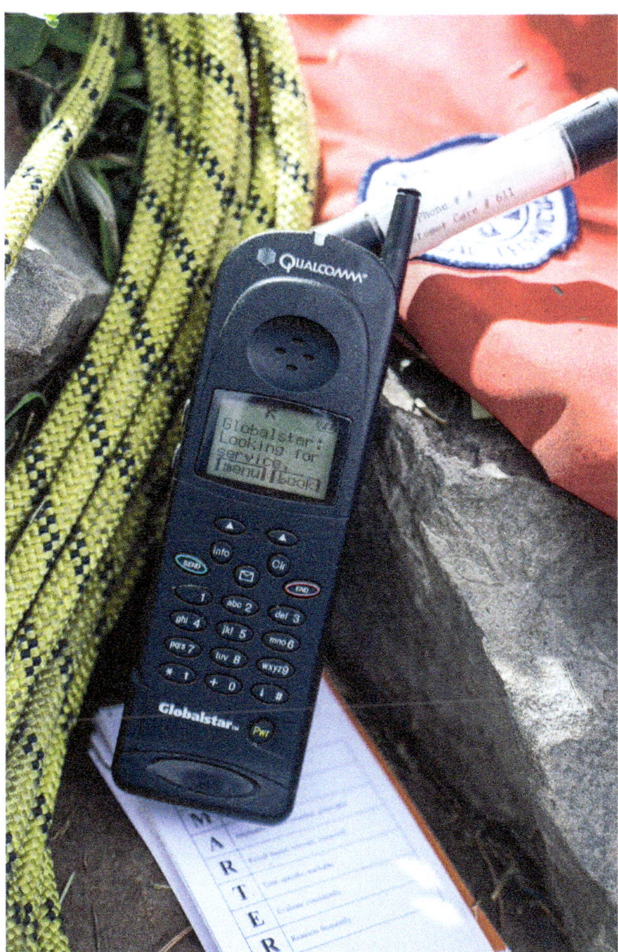

FIGURE 11-11 A satellite telephone or "sat phone" is a type of wireless, mobile phone that connects to geosynchronous or low Earth-orbiting satellites instead of terrestrial cell sites.

confined spaces. The wire carries the signal and virtually ensures that a rescuer can be heard at any time. Many rescuers find the greatest advantage of these systems is the psychological reassurance of knowing that they will always be able to communicate, especially when they are out of visual contact with nonentry personnel.

Several hard-wired units have emergency buttons that can be activated if a rescuer needs assistance but is unable to talk. Some are intrinsically safe, making them useful at incidents where the atmosphere is flammable or explosive, such as silos, sewers, vats, storage tanks, or ship hulls. The main power supply for intrinsically safe units remains outside the explosive environment. The fully shielded wire carries only a few millivolts. Most hard-wired systems are also insulated from outside electrical signals that can create interference or static.

Hard-wired communications systems can also be used by divers. Underwater communication is particularly important in dark or dirty water where visibility is severely restricted. This technology allows divers to communicate and coordinate their efforts. It also allows divers to communicate with rescue personnel on the surface. These systems give psychological reassurance to divers.

The major limitation with any hard-wired system is the length of the wire. Depending on the system, the wire is generally limited to 500 to 1,500 feet (152 to 457 meters). For longer distances, a repeater may be necessary to boost the signal. Most hard-wired systems are also limited to four or five users, unlike RF systems that can accommodate thousands of users. However, sometimes two hard-wired systems can be connected at the control console to increase the number of users.

Users of hard-wired systems must also deal with dragging wire, which may become snagged or tangled. One approach to this problem involves feeding the line or lines (including additional lines such as air hose and power lines) into 2-inch (5-cm) tubular webbing. This webbing system can be made into various length sections that can be combined as needed for extension. The slick texture of the nylon webbing makes it less vulnerable to becoming stuck or jammed on obstacles or bends within a confined space.

Communications Wire/Rope

Many rescue incidents require a safety line to be attached to rescuers at all times. Rescuers involved with confined space entry, diving (especially under ice and in caves), rappelling, or swiftwater entry often must use safety lines. Sometimes the rescuers also need to take a hard-wired communication line with them. Additionally, they may have to take an air hose for air supply (surface supplied air). The three separate lines may present a hazard to the rescuer if they become tangled, twisted, or caught.

Communications wire/rope is a technology that combines two of these lines into one to reduce the risk of tangling. It is usually made as a kernmantle (core in sheath), with a wire running through the inside of the rope's core. Rope strength is not significantly compromised by the encased wire, allowing it to serve as a safety line. Each end of the wire/rope has a locking coaxial-type connection so that it can be attached to a radio, headset, or other communications console.

Most communications wire/rope has a breaking strength around 5,000 pounds (2,268 kilograms), depending on the diameter of the rope. However, military-grade wire/rope is rated as high as 9,000 pounds (4,082 kilograms). The rope is made from synthetic fibers and is waterproof. Since the wire runs through the center of the rope, it is intrinsically safe for rescue operations in flammable environments. Under high stress, however, the wire portion of the rope could be damaged by the greater elasticity of the rope. Communications wire/rope is available in various diameters and lengths and generally costs approximately $3 per foot if it is encased in kernmantle rope.

Satellite Emergency Notification Devices

Satellite emergency notification devices (SEND) are non-Cospas-Sarsat type, commercial distress alerting devices that have become increasingly available in recent years. These devices are readily available to the general public and require an annual subscription to enable all the features. Their 911 function does not alert traditional emergency services. These alerts are forwarded to a commercial call center, which uses a public safety answering point (PSAP) database to alert police, fire, or emergency medical services in the area of the alert. These alerted agencies may or may not be the agency having jurisdictional authority for SAR in that area (NSARC, 2011).

Additional Resources

Of course, there are many other specialized equipment resources with which SAR personnel might come in contact. For instance, many specialized pieces of equipment used by the military might come in handy in SAR situations. Mine detectors, for example, have been used in avalanche rescue. The same might be said for thermistors, which are sensitive to changes in temperatures in the medium over which they are passed. Ground penetrating radar (GPR) uses radar pulses to "see" what is buried underground. Mechanical sniffers are sensitive to odors and have been used to detect bodies in disaster settings, and magnetometers, which work on deviations in the Earth's magnetic field, have been used to find rocks, metal, and even bodies covered in snow.

If the potential exists for resources to be required, especially of the expensive and/or highly technical type, it is up to SAR personnel to seek out reliable sources and confirm availability. First notice of an incident is not the time to investigate resource availability or effectiveness. Plan ahead, know where to go, know who to ask, and know whether what you need is available—all before anything is needed.

SAR responders require a communications plan that effectively addresses interoperable communications for events of any potential scope. In assessing communications needs, a good starting place is the National Interoperability Field Operations Guide (NIFOG), which provides a framework for interoperable communications. NIFOG is a pocket-sized guide of technical reference material for technicians responsible for radios that are used in SAR response applications. The NIFOG covers regulations on interoperability, available channels, and commonly used emergency frequencies. Although not a replacement for a communications plan, the NIFOG does provide the basis for constructing a mission-specific plan (NSARC, 2011).

Resources available to SAR personnel are limited only by the imaginations of those working in the field. Improvising or adapting existing equipment to invent new solutions to challenges is the hallmark of many SAR operations (**FIGURE 11-12**), so do not allow limited resources to obstruct progress. Find a way to make what you have work, and you will have continued a long tradition of the imaginative innovation that is often necessary to save lives and reduce suffering.

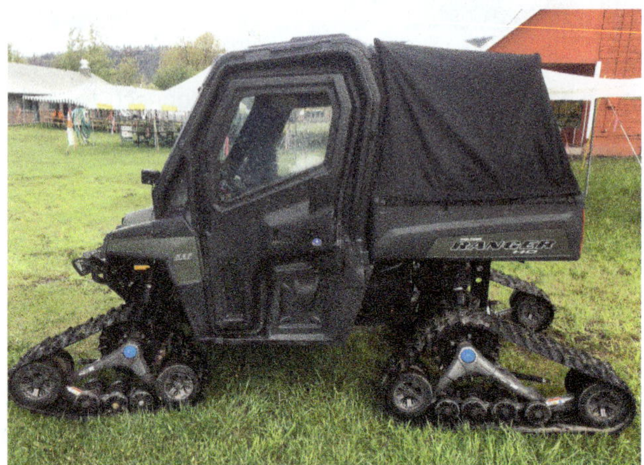

FIGURE 11-12 Improvising or adapting existing equipment to invent new solutions to challenges is the hallmark of many SAR operations.
Courtesy of Donald Cooper.

Wrap-Up

READY FOR REVIEW

- A resource, in regard to search and rescue, refers to a person, group, or piece of equipment that has the ability to contribute to an operation or organization.
- Human search resources (ground searchers) include rapid (hasty) search teams, area searchers, and human trackers.
- Rope rescue is a very specialized discipline that involves equipment such as ascenders, pulleys, friction devices, and carabiners; it includes skills such as tying knots, rigging a mechanical advantage system, and rappelling.
- Management resources are often among the most important to the success of an incident, especially when extended operations and planning are required.
- Specialized groups have evolved to meet SAR operational objectives in harsh and hazardous environments. They are trained to overcome both environmental and operational challenges simultaneously.
- Animals used in SAR generally need the same support as their human counterparts.
- Informational resources are those databases and technical information sources that can be accessed when research is necessary for both planning and operational decision making.
- Specialized transportation such as aircraft and specialty vehicles, electronic devices, and extraordinarily capable communications equipment are just a few examples of this constantly expanding realm of resources being applied to meet SAR objectives.

SEARCH AND RESCUE TERMS

Coverage (coverage factor) "The ratio of the search effort (Z) to the area searched (A); C = Z/A. For parallel sweep searches, it may be computed as the ratio of sweep width (W) to track spacing (S). C = W/S" (NSARC, 2011, p. xv). Coverage may be thought of as a measure of "thoroughness." The probability of detection (POD) of a search is a function of coverage.

Grid search Search method in which human, visual search crews systematically line search a bounded, well-defined, usually relatively small segment.

Ground searchers Searchers used to conduct confinement, attraction, rapid (hasty), and area searches (NSARC, 2011).

Mobilization center Off-incident location at which emergency service personnel and equipment are temporarily located pending assignment, release, or reassignment.

Rapid (hasty) search teams Small (usually three members), well-trained, highly mobile, rapidly deployable, self-sufficient, clue-conscious search teams.

Search lanes The areas an individual searcher is assigned to scan during a search.

Sign Discoverable evidence located in an area where a subject would likely have passed.

Sign cutting The process of looking for the first piece of evidence from which to track.

REFERENCES AND SUGGESTED READING

American Rescue Dog Association. 2002. *Search and Rescue Dogs: Training the K-9 Hero*, 2nd edition. Indianapolis, IN: Howell Book House.

ASTM International. 2017. Search and rescue operations standards: List of search and rescue standards developed by ASTM. https://www.astm.org/Standards/search-and-rescue-operations-standards.html.

Brown, Mike G. 2006. *Engineering Practical Rope Rescue Systems*, Second Edition. Clifton Park, NY: Delmar Learning.

Durkee, George, and Vanessa Glynn-Linaris. 2012. *Using GIS for Wildland Search and Rescue*. http://www.mapsar.net/files/gis-for-wildland-search-and-rescue-ebook.pdf.

Federal Aviation Administration. 2018. Unmanned aircraft systems. https://www.faa.gov/uas/.

Frank, James A., ed. 2017. *CMC Rope Rescue Manual*, revised 5th edition. Santa Barbara, CA: CMC Rescue.

Linxweiler, Eric and Mike Maude, Editors. 2017. *Mountaineering: Freedom of the Hills*, 9th edition. New York: Mountaineers Books.

Goodrich, Michael A., Bryan S. Morse, Damon Gerhardt, Joseph L. Cooper, Morgan Quigley, Julie A. Adams, and Curtis Humphrey. 2007. Supporting wilderness search and rescue using camera equipped mini UAV. *Journal of Field Robotics* 25, no. 1-2, 89–110. doi:10.1002/rob.20226.

Grabianowski, Ed. 2017. How stuff works: How many skin cells do you shed every day? http://health.howstuffworks.com/skin-care/information/anatomy/shed-skin-cells.htm.

Hawley, Chris. 2000. *Hazardous Materials Response and Operations*. New York: Delmar Learning.

International Association of Fire Chiefs, and National Fire Protection Association. 2011. *Fundamentals of Technical Rescue*. Sudbury, MA: Jones & Bartlett Publishers.

Judah, Christy. 2014. *Training a Search and Rescue Dog for Wilderness Air Scent Detection*. NC: Coastal Books.

Landau, Elizabeth. 2015. NASA technology: FINDER search and rescue technology helped save lives in Nepal. https://www.nasa.gov/jpl/finder-search-and-rescue-technology-helped-save-lives-in-nepal.

Mine Safety and Health Administration, U.S. Department of Labor. 2017. Mine Safety and Health Administration. https://www.msha.gov.

Mitchell, Jeffrey T., and George S. Everly. 2001. *Critical Incident Stress Debriefing: An Operations Manual for CISD, Diffusing and Other Group Intervention Services*, 3rd edition. Ellicott City, MD: Chevron Publishing Corporation.

Mountain Rescue Association. 2017. Mountain Rescue Association: Home. http://mra.org.

National Cave Rescue Commission. 2017. National Cave Rescue Commission: Home. http://ncrc.info.

National Fire Protection Association. 2017a. NFPA 1670, *Standard on Operations and Training for Technical Search and Rescue Incidents*. Batterymarch, MA: NFPA.

National Fire Protection Association. 2017b. NFPA 1006, *Standard for Technical Rescue Personnel Professional Qualifications*. Batterymarch, MA: NFPA.

National Oceanic and Atmospheric Administration National Weather Service. 2017. Industrial meteorology: Commercial weather vendor websites serving the U.S. http://www.nws.noaa.gov/im/more.htm.

National Search and Rescue Committee. 2011. Land Search and Rescue Addendum to the National Search and Rescue Supplement to the International Aeronautical and Maritime Search and Rescue Manual, Version 1.0. https://www.hsdl.org/?abstract&did=715465

National Ski Patrol. 2017. National Ski Patrol: Safety. http://www.nsp.org/NSPMember/Safety/NSPMember/Safety/Safety.aspx?hkey=bc91235b-7ce3-4d11-8e27-8b18b3c09a94.

National Speleological Society. 2017. National Speleological Society: Home. https://caves.org.

Ray, Slim, and Bechdel, Les. 2009. *River Rescue: A Manual for Whitewater Safety*, 4th edition. Asheville, NC: CFS Press.

Roop, Michael, Tom Vines, and Richard Wright. 1998. *Confined Space and Structural Rope Rescue*. St. Louis, MO: Mosby, Inc.

Silvagni, Mario, Andrea Tonoli, Enrico Zenerino & Marcello Chiaberge. 2016. Multipurpose UAV for search and rescue operations in mountain avalanche events, Geomatics, Natural Hazards and Risk, 8:1, 18-33, DOI: 10.1080/19475705.2016.1238852.

Speiden, Robert. 2009. Foundations for Awareness, Signcutting and Tracking. Christiansburg, VA: Natural Awareness Tracking School, LLC.

Syrotuck, William G. 2000. *Scent and the Scenting Dog*. Mechanicsburg, PA: Barkleigh Productions.

Taylor, Albert S., and Donald C. Cooper. 2014. *Fundamentals of Mantracking: The Step-by-Step Method*. 3rd edition, New York: Skyhorse Publishers. Available at www.NASAR.org.

U.S. Department of Labor Occupational Safety and Health Administration. 2017a. Occupational Safety and Health standards, toxic and hazardous substances, hazard communications, 29 CFR 1910.1200. https://www.osha.gov/pls/oshaweb/owadisp.show_document?p_table=standards&p_id=10099.

U.S. Department of Labor Occupational Safety and Health Administration. 2017b. Occupational Safety and Health standards, toxic and hazardous substances, hazardous waste operations and emergency response, 29 CFR 1910.120(q)(6)(i). https://www.osha.gov/pls/oshaweb/owadisp.show_document?p_table=standards&p_id=9765.

Vines, Tom, and Steve Hudson. 2016. *High Angle Rescue Techniques: Levels I & II*, 4th edition. Burlington, MA: Jones & Bartlett Learning.

Waharte, Sonia and Niki Trigoni. 2010. *Supporting Search and Rescue Operations with UAVs*. Presentation at 2010 International Conference on Emerging Security Technologies, September 6-7, 2010. The Institute of Electrical and Electronics Engineers, Inc. [IEEE]. https://www.cs.ox.ac.uk/files/3198/submission_waharte.pdf.

Walbridge, Charles, and Wayne A. Sundmacher. 1995. *Whitewater Rescue Manual: New Techniques for Canoeists, Kayakers and Rafters*. New York: International Marine/Ragged Mountain Press.

Chapter Opener: © Ivabalk/Shutterstock; Rescue K-9: © C. Lee Parrish/Shutterstock; Rescuer(s) climbing mountain: Courtesy of NASAR.

CHAPTER 12

Foot Travel for SAR Personnel

OBJECTIVES

Upon completion of this chapter and the related course activities, the student will be able to meet the following objectives:

- Explain the difference between technical and nontechnical travel.
- List three considerations the search and rescue (SAR) professional should consider in preparing for the rigors of the SAR environment.
- Describe the importance of route and pace as they relate to walking technique.
- Describe several alternatives to consider when confronted with traveling through thick brush.
- Describe at least three points to consider when selecting a crossing site on a fast-moving stream or river.
- Discuss considerations for safe uphill and downhill foot travel.

Travel Considerations

Just because you have good motor skills and balance does not ensure your capability to travel in the wilderness or work in the rigorous environments posed by a search and rescue mission. There are many "tricks of the trade" that not only ensure comfort and optimal speed but, most importantly, provide the degree of safety required for search and rescue (SAR) work.

To get from one place to another in SAR, there are many guidelines to consider that will make the mission safer and easier for everyone in the field.

Technical and Nontechnical Travel

Foot travel may be required in one of two forms during a SAR incident: nontechnical and technical. SAR personnel have very little control over where or when this type of travel takes place. Assignments are made, and SAR personnel simply carry them out. Specific skills and knowledge of proper travel technique can increase comfort and reduce injury.

Walking and nontechnical travel (searching, getting to the search area, etc.) may be necessary in one or more general environments (desert, mountain, arctic, river, tropical, forest, etc.).

Climbing or other technical travel (accessing a search area, examining a high-risk area, technical rescue, etc.) may also involve one of many environments (ice, rock, talus, etc.). Again, proper technique improves safety and ease of travel.

Recreation

Traveling on foot for recreational purposes can also involve technical and nontechnical actions but with far different motivations and goals. Here, the traveler has total control over where and when travel takes place. This is a distinct advantage in terms of safety. Technique still plays a large part, but planning is far more important because it is not nearly as rushed as during a SAR incident. Dangerous routes can be avoided by planning around them.

Walking, hiking, hill walking, or nontechnical travel is most often used to easily and safely move through an area chosen for aesthetic characteristics (pretty sights, nice views, good camping or picnic areas) or because it offers a desired physical or mental challenge or benefit.

Urgent or Emergency Situation

Walking may be the only way out of a dangerous situation for SAR personnel, especially if the individual is lost. For example, a hiker with an injury may be in danger of exposure or infection without definitive medical care. Since care is rarely available in the hiking environment, travel is required to transport the individual to the care. If the hiker is lost, travel is complicated substantially, even if he or she physically can walk. Motivation in this situation comes from survival senses and is rarely related to travel skill and knowledge. Considerations regarding travel in an emergency (to travel or not to travel) are covered in Chapter 6, *Survival and Improvisation*.

Walking

As mentioned in Chapter 5, *Physiology and Fitness*, conditioning is an important component of SAR involvement. Since walking is the primary mode of transportation in a SAR incident, being conditioned to walk or hike for long distances may mean the difference between effectiveness and futility. Conditioning should include nutrition and hydration for a comprehensive approach to being prepared for travel in SAR work.

Five things are needed to prepare for traveling in SAR work: fitness (cardiovascular and muscular endurance, muscular strength, and flexibility), energy, water, rest, and technique. The first four of these topics are discussed in detail in Chapter 5. However, because technique can influence so many other aspects of outdoor travel, some basic guidelines are provided here.

Physical Fitness

Physical preparation for travel is straightforward. Under ideal conditions, SAR personnel are in excellent physical shape, fueled with nutritious food, well hydrated, and well rested before an arduous mission. While that is not quite realistic, good rest and nutrition substantially improve performance over those in poor condition, who eat and drink poorly, and who get little or no rest before call-out. In fact, maximum performance in SAR is only one of the many benefits of proper health, nutrition, rest, and exercise.

Gear

SAR personnel also need to be prepared for traveling by knowing how to dress, pack, and plan. Clothing for specific environments is covered in Chapter 7, *Search and Rescue Clothing*. It is important to note that proper dress is mandatory for effective and safe travel. SAR personnel should wear their clothing in layers and adjust for climate, temperature, and precipitation. How to pack is covered in Chapter 9, *The Ready Pack and Personal Equipment*.

Planning

Planning a trip and route finding are also important, but this, of course, is not something that can often be done before a SAR incident. After receiving an assignment in a SAR mission, there may be a brief opportunity for planning. Whether traveling to an assigned area or traveling within an area requiring SAR, the route should be carefully planned. Once you determine that travel on foot is required, it is your responsibility to identify the best type of travel (snowshoe, ski, hike, climb, etc.) and plan the best route. Maps and experienced individuals can be valuable tools for travel planning, but keep in mind that no matter what you use, you must plan your travels, know the route, and follow your plans.

Being Prepared

The following points summarize how SAR personnel prepare for the rigors of traveling in a SAR environment:

- A SAR incident could occur at any time, so you should be in a state of readiness at all times.
- Maintain a level of physical conditioning commensurate with your specific SAR responsibilities. In other words, field personnel should maintain a high level of conditioning.
- Eat proper foods in appropriate amounts and get plenty of rest.
- Maintain hydration by drinking plenty of water before and during a mission.
- Be properly clothed for the type of travel anticipated.
- Pack and carry the appropriate equipment for the type of travel anticipated.
- Before traveling in a SAR mission, plan your travels and know your route.

Walking Technique

Land travel techniques are based largely on experience. However, experience can be partially replaced by practices learned through instruction and observation.

Skill and technique are as important for SAR travel as fitness. Without the proper techniques, the best conditioned person in the world could easily reach his or her limits while traveling. After your physical limits are reached, you tend to lose effectiveness as a searcher, so there is a direct relationship among conditioning, skills, and effectiveness in the field.

On short journeys, it is not essential to walk properly or efficiently. However, walking for several miles during a SAR mission with a heavy load, where lives depend on your ability to travel, is another matter.

Route

When the exact route or approach to an objective is not important to the desired outcome, SAR personnel can improvise and travel the easiest and simplest route. When deciding exactly which path to take (route finding), several options are usually available. A compass heading is often used to get from one place to another but can be difficult in rugged terrain. Novices could stick to this type of route because it is easy and requires little thought, but the terrain could be difficult. SAR personnel who have some experience first determine their objective, and then figure an easy route to that goal by finding the path of least resistance.

Often, a curved route of greater distance can be easier and faster to travel than a straight path. Following a route of constant elevation (contour line) is easier because it requires less energy than moving uphill and downhill. Traveling by altimeter uses this approach and can be a valuable skill in your navigational arsenal. Game trails, roads, and human-made trails may take the traveler a greater distance but also may allow quicker walking and, therefore, less overall travel time.

Factor terrain, weather, and vegetation into the decision to take a longer but quicker and easier route to an objective. Whatever the situation, consider everything, and you can almost always find a better path.

Pace

Pace and rest are crucial to efficient travel. Maintain a realistic pace to save energy. It increases durability and keeps body temperature stable because it reduces the practice of quick starts and lengthy rests. More importantly, a moderate, realistic pace is essential in high altitudes to avoid hypoxia (lack of oxygen), which can lead to lapses of judgment and hallucinations. In addition, practice rhythmic breathing to prevent headache, nausea, lack of appetite, and irritability. Rhythmic breathing is simply a consistent breathing cycle to a set pace. Maintaining a regular breathing and pace ratio allows for more relaxed walking and often takes the mind off the drudgery of monotonous travel.

Fatigue in the SAR environment is dangerous. It increases the chances of accident and injury, and it weakens judgment. Everyone needs to rest, no matter how physically fit. Do not force rest; enjoy it. If you are barely making it to the next rest stop before collapsing, you need to rest more often. Inexperienced travelers tend to rest too often and underestimate their abilities. Rest stops should be short, as it requires added energy to begin again after cooling off. A rest of about 10 minutes per hour while traveling over easy terrain is usually acceptable.

Occasionally, the terrain may be so difficult and the energy required to travel so great that rest is required between each step. This is when you can use the "rest step" (**FIGURE 12-1**). Adopted from mountaineering, the "rest step" is a technique of taking small steps, locking each knee, and synchronizing the breathing. This allows for a brief respite before taking the next small step. This technique is slow, but it may be the only way to travel over difficult terrain, especially at high altitude. Think of it as steady, consistent, and slow travel instead of erratic stop-and-go movement. A novice SAR hiker can virtually eliminate all long rest stops with this technique and actually make very good travel time.

SEARCH AND RESCUE TIP

The rest step, adapted from mountaineering, is a method of allowing respite between steps. Lock each knee and synchronize the breathing in between each small step.

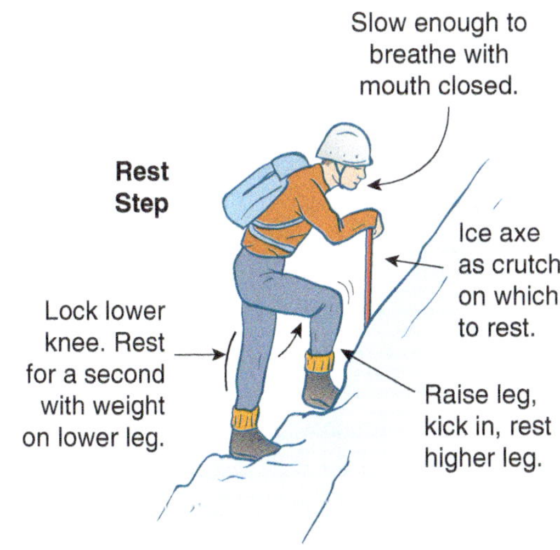

FIGURE 12-1 The rest step is a mountaineering technique developed to maintain pace with heavy loads, at high altitudes, or in rough, steep terrain. The technique is slow, but in rough, steep terrain, especially at altitude, it provides for good footing and minimal waste of energy.

Too often, novice SAR personnel make the mistake of walking too fast, usually thinking of the distance to be covered, the urgency of the situation, or the perceived shame of traveling slower than others. Speed of travel is dictated by the area to be covered, the time available (or assigned), and the capability of the slowest member of the team. Walking too fast decreases the **probability of detection (POD)** and reduces energy stores. One well-respected mountaineering reference suggests that if a pace cannot be sustained hour after hour, it is too fast. In addition, the authors state that you are going too fast when it takes great effort to take the next step or when the lungs are gasping for air (Gawel et al., 2010). Whatever the problem and whatever the cause, walking fast may be common in recreational hiking, but it is inexcusable and unsafe in SAR work.

In a group, pace is determined by the slowest traveler. Retaining excess energy is far better than dealing with severe fatigue. Spacing between individuals in a group is also important while walking. When distance has not been dictated by the search assignment or desired coverage, the rate of travel and the terrain determine the distance between travelers. On most trails, at average walking speeds, this distance is about 6 to 10 feet (1.8 to 3 meters) apart. Unless directed to do otherwise for operational purposes, SAR team members should typically maintain visual contact with other team members and should certainly stay within earshot of each other.

Downhill Travel

Even though downhill walking is less fatiguing than uphill, traveling downhill is not without its challenges. Toes are jammed into the front of the shoes, knees are jarred, and the entire body begins to ache from dropping the weight of the body onto a locked knee and leg at each step. Blisters seem to multiply as the best fitting footgear is tested, and energy is expended preventing a steady speed increase. What do you do? Start by tightening your laces to decrease the movement of the foot inside your footwear. This reduces blisters but also reduces circulation to the feet. Taking this approach in cold weather requires constant monitoring of the feet to make sure circulation is maintained. Second, fill the toe area of the footgear with socks or other padding to cushion the impact of the feet, and place the foot lightly on the ground during walking. Placing the feet lightly takes much muscle energy and requires resting just as much as traveling uphill.

Generally, tighten shoelaces or bootlaces for any travel over terrain where the foot inside the shoe can put pressure in any direction except down. Pressing the foot in any direction but down subjects the feet to stress for which they may not be prepared (no calluses) (see Chapter 7).

A walking stick or an ice axe can be valuable adjuncts to the SAR traveler. The walking stick, in addition to being useful for support during travel, can be substituted for everything from a tent pole to a weapon. One of the more common uses of a walking stick in SAR work is as a tracking stick (see Chapter 13, *Tracking*).

General Wilderness Travel

Wilderness travel requires constant awareness. A novice views a landscape from the top of a hill with care and interest, and says, "Let's go." The experienced person carefully surveys the surrounding countryside. A distant blur may be mist or smoke; a faint, winding line on a far-off hill may be human-made or an animal trail; a blur in the lowlands may be a herd of deer or cattle. One—or perhaps all—of the information gathered visually could serve to make traveling easier and safer.

Two fundamental rules regarding wilderness travel need to be mastered to expend a minimum of energy and time when moving across the ground. First, keep the weight of the body directly over the feet. Second, keep the sole of the foot flat on the ground to improve traction. These fundamentals are most easily accomplished by taking small steps at a slow, steady pace. When crossing sloped ground, avoid an angle of descent that is too steep, and use to your advantage any indentations or ground protrusions, however small, to improve traction.

Consider hard ground to be firmly packed dirt that does not give way under the weight of a person's step. When ascending, apply these fundamentals with the addition of locking the knees on every step to rest the leg muscles. When encountering steep slopes, traversing them is easier than climbing straight up. Turn at the end of each traverse by stepping off in the new direction with the uphill foot. This prevents crossing the feet and possible loss of balance. In traversing, the full-sole principle is accomplished by rolling the ankle away from the hill on each step. For narrow stretches, the herringbone step may be used; that is, ascending straight up a slope with toes pointed out and using the principles stated previously. Where the

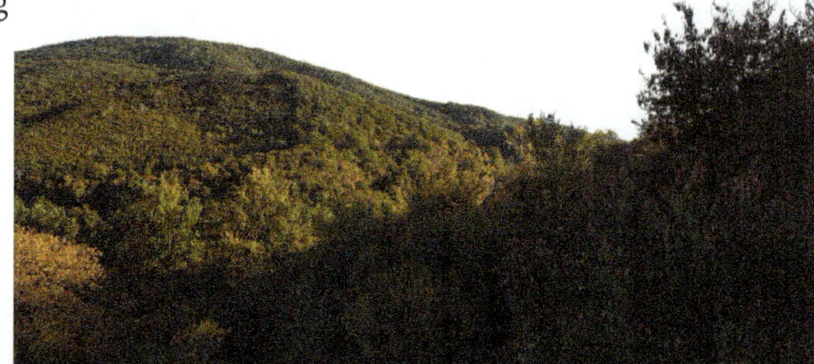

terrain allows, descending is usually easiest by coming straight down a slope without traversing. Keep your back straight and your knees bent in such a manner that they take up the slack of each step. Again, remember that the weight must be directly over the feet, and place the full sole on the ground with every step.

SEARCH AND RESCUE TIP

There are two basic rules of wilderness travel:

1. Keep the body weight directly over the feet.
2. Keep the sole of the foot flat to improve traction.

When confronted with obstacles within your route of travel, such as rocks and downed trees, the preference is to step over them rather than on them, especially in uphill travel, unless you want to check for snakes or critters on the other side. Even walking around such obstacles is occasionally preferred to walking onto a rock or tree and then over. It usually takes more energy to step onto the obstacle, then over it, than it does to simply step over it altogether.

In hot environments, rest where shade offers relief from the sun. Look for areas where leaves or low-lying (waist-high) brush and weeds flutter, indicating air movement. This may offer a cooling effect and reduce the presence of insects during a brief rest or food stop. In cold environments, rest where trees or terrain offer relief from the wind and precipitation.

Trails

A trail is evidence of the frequent travel of either humans or animals. However, trails can vary from small, well-traveled highways to barely visible, rarely used paths. Animals other than humans can be responsible for creating these throughways and can often be credited with producing the only passable paths through environments too difficult for human passage. Human-made trails usually have markings that allow easy trail identification, but these marks can be lost or unreadable and, therefore, should not be depended on for navigation. SAR personnel should keep in mind that trails are rarely designed for rescue operations. They should look at trails as opportunities to use avenues of least resistance, not as the only avenues available. Trails also provide likely spots for clues, since a lost subject may also have taken the path of least resistance.

Traveling on trails is easy and deserves little time dedicated to technique, but some guidelines can be helpful. Recall the importance of spacing when traveling in a group. Give fellow travelers room to move and room to stop without being trampled. Loosen laces to facilitate foot circulation while traveling on good, flat trails, and tighten them when on more severe and sloped terrain. Take rest breaks off the trail so that others can easily pass. Keep your eyes open for evidence left by other people, which may include footprints, sign, and discarded materials left by the lost subject.

Brush

Technique for traveling through brush is not nearly as important as learning to avoid it altogether. Proper travel technique through brush is directed at getting through it quickly or traveling around it—unless, of course, it needs to be searched. This type of vegetation is usually found in gullies and drainages where water and rich soil are prevalent. Brush can be small trees, shrubs, or vines that cause difficulty in travel because they prevent thorough examination of the ground and impede walking. When walking downhill, brush can be dangerous because a foot may catch the vegetation and cause a fall. Thorns may also be present in this type of vegetation, which can cause injuries ranging from minor abrasions to major impalements that can lead to dangerous infections in the field.

When you cannot avoid brush, following these suggestions may be helpful:

- Walk around the brushy area, if possible. Even walking miles (kilometers) on a trail or road can be easier and safer than several hundred feet (or meters) of heavy brush.
- Avoid areas where brush flourishes, such as ravines, drainages, and second-growth, short-timbered areas. Learn where brush usually grows and be able to identify it on a map. Searching these types of areas may involve more sign cutting than area search. Someone passing through brush usually leaves a great deal of evidence of his or her passing.
- Heavily timbered areas usually have sparse underbrush. Travel in these areas, if possible.
- If travel in drainage or a creek bed area is necessary, consider walking right in the creek or stream. It may be safer than the alternative.
- Find game trails. Animals have the same problems with brush as humans. They rarely travel through dense brush, and if they do, the trails they leave are much easier for human passage.
- Brush usually does not flourish on scree, ridgelines, and where snow is always present. Consider these routes if they can be traveled safely.

Grassy Slopes

Grassy slopes are usually made up of small tussocks of growth rather than one continuous field. In ascending, techniques should include taking advantage of any indentations or protrusions for traction. It is better, however, to step on the upper side of these protrusions or tussocks where the ground is more level than on the lower side. Descending on grassy slopes is best accomplished by traversing with care taken to visualize every step so as not to twist or turn an ankle. Be especially careful because wet, grassy slopes can be treacherous regardless of the type of boot sole.

Grassy areas tend to readily show signs of human passage. Make sure to look for subtle evidence of travel on grassy areas to determine a direction of travel.

Scree and Talus

The word *scree* comes from the Old Norse word for *landslide* (Harper, 2017). **Scree slopes** consist of small rocks and gravel that have collected below rock ridges and cliffs. The size of the scree can vary from small particles to rocks the size of a fist (**FIGURE 12-2**). Occasionally, it is a mixture of all sizes of rocks, but most scree slopes comprise rocks the same size.

Ascending scree slopes is difficult and tiring and should be avoided when possible. All principles of ascending hard ground apply, but each step must be picked carefully, so the foot does not slide down when weight is placed on it. This is best done by kicking in with the toe of the upper foot, forming a step in the scree. After determining the step is stable, carefully transfer weight from the lower foot to upper and repeat the process. The best method for descending scree is to come straight down the slope with feet in a slight pigeon-toed position, using a short shuffling step, with the knees bent and back straight. When several travelers descend a scree slope together, they should be as close together as possible, one behind the other, to prevent injury from dislodged rocks. Since there is a tendency to run down scree slopes, care must be taken to ensure that this is avoided, and control is not lost. When traversing a scree slope with no gain or loss of altitude, use the hop-skip method, which is simply a hopping motion in which the lower foot takes all the weight and the upper foot is used for balance.

The word *talus* comes from the French word for *slope* (Harper, 2017). **Talus** is the term sometimes used by climbers to describe something similar to scree, except the rock pieces are larger, and the rocks do not slide as much. Geologists use the term to describe the slope on which scree is found. The technique of walking on talus or large scree is to step on top of, and on the uphill side of, the rocks. This prevents them from tilting and rolling downhill. All other previously mentioned fundamentals apply. Usually talus is easier to ascend and traverse, whereas scree is a more desirable avenue of descent.

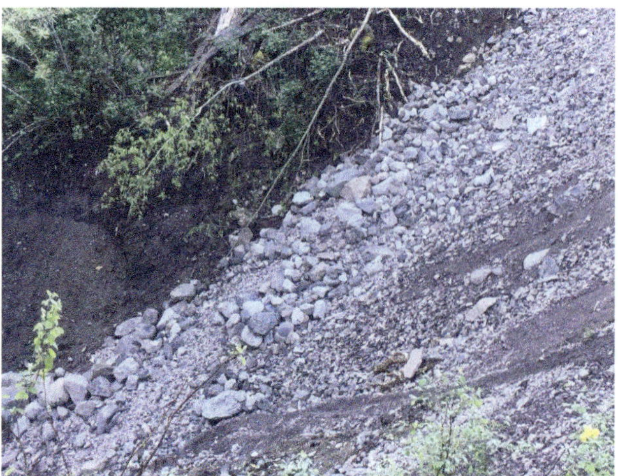

FIGURE 12-2 Scree slopes consist of small rocks and gravel that have collected below rock ridges and cliffs. The size of the scree varies from small particles to the size of a fist.
Courtesy of Donald Cooper.

Streams and Rivers

SAR personnel may find it necessary to cross a stream or a river when traveling through some terrain. These rivers and streams can range from small, ankle-deep brooks to large rivers that may be so swift that a person can hear boulders on the bottom being crashed together by the current (**FIGURE 12-3**).

Safely crossing any waterway at a recognized ford (a shallow place in a river or stream allowing one to walk or drive across) is always the preferred approach, but this may be impossible. Take time to examine the possibilities before deciding to jump into any stream.

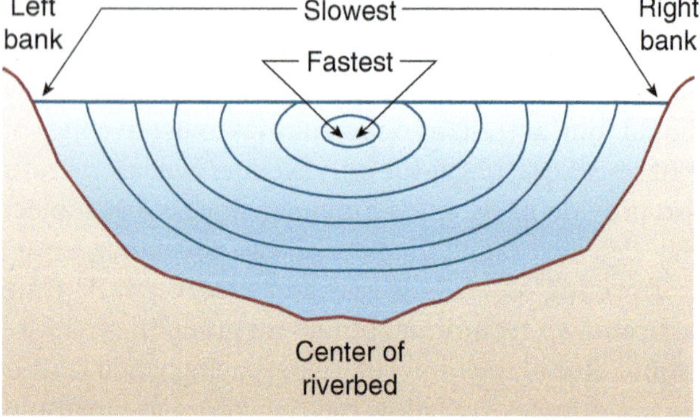

FIGURE 12-3 Cross section of a river showing relative current speed.

Careful study is required to locate the best place to safely cross a stream. If there is a high vantage point beside the river, a team member should climb the rise and look over the river. Do not be afraid to move parallel to the river to find a safe crossing point. Finding a safe crossing may be easy if the river breaks into several small channels. Survey the area on the opposite bank to make sure travel will be easier after crossing. If the waterways are of glacial origin, postpone crossing until early morning when the flow is likely to decrease.

When selecting a crossing site on a fast-moving river, the traveler should do the following:

- When possible, select a travel course that leads across the current at about a 45-degree angle downstream.
- Never attempt to ford a stream directly above or close to a deep or rapid waterfall or a deep channel. Cross the stream where the opposite side comprises shallow banks or sandbars.
- Avoid rocky places, since a fall may cause serious injury. However, an occasional rock that breaks the current may be of some assistance. The depth of the water is not necessarily a deterrent. Deep water may run more slowly and be safer than shallow.
- Have a plan of action for making the crossing before entering the water. Use all possible precautions, and if the stream appears treacherous, cross using a technique that stabilizes the traveler in the water. Some of these techniques include rope assistance, pole assistance, and team crossing (**FIGURE 12-4**).
- Point feet upstream and avoid pointing the feet downstream. A foot or an ankle can easily be trapped under a rock or in a root, causing a fall and entrapment. Falling in moving water with a foot entrapped can quickly lead to death.

Before attempting any crossing of any water at all, unfasten the waist strap to any pack and remove one arm from the shoulder straps to facilitate an expedient ditching of the pack should swimming be required after a fall. This might also be a good time to make sure any vulnerable pack contents will be kept dry should you have to ditch the pack.

Examine the exact route carefully before crossing. If making a rock-to-rock jumping attempt, be sure of the route and be careful of slippery footing. Perhaps sand could be thrown on the slippery spots. An ice axe or a walking stick can make the difference between a safe crossing and a tragedy. Poke the axe or stick into the water ahead of you, searching for dangerous holes in the bottom, or lean upstream onto the shaft as an added point of support during crossing. A tripod (two legs and a walking stick) is a much more stable platform when trying to cross moving water.

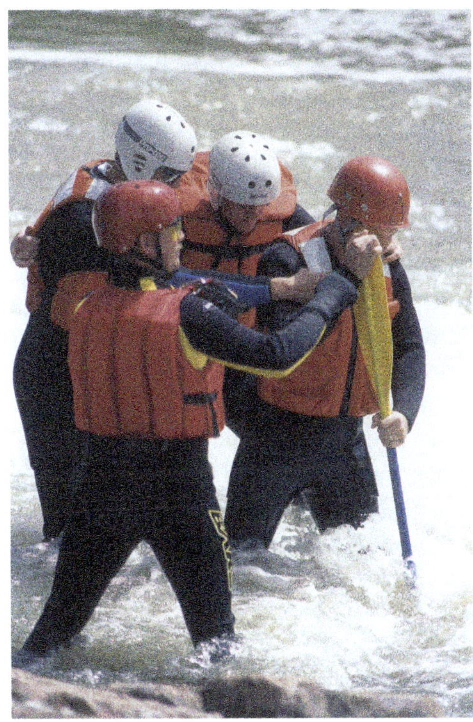

FIGURE 12-4 If the stream appears treacherous when attempting a crossing, cross using a technique that stabilizes the traveler in the water, such as rope, pole (shown), or team crossing (shown).

The speed and force of water is quite easy to underestimate. The sound of flowing water coupled with calm surroundings tends to make rivers and streams seem almost serene. However, the power of moving water is one of the strongest forces in nature and should not be taken lightly. Never work against that power; work with it. In a battle against powerful natural forces, you can never win.

Never affix a rope to the river crosser. If a belay is desired, the line should be held in the hand so it can be dropped should the rope impede travel or cause entrapment. When possible, a rescuer should be positioned downstream with a throw bag in case the river crosser drops the rope.

If you do find yourself in fast-moving water swimming downstream after a fall, make sure to put your feet downstream with toes up and out of the water, swim on your back, and ditch your pack. Facing downstream, feet first, allows you to see objects and to use your legs to push off an obstacle or climb over a **strainer** rather than being sucked into it or becoming entangled. Paddle with your hands toward shore and do not attempt to stand until reaching shallow water near shore. Attempting to walk in fast-moving water can entrap a foot and force you underwater with very little chance of survival.

When walking in water, consider taking off your footgear and even your socks. It may be cold, but the brief discomfort during the crossing is usually better than cold, wet feet for the rest of the day from soaking wet boots and socks. If removal of the footgear is impractical, try inserting a vapor barrier (e.g., plastic bags) inside your boots or shoes and over your socks. This will aid in keeping your feet warm during the crossing. Never try to put bags over your boots or shoes for a water crossing. It is a waste of time because the first step may break a hole in the material, rendering it far less than waterproof. In addition, the material may get caught underwater and cause an unexpected fall.

Whatever method is used to cross a stream or river, tailor the approach to the weakest member of your group. Look long and hard before attempting a wet crossing, and be sure to exhaust all chances of a dry ford.

Desert

Before traveling in the desert, weigh the decision to travel against the environmental factors of terrain and climate, condition of SAR personnel, hazards, and the amount of water and other resources required (**FIGURE 12-5**).

The time of day for traveling is greatly dependent on two significant factors. First and most obvious is temperature, and second is type of terrain. For example, in rocky or mountainous deserts, the eroded drainages and canyons may not be seen at night and could result in a serious fall. Additionally, human-built features such as mining shafts or pits and irrigation channels could cause similar problems. If the temperature is not conducive to day travel, and the option is available, SAR team members should travel during the cooler parts of the day (in early morning or late evening). During the winter in the mid-latitude deserts, the cold temperatures make day travel most sensible.

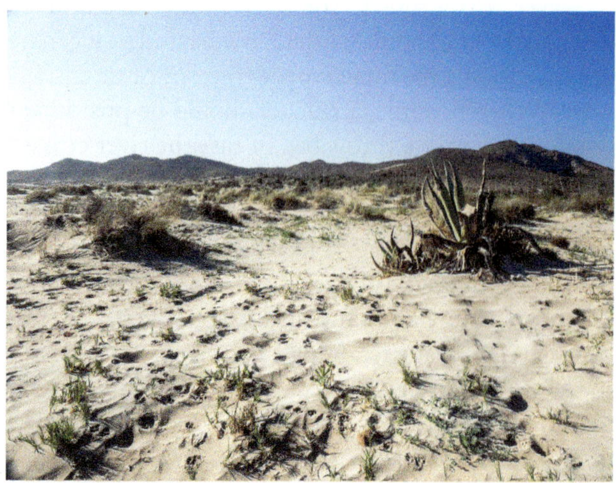

FIGURE 12-5 The decision to conduct SAR operations in the desert must be carefully weighed against the numerous risks and hazards that exist.

There are three types of deserts: mountain, rocky plateau, and sandy or dune deserts. All of these can present difficult travel problems.

Mountain deserts are characterized by scattered ranges or areas of barren hills or mountains, separated by dry, flat basins. High ground may rise gradually or abruptly from flat areas to a height of several thousand feet above sea level. Most desert rainfall occurs at high elevations, and the rapid runoff causes flash floods that erode deep gullies or ravines and deposit sand and gravel around the edges of the basins. Basins without shallow lakes have alkaline flats, which can cause problems with chemical burns and can destroy clothing and equipment.

For desert travel, a compass is a valuable piece of equipment. Without a compass, you must use landmarks for local navigation, and this can lead to difficulties. Mirages can cause considerable challenges. Ground haze throughout the day may obscure vision. Distances are deceptive in deserts; travelers have reported difficulty in estimating distances and the size of objects. Objects have a way of vanishing in some cases when the eye is moved for an instant, and in other cases, many peaks or hills look alike, causing difficulties in determining the original object.

The persistent winds of desert areas seem to provide no cooling effect, and some experienced desert travelers have reported that the wind "got on their nerves." More significant is the fact that the constant wind usually carries an amount of sand or dirt particles that can irritate the eyes, ears, nostrils, and mouth and can cause abrasions that are often severe.

There is no question that those who are familiar with working in hot areas are more likely to tolerate the heat of the desert. However, it is the nature of SAR work that teams are mobilized with little notice and are exposed to extreme environmental conditions without adequate time to acclimate. This poses quite a problem for SAR leaders. Ideally, they should draw their personnel from acclimatized teams, but this is rarely possible. Everyone operationally involved in these types of missions must understand the hazards and how to handle them. Everyone needs to be mindful of the extreme threat that heat can pose. Any group preparing itself for SAR work in hot climates should undergo specialized training prior to engaging in such work. This training should progressively increase in difficulty until members learn the necessary skills for operations within their area.

Specific skills and knowledge necessary for desert SAR work should include, but not necessarily be limited to, the following:

- *Knowledge of heat stress and its impact on the body and mind.* The effects of heat stress are cumulative.

Working day after day, even with intermixed rest, catches up to you.

- *Energy conservation and discipline for desert work.* SAR assignments must be conservative, especially prior to acclimatization. If unacclimated SAR personnel must work hard in the heat for one hour, then they must rest for the next two hours.
- *Pacing.* Rest before you need to, start up slowly and wind down slowly, rest during the hot part of the day, work at night, and get sufficient sleep.
- *Water and electrolyte management.* It is important to consume both water and electrolyte replacements (e.g., sports drinks) at the same time; one without the other may only worsen the situation.
- *Avoiding dehydration and heat problems.* Adequate hydration helps you avoid heat stroke, heat exhaustion, heat cramps, heat weakness, sun blindness, electrolyte imbalance, and other problems.

Jungle

The inexperienced person's view of jungle travel may range from difficult to nearly impossible. However, with patience and good planning, the best and least difficult route can be selected. In some cases, the easiest routes are rivers, trails, and ridgelines. However, there may be hazards associated with these routes.

Rivers and streams may be overgrown, difficult to reach, impossible to raft or ford, and may also be infested with leeches and other parasites. Trails may lead to a dead end or into thick brush or swamps. Ridges may end abruptly at a cliff. Vegetation along a ridge may also conceal crevices or extend out past cliffs, making the cliff unnoticed until it's too late.

The machete is a good aid in the jungle, but SAR personnel rarely carry such a device. Brush is better parted than cut, but if the machete is required, it should be used in a down-and-out angle, instead of flat and level, as this method requires less effort.

In a jungle-like environment, team members should take their time and not hurry. This should allow them to observe their surroundings and get a better insight as to the best route of travel. Individuals should pay attention to the ground for the best footing locations as well as evidence from the passage of others, that is, the missing subject. Avoid grabbing bushes or plants when walking because some vegetation is poisonous, and these actions may disturb animals. Step carefully; falling can be a painful experience because of the many plants that have razor sharp edges, thorns, and hooks. In jungle-like areas, wear gloves and fully buttoned clothes for protection from the same hazards.

Quicksand may be a problem. In appearance, quicksand looks just like the surrounding area with an absence of vegetation. It is usually located near the mouths of large rivers and on flat shores. The simplest description of quicksand is that it is a natural water tank filled with sand and supplied with water. The bottom consists of clay or other substances capable of holding water. The sand grains are rounded, as opposed to normal sharper-edged sand, which is caused by the same water movement that prevents it from settling and stabilizing. The density of this sand-water solution often supports a person's body weight, but there is a danger of drowning if a person panics. In quicksand, use the spread-eagle position to help disperse the body weight to keep from sinking and use a swimming motion to gain solid ground. Avoid panicky, quick movements. Don't struggle! Just spread out and swim or pull yourself along the surface.

Snow

SAR personnel are frequently required to travel in snow and ice. The greatest hazard in snow and ice areas is the intense cold and high winds. Both can lead to physical problems such as hypothermia and frostbite as well as a loss of dexterity and coordination. Judging distance can be difficult because of the lack of landmarks and the clear, cold air. Image distortion is a common phenomenon.

Where strong winds prevail and fresh snow has recently fallen, white-out conditions may exist, making safe travel impossible. A white-out condition occurs when there is complete snow cover and wind-driven snow, or humidity causes uniform light to be reflected from both the ground and the sky. The result is little or no depth perception, so everything appears white. If traveling during bad weather in the snow, take great care to avoid becoming disoriented or falling into crevasses, over cliffs, or over high snow ridges.

In arctic areas, strong winds often sweep unchecked across tundra areas (due to lack of vegetation), causing white-out conditions. Because of blowing snow, fog, and lack of landmarks, a compass is a must for travel, yet it still may be difficult to navigate a true course because the magnetic variation (declination) in the high latitudes (polar areas) is often extreme. During the summer months in these same arctic regions, the terrain

SAFETY TIP

Snow travel can create the following problems:

- Depth perception is impeded.
- Footing in steep terrain is compromised.
- High wind creates white-out conditions.
- Glacial snow may have crevasses.
- Conditions vary throughout the day.
- Extra equipment is required (e.g., snowshoes, skis).
- Energy expenditure increases.

is usually a mass of bogs, swamps, and standing water, and crossing them is difficult at best. Rain and fog are common, and insects such as mosquitoes, midges, and black flies can be significant problems. If the skin is not completely covered, or if travelers do not use a head net and insect repellent, insect bites may be a major threat to health and mental well-being.

Summer travel in timbered, subarctic environments should not present any major problems. However, travel on ridges is preferred because the terrain is drier, and there are usually fewer insects. During the cold months, snow may be deep, and travel is difficult without some type of snowshoes or skis. Travel is generally easier on frozen rivers, streams, and lakes, which may have less snow, making them easier to walk on.

In mountainous country, it is often best to travel along ridgelines because they provide a firmer walking surface, and there is usually less vegetation with which to contend. High winds make travel impractical if not impossible at times. Glaciers have many hidden dangers. Glacial streams may run just under the surface of the snow or ice, creating weak spots, or they may run on the surface and cause slick ice. Crevasses running across glaciers can be a few feet to several hundred feet deep. A thin layer of snow often covers crevasses, making them practically invisible. Unwary team members can fall into crevasses and sustain severe injuries or death. If glacial travel is required, it is best to use a probe pole or an ice axe to test the footing ahead.

In ice and snow conditions, river and stream travel can be hazardous. Comparatively straight rivers are that way because of the volume of water flow and extremely fast currents. These rivers tend to have very thin ice in the winter, especially where snow banks extend out over the water. If an object protrudes through the ice, the immediate area may be weak and should be avoided. Where two rivers and streams come together, the current is swift, and the ice may be weaker than on the rest of the river. Very often after freezing, the source of the river or stream dries up so rapidly that air pockets form under the ice and can be dangerous. During the runoff months (spring and summer), rivers and streams usually have a large volume of very cold water that can cause cold injuries. Stream banks are often choked with alder, devil's club, and other thick vegetation, making traveling very slow and difficult.

In snow environments, optimum travel conditions may vary from hour to hour. Certain indicators may show the best method of travel, such as depth that a person sinks into the snow. The best snow condition is one that supports a person on or near the surface when wearing boots, and the second best is calf-deep snow conditions. If possible, avoid traveling in thigh- or waist-deep snow, and wear snowshoes when conditions dictate.

South and west slopes offer hard surfaces late in the day after exposure to the sun has melted the snow slightly and the surface is refrozen. East and north slopes tend to remain soft and unstable. Walking on one side of a ridge, gully, clump of trees, or large boulders is often more solid than the other side. Dirty snow absorbs more heat than clean snow; slopes darkened by rocks, dust, or uprooted vegetation usually provide more solid footing. Travel can be best in the morning to take advantage of stable snow conditions. Since sunlight affects the stability of snow, travel may be best when done in shaded areas where footing should remain stable.

In areas covered by early seasonal snowfall, travel cautiously between deep snow and clear ground. Snow on slopes tends to slip away from rocks on the downhill side, forming openings. These openings, called moats, are filled by subsequent snowfalls. During the snow season, moats below large rocks or cliffs may become extremely wide and deep, presenting a hazard to any SAR personnel.

Using an Ice Axe to Arrest a Fall

The use of the ice axe in SAR is derived from its roots in mountaineering (**FIGURE 12-6**). The axe is carried primarily for use in mountainous conditions, usually at higher elevations, when ice and snow conditions are coupled with severe terrain. Classically, carry the ice axe to aid in balance while walking (downhill, uphill, glissading, etc.), as a braking device during a fall or glissades, or as an anchor in snow. When using the device properly, it can save your life and aid in rescuing others.

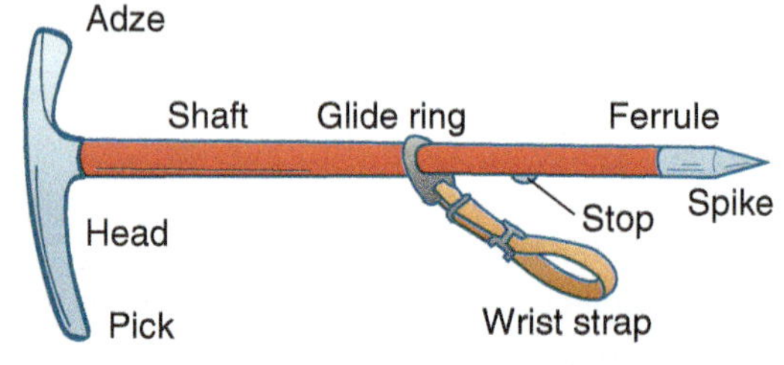

FIGURE 12-6 Parts of an ice axe.

On any slope where a slip may lead to a quick descent or a slide down a mountainside, carry the ice axe in a position ready to make an arrest. The ready position is as follows:

1. Place one hand, preferably the stronger one, on the head of the axe with the thumb under the adze and the fingers over the pick.
2. Place your other hand on the shaft next to the spike.

If walking with the axe in one hand, use your stronger hand. If you slip, your immediate action is to grasp the shaft with the free hand and go into the arrest position (**FIGURE 12-7**). When the fall occurs, the faster you brake, the better your chances of stopping. Move quickly! The faster you slide, the harder it is to stop. Immediately press the pick into the slope just above the shoulder so the adze is near the angle formed by the neck and the shoulders.

The shaft should cross the chest diagonally with the spike held firmly close to the opposite hip. Hold a short axe (for ice climbing) in the same position, although the spike will not reach the opposite hip. Your chest and shoulders should press strongly on the shaft, and your spine should be arched slightly to distribute weight primarily at the shoulders and toes. Legs should be stiff and spread apart, toes digging in (if wearing crampons, keep your toes off the surface until almost stopped), and hang on the axe. Basically, the ideal arrest position is sliding on the stomach, feet downhill, with the weight on the pick (shoulders) and the toes. The hand on the shaft must be toward the spike end so that the axe does not pivot on the pick and cause injury.

Additional guidelines for using an ice axe to arrest a fall include the following:

- Do not try to lift your body off the ice while pressing the pick into the ground. Keep the axe close to the chest and keep your face down. The ice and snow at that level is uncomfortable, but lifting the body can decrease control.
- Do not press the spike end into the ice to attempt an arrest because this could rip the axe out of your hand or pivot the shaft over your head and make it useless for arresting.
- Keep the axe below the shoulders at all cost. The pressure that one can apply for braking is substantially decreased when holding the axe over the shoulders.
- If you fall onto your back with feet downhill, grasp the axe properly and turn toward the hand that

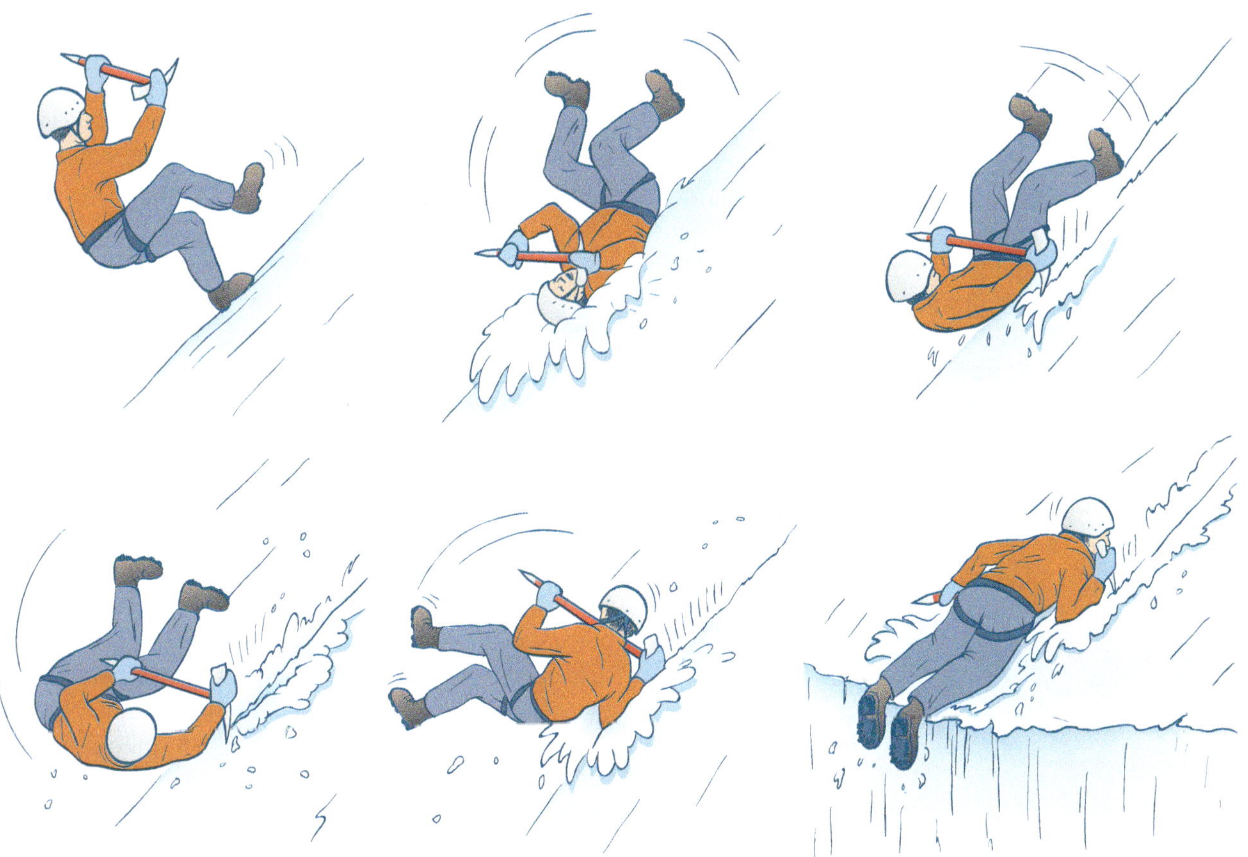

FIGURE 12-7 Use of an ice axe to arrest a fall.

holds the pick end of the axe. Assume the prone, feet downhill, arrest position.

- If you fall onto your back with your feet uphill, press the pick into the ice beside your hip with the shaft held across your body. Use the pick as a pivot and turn your body to the head-uphill position by rolling onto your stomach. Pull the pick into the proper shoulder position and continue to press into the ice until stopped.
- Hold onto the axe. Losing your axe in mountainous terrain where ice and snow impede safe travel is paramount to throwing away your clothes. In both, you are in a dangerous environment without the tools necessary for safe travel.

Snowshoes

Use a striding technique for movement with snowshoes (**FIGURE 12-8**). In taking a stride, lift the toe of the snowshoe upward to clear the snow and thrust forward. Conserve energy by lifting the snowshoe no higher than is necessary to clear the snow. If the front of the snowshoe catches, pull the foot back to free it and then lift it before proceeding with the stride. The best method of travel that requires the least exertion is a loose-kneed, rocking gait in a normal rhythmic stride. Take care not to step on or catch the other snowshoe.

On gentle slopes, ascend by climbing straight upward; traction is generally very poor on hard-packed or crusty snow. Ascend steeper terrain by traversing and packing a trail similar to a shelf. When climbing, place the snowshoe horizontally in the snow. On hard snow, place the snowshoe flat on the surface with the toe of the upper one diagonally uphill to get more traction. If the snow supports the weight of a person, it may be better to remove the snowshoes and temporarily proceed on foot. In turning, the best method is to swing the leg up and turn the snowshoe in the new direction of travel.

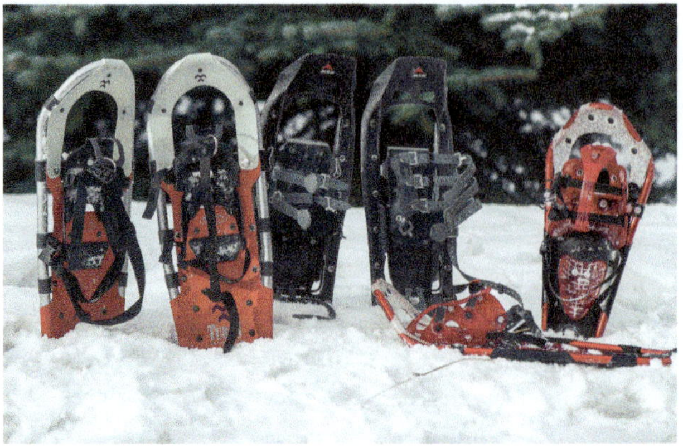

FIGURE 12-8 Examples of modern snowshoes that could be used in SAR operations.

Step over obstacles such as logs, tree stumps, ditches, and small streams. Take care not to place too much strain on the snowshoe in shallow snow. There is danger of catching and damaging the webbing on tree stumps or snags. Wet snow frequently builds up under the feet, making walking uncomfortable. Knock this snow off with a stick or pole.

Generally, ski poles are not used in snowshoeing; however, one or two poles are desirable when carrying heavy loads, especially in mountainous terrain. Do not fasten the bindings too tightly, or circulation may be impaired and cause frostbite. During stops, check the bindings for fit and possible readjustment.

Uphill Travel

Maximum altitude may be obtained with less effort by traversing a slope. A zigzag or **switchback** route used to traverse steep slopes places body weight over the entire foot as opposed to the balls of the feet as in a straight line uphill climb. An additional advantage to zigzagging or switchbacking is alternating the stress and strain placed on the feet, ankles, legs, and arms when making a change in direction.

When making a change in direction, the body is temporarily out of balance. The proper method for turning on the steep slope is to pivot on the outside foot (the one away from the slope). With the upper slope on the right side, kick the left foot (pivot foot) directly into the slope. This transfers the body weight onto the left foot while pivoting toward the slope. The slope is then positioned on the left side, and the right foot is on the outside.

In soft snow on steep slopes, stamp in pit steps for solid footing. On hard snow, the surface is solid but slippery, and level pit steps must be made. In both cases, make the steps by swinging the entire leg in toward the slope, not by merely pushing the boot into the snow. In hard snow, when one or two blows do not suffice, use crampons. Space steps evenly and close together to facilitate ease of travel and balance. Additionally, the lead traveler must consider the other team members, especially those who have a shorter stride.

A team should travel in single file when ascending, permitting the leader to establish the route. In this configuration, the physical exertion of the leader is greater than that of any other team member. The leader must remain alert to safeguard other team members while choosing the best route of travel. Rotate the leader frequently to prevent exhaustion of any one individual. Team members following the leader should use the same leg swing technique to establish foot positions, improving each step as they walk. Each foot must be firmly kicked into place, securely positioning the boot in the step. In compact

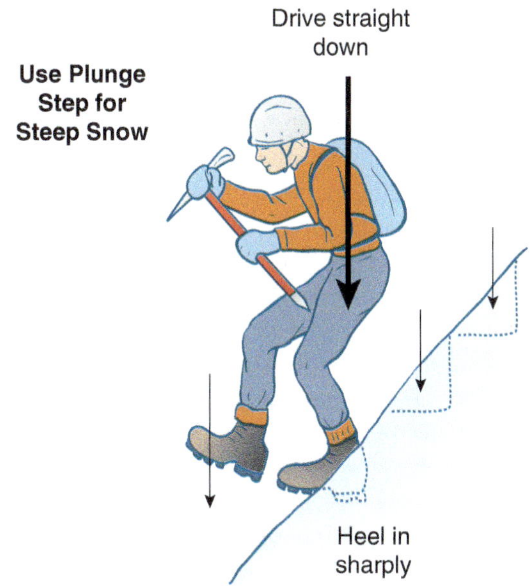

FIGURE 12-9 The plunge step is used to descend scree or snow.

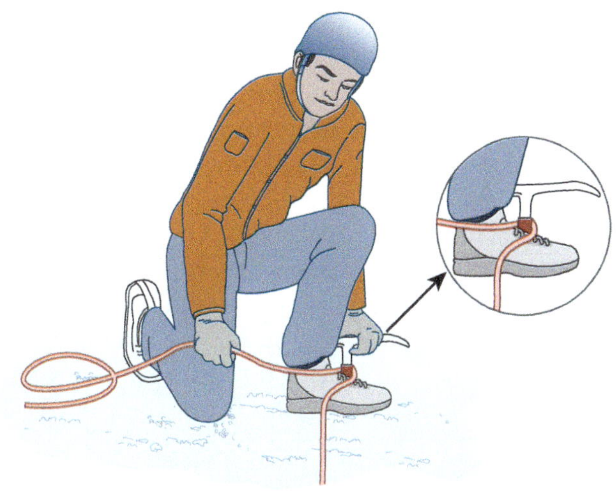

FIGURE 12-10 The boot axe belay requires that the full length of the ice axe penetrates firm snow. The brake is applied by wrapping the rope around the heel of the boot.

snow, the kick should be somewhat low, shaving off snow during each step, thus enlarging the hole by deepening. In very soft snow, it is usually easier to bring the boot down from above, dragging a layer of snow into the step to strengthen and decrease the depth of it.

When it is necessary to traverse a slope without an increase in elevation, the heels rather than the toes form the step. During the stride, the climber twists the leading leg so that the boot heel strikes the slope first, carrying most of the weight into the step. The toe is pointed up and out. Like the plunge step, the heel makes the platform secure by compacting the snow more effectively than the toe (**FIGURE 12-9**).

Descending

The route down a slope may be different from the route up a slope. Route variations may be required for descending different sides of a mountain or moving just a few feet from icy shadows onto sun-softened slopes. A good surface snow condition is ideal for descending rapidly since it yields comfortably underfoot. The primary techniques for descending snow-covered slopes are plunge stepping and descending step by step.

The plunge step (see Figure 12-9) makes extensive use of the heels of the feet and is applicable on scree as well as snow. Ideally, the plunging route should be at an angle, one that is within the capabilities of the team and affords a safe descent. The angle at which the heel enters the surface varies with the surface hardness. On soft snow slopes, almost any angle suffices; however, if the person leans too far forward, there is a risk of lodging the foot in a rut and inflicting injuries.

On hard snow, the heel cannot penetrate the surface unless it has sufficient force behind it. Failure to firmly drive the heel into the snow can cause a slip and subsequent slide. The quickest way to check a slip is to shift the weight onto the other heel, making several short, stiff-legged stomps. This technique is not intended to replace the "ice arrest" technique, which is usually more effective. When roped, plunging requires coordination and awareness of all team members' progress. Limit the speed of the team to the slowest member. Plunging may not work when wearing crampons due to the snow compacting and sticking to them.

Use the step-by-step descending technique when the terrain is extremely steep, the snow is significantly deep, or circumstances dictate a slower pace. On near-vertical walls, it is necessary to face the slope and cautiously lower oneself step by step, thrusting the toe of the boot into the snow while maintaining an anchor or hand-hold with the axe. Once the new foothold withstands the body's full weight, repeat the technique. On moderately angled terrain, the team can face away from the slope and descend by step-kicking with the heels.

A belay, or anchor, can be set up in several different ways using the ice axe and your body. One of these is termed the *boot axe belay* (**FIGURE 12-10**). The boot axe belay can be set up rapidly and used when a team is moving together, and belaying is required only at a few spots. Practice the boot axe belay until a sweep and jab of the ice axe can set up the stance within a couple of seconds. The axe provides an anchor to the slope, and the slope and the boot brace the axe. Both give a friction surface over which the run of rope is controlled.

To prepare a boot axe belay, stamp out in the snow a firm platform, large enough for the axe and uphill boot. Jam the ice axe shaft as deeply as possible, at a slight uphill angle (against the anticipated fall), into the snow at the rear of the platform. The pick is parallel to the fall line, pointing uphill, thus applying the strongest dimension of the shaft against the force of a fall. The length of the pick prevents the rope from escaping over the top of the shaft.

The belayer stands below the axe, facing at a right angle to the fall line. Stamp the uphill boot into the slope against the downhill side of the shaft at a right angle to the fall line, bracing the shaft against downhill pull. The downhill boot is in a firmly compacted step below the uphill boot so that the leg is straight, stiffly bracing the belayer. The uphill hand is on the axe head in arrest grasp, bracing the shaft against downhill and lateral stress. From below, the rope crosses the toe of the boot, preventing the rope from trenching into the snow. The rope bends around the uphill side of the shaft, then down across the instep of the bracing boot, and is controlled by the downhill hand. To apply braking through greater friction, the downhill or braking hand brings the rope uphill around the heel, forming an "S" bend.

Crampon Technique

Crampons are a lightweight frame of steel spikes that can be attached to one's boots. Special care must be taken to attach the crampons tightly to the boots, running the strap through each attachment point. If crampons do not have heel loops, ankle straps should be long enough to be crossed behind the boot before being secured to prevent boots from sliding backward out of the crampons. Crampons can be lost if this precaution is not taken. When measuring new straps, make allowance for gaiters, which sometimes cover the instep of the boot. When putting on the crampons, lay each crampon on the snow or ice with all rings and straps outward, then place the boot on the crampon and tighten the straps. Even modern synthetic straps should be checked from time to time to make sure they are tight, have not been cut, and are not trailing loop strap ends that could cause the wearer to trip.

If crampons might be needed, they should be carried. Weather conditions change rapidly; an east-facing slope may be mushy enough for step-kicking during the morning but can become a smooth sheet of ice in the afternoon shade. Furthermore, using crampons may contribute directly to the team's safety by enabling the team to negotiate stretches of ice faster and with less fatigue than having to chop steps. Your situation determines whether to wear crampons. Wearing crampons should not be considered mandatory because of venturing onto a glacier; neither should a team attempt to save time by never wearing crampons on steep, exposed icy patches just because they are fairly short. Another important guideline is to don crampons before they are needed to avoid teetering in ice steps. On mixed rock and ice climbs, constant attaching and removing crampons takes so much time that the objective may be lost.

Wear crampons throughout the entire climb if the terrain is 50% or more suitable for crampons (crampons may skid or be broken on rock surfaces). Crampons may not be required if the snow or ice patches are fairly short, good belays are available, and rock predominates. These alternatives are merely suggestions, and the decision must be based on the conditions at hand.

Take crampons off when the snow begins to ball up badly in them and no improvement in snow conditions is anticipated. On the ascent, it may be possible to clear away the soft surface snow and climb on the ice below, but this is usually impractical and futile on the descent. Occasionally, the climber should kick the crampons free of accumulated snow. The time-worn practice of striking the ice axe shaft against the crampons to knock out the snow is effective but hard on the axe and perhaps the ankle. In situations where the crampons must be worn even though the snow balls up in them, shuffling the feet through the snow instead of stepping over the surface tends to force the accumulated snow through the back points. The normal kicking motion of the foot generally keeps the crampons snow-free on the ascent and while traversing.

On the descent, drive the toe of the boot under the surface of the snow ahead of the heel, walking on the ball of the foot. Keep the weight well forward and use short skating steps, allowing the foot to slide forward and penetrate the harder sub-layers.

Flat-footing involves a logical and natural progression of coordinated body and ice axe positions to allow the climber to move steadily and in balance while keeping all vertical points of the crampons biting into the ice. The weight is directly over the feet, the crampon points stamped firmly into the ice with each step, with the ankles and knees flexed to allow boot soles to remain parallel to the slope.

On gentle slopes, the climber walks straight up the hill. Normally, the feet are naturally flat to the slope, and the axe is used as a cane. If pointing the toes uphill becomes awkward, they may be turned outward in duck-fashion. As the slope steepens, the body is turned to face across the slope rather than up it. The feet may also point across the slope, but additional flexibility and greater security are gained by pointing the lower foot downhill. Use the axe to maintain balance, and carry it in the cane position or the arrest grasp with either the pick or point touching the slope. Movement is diagonal rather than straight upward, and the climber takes advantage of terrain irregularities and graded slopes. Change your direction as in step-kicking on snow by planting the downhill foot, turning the body toward the slope to face the opposite direction, and stepping off with the new downhill foot.

SEARCH AND RESCUE TIP

Crampons have often been lost because the precaution of securing them to the boots was not taken. If the crampons do not have heel straps, use the ankle straps to cross behind the boot to prevent boots from sliding backward out of the crampons.

On gentler slopes, use the flat-footed approach throughout. On steeper slopes, it is more secure and easier to initiate the turn by kicking the front points and briefly front-pointing through the turn. At some point in the turn, the grip on the axe must be reversed. The exact moment for this depends on the climber and the specific situation. However, the climber's stance must be secure when temporarily relinquishing the axe as the third point of support.

On steep slopes, which approach the limit of practical use of this style of ascent, the climber relies on the axe for hold security as well as for balance. Hold the axe in the arrest grasp with one hand on the head and the other on the shaft above the point. Plant the well-sharpened pick firmly in the ice at about shoulder height to provide one point of suspension while a foot moves forward, and the crampons are stamped.

Descent follows the same general progression of foot and axe positions; descend the fall line, gradually turning the toes out as the slope gets steeper. As the slope steepens, widen the stance, flex the knees, lean forward to keep weight over the feet, and finally, face sideways and descend with the support of the axe in the arrest position. On very steep or hard ice, it may be necessary to face the slope and front-point downwards. When walking flat-footed downhill, all crampon points should be stamped firmly into the ice. It may be necessary to strive to take small steps, allowing the climber to maintain balance during moves; long steps require major weight shifts to adjust balance.

Climbing

Balance climbing is the type of movement used to climb rock faces. It is a combination of the balance movement of a tightrope walker and the unbalanced climbing of a person ascending a tree or ladder. During the process of route selection, climbers often visualize the route and mentally climb it to learn what might be expected. Climbers should not wear gloves when balance climbing.

Body Position

The climber must keep good balance when climbing (the weight placed over the feet during movement). The feet, not the hands, should carry the weight (with rare exception). The hands are for balance (**FIGURE 12-11**). The feet do not provide proper traction when the climber leans in toward the rock. With the body in balance, the climber moves with a slow, rhythmic motion. Whenever possible, use three points of contact with the climbing surface, such as two feet and one hand. The preferred handholds are waist to shoulder high. Resting is necessary when climbing because tense muscles tire quickly. When resting, keep the arms low, where circulation is not impaired. Use of small intermediate holds is preferable to stretching and clinging to widely separated big holds. Avoid a spread-eagle position, where a climber stretches too far and cannot let go.

Due to balance and body position issues, SAR personnel may not want to carry their SAR packs while climbing. A pack can be roped and lifted separately after a climb, as needed.

Types of Holds

Push holds are desirable because they help the climber keep the arms low. However, they are more difficult to hold onto in case of a slip. A push hold is often used to advantage in combination with a pull hold. Pull holds are those that are pulled down and are the easiest holds to use. They are also the most likely to break out.

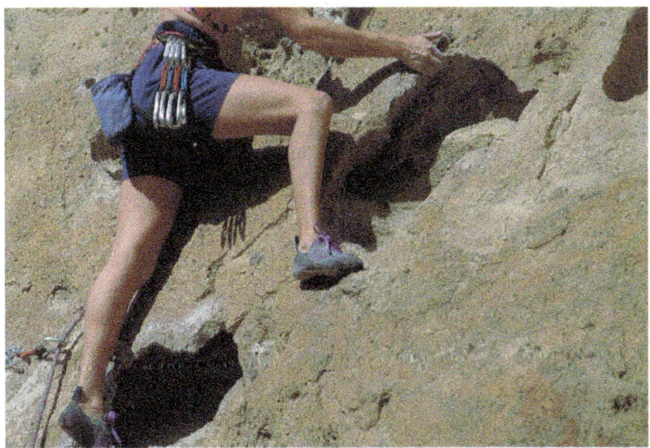

FIGURE 12-11 When climbing, the feet, not the hands, should carry the weight (with rare exception). The hands are for balance.

Jam holds involve jamming any part of the body or extremity into a crack. This is done by putting the hand into the crack and clenching it into a fist or by placing the arm into the crack and twisting the elbow against one side and the hand against the other side. When using the foot in a jam hold, take care to ensure placing the boot so it can be removed easily when climbing is continued; there are limits to how far the foot and ankle can flex.

The holds mentioned previously are considered basic, and from these, any number of combinations and variations can be used. The number of these variations depends only on the limit of the climber's imagination. Following are a few of the more common variations:

- The lay back (lieback) is done by pulling with arms to the side and pushing with the feet in the opposite direction (rockclimbing.com, 2017). Lay backing is a classic form of force or counterforce where the hands and the feet pull and push in opposite directions, enabling the climber to move up in a series of shifting moves. It is very strenuous.
- An undercling (undercut) is a hold that requires fingers to face upward rather than downward (rockclimbing .com, 2017).
- Mantleshelving, or manteling, is a climbing technique involving the transfer of upward force from a pulling action to a pushing action, much like a child would climb the kitchen counter to reach the cabinets above (rockclimbing.com, 2017). This move takes advantage of down pressure exerted by one or both hands on a slab or shelf. Straightening and locking the arm raises the body, allowing a leg to be placed on a higher hold before standing (**FIGURE 12-12**).
- A chimney is a parallel-sided crack wider than body width. Chimney climbing is done by using the arms and the legs to apply pressure against the opposite faces of the rock in a counterforce move. The outstretched hands hold the body while the legs are drawn as high as possible. Flexing the legs forces the body up. Continue this procedure as necessary. Another method is to place the back against one wall and the legs and the arms against the other and "worm" upward.

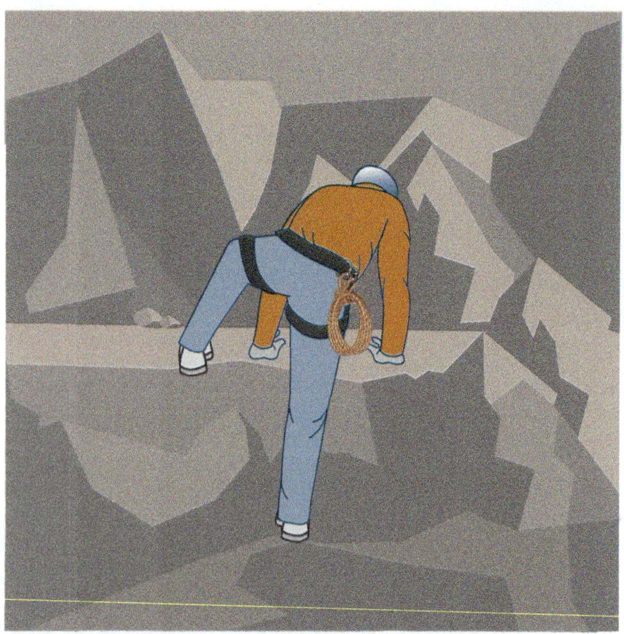

FIGURE 12-12 An example of manteling.

Friction Climbing

A slab is a relatively smooth portion of rock lying at an angle. When traversing, point the lower foot slightly downhill to increase balance and friction of the foot. Use all irregularities in the slope for additional friction. On steep slabs, it may be necessary to squat with the body weight well over the feet, with hands alongside for added friction. Use this position for ascending, traversing, or descending. A slip may result if the climber leans back or lets the buttocks down. Wet, icy, mossy, or scree-covered slabs are the most dangerous.

Friction holds depend solely on the friction of hands or feet against a relatively smooth surface with a shallow hold. They are difficult to use because they give a feeling of insecurity, which the inexperienced climber tries to correct by leaning close to the rock, thereby increasing the imbalance. They often serve well as intermediate holds, giving needed support while the climber moves over them. However, they would not hold if the climber decided to stop.

Wrap-Up

READY FOR REVIEW

- Walking and nontechnical travel (searching, getting to the search area, etc.) may be necessary in one or more general environments.
- Climbing or other technical travel (accessing a search area, examining a high-risk area, technical rescue, etc.) may also involve one of many environments.

- Traveling on foot for recreational purposes can also involve technical and nontechnical actions but with far different motivations and goals.
- Since walking is the primary mode of transportation in a SAR incident, being conditioned to walk or hike for long distances may mean the difference between effectiveness and futility.
- Five things are needed to prepare for traveling in SAR work: fitness, energy, water, rest, and technique.
- Two fundamental rules regarding wilderness travel need to be mastered to expend a minimum of energy and time when moving across the ground. First, keep the weight of the body directly over the feet. Second, keep the sole of the foot flat on the ground to improve traction.
- The climber must keep good balance when climbing (the weight placed over the feet during movement). The feet, not the hands, should carry the weight (with rare exception). The hands are for balance.

SEARCH AND RESCUE TERMS

Crampons A lightweight frame of steel spikes that can be attached to one's boots; for walking or climbing on ice.

Jam holds Climbing holds that involve jamming any part of the body or extremity into a crack. This is done by putting the hand into the crack and clenching it into a fist, or by placing the arm into the crack and twisting the elbow against one side and the hand against the other side.

Probability of detection (POD) "The probability of the search object being detected, assuming it was in the areas that were searched. It is a function of coverage factor, sensor, search conditions and the accuracy with which the search resource navigates its assigned search patterns. Measures sensor effectiveness under the prevailing search conditions" (NSARC, 2011, p xxi).

Scree slopes Areas consisting of small rocks and gravel that have collected below rock ridges and cliffs.

Strainer In swift water, an obstacle that moving water can flow through, but that a swimmer or boat cannot. It is formed by natural or human-made objects, such as storm grates over tunnels, trees that have fallen into a river (log jam), bushes by the side of the river that are flooded during high water, wire fence, rebar from broken concrete structures in the water, or other debris.

Switchback A zigzag pattern used to traverse steep slopes.

Talus The term sometimes used by climbers to describe something similar to scree, except the rock pieces are larger, and the rocks do not slide as much. Geologists use the term to describe the slope on which scree is found.

REFERENCES AND SUGGESTED READING

Harper, Douglas. 2017. Online etymology dictionary. http://www.etymonline.com/index.php.

Johnson, Mark. 2003. *The Ultimate Desert Handbook: A Manual for Desert Hikers, Campers, and Travelers*. New York: Ragged Mountain Press/McGraw Hill.

Linxweiler, Eric and Mike Maude, Editors. 2017. *Mountaineering: Freedom of the Hills*, 9th edition. New York: Mountaineers Books.

Manning, Harvey. 1986. *Backpacking: One Step at a Time*, 4th edition. New York: Vintage Books.

McManners, Hugh. 2007. *The Complete Wilderness Training Book*. 2nd revised edition. New York: DK Publishing.

National Search and Rescue Committee. 2011. Land Search and Rescue Addendum to the National Search and Rescue Supplement to the International Aeronautical and Maritime Search and Rescue Manual, Version 1.0. https://www.hsdl.org/?abstract&did=715465

Petzoldt, Paul. 1974. *The Wilderness Handbook*. New York: W.W. Norton & Company, Inc.

Rawlins, Chip, and Fletcher, Colin. 2002. *The Complete Walker IV*, revised edition. New York: Alfred A. Knopf, Inc.

Ray, Slim, and Les Bechdel. 2009. *River Rescue: A Manual for Whitewater Safety*, 4th edition. Asheville, NC: CFS Press.

Rockclimbing.com. 2017. Climbing dictionary. http://www.rockclimbing.com/Articles/Introduction_to_Climbing/Climbing_Dictionary_528.html#l.

CHAPTER 13

Tracking

OBJECTIVES

Upon completion of this chapter and the related course activities, the student will be able to meet the following objectives:

- Identify and define the following terms useful in understanding the tracking process:
  - Track aware
  - Tracking
  - Sign
  - Sign cutting
  - Step-by-step method of tracking
  - Medial
  - Lateral
  - Supination
  - Pronation
- Describe the method and proper use of a sign-cutting or tracking stick.
- Describe the method of labeling partial and complete tracks and right and left tracks.
- Describe the responsibilities of each of the members of a tracking crew (point, flankers).
- Describe the visual cues a tracker should be able to discern.

The contents of this chapter are excerpted with permission from *Fundamentals of Mantracking: The Step-by-Step Method*, 3rd edition, by Albert "Ab" Taylor and Donald C. Cooper, Skyhorse Publishing, © 2014 Donald C. Cooper, All Rights Reserved. Available through the NASAR bookstore (www.nasar.org).

Tracking in Perspective

Tracking, by simple definition, is following signs of track left by someone or something. It is used to detect the path (direction, movement) of someone or something. However, tracking, when applied to search and rescue (SAR) missions, becomes a more complex skill. It not only concerns itself with detection but with interpretation of clues as well. Tracking is both an investigative (strategy) and an operational (tactics) SAR tool.

Unfortunately, tracking is underutilized in SAR situations. Often, SAR personnel ignore sign and track because they are unaware of its potential. Too often, SAR personnel and managers unknowingly walk on the very **evidence** for which they search while distracted by their computers and reference books. A story has been printed on the ground and we, as **track aware** searchers, must discover its existence, then learn to read it (**FIGURE 13-1**). This is not to say that once tracking is applied to SAR situations, every missing subject will be found. Rather, tracking gives the subject a much better chance of survival, and it can help prove (or disprove) that a missing person is within a designated geographical area.

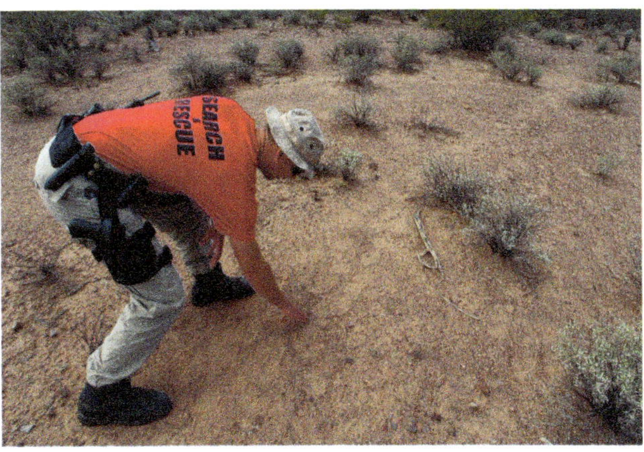

FIGURE 13-1 A story has been written on the ground, and we, as track aware SAR personnel, must discover its existence and learn to interpret it.
© David McNew/Staff/Getty.

SEARCH AND RESCUE TIP

Qualities of a good tracker include the following:

- Patience
- An inquisitive mind
- Honesty
- Perseverance
- Good observation skills
- Honed senses (all five)
- Endurance
- Good field craft skills
- Determination (mental and physical)
- Knowledge of fauna and flora
- Curiosity

Definitions and Terminology

A **track** or **print** is an impression left from the passage of a person that can be positively identified as being human. Further, a track may be complete, meaning that the entire impression is visible; **partial**, meaning that it is not visible in its entirety; and/or identifiable, meaning that, complete or partial, it has at least one characteristic that differentiates it from others like it. **Tracking** is simply defined as following someone, or something, by stringing together a continuous chain of their sign. **Sign** is any evidence of change from the natural state that is inflicted on an environment by a person's passage. A track, whether complete or partial, is many individual pieces of sign combined in such a way as to form a print. The technique is first to find some sign, then interpret it, and ultimately act on it. Simply put, tracking is the ability to discover and combine sign in chronological order, consider its meaning after investigation, and do this over a large area.

To be of any use, sign must be discovered. Seeing it is usually fairly easy because there is so much of it. A walking person leaves sign approximately every 18–20 inches, or over 3,000 times per mile, so catching even a small percentage of it should not be much trouble. The problem lies not in finding sign but in determining which is relevant and which is not. The novice tracker, for example, often sees plenty of relevant sign, yet disregards it because he or she thought it to be insignificant. The experienced tracker sees the same information but has learned to interpret its meaning.

SEARCH AND RESCUE TIP

A walking person leaves sign approximately every 18–20 inches, or over 3,000 times per mile.

If sign is considered evidence, then common law enforcement terms can be applied to distinguish different types. Sign can be separated into two categories: conclusively human and corroborant. **Conclusively human sign** is a disturbance that, on its own, can positively be said to have been caused by a person and not an animal. The use of the SAFE test (see the Tip box) can be helpful in determining whether a print is conclusively human. **Corroborant sign** is a disturbance that is not decisively human and could have been caused by an animal. This type of sign may corroborate other evidence but, when considered on its own, is not conclusive. It cannot be positively determined to have been caused by a person but may confirm or substantiate other evidence with which it may be found.

SEARCH AND RESCUE TIP

Use the SAFE test to determine whether a print is human:

S—Is it the size and shape of a human print?

A—Does it include one or more 90-degree angles?

F—Is there significant flatness, especially in the size and shape of a human print?

E—Does it have one or more clear edges that incorporate sharp or 90-degree angles?

Sign cutting is looking for sign to establish a starting point from which to track. Tracking involves following a chronology of sign, or consecutive tracks, step-by-step. Sign cutting is searching for the first sign or track. Another principal difference between tracking and sign cutting is that tracking is done by traveling the same direction as the person who laid the track; sign cutting is done traveling (ideally) perpendicular to the direction of travel of the person being followed. Sign cutting is done by looking for sign in a path that would intersect that of the person who laid the track. It is most effective when performed in an area where the sign being sought is most visible and easily seen. An area that is particularly good for finding sign, such as wet sand, mud, soft dirt, or snow, is sometimes called a **track trap** or **cuttable area**. Track traps can also be human-made by scraping an area clean to show sign easily.

Sign cutting can substantially reduce the search area by detecting sign that indicates direction of travel. This can be a very efficient application of resources, particularly at the onset of an incident when urgency is high, and the quantity of searchers/trackers is low.

Jump tracking is a form of tracking that involves finding a big, obvious footprint, then proceeding along the presumed direction of travel until another obvious track is found. Jump tracking involves guesswork, luck, essentially no skill, and can be dangerous when a life depends on skillful tracking. One of the biggest problems in tracking has always been the destruction of sign by unknowing, energetic, and well-meaning searchers. Jump tracking offers great potential for this type of clue erasure. Since virtually all humans can jump track without training, this is not the type of tracking that will be discussed here.

Although there are multiple ways to describe it, in this text *stride* is the measured distance between the rear margin of the heel of one footfall and the rear margin of the heel of the following footfall. **Step-by-step tracking** is a disciplined tracking methodology and teaching system where a tracker sees each step in sequence and proceeds no farther than the last visible track, using the stride to determine where next to look for sign. This system, above all, makes searchers of all types **clue conscious** and track aware (aware that track and sign exist). It is the standard for which an experienced tracker strives at all times. In theory, a tracker attempts to find every piece of evidence left by his or her **quarry**. In a real situation, this is not always possible, and even the best trackers must accept small gaps in the continuous chain of evidence. The words *small gaps* best distinguish the step-by-step method from jump tracking.

Bracketing is an occasionally acceptable method of interpolation between tracks that can be used when standard step-by-step approaches fail to produce. Bracketing is meant as a stopgap measure that uses a predetermined stride to skip one step in sequence to find the next, and then use it to find the one skipped. In terms of the step-by-step approach, bracketing is cheating because it involves moving past the last visible sign to continue the track. Bracketing is not a license to jump track and should be used only infrequently to maintain continuity on an important track. Students may come to this on their own but will never receive permission to do it from an instructor.

Programs that teach the step-by-step method do not teach tracking, as such. They teach an approach that offers the tools to teach oneself tracking. Anyone can learn to track. All it takes beyond learning the basics of the step-by-step approach, if you are motivated, is practice—hours and hours of practice. You may never become an expert tracker, but, at the very least, the step-by-step approach makes you track and sign aware and, therefore, a better searcher.

Using common terms to describe the various parts of the foot can be useful while tracking (**FIGURE 13-2**). Generally, the **heel** is the back part of the foot below the ankle, and the **forefoot** is the larger part of the foot forward of the ankle. **Medial** is a medical term that is often used to describe something that is situated toward the middle or midline of the body. **Lateral** is the term used to describe something situated away from the middle or to the side, usually to the left or the right. On most feet, the little toe is lateral, and the big toe is medial. The term **anterior** is used to refer to something toward the front of the body or toward the head, and **posterior** is used to describe something toward the back of the body. The **arch** of the foot usually refers to the bottom, medial part of the foot, just forward of the ankle, that curves above the ground. It stretches from the heel bone (the calcaneus) to the three medial metatarsals (five middle, long bones of the foot). Medical practitioners also refer to this arch as the *medial longitudinal arch*. The bones of the toes are called **phalanges**, and the big bones of the foot below and including the ankle and the calcaneus are called the **tarsals**.

Supination of the foot is a movement of the foot and leg in which the foot rolls outward with an elevated arch so that in walking the foot tends to come down on its outer edge (**FIGURE 13-3A**). When the foot falls flat on the ground, striking both the outer edge and the inner margin at the same time, this is considered *neutral* movement of the foot (**FIGURE 13-3B**). **Pronation** of the foot is rotation of the medial (middle) bones in

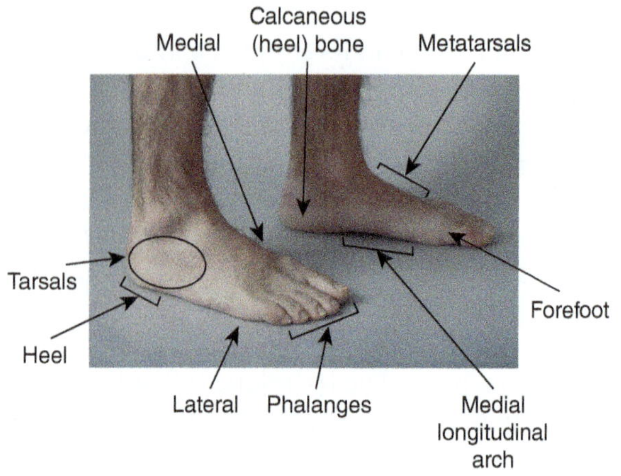

FIGURE 13-2 Parts of the foot.
© Bruno Boissonnet/Science Source.

the midtarsal region of the foot inward and downward so that in walking the foot tends to come down on its inner margin (**FIGURE 13-3C**). These terms can be useful when trying to describe how a foot struck the ground to produce a track.

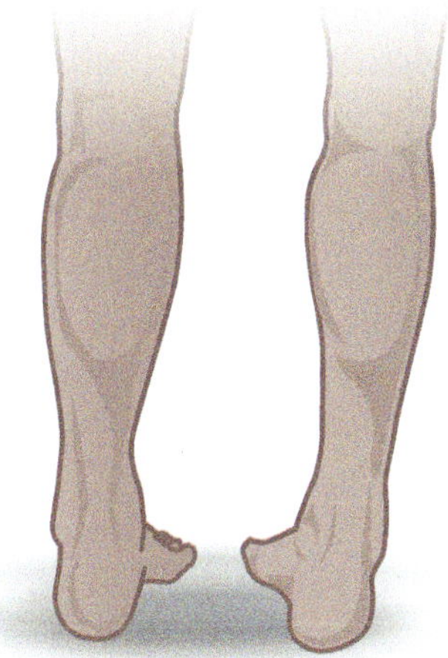

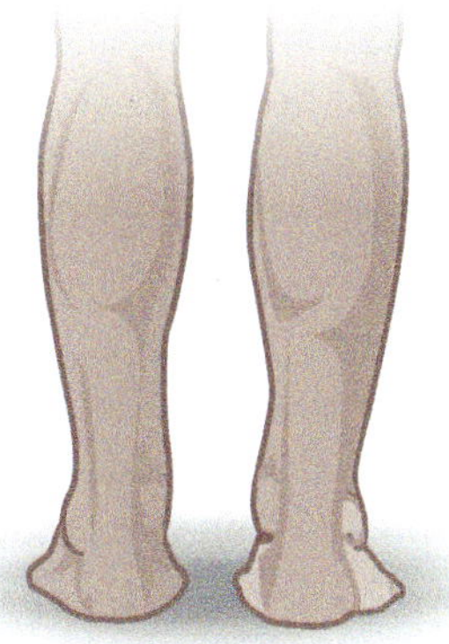

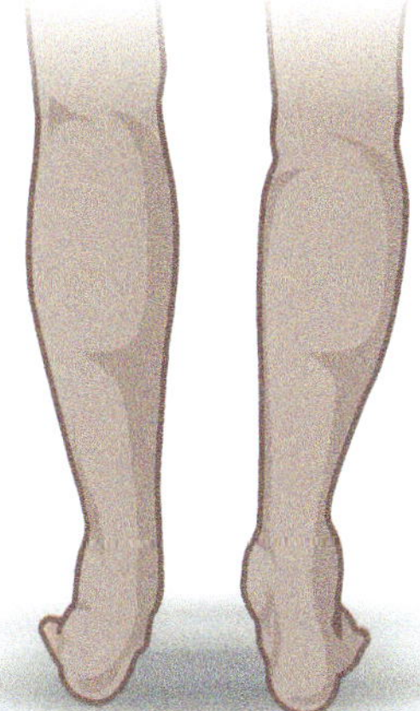

FIGURE 13-3 Common movements of the foot and the leg. **A.** Supination. **B.** Neutral. **C.** Pronation.

The pattern of how a person walks is called **gait** and may vary depending on the medical or physical condition of the subject. **Steppage gait** is when one walks with a footdrop where the foot hangs with the toes pointing down, causing the toes to scrape the ground while walking and requiring the walker to lift the leg higher than normal when walking. **Waddling gait** is a duck-like walk where the lateral distance between footfalls can be larger than a normal gait. The lateral distance between footfalls, perpendicular to the direction of travel, is referred to as **straddle** and can be measured just like stride. Straddle can increase when one carries a heavy load.

When one walks with the toes pointed inward (medially), this is sometimes called **pigeon toed** or **intoeing**. In medical terminology, the terms *metatarsus varus* or *metatarsus adductus* may be used. The opposite of intoeing is **toe out** or **splayed feet**, which is when the toes point outward (laterally) when walking.

Equipment for Tracking

Tracking, essentially, requires very little equipment. A pair of eyes which, aided or not, provide nearly 20/20 vision is tracking's only prerequisite. However, experience has indicated that some items can be quite helpful.

1. Clothing should be appropriate for the terrain and the weather and durable enough to withstand ventures into dense brush and rugged terrain. A broad-brimmed hat may be handy for protecting the eyes from the sun or shading tracks when the sun is high in the sky. Above all, the tracker must be able to work comfortably in whatever environment he or she is thrust.
2. A walking or **sign-cutting stick** is a must, especially for novice trackers. A light, durable stick, approximately 40 inches long, is best, but longer may be preferred. This stick, which is used to focus the attention of a tracker, should have at least two O-rings or rubber bands on it for measuring distance and stride (some trackers use many more than two rings).
3. A measuring device, such as a tape measure, can be valuable when measuring print size or stride. Some attach a measuring tape to their stick, but most simply carry a metal, carpenter's-type tape measure in their pocket. One that indicates both metric (centimeters) and imperial (inches) measurements is a good idea.
4. A small notepad and pencil are needed to record measurements and fill out track reports. A good drawing of a print is indispensable.

5. Trail tape can be carried to cordon off evidence or sign or to prevent the trampling of a good track. Plastic surveyor's tape works well, but care must be taken to see that it is retrieved after it has served its purpose. A bright, high-visibility color is best for this purpose.
6. A flashlight can be important when light is not at an optimum. Since light plays such an important part in seeing, it is easy to appreciate how an artificial light source could be helpful.
7. A mirror can be used to redirect natural light low across sign when the sun is high in the sky.

Some have also found it helpful to include as part of one's tracking equipment knee pads, to make crawling on the ground more comfortable, and colored hair bands, to use on the sign-cutting stick.

Tracking is not an equipment-intensive pursuit. Sight, patience, perseverance, and determination are the only real requirements to be a tracker. The above-mentioned specific equipment is helpful, but the brain and the body are the primary tools of the trade.

Credo of the Novice Tracker

The fundamental principle on which tracking is based is sound training. The rules upon which all future tracking experience is based lie within the following credo. These very basic rules also serve as the ABCs of the step-by-step method of tracking.

1. Do not advance beyond the last print until you find the next one.
2. Do not destroy the evidence.
3. Use a sign-cutting stick.
4. See rules 1 and 2.

Any track or sign is considered evidence until proven otherwise. Treat all track and sign as if it were positively identified as being that of the person being sought. Once a track or sign has been destroyed, it cannot be reconstituted. It is lost forever. The destruction of a track, clue, or any sign not only chips away at the finite body of available information, it reduces the chances of meeting your objective. If that objective is finding a lost person, destroying tracks, clues, or any sign can literally mean the difference between life and death.

Beyond simply finding and interpreting sign, a tracker is obliged to protect it. Remember, any clue is important, no matter how small or seemingly insignificant. Do not move from one place to another without being track aware. An untrained person stepping on good sign or track is unfortunate. A tracker or searcher doing the same is inexcusable.

Light

Since tracking is an intensely visual skill, it is easy to see how light plays an important role. Tracking is far simpler when the light is of the proper intensity and from the right direction (**FIGURE 13-4**). However, the natural environment does not always supply the optimum lighting conditions required for tracking during a SAR incident. When learning to track, using the sun properly is one of the most important things to learn. Tracks are easiest to see when the sun is at a low angle (e.g., early in the morning and late in the afternoon). When the sun is low, it causes longer shadows that bring out the details of any depression on the ground, making sign easier to see. Clouds, diffuse light (through pollution or clouds), and the sun high overhead all diminish the shadow effect. Put simply: Sign and track—impressions

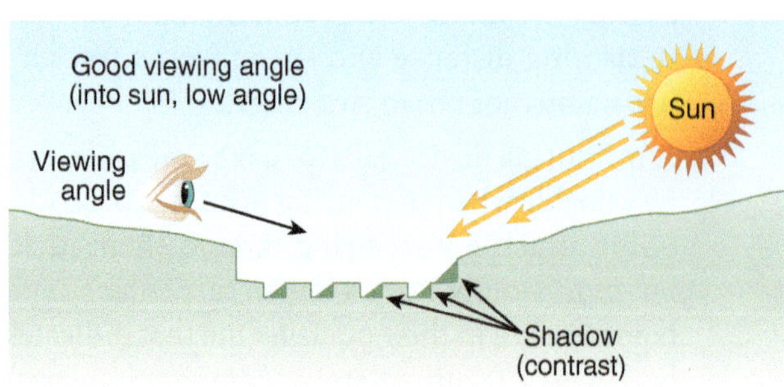

A

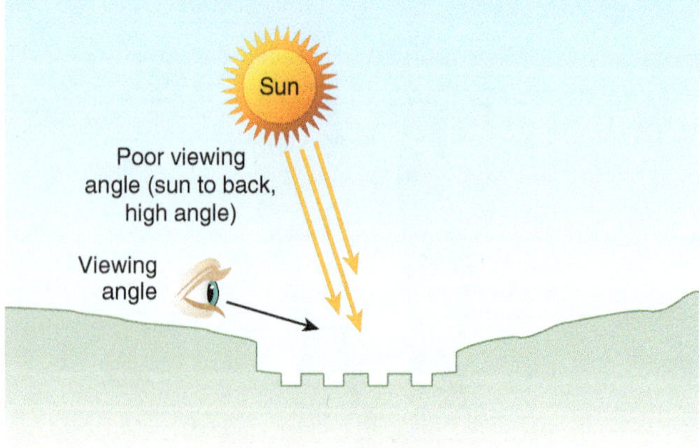

B

FIGURE 13-4 **A.** When viewing even the slightest impression on the ground, keep the light source facing you and at a low angle to enhance the use of shadows that contrast and outline details within the track. **B.** Viewing with the light at your back or at a high angle is far less effective.

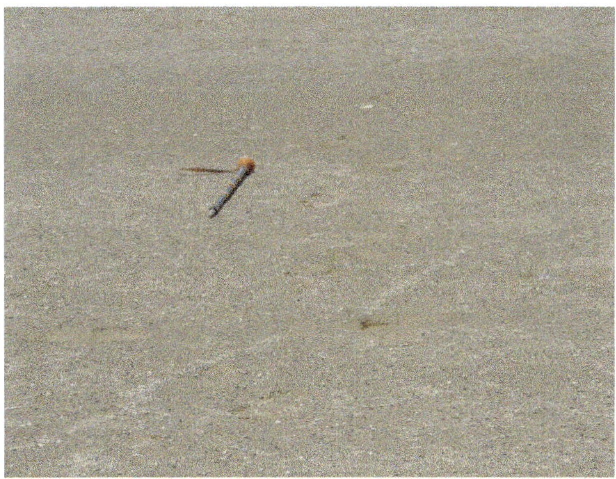
A

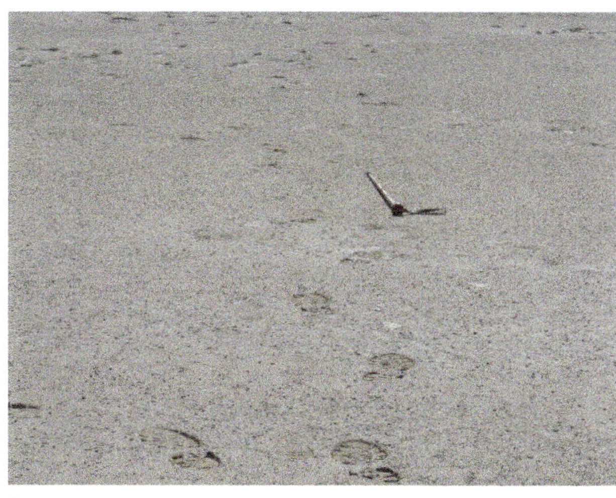
B

FIGURE 13-5 **A.** Track viewed in unfavorable light (sun at back, high angle). **B.** Same track viewed in more favorable light (sun to front, low angle).
Courtesy of Donald Cooper.

in the ground—are usually easier to see while facing the light source and with that source at a low angle to the ground.

Since facing the light source can make tracks easier to detect, moving around into a position to optimize the angle to the sun is to be encouraged (**FIGURE 13-5**). Be careful, however, that you do not trample evidence in your search for the proper light angle. The angle does not matter if you have nothing to look at but your own footprints.

SEARCH AND RESCUE TIP

Using the sun (light) properly is very important when learning to track. When the sun is low, long shadows bring out details of tracks on the ground.

Tracking at Night

Because light plays such an important role in tracking, it is easy to see how tracking can be performed at night when the light source is completely under the control of the tracker. An artificial light source can be rotated completely around the track from a low angle to allow for the best view, thus emphasizing otherwise unnoticed sign. An additional benefit of tracking at night can be realized if the missing individual stops moving (to sleep, for instance), thereby allowing night trackers to catch up.

In addition, since darkness at night hides most of the distractive nuances seen during the day, your light source can serve to focus your attention and concentration where it should be.

A diffuse hand lantern works best when tracking at night. Some success has been achieved with white gas lanterns, such as Coleman® lanterns, with deflectors that keep the light out of the tracker's eyes. Also, battery-powered fluorescent lanterns have been used effectively. The key, however, is not brightness. The large flashlights commonly carried by law enforcement personnel are generally worthless as tracking lights. These bright lights diminish night vision and are too intense to bring out subtle sign on an otherwise dark night. LED lights may work, but the color of the light is key. Avoid too many LED bulbs in the light source, and test the color at night to see how well it works. The ideal night tracking light should not be so bright as to ruin night vision yet lasts a long time (good battery life), is light and durable, and offers a diffuse beam.

Some experienced trackers have attached headlamps to their lower legs, just below the knee, or to their **tracking stick** to obtain the best angle while walking. The U.S. Border Patrol often uses lights attached low on a vehicle for cutting sign on a road. The proper light attached at the correct angle can allow a driver or an observer/spotter to follow track on the side of the road for a great distance at a faster speed than could be achieved on foot.

Be imaginative and try night tracking yourself. You will be amazed at how well it works.

Sign-Cutting Stick and the Step-by-Step Method

Most trades have their specialized tools. In tracking, it is the sign-cutting stick. It is hard to believe that such a simple tool can be so effective, but it is true. When properly used, a sign-cutting stick can seem to make sign pop out of thin air. In reality, all it does is force you to look where you want to be looking instead of everywhere else.

The step-by-step method of tracking is stride-based. That is, a tracker gets from one track to the next by determining **stride** (measured distance from the heel of the rear print to the heel of the front print), then searching one stride from the last track found. This requires some type of device for measuring stride; for this, the sign-cutting (or tracking) stick works well.

Stride can be marked on the sign-cutting stick with an O-ring or rubber band (a marker) by measuring an existing track from the heel of one track to the heel of the next track. When the marker is placed near the heel of the last track and pointed in the direction of travel, the stick becomes a pointer toward where the next sign or track is expected to be found. The stick causes the tracker's attention to be focused on a small piece of ground rather than a large area. Finding sign is easier when the search area is limited. A sign-cutting stick does just that.

To use the sign-cutting stick, do the following:

1. Find or make a stick that is approximately 40 inches long, or longer. On it, place at least two rubber bands (or rubber O-rings or other rubber or elastic rings—colored bands work well) that can be moved on the stick but stay in place if desired. For one-time uses, a large twig can be procured from the environment and marked with a knife, pencil, or other marker.
2. At the earliest opportunity while tracking someone, determine his or her stride by measuring the distance from the heel of the rear print to the heel on the front print. Position a marker on your sign-cutting stick (rubber band, O-ring, or other mark) so that the distance from the tip of the stick to the marker is the same distance as the stride.
3. On the last print found, hold the stick so that the stride mark is held close to, but above, the rear of the heel. Move the tip of the stick through an arc that covers the area where the next track should occur.
4. While sweeping the stick very slowly, study the area directly in front of the tip for sign. Take about 20 seconds to sweep from 10 o'clock to 2 o'clock, focusing primarily to the left for a left print (10 o'clock) or to the right for a right print (2 o'clock). Somewhere during the sweep, the tip of the stick should be pointing to the heel of the next print (**FIGURE 13-6**). It may be obvious, or it may be difficult, but it is there. If you do not find anything during the first sweep, make the next sweep even slower. Constantly be alert to the possibility that the subject being tracked may abruptly change direction or alter his or her stride.

Use of Tracking Stick

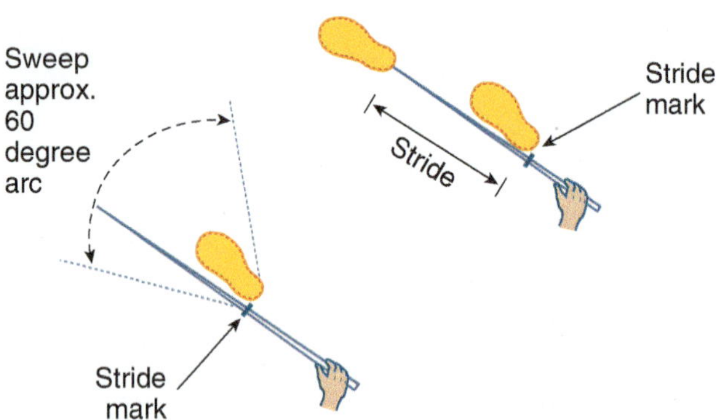

FIGURE 13-6 Using the sign-cutting stick to find the next sign. Measure a known stride and mark the length with the O-ring or rubber band on the stick (from the tip). Take 20 seconds to sweep from 10 o'clock to 2 o'clock, looking for sign at the tip of the stick. If you do not find anything, make the next sweep even slower and wider.

A person's eyes are accustomed to wandering as they choose, without the owner/operator being consciously aware of the mechanics involved. Basically, the eyes do as they please unless directed to do otherwise, which is why we need the assistance of our most valued tool (and friend), the sign-cutting stick. This potent tracking aid assists us in training the eye to concentrate on the small piece of real estate, about 1 square foot, where the next track may fall. As simple as this procedure seems, it is extremely difficult to learn because the eyes are in intimate contact with the brain, which (for most) can perform several functions at once. The eyes, however, can look only at one spot at a time. While most of us use and move the stick as we are taught, we too often allow our eyes to nervously dart several steps ahead or to the side, hoping to get lucky and find that big, easy sign (proving that you are related to Daniel Boone after all). The point is this: you are probably cursed with a cheating mind and a wandering eye, and if you let them control your actions, you will never learn to track. Force your eyes to return to finding that difficult sign in front of the stick and concentrate there ONLY. This is where you will learn the trade.

Try this exercise: In the middle of a regular 8.5- by 11-inch piece of paper, cut a square hole 2 inches by 2 inches, and lay the paper on the ground. Point your sign-cutting stick at the square and spend the next 30 minutes or so examining every minute detail within this square. Do you see pebbles or grains of sand? Count them. Note their color, texture, and location within the area. Is there any vegetation in the area? How big? What color? Any insects? What do they look like? You get the idea. Take notes and document everything you learn about this small area, and, after a short break, have your partner repeat the process in the same area. Afterwards, compare notes and learn from each other. This level of scrutiny is often required when sign cutting.

Labeling Tracks

It is important when using the sign-cutting stick to know if the track being sought is a right footprint or a left one. By marking the last track found, a tracker can immediately tell which (left or right) should be next.

Tracks should be marked in two ways: indicate whether they are right or left, and circle them if they are fully identifiable. To mark a track or partial track left or right, start by using the sign-cutting stick to etch a semicircle to the rear of the track. To a tracker, this arc should indicate that there is a track immediately ahead, STAY OFF. A short hash mark is placed at the right end of the arc to indicate right, and at the left end of the arc to indicate left (**FIGURE 13-7**).

Trackers are rarely lucky enough to get a series of full prints to follow. They must depend on chaining together a collection of sign. When a print is found that is positively identifiable—that is, there is enough print visible to indicate shoe type and sole pattern—it should be completely encircled. This should indicate to others that they are to stay away so that a drawing can be made, and the evidence preserved.

Tracking Team

A common approach to following a track by the step-by-step method is to use three-person teams (**FIGURE 13-8**). The three-person team, comprising a **point person** and two **flankers**, has several advantages (**FIGURE 13-9**):

Labeling Tracks

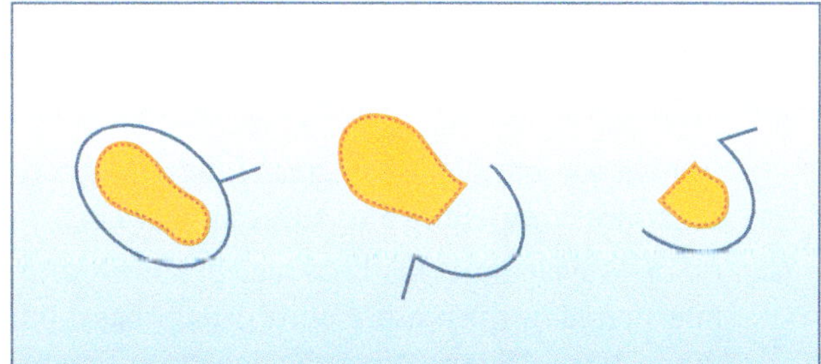

FIGURE 13-7 Circle complete, fully identifiable tracks (left). Place a semicircle behind a partial print with a hash mark on the left to indicate a left print (center) or on the right to indicate a right print (right).

Tracking Team

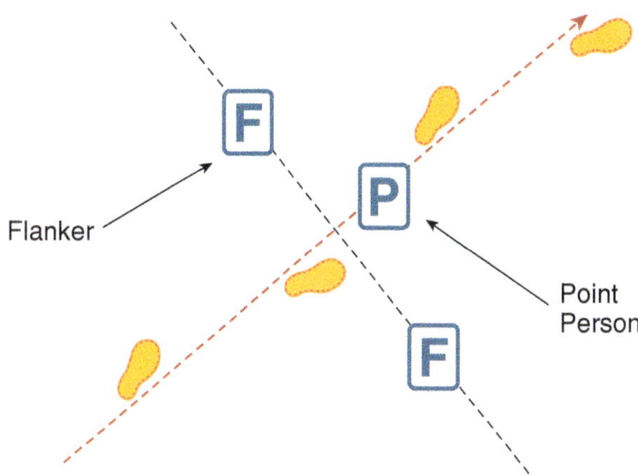

FIGURE 13-8 Three-person tracking team. Flankers work on either side of, and slightly behind, the point person. The point focuses on finding the next track (using the tracking stick) while the flankers take a wider view.

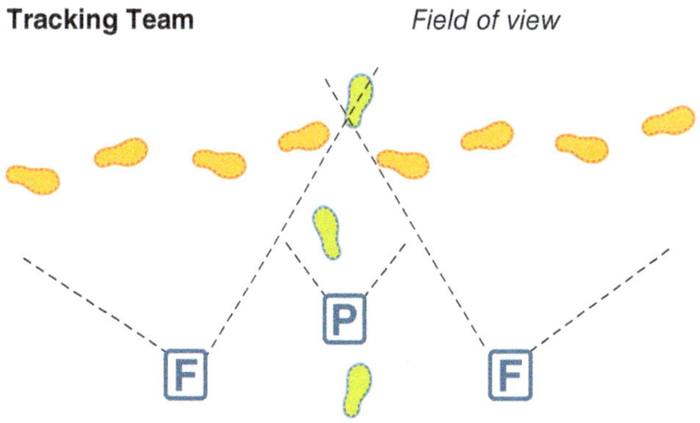

FIGURE 13-9 Field of view for three-person tracking team. Flankers look ahead and to the side for converging tracks while the point concentrates on the area immediately in front of the team.

1. It allows for consultation in difficult situations because three heads are better than one. If you can convince another hard head that what you are seeing is sign, then you are twice as likely to be right.
2. When training, it builds confidence, reduces errors, and benefits students by allowing a verbal exchange of the details of what is seen rather than just mutual observation of a clue.
3. It allows rotation of the point person who is physically on the ground searching for sign. Point is a tiring position, especially when sign is limited.
4. It allows the team to split up if several trails diverge. Any team member can call the team back together when one finds that he or she is

on the correct track. Actually, this is sign cutting and can lead to bad habits during learning the phase, so be careful.

The general responsibilities of the team members are as follows:

- Point person
  - Stays just behind the last track found and uses a sign-cutting stick to search for the next one and mark the tracks as the team progresses
  - Keeps the flankers from obliterating sign by getting ahead and informs them if they do
  - Coordinates the efforts of the team
- Flankers
  - From more of an upright position, watch the side for incoming tracks that might confuse the situation
  - Watch for a sudden turn of the trail being followed
  - Help the point find the next track from their vantage positions

Tracking, like other types of searching, is not something that can be done all day long without rest. For a tracker to be effective, he or she must rest at regular intervals and rotate through the point position with other trackers. Searching for anything while exhausted and fatigued is detrimental to the search effort. Sign or track, like all evidence in a search, must be discovered to be useful. Pressing on while fatigued is admirable, but a tired tracker may miss things that could affect the entire effort. When lives may weigh in the balance, this is unacceptable.

A component of the **tracking team** that is often misunderstood is the continuous exchange of ideas and information that should take place among team members. An interplay of opinion between the point and flankers allows ideas that one may have to be filtered through the thoughts of the others. This interaction could be as simple as the point continuously talking about what is seen and can include each of the flankers challenging the point so that all opinions on any discovery can be considered. After everyone has spoken their piece, a consensus can be achieved. This ends up being an efficient way of preventing an overbearing individual from pushing the team in an undesirable direction. When everyone is involved in what is going on, there is a better chance that the team is heading the right way. Do not construe this to mean that silence is never desirable, however. Occasionally, when great concentration is required, silence may indeed be golden.

If you take the time to describe, in detail, what you see and why you think it relates to your subject's track, you will be much less likely to con yourself into moving to the next step without just cause.

Detecting Sign

Whenever a person walks through an area, whether it be at home or in the wilderness, evidence is left of that passage. A person must contact his or her environment to travel by foot. In fact, walking, the most common type of unaided travel, requires a person to come into contact with his or her environment approximately once every 18 to 20 inches. Some disturbance (sign) is made through that contact, and the first phase of tracking incorporates detecting this sign. The next phase of tracking includes following a track after finding the initial sign.

If a tracker looks for certain signals or visual cues (a *cue* is a stimulus that guides behavior) that catch the eye, rather than tracks or prints, then, in the end, far more is seen. When a tracker has a preconceived notion of what he or she is looking for, much of what could be helpful is disregarded. A tracker must keep an open mind and look at everything that might possibly be of assistance. From there, bits of information can be objectively disposed of, rather than unintentionally ignored.

Common Visual Cues

To see a track or a print, a tracker first needs to be able to discern one or more of certain common **visual cues**. These cues not only offer a specific attraction to seek, they serve well as general categories of sign. These items are what a tracker should be seeking:

1. *Outline*: Boundary or perimeter line around an area, delineating it from its surroundings. May be a small line or a complete track perimeter.
2. *Shape*: Large enough to be human; usually involves flattening, which can be unusual for the environment.
3. *Contrast*: Difference in color, texture, or shape from its surroundings; the greater the difference, the more compelling and attractive the cue.
4. *Color*: Wavelength of light as seen by the eye and interpreted by the brain. Nature usually has mild tones, but differences can be detected. This is not nearly as important in natural environments as in human-made ones.
5. *Texture*: Rough or smooth; the consistency or smoothness of a surface.

If the tracker looks for these cues rather than just tracks or prints, much more is seen, and much more information is available to the tracker for interpretation. Don't look for the whole; look for the parts. When the parts are found, the whole can be compiled.

Note that most of the visual cues described are simply different ways of saying, "look for something that does not belong." When something out of the ordinary is seen, there is a good chance that it can be valuable to a tracker. Thus, all cues listed are essentially different types of contrast in that they all have the tracker looking for abnormalities (i.e., differences in shape, in color, in texture).

"Looking" Guidelines

These guidelines can help the searcher get the most out of his or her sight when it is needed:

1. Change views from the big, overall picture to the small objects regularly. Varying the focus can stimulate the eyes as well as thc mind and help prevent unconscious, passive viewing and promote active, aggressive vision. The point of a tracking team can quickly tire from examining small evidence intensely over long periods of time. Looking up and away from the microenvironment can bring back perspective and allow the tracker to see what was invisible just a moment ago.
2. Look for visual cues, not for preconceived shapes or objects. Move in and inspect more closely anything that seems out of the ordinary or falls into a category of sign (i.e., outline, shape, contrast, color, texture).
3. Avoid any preconceptions and look at everything. Take your time. There is usually a lot to see.
4. Do not look for the whole; look for parts of the whole. There are more of them, and they can lead directly to a desired objective.

Sign: The Specifics

The subtle details of sign are beyond the scope of this text, but much can be learned from one single footprint. Some of the information available from a single print includes the following:

1. Length and width can help identify the print and distinguish it from others that may be similar. Size of a print can also give a rough idea of the person's size.
2. The general type of sole (if discernible) can help distinguish it from others as well as offer an aid in describing the print to searchers.
3. Measurements of specific parts of a sole pattern can help positively identify a print. That is, lug sizes, areas of wear, or pattern dimensions can help distinguish one print from others.
4. Several prints in a row can help determine direction of travel and stride, which can aid in finding subsequent prints.

Even though it is rare to find a complete, clear print, fragments of prints and sign are common in most terrain. Because of this, as much information as possible must be learned from each piece of sign. Tracking is not a race to see who finishes first; it is an exercise in accuracy and efficiency. There is no excuse for losing the trail. Getting there quickly is worthless if you end up at the wrong place.

Drawing a print, particularly a complete and identifiable one, can help the artist become more familiar with the details of the print and can be used to help others to know what print to seek (**FIGURE 13-10**). The drawing can be copied and handed out to searchers so that one specific print can be sought, thus lessening the possibilities. When time allows, drawing a print, or a part thereof, is always a good idea. A standard track report form that offers an area to draw and describe a print is good for this purpose (see form in Appendix A). Of course, photographing a print is often an option, especially given technology available as close as one's mobile phone, but a camera phone used to photograph evidence may itself become evidence and may then have to be seized and preserved like any other evidence. Therefore, carrying

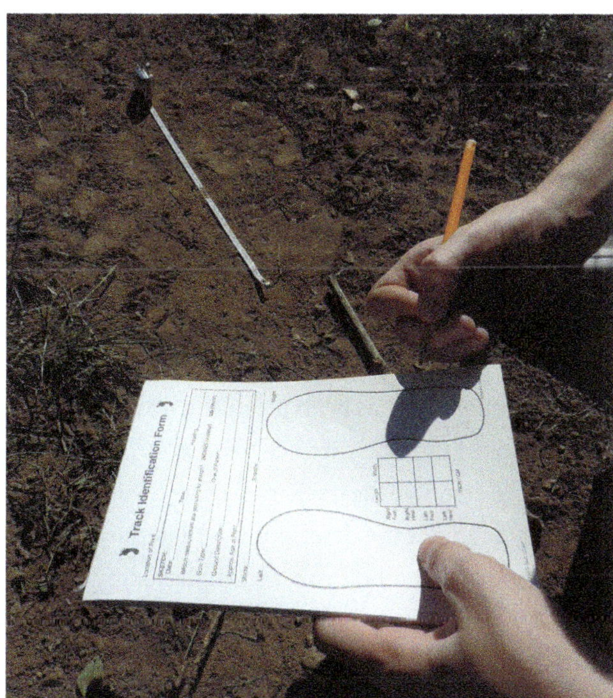

FIGURE 13-10 Drawing a footprint, particularly a complete and identifiable one, can help others to know what print to seek. Document every conceivable measurement as well as every distinctive mark.
Courtesy of Donald Cooper.

a separate camera may be a good idea and drawing a print may be a low-tech, attractive option.

It would be impossible to mention all the different types of sign that exist because sign varies so much with terrain, weather, time of day, vegetation, and more. Sign depends mostly on the environment in which it is produced. A marsh may produce completely different sign than would a desert, for instance, but some similarities do exist. These similarities must be understood by all trackers, but it's still important that a tracker be familiar with the sign most common to his or her region.

In addition, as mentioned previously, sign can be conclusively human or corroborant. Conclusively human sign is a disturbance that, when considered on its own with no other evidence, can be said to have been definitely caused by a person and not an animal. Corroborant sign, on the other hand, is disturbance that is not decisively human and could have been caused by an animal. This type of sign may corroborate other evidence but, when considered on its own, is not conclusive. It cannot be determined to have been definitely caused by a person, but it may confirm or substantiate other evidence with which it may be found. While conclusively human sign is often discovered by very unskilled trackers (jump tracking), corroborant sign is not. Frequently, corroborant sign is obvious to a skilled tracker yet invisible to the novice, and when a novice does discover such disturbance, it is often misinterpreted. Also, corroborant sign, which by itself proves nothing, would most certainly have been caused by the person being tracked if it were to fall exactly between two other pieces of sign at approximately a stride's distance. Because of this, corroborant sign can be as important in the long run as conclusively human sign and should never be overlooked or ignored.

Communicating Prints: Track ID

It is essential for a tracker to be able to do three things with a print once it has been positively identified:

1. Communicate the track to others.
2. Differentiate the track from other similar tracks.
3. Document the description for later use.

The last two can be easily accomplished by simply studying the print, measuring it, and then drawing it (**TABLE 13-1**). Photographing the track can be important, but much more can be learned by drawing it. Drawing the print can bring details to the attention of the tracker that otherwise might have been missed and can emphasize subtle marks that might be difficult or impossible to see in a photograph. Photographing a track is a good idea, but it should supplement, not replace, a sketch.

TABLE 13-1 Classification of Prints

Classification	Difficulty	Description
Class 1	Very easy	Perfect, complete
Class 2	Easy	Complete
Class 3	Moderate	ID but partial print
Class 4	Hard	Human but no ID
Class 5	Severe	Sign only

Reproduced from *Fundamentals of Mantracking: The Step-by-Step Method*, Third Edition, by Albert "Ab" Taylor and Donald C. Cooper, Skyhorse Publishing, © 2014 Donald C. Cooper, All Rights Reserved.

Study and measure every aspect of a print and indicate the measurements on the drawing. As a minimum, measure the length of the track; the widest part of the sole and the heel; the length of the heel; the stride (heel to heel), if possible; widths of any lines or marks; distances between lines or marks; number and size of any geometric shapes; and the number of lugs or other sole characteristics. Be careful to note any nail holes or stitches that are evident in the print, as well as the number and sizes of any marks or lines. Search for and note any cuts, worn spots, or other details unique to the print. Everything visible should be noted and documented on the sketch. Any one of these characteristics might be what differentiates this track from others and is, therefore, important.

Beware of suggesting a size for the print (e.g., size 3 or 4) from measurements made in the field. Manufacturers vary widely in their approach to sizing footgear, and no standards really exist. Rather than convey an estimated size, relate the measurements (length, width, etc.). In addition, take a digital photo that includes a measuring device (ruler or tape measure) in the photo to provide scale. With today's technology, this can also be quickly conveyed to others with a smart phone, if approved by the incident commander, but be aware that a phone used in this way may become evidence and could be confiscated as such.

The drawing and/or photo can be copied and distributed to other searchers, but occasionally the print may need to be described via radio or telephone. Tracking is almost entirely visual, whereas voice communication is entirely verbal. The skills required to perform both well are related but not the same. Practicing both is important.

When verbally communicating a track, certain ideas should be kept in mind to minimize confusion and maximize efficiency:

- Make sure to identify yourself and give your location, if necessary, as well as the direction of travel (with compass) of the track.
- Keep it simple. Paint a mental picture by using words that are familiar to everyone and to which everyone can relate. Use words that are easy to understand and whose meaning is limited.
- Begin with a general description. Is it a flat (no heel) or a heel (a distinct heel)? Continue with a term that describes the general class of footgear, if possible. (e.g., athletic shoe, sandal, work boot, hiking boot, dress shoe, cowboy boot). Beware of speculation as to the type, and know the differences before using the terms.
- As a secondary consideration, briefly describe the type of terrain and ground conditions as well as the age of the track, if you can. This might give an indication of the detail to expect.
- Give the specific details describing the sole pattern starting at one end of the print (tell which). Such details should include, but not necessarily be limited to, the following:
    - Although all measurements should be documented, in the interest of clarity and brevity, only the length and width of the print and the length and width of the heel should be conveyed over the air. Consider using descriptive terms rather than exact measurements for radio communication. Terms like "as wide as a pencil" might be understood better than "1/4 inch."
    - Number or type of lugs (shape, measurements, etc.).
    - Number or spacing of any nail holes and/or stitches.
    - Shape of the leading edge of the heel (e.g., straight, concave, V-shaped).
    - Shape of the toe (e.g., sharply pointed, round, square).
    - Specific shape of marks in the pattern (e.g., circle, square, diamond, oval, line, thick line, broken line, wavy line, herringbone). Avoid using ambiguous terms such as "round" and "flat," and stick to more visual terms.
    - Specific way of walking. Look for dragging of feet, scuffing, toes pointing out or in, wide straddle (feet placed widely apart), consistently shorter stride with one foot, long stride (runner or jogger), or anything that may make this track unique.
    - Look for tendencies or trends in where the subject walks and convey them. Does the subject always walk at the side of the road? Does the subject step over logs rather than on them? Does the subject tend to walk drainages rather than ridges? Does the subject avoid brush? Does he or she walk in a straight line no matter what? If not, what tends to change the direction of travel? Fences? Wooded areas? Water?
- In sensitive situations where the details conveyed via radio are immediately important, have the receiving party confirm your description by repeating it back to you. In practice, this may be a good idea every time a print is described over the radio or phone.
- Use a standardized track report to record your findings.

Strategy

If a SAR incident is managed properly, trackers will be called to participate early in the plan. Trackers need to know their place within the structured hierarchy and to whom they answer. These topics, as well as others that are important to the tracker, are covered in any of the fine educational programs dealing with search management. Only the considerations of approach and strategy that facilitate a tracking team's specific tasks are discussed within this text.

Initially, after dealing with any administrative details, a tracking team called to a SAR incident should attempt to determine where the lost subject was last seen or known to have been. This information may be conveyed through the command structure, or it may have to be determined by the trackers themselves. Where was the person last seen? Where did they pass or what did they do? The area where the victim was last known to have been has the highest chance of containing tracks or other evidence that can be used by a tracker to determine a direction of travel. It takes only three prints to determine direction of travel, and if you can accomplish just this much, you have contributed more to the search than most could ever hope.

From a subject profile, a tracker should be able to guess what size print is being sought (small child, small adult, large adult, etc.) and the approximate length of the stride. If you are lucky, the profile could offer a specific, **complete print**. When you have an idea what is being sought, and once an area is identified as "hot" for sign, other people should be kept away to avoid confusion or destruction of the evidence. This cannot be overemphasized. Next, cut sign around the area (perimeter cut), trying to determine a direction of travel, and note any specific additional evidence such as a complete print. Better yet, carefully approach the last known point and examine the entire area without moving around unnecessarily. If a scuff, track, or other sign is visible, stand behind it and scrutinize the area in front of it for additional evidence that might suggest a general direction of travel. Look beneath your own feet to see how they impact the area and look for this specific type of sign. Once the direction of travel has been determined from the last known point, another tracking team could cut an intersecting line. Be extremely careful not to damage any existing sign. This may be all anyone

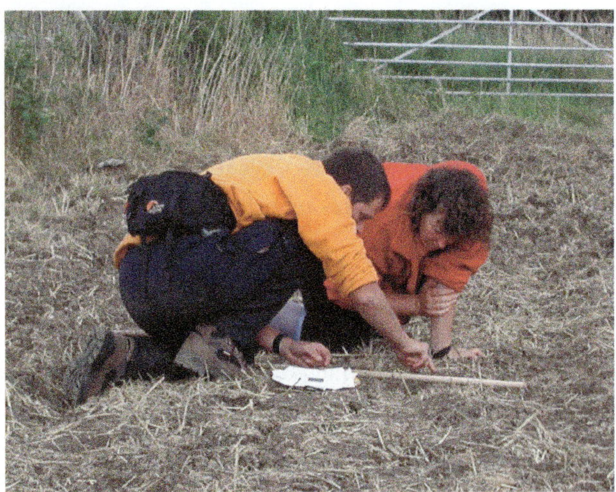

FIGURE 13-11 Once a direction of travel is determined, one tracking team always stays on the trail, following it step-by-step.

has to go on. Take every precaution necessary to preserve any prints found, then see that they are documented and communicated to others involved in the search.

Once a direction of travel is determined, one tracking team always stays on the trail, following it step-by-step (i.e., never going past the last conclusive sign) (**FIGURE 13-11**). This means that there is always someone on the trail. Other strategies can be applied to speed up the process, some of which is discussed, but the importance of keeping someone on the last track cannot be overemphasized.

The most time-consuming project is usually finding the first track. This is why it is important at the onset to keep everyone (nontrackers) away until sign can be cut and certain basic information gathered (print specifics, direction of travel, etc.). It is important to be able to find a track and be reasonably sure that it belongs to the lost subject. Accuracy is more important here than speed. Once the track is positively identified and a direction of travel is determined, then the pace can pick up quite a bit in most situations.

To improve the quality of service trackers can offer when involved in a search effort, it is worth referring to the following guidelines. After all, it is far better to learn from mistakes of others than from your own!

1. Get the most recent copy of the best map available for your area. A USGS 7.5-minute topographical map is best for foot travel. Maps can now be printed or displayed as needed in almost any scale from a laptop, tablet, or smart phone.
2. Make sure that both vehicular and foot traffic is kept to a minimum for the best sign-cutting results within the high probability area(s).
3. Check for sign and track along trails and roads on the approach to the search area. Be track aware.
4. Get as much information as possible about the missing subject(s) before going into the field. Try to obtain a detailed subject profile.
5. Only one or two of the most experienced trackers should investigate the area (cut sign) initially. This minimizes conflicting sign.
6. Preserve evidence found at all cost. Document and catalog all likely tracks and sign while traveling into the search area, and be particularly aware of tracks that travel in unusual or erratic patterns. Establish a system for sorting and discarding prints, and make sure the tracking team's prints can be easily distinguished from any others. One way to accomplish this is to put an identifying mark on the footgear of every member of the tracking team.
7. Since hazards in an area are likely spots to find the subject, they are also good areas to look for sign: look first in caves, mines, near cliffs, in holes, in ponds, etc. within the search area.
8. Make sure that a perimeter has been established beyond which a person could not pass without being noticed. In search management lingo, this is known as *confinement*.
9. Cut the perimeter within the confined area, but beware of presuming that no sign on a perimeter cut means that a sector can be ruled out. The subject may have traveled into the sector after the cut.
10. Talk to everyone confronted while traveling within the search area. Presume that everyone is suspect (e.g., the missing person) until proven otherwise.
11. Look for clues and the lost subject, call out the subject's name at regular intervals, and then listen for a response. Bear in mind that, depending on the individual and the situation, some subjects may not answer. This includes children.
12. Use the step-by-step method of tracking.

Perimeter Cutting

If following the trail from the last known point is not possible, another method of speeding up the pace is to employ **perimeter cutting** (similar to sign cutting). When initially cutting sign in an area, or when tracking becomes particularly slow, trackers can cut sign in a perimeter around an area where there is a good chance the subject has been. The purpose of such an effort is simply to discover sign at a farther distance from the last sign. If this perimeter team can positively identify the track and direction of travel, they can become the step-by-step team and allow the rear team to perimeter cut around them. The perimeter cut can range from several yards to several miles, depending on the terrain and how long the victim has been missing.

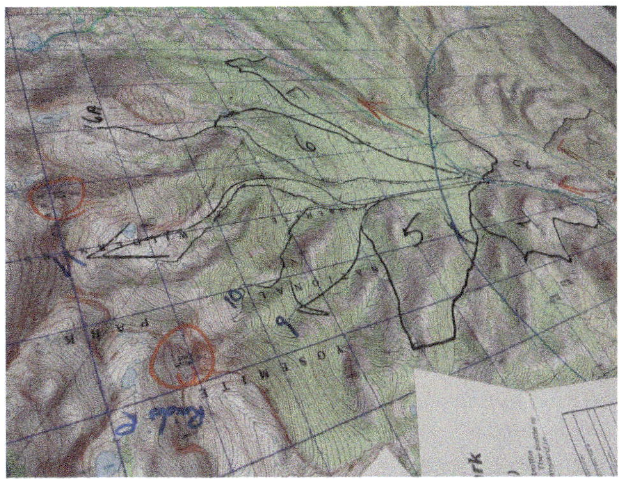

The shape of the perimeter can be square, triangular, circular, or any shape. It can even follow compass headings. The only requirement is that, no matter which shape is chosen, the loop must be completed. Two trackers can cut sign in opposite directions, meeting to close the perimeter, or one team can cut sign continuously until they reach their starting point again. The only exception to this rule would be when sign is found, and urgency is very high, but resources are limited. If no sign is found, consideration should be given to the fact that no one has entered the area.

If careful thought is put into where to cut a perimeter, much time and energy can be saved. Use natural barriers such as cliffs, large rivers, and thick brush where a person would not likely pass to limit the perimeter. Use areas where track and sign are easily seen to complete the perimeter (e.g., river banks, dry stream beds, plowed fields, tall grass, steep banks, trails, road edges). Pick areas that would allow you to be certain if someone passed. Now the entire perimeter is either easy to cut or impossible to pass through.

SEARCH AND RESCUE TIP

When cutting a perimeter, use natural barriers such as rivers or thick brush to limit the perimeter space, saving much time and energy.

The same rules that apply for sign cutting apply for perimeter cutting with the following additions:

1. Do not allow anyone to walk or drive within the perimeter being cut, with the possible exception of the trackers on step-by-step who must stay with the track they are working. The most common destroyer of sign and track is people, on foot or in a vehicle.
2. Each successive perimeter cut should be made just as carefully as the first.

If a perimeter cut is unsuccessful, it can mean that the cutting team missed something or that the subject has been passed and is between the two teams. In either case, it is extremely important that once a team gets on a track, they stay there until another positive ID is made. Close is not good enough. Someone must always be on the last track after a positive ID has been made.

Further Considerations

Now that we have reduced tracking to simple terms, it is time for an injection of reality. Tracking, although constructed of simple components, can involve some of the most complex issues in life. It deals with mysteries, grief, death, love, loss, and so much more. No dealings with such emotion-wrought topics could possibly be simple. Tracking works because it is a logical, analytical process that deals only with facts, not conjecture, hearsay, or emotion.

When a tracker is confronted with influences that do not contribute to the factual, logical input required, then confusion occurs. Tracking is not gauged by miles per hour, so when a tracker is rushed, effectiveness suffers. Tracking is very sense-intensive, so when a tracker is overwhelmed with sounds, sights, and unrelated thoughts, effectiveness suffers (**FIGURE 13-12**). As a tracker, try to concentrate on what you can control. Deal with the facts. Deal with them logically and take your time.

Where tracking is required during an incident, situations may arise that have not been broached in this text. Incident commanders may not call out trackers because they believe, many times without a

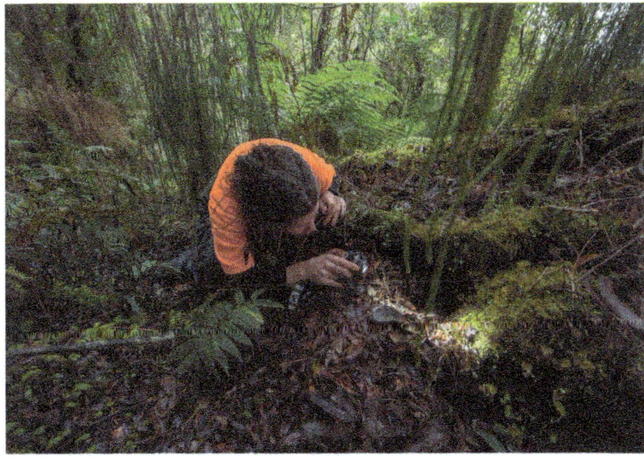

FIGURE 13-12 Tracking is not an equipment-intensive pursuit. Sight, patience, perseverance, and determination are requirements.

working knowledge of tracking, that tracking "will not work here." Good trackers may not be able to get to the subject in time to find them alive. External influences may apply undue pressure, most without an understanding of the tracker's art. Lost subjects may not be found. Clues may be misinterpreted. Lives may be lost.

Before you become totally disillusioned, however, take comfort in this fact: the same things occur in searches every day where tracking is not employed. Lives are lost, and problems arise even when tracking plays no part. Tracking is only a tool that can be used to reach an objective. It is not a panacea, but it may offer an effective option when used properly. Without tracking and its associated skills, are we really doing all we can as search and rescue personnel? Are we missing something? Could we do better?

Stay Focused on the Fundamentals

Consider these thoughts when you are confronted with situations that cause you to hurry or improvise:

1. Only a tracker can determine whether tracking can be effective in any given situation. A "jump-tracker" is not a tracker.
2. Only trackers can decide when, how, and how thoroughly to search for subtle sign and track. Do not be pushed into hurrying. It does not work. Do not be rushed into making mistakes.
3. Tracking is most effective when applied within an effective management scheme. Organization and leadership are always important.
4. Always be track aware. Be aware that for every mile a person walks, there are thousands of clues. Find them!
5. Do not concentrate on determining if and when tracking will NOT work. Rather, concentrate on how tracking can work every time. Make it happen. Think that it will work. Occasionally, you may be wrong.
6. Deal only with the facts. When inundated with theories, write down the facts and use them to develop a theory rather than searching for facts to substantiate one.

Wrap-Up

READY FOR REVIEW

Anterior A medical term used to refer to something toward the front of the body or toward the head.

Arch The bottom, medial part of the foot, just forward of the ankle, that curves above the ground. It stretches from the calcaneus to the three medial metatarsals and is sometimes referred to as the medial longitudinal arch.

Bracketing An occasionally acceptable method of interpolation that uses a predetermined stride to skip one step in sequence to find the next, and then use it to find the one skipped.

Clue conscious Aware that clues exist.

Complete print The entire impression is visible.

Conclusively human sign Evidence (sign) that, on its own, can be said to have been definitely caused by a person and not an animal.

Corroborant sign Disturbance that is not decisively human and could have been caused by an animal. It cannot be determined to have been definitely caused by a person, but it may confirm or substantiate other evidence with which it may be found.

Cuttable area A reasonably good area for cutting sign.

Evidence Something legally acceptable before a court, such as an object or a witness, that bears on or establishes an issue. In tracking, evidence is divided into physical and incorporeal.

Flankers Members of a three-person tracking team standing on either side of the point person who help discover sign, usually from a standing position.

Forefoot The larger part of the foot, forward of the ankle.

Gait The pattern of how a person walks.

Heel The back part of the foot below the ankle.

Identifiable A complete or partial print that has at least one characteristic that differentiates it from others similar to it.

Intoeing See *pigeon toed.*

Jump tracking An unskilled form of tracking that involves finding an obvious footprint, then proceeding along the presumed direction of travel until another obvious track is found.

Lateral A medical term used to describe something situated away from the middle or to the side of the body; usually to the left or the right.

Medial A medical term that describes something that is situated toward the middle or midline of the body.

Partial Only part of the impression is visible.

Perimeter cutting Sign cutting around the boundary or outer edge of an area.

Phalanges The bones of the toes (and fingers).

Pigeon toed When one walks with the toes pointed medially. This is sometimes called *intoeing*, and the medical terms *metatarsus varus* or *metatarsus adductus* may also be used.

Point person Member of a three-person tracking team that leads the act of sign discovery, usually from a position just ahead of, and between, the flankers.

Posterior A medical term used to describe something toward the back of the body.

Print Impression left from the passage of a person that can be positively identified as being human.

Pronation Rotation of the medial bones in the midtarsal region of the foot inward and downward so that in walking the foot tends to come down on its inner margin.

Quarry Anything being pursued.

Sign Any evidence of change from the natural state that is inflicted on an environment by a person's or an animal's passage.

Sign cutting Looking for sign to establish a starting point from which to track. Usually performed perpendicular to the direction of travel of a subject. Also called *cutting sign*.

Sign-cutting stick A walking stick-type device used by trackers to measure stride. Furthermore, it assists in focusing attention where the tracker should be looking for sign and not everywhere else. Also called a *tracking stick*.

Splayed feet When the toes point outward (laterally) when walking; the opposite of intoeing. Sometimes referred to as *toe out*.

Step-by-step tracking A disciplined tracking methodology and teaching system where a tracker sees each step in sequence and proceeds no further than the last visible track, using the stride to determine where next to look for sign.

Steppage gait When one walks with a footdrop where the foot hangs with the toes pointing down, causing the toes to scrape the ground while walking and requiring the walker to lift the leg higher than normal when walking.

Straddle The lateral distance between footfalls, perpendicular to the direction of travel.

Stride Measured distance from the heel of the rear print to the heel of the next front print.

Supination A movement of the foot and the leg in which the foot rolls outward with an elevated arch so that in walking the foot tends to come down on its outer edge.

Tarsals The big bones of the foot below and including the ankle and the calcaneus.

Toe out See *splayed feet*.

Track An impression left from the passage of a person or an animal.

Track aware Conscious that sign, tracks, and prints exist and may be useful.

Tracking Following someone or something by stringing together a continuous chain of their sign. Following a chronology of sign.

Tracking stick See *sign-cutting stick*.

Track trap An area particularly good for detecting sign (e.g., sand, mud, snow). May be human-made by clearing off an area so that sign would be more easily detected if a subject subsequently passed through.

Tracking team A three-person group, comprising a point and two flankers, and organized specifically to track.

Visual cues Visible indications that something does not belong and may be part of a track (sign). There are five common visual cues: outline, shape, contrast, color, and texture.

Waddling gait A duck-like walk where the lateral distance between footfalls can be larger than a normal gait.

REFERENCE

Taylor, Albert S., and Donald C. Cooper. 2014. *Fundamentals of Mantracking: The Step-by-Step Method*. 3rd edition, New York: Skyhorse Publishers. Available at www.NASAR.org.

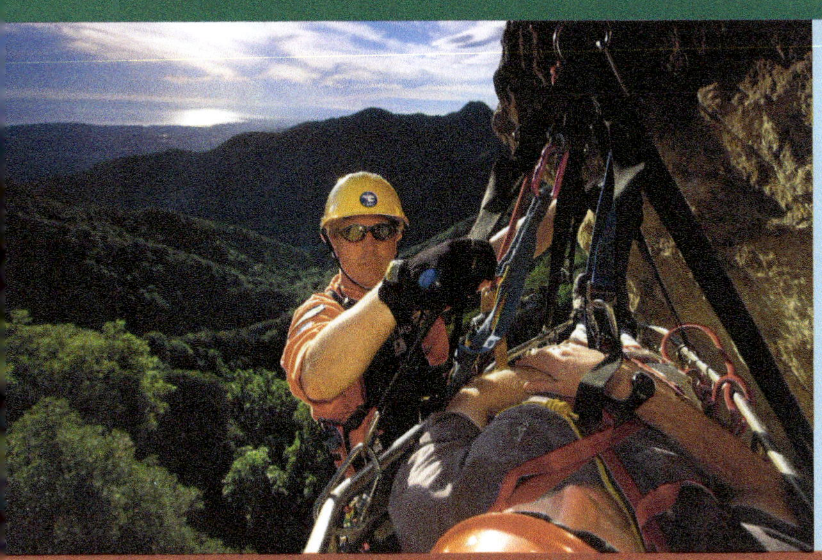

SECTION 3

Search and Rescue Operations

CHAPTER 14

Principles of Search and Related Issues

OBJECTIVES

Upon completion of this chapter and the related course activities, the student will be able to meet the following objectives:

- Describe the attitude that aggressive searching requires.
- List and describe at least three of the five rudiments of search (the "crucials").
- Explain the concept and the relevance of clue consciousness.
- List the three things on which any measure of detection is based.
- Explain the difference between a region of probability and a search segment.
- Describe the conventional notation of search theory and the meaning of each of the three variables.
- Explain the most significant contribution that field searchers can make in a search.
- Explain generally why input from search crews is critical to effective search planning.
- Describe how field search and rescue (SAR) personnel should handle a confrontation by news media, political entities, or the friends and family of the subject.
- Describe how information regarding lost person behavior can be used by search crews.
- Explain the difference between physical and incorporeal evidence.
- List and describe at least three considerations after discovering a deceased person during a search.

Attitude and Philosophy

It is important that the motivation of the search and rescue (SAR) personnel be consistent with the search and rescue community's motto—". . .these things we do, that others may live"—if satisfaction and any level of success is expected.

SAR exists for one reason only: to reduce suffering and pain for the missing or injured subject. There is little or no money in SAR, and there is rarely acclaim. It is tiring work that is often uncomfortable, unnerving, frustrating, smelly, hot, cold, sweaty, and rarely required when responders would find it convenient. Only on occasion is there is a thank you, and injuries or even death are common. People involved in SAR must be focused, dedicated, skilled, confident, and thick-skinned.

That said, one can experience no greater satisfaction than is received from helping others. It is rare that a person accepts such a challenge, and rarer yet when a person who wants to help has the skill and the knowledge necessary to offer assistance in a SAR situation.

Discipline is important in SAR because of the miserable conditions that often prevail when effective operations are so important. Bad weather, cold, heat, fatigue, lack of success, etc., are all conditions that can erode one's attitude. If a proper attitude cannot be maintained in less than ideal conditions, perhaps the searcher should reconsider his or her position in the organization.

SAR is hard work. Without discipline, SAR personnel may not only be ineffective but also dangerous. Worse than not being sufficiently disciplined to handle difficulties encountered during a SAR incident is not recognizing that problems exist. SAR personnel must be able to recognize when their own limits have been reached, whether they be physical, mental, or both. Physical limitations involve fatigue, pain, injury, etc., and mental limitations can range from fear to mental fatigue and may include boredom, apathy, and a lack of motivation.

Very often, coping with a physical or mental limitation means removing oneself from the environment that is causing the problem. Quitting or changing one's involvement in the search effort is much preferred to continuing in a useless—or worse, detrimental—role. Acting as though you can handle it not only wastes time, it is also counterproductive and may be dangerous. No one will ever fault a searcher for admitting that he or she has reached a personal physical, mental, or capability limit. However, there may be grave consequences for ignoring the same.

Four to six hours of actual searching (excluding travel and rest time) is generally considered the average usefulness of a field searcher per operational period, although the time may vary depending on the situation. Effective searching is strenuous and sensory abusive. The senses that are required to search effectively need rest if they are expected to be effective. Searching requires an alert mind, an able body, and acute senses. A searcher must be rested, well conditioned, and well nourished. All senses are required for effective searching: sight (eyes), hearing (ears), smell (nose), and common sense (thinking and judgment). Effectiveness diminishes when a searcher works for long hours without relief or rest. Attention to detail is important. Just looking—passive vision without recognition and interpretation—isn't always enough when you need to *see*.

Aggressive searching requires a positive attitude about finding clues as well as the subject of the search (**FIGURE 14-1**). The searcher must believe that there is a clue behind every stump and rock pile. Optimism must be dominant. "The subject needs our help and I'm the one who is going to find the clue that leads to success!"

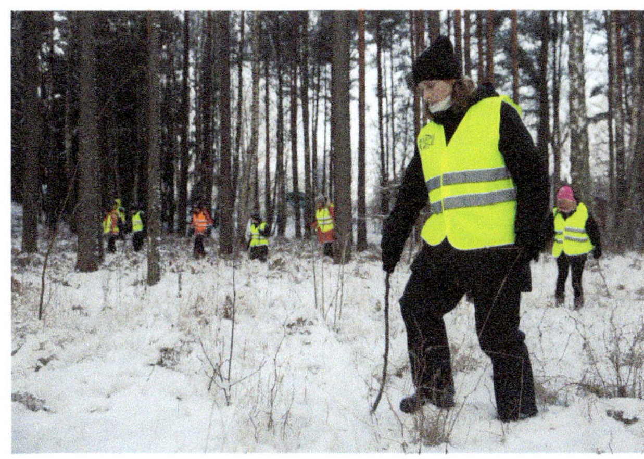

FIGURE 14-1 Aggressive searching requires a positive attitude about finding clues as well as the subject of the search.

It is very easy to think negative thoughts during a search. Some inexperienced searchers think that their effort is unsuccessful or wasted if the subject is not found immediately. "After all, if we were successful, we would have found the subject, right?" This type of attitude is at best self-defeating and at worst flat wrong. Not finding a clue or the subject can be very helpful to the skilled search planner. A search resulting in no clues can be as good as a pile of clues—they both have meaning and can help lead us to the lost subject. It is far more fruitful to maintain a positive outlook while dismissing negative thoughts as fantasies of an idle mind. A good searcher thinks positively and avoids the alternative.

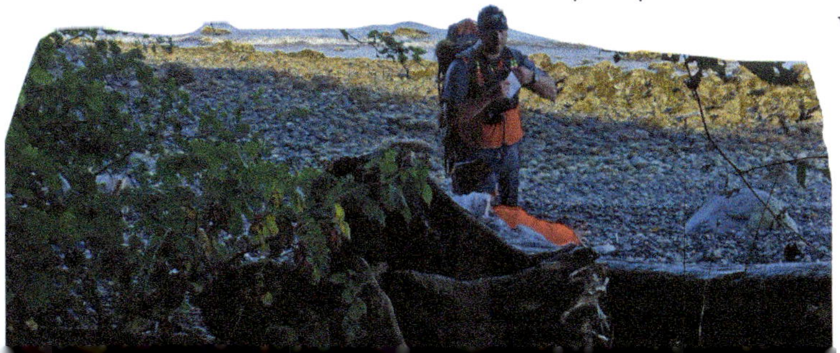

Rudiments of Search: The Crucials

The fundamentals of land search are based on principles that have long been accepted by search managers and planners, but they are also important to field searchers. These principles, collectively termed *crucials* here, are described in six statements that summarize the minimum requirements for effective searching.

Search Is an Emergency

Search is an emergency because the subject may need emergency care, and the subject may need protection from himself or herself and/or the environment. Time and weather destroy clues, and an urgent response lessens the search difficulty. Urgency is sometimes difficult to justify because, left alone, lost people often survive and walk out without assistance. Because the difficulty of a search is often directly related to the size of the area to be searched, a fast response can minimize the travel time of the lost subject, keep the **search area** smaller, and more quickly lead to success.

To respect the search subject's emergency (and that of the subject's family), searchers must respond urgently (search is an emergency until proven otherwise), search at night (the subject is probably immobile), maintain a visible effort (never quit), and create an atmosphere of positive urgency (everyone should act as if their actions will resolve the search). However, all SAR personnel must continue to approach the problem in an organized, disciplined manner. The sense of urgency should not be allowed to degenerate into disorganized, helter-skelter scrambling. In general, initial strategies that offer the maximum potential for locating a responsive, conscious subject should be used.

Search Is a Classic Mystery

Search is a classic mystery, and, therefore, searchers must act and feel much like the fictional character, Sherlock Holmes, who said, "What one man can invent another can discover" (Doyle, 1903, p. 25). Searchers and search managers must know what clues to look for and how to discover them.

Search for Clues and the Subject

Search for clues as well as the subject(s) because there are many more clues than subjects, and clue detection can substantially reduce search difficulty. Every person who travels on land leaves clues such as tracks, scent, and other discoverable evidence of his or her passing. Even not finding a clue can be a clue in itself.

Focus on Aspects Important to Success

Concentrate on aspects that are important to search success and under your control. Doing otherwise is simply a waste of time, effort, and money. For example, repeatedly questioning the assignment given you as a searcher is much less productive than trusting that the assignment is necessary and appropriate before performing the assigned task.

Know if the Subject Leaves the Search Area

Know if the subject leaves the search area because a search without a subject is nonsense. Unless the subject is contained early, search difficulty increases rapidly. This is more a management than an operational concern, but searchers must still understand the importance of discovering and reporting any evidence that the subject left the search area.

Grid Search as a Last Resort

Use high-coverage grid searching only as a last resort because the cost and risks are greater than many alternative techniques. High-coverage grid searching (line searching) takes many people, much organization, a great deal of support, and often too much time for the benefits derived. It is also extremely damaging to the environment and clues that were not detected, and it may make subsequent searches almost impossible. Other techniques are frequently a better use of resources and should often be employed first before attempting to do a very thorough grid search.

Field personnel need to know something about what it is that compels those in charge to act in certain ways (e.g., acceptance of the "crucials"). Searchers need not possess all the knowledge of the search manager or planner, but they should understand the basic principles involved in managing and planning a search. With this basic knowledge, field searchers might better understand why they are asked to perform certain tasks, what is expected of them, and why. This can also help searchers provide better information back to the search management team.

Clue Consciousness

Recall from the "crucials" that searchers must search for clues as well as lost subjects. There are more clues than subjects, the detection of clues reduces the search area, and the value gained from the detection of certain clues approaches that of the lost subject. In other words, be conscious of clues, not just the subject of the search.

Clue seeking is the major job of field personnel, and following certain guidelines allows this job to get done more effectively. Clue seeking is an ongoing process that starts before callout and ends only after the final critique. Important clues can be found in the field as well as in the command post. Clues can be found, discovered, deduced, stumbled upon, assumed, etc., and there are as many ways to find clues as there are clues to be found.

Good clue seeking is learned. The art of clue seeking must be practiced frequently to develop and maintain a high level of skill. Experience is necessary to develop a sense of what information is important to the search and what is not. Experience also makes it easier to recognize or discover clues.

Regarding the interpretation of a clue, an opinion should be formed based solely on the information available. What must be avoided is forming an opinion and then gathering information to support that opinion. Do not immediately form an opinion about the value of a clue. Sometimes a clue, especially when clues are scarce, may seem more important than it actually is.

Clues should be sought and gathered from all available sources. Basing any theory or hypothesis on one source or one piece of information is, at best, questionable and at worst dangerous. It is better to gather all the information possible, such as assembling a complete subject profile and then letting the totality of the information offer direction.

Clue Orientation and Detection

State-of-the-art search techniques are "clue orientated," that is, they are dependent on the detection of clues, which can lead to the location of the subject.

Any measure of detection is based on the unique combination of the characteristics of three things: the **sensor** (searcher), the **search object** (subject or clue generator), and the environment in which the detection opportunity takes place. Changing any one of these variables can significantly affect how easy or difficult an object is to detect. For example, a human, visual searcher (sensor) looking for a green golf ball (search object) on an open field with short, green grass on a cloudy day (environment) suggests some unique level of detectability. Changing the characteristics of any one of the three variables (sensor, object, or environment) could significantly change the detectability of the object sought. For example, if the environment is changed to nighttime, or the search object is changed to something smaller and more difficult to see, or if the searcher has poor, uncorrected vision, the search becomes far more difficult. On the other hand, if the golf ball were changed to a beach ball, or if the grass were brown and contrasted with the green golf ball, detection would likely be easier.

SEARCH AND RESCUE TIP

Clue detection is based on the unique combination of the characteristics of:

- The sensor
- The search object
- The environment

The Sensor

Searchers (sensors) must be able to detect what they seek when given a detection opportunity. This requires that they know what to look for (potential clues) and know what to do when they find it. This is accomplished through training and practice. When a clue is discovered, searchers must know exactly what to do about it. Ideally, this should be determined during the assignment **briefing** prior to entering the field.

The characteristics of the sensor are important to detection. Untrained, fatigued, or distracted searchers are less likely to discover clues. The best search dog has only limited effectiveness if its handler cannot interpret the dog's signals. Certain sensors are better in certain environments, searching for certain search objects, than others. A skilled human searcher may be able to find a person lying in a field, but he or she may not be able to detect human scent from a subject who cannot be seen. In the latter situation, an air scent dog is the better "sensor."

How sensors are applied is also important. When looking for a lost person, the specific tactics chosen should be appropriate for the situation. For example, if the subject is likely to be responsive, attraction techniques may be effective. If the subject is not likely to be responsive, attraction techniques may be a waste of time. A specific sensor should be carefully matched to the situation in which it is applied. To do otherwise may lead to a missed detection opportunity and may even destroy the evidence altogether.

The Search Object

The characteristics of the search object are important to detection. A large, brightly colored object that contrasts with its environment is easy to detect visually. A small or camouflaged object is harder to detect. In daytime visual searches, the type, size, color, and shape of the search object are important factors, whereas for night visual searches, search object illumination and reflectivity are important. When possible, searching should be conducted from a direction in which the search object receives the best illumination, color brightness, or contrast (IMO/ICAO, 2016).

Human subjects can do things that make them easier or harder to detect. They can start fires, deploy signals, discard rubbish, leave tracks, and wear brightly colored clothing. They can also evade detection, leave few tracks, discard nothing, and otherwise leave little evidence of their passing. The more a searcher knows about the subject (e.g., capabilities, equipment), the easier it is to predict the type and quantity of clues the subject might leave. A comprehensive subject profile is essential to make this happen.

Human subjects leave predictable clues. Virtually every person who moves through an area impacts his or her environment thousands of times and potentially leaves thousands of pieces of the evidence of his or her passing: tracks, scent, discarded material, etc. Thus, the most common problem is not a lack of clues but too many of them and distinguishing between which are relevant and irrelevant. A detailed subject profile can enable both searchers and managers to either relate a particular clue to the subject or discount it altogether.

The five general categories of search clues include the following:

- Physical (footprints, discarded material)
- Documentary (summit log, trail register)
- Testimonial (witnesses, family, friends, people in search area)
- Events (flashing lights, whistle, yell)
- Analytical (the results of reasoning; e.g., if the subject wanted to get from A to B, he or she would have to go through location C)

The key to effective clue-oriented search is to identify and interpret clues left by the lost subject and constantly monitor the search area for changes.

A good searcher must be able to distinguish between relevant and irrelevant clues, that is, those left by the subject versus those left by others (searchers, bystanders, wildlife, etc.), and be able to interpret the numerous potential messages conveyed by them.

There are at least four pieces of information that human subjects may convey through the clues they leave:

1. *The present location of the subject.* A yell, a whistle, a flash of light
2. *The previous location of the subject.* Evidence of where the subject was
3. *The destination of the subject.* Evidence of where the subject is going
4. *The subject was not here.* A total lack of clues

Searchers must be open to, and capable of, detecting clues that would lead to the discovery and development of this information.

All clues were generated at a specific point in time. If this time can be precisely established, multiple clues can indicate direction of travel. This chronology or timeline of clues can be extremely helpful to search planners. Therefore, searchers should be sure to document exactly when their discovery was made and determine as best they can exactly when the clue was generated.

The Environment

The characteristics of the environment in which a detection may occur also play an important role (**FIGURE 14-2**). Meteorological visibility—potentially reduced by fog, smog, haze, low clouds, and precipitation—directly affects visual searchers in the field. The time of day is also important. Adequate ambient light is vital for visual searchers, and the best time of day for searching is usually when the sun is at a relatively high elevation,

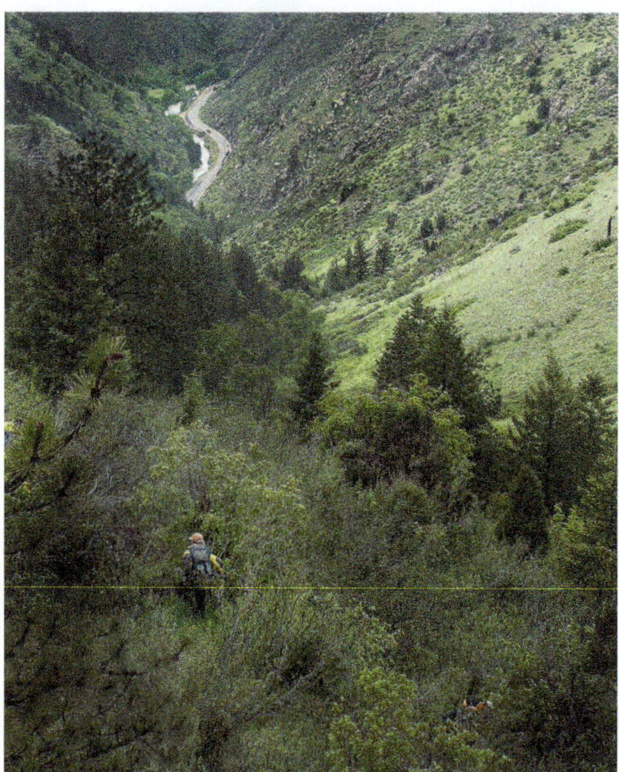

FIGURE 14-2 The characteristics of the sensor, search object, and environment in which a detection may occur all play an important role in how easy or hard detection may be.

which is different than for trackers who prefer early morning and later afternoon, when the sun is at a low angle to the ground. Night searches require that searchers carry and use additional lighting equipment, and when meteorological visibility is poor, night searching may not be effective at all, even with the best lighting equipment.

The type of terrain can also affect detection. A search object may be seen easily in a flat area with little vegetation, but the same object may be very difficult to see in mountainous terrain that is heavily forested or covered in boulders. Obstructions in the terrain—such as trees, bushes, and rocks—all can prevent the detection of a search object. Difficult environmental conditions that make travel difficult could also have a detrimental effect on searchers (the sensor), thus reducing their ability to detect.

It is also important that searchers know what to do about the discovery of clues before the discovery is made. The best time to determine this is at the briefing, before a search assignment is carried out, when responses to clue discovery can be planned and agreed upon.

Clue Specifics

There are several pieces of information that can help the searcher by providing clues, and almost all of these can be discerned during the completion of a missing person questionnaire (see Appendix A). When the following information is used as a basis for ongoing clue detection, a sound foundation for discovery is laid.

1. What general category does the subject fit into (child, hunter, fisherman, hiker, climber, photographer, berry picker, despondent, etc.)? Using categories described in the latest lost person behavior literature may be the most helpful (Koester, 2008).
   - What is the detectability of the particular category? For example, hunters wear bright colors, whereas hikers may not.
   - Does the category indicate whether the subject might be on or off the road? Hikers might be on a trail, whereas climbers could be on the rocks.
   - Can the category indicate how far or over what terrain the subject may travel? Climbers may climb a cliff, but an elderly berry picker will probably not.
   - Does the category of the subject indicate how far they might travel? Hikers may travel far, whereas elderly people may not.
   - How does the category of the subject affect their survivability? For example, a hunter may be much better prepared for bad weather than a photographer.
2. Identifying and studying the **point last seen (PLS)** or **last known position (LKP)** of the subject may uncover important clues.
   - What are the geographical restrictions encountered by the subject when he or she attempts to travel? Recreate the scene and put yourself in their shoes. Identification of the LKP or PLS is important because it forms the starting point for all physical clue detection. Accuracy is important.
3. Investigating the circumstances of the loss of the subject can indicate his or her starting location, where he or she was going, how he or she got there, and how he or she may behave while lost. Using information described in the latest lost person behavior literature may be helpful here (Koester, 2008).
   - What was the subject supposed to be doing when the loss occurred?
   - Was the subject en route somewhere? To where? By what route?
   - Was the subject expected somewhere? Where? When? How prepared was the subject for the trip?
   - What was the attitude and personality of the subject(s) (aggressive, anxious, etc.)?
   - In the sequence of events, when did the searchers begin to search and where did they start?
   - What does the literature say about how the specific category of subject might behave?
4. The physical and mental health, as well as the general condition of the subject, can mandate urgency or offer other important guidance.
   - What is the subject's general capability? What can he or she do, and what can't he or she do?
   - What is the subject's state of health at the time of loss? Is he or she an alcoholic, or a drug user or abuser? Does he or she have high blood pressure? Does the subject take any medications regularly? What will happen to him or her without the medications? What are the side effects of the medications? Are major medical problems involved, such as heart or lung problems or diabetes? Does the subject have mental problems such as depression, phobias, or senility?
5. The subject's personality can be a factor in determining how he or she might handle certain situations and, therefore, can indicate how he or she acts and what he or she does.
   - Personality traits may include aggressive or pondering; loner or gregarious; self-sufficient or dependent; irritable or upset easily; despondent or depressed; independent, persevering, or realistic; neglectful; perfectionist.
6. Equipment that the subject was carrying not only can indicate his or her skill level, but it can turn into a clue if dropped or lost by the lost subject. A complete subject profile indicating all equipment carried by the subject can be invaluable for related clue identification. It is also easy to assess preparedness of the subject by evaluating equipment carried. Footgear can be important in identifying tracks as those of the subject.
7. Terrain evaluation (in the search area) is important not only as an indicator of where and how the subject may travel, but also as an indicator of how long the subject(s) may survive.
   - Are there forks in the road or trail that may have confused the subject?
   - What sights or sounds might have been seen or heard (from the point last seen) that may have attracted the subject?

- What barriers may limit the search area? These include rivers, natural routes that offer less resistance to travel, etc. Conversely, are there areas where the subject is not cut off by barriers?

8. The post-mission critique has much to offer in the way of identifying clues that were overlooked or overly emphasized. Many clues may be discovered after a mission when the **scenario** is fully disclosed. Analyzing these can offer information on how not to miss similar clues next time, and reasons for overlooking clues can be studied to identify better search methods or problems in the next search.
   - What was done wrong? What was done right?
   - Often, too much weight is put on a lone clue or group of clues because there is little else to go on or the clue detector is not open-minded about his or her discovery. Recall that clues should never be considered simply at face value. Some thought should be put into whether any clue is relevant and then to its appropriate interpretation.
   - This new knowledge from the critique regarding clue detection, interpretation, and analysis should be cataloged and well documented so that lessons from them can be relayed to new generations of clue detectors.
9. Tracking is the art of following someone or something by stringing together a continuous chain of their sign (see Chapter 13, *Tracking*). It can be quite effective when there is a positive last known point or point last seen. *Sign cutting* is defined as looking for sign to establish a starting point from which to track. *Sign* is any evidence of change from the natural state that is inflicted on an environment by a person's (or animal's) passage (**FIGURE 14-3**).
   - Tracking is a very intense, mental, analytical discipline that takes much practice. Tracking can be invaluable in a SAR incident when it is performed by skilled trackers, but it can also be a waste of time and even harmful if those practicing it are unfamiliar with its subtleties. The use of tracking in SAR has increased over the years, and the results have been quite remarkable.
   - Sign cutting alone is worthy of study because its essence is the identification and analysis of discoverable evidence, which is an appropriate definition of clue consciousness.

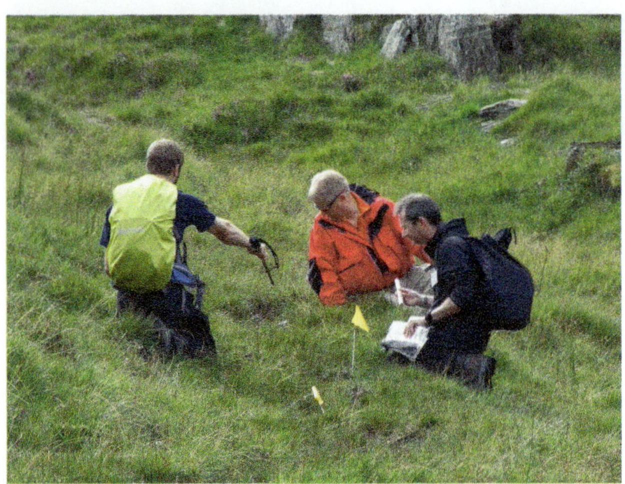

FIGURE 14-3 Tracking is the art of following someone or something by stringing together a continuous chain of their sign. It can be quite effective when there is a positive last known point or point last seen.

Courtesy of Donald Cooper.

SEARCH AND RESCUE TIP

Sign is any evidence of change from the natural state that is inflicted on an environment by a person's (or animal's) passage.

Key Search Concepts

The *search area* (sometimes referred to as the **possibility area**) is the term used to describe the smallest area to be searched, consistent with all available information, containing all the possible **search subject** or object locations (IMO/ICAO, 2016). To keep this area as small as possible, and thus keep the search as easy as possible, steps must be taken to ensure that the subject does not leave the search area (called **containment**) and that all possible search subject/object locations are included in the search area. Both are primarily search management and planning concerns; however, field personnel must understand their operational role in the process. Searchers may be used as containment resources that help detect if or when the subject leaves the search area. Searchers may be asked to serve as a lookout on a road, trail, or elevated position to keep an eye out for the subject, or they may be tasked to work with a search crew to actively search a bounded search segment. Searchers must remain confident that search planners will provide them numerous detection opportunities because the confidence and optimism of searchers drives the quality of their search.

A **region**, also called a *region of probability*, is a delineated, geographic subset of the search area within which there is a uniform likelihood of containing the search object or subject. That is, the subject is equally likely to be in any particular location within the same region—the **probability density (Pden)** is the same in all parts of any given region. Region boundaries and the size of regions are based only on factors that affect the location and probability of area (POA) of the search object (i.e., where to search), not on suitability for assigning search resources (i.e., how to search). A region boundary means that a search planner believes there is a different likelihood that the search object is on one side of the boundary versus the other. Often, regions are further subdivided into segments to be effectively searched (NSARC, 2011). A region may contain searchable segments, or a region itself may be a searchable segment. In short, regions are based solely on issues related to POA, or where the subject is more or less likely to be. Although regions of probability are more relevant to search planners, search crew members should know what they are when they are mentioned.

In contrast to a region, a **segment**, or **search subarea**, is a delineated, geographic subset of the search area based on operational factors that affect searchers. Boundaries of a segment and the segment size are not based on where the subject is likely to be. They are based on whether it can be searched by the intended SAR resource to an acceptable level of thoroughness in a specified length of time. For example, aircraft segments are generally larger than segments intended for ground teams, and the size of aircraft segments must be dependent on how long the aircraft can stay on scene before refueling. Segments are based solely on issues related to how the segment will be searched—that is, searchability, not probability—and are concerns of field personnel because searchers are assigned segments to search. The boundaries of a segment must also be identifiable both in the field and on a map so search crews know when they have reached it.

At most organized SAR incidents, before starting their assignment, search crews going into the field are briefed by a member of the incident management team. That is, information is conveyed to field personnel concerning such things as situation status, subject information, terrain in the search area, safety procedures, hazards to expect, how to handle discovered clues, and much more. This is referred to as the *briefing* (**FIGURE 14-4**). After an assignment is completed, the same search crew is *debriefed*, which is where the crew's observations and activities during their assignment are communicated to the incident management team (**FIGURE 14-5**). This is referred to as the **debriefing** and is considered the most critical information exchanged during any SAR operation. Without it, search planners will not have the information they need to determine where best to search and to what extent the search has been successful.

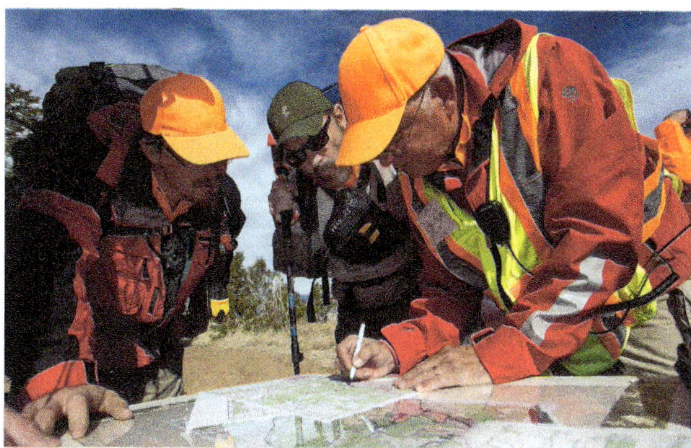

FIGURE 14-4 Team briefing. Prior to going into the field, a search team is briefed on information regarding situation status, subject information, terrain in the search area, safety procedures, hazards to expect, how to handle discovered clues, and much more.

© 2016 Howard Paul, Photography for Communication and Commerce.

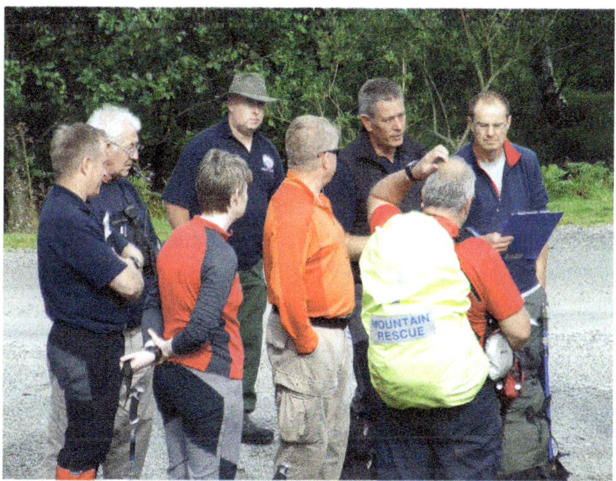

FIGURE 14-5 Team debriefing. After an assignment is completed, the search crew is debriefed, which is where the crew's observations and activities during their assignment are communicated to the incident management team.

Courtesy of Donald Cooper.

Search Theory

In the most general sense, a successful search requires two things: that we look in the right place, and that we can detect that which we seek. Another way to say this is that the likelihood that a search will be successful depends on two related probabilities: the probability that the search object is in the area searched and the probability of detecting the search object, presuming it is in the area being searched. So, what is "probability?"

Probability theory is a branch of mathematics with which a person may systematically deal with uncertain events. Probability, usually described as a percentage (%) that falls between 0 and 100%, describes the chances something will happen. Contemporary probability theory is well established and finds application in almost every area of scholarly activity from music to physics and in daily experience from weather prediction (e.g., chances of rain) to predicting the risks of new medical treatments (e.g., mortality and morbidity). In a SAR event, uncertainties are prevalent. Having a way to quantify these uncertainties and represent them more precisely with numbers is useful, especially when comparing one search plan or one option to another.

There are three important probabilities used in the application of search theory that can help search planners determine where and how to search: the **probability of detection (POD)**, the **probability of area (POA)**, and the **probability of success (POS)**. Some of these concepts are more important to operational personnel than others, but an understanding of the general ideas can significantly improve operational effectiveness and communications between search planners and search crews.

POD represents the chances the search object will be detected, assuming it was in the area searched. POD is considered a measure of the effectiveness of the sensor (e.g., human searcher, electronic sensor, dog team). The search activities undertaken in the search area by searchers affects POD. It is important after a search that searchers accurately and completely describe what they did so search planners can use the information to compute POD.

POA describes a measure of the chances the search object is contained within the boundaries of any region within the search area. POA describes where the search object or subject is more or less likely to be. Maritime search planners refer to POA as *probability of containment (POC)*; the terms have identical meanings. Although it is an important element of search planning, POA is rarely of concern to searchers.

POS describes a measure of the chances of finding the search object with a particular application of search resources and is considered a measure of overall search effectiveness. In the end, the objective of all search planning, and indeed search theory itself, is to maximize the POS in the least amount of time with the given (usually limited) search resources. Mathematically, this is represented by the conventional notation of search theory:

$$POS = POA \times POD$$

This equation shows that POS is dependent on two factors—POA and POD—neither of which is more important than the other. Although field searchers may focus on the detection part of the equation, they should never lose sight of the fact that the overall goal of search planning is to maximize POS, not POD. Search planners and managers determine how this is best achieved, and field search operations play a key role, but success depends on everyone doing their part.

SEARCH AND RESCUE TIP

The object of all search planning, and indeed search theory itself, is to maximize the probability of success in the least amount of time with the given (usually limited) search resources.

Very often the best distribution of search resources within the search area (i.e., optimal effort allocation) is not obvious or intuitive. Searchers rarely have access to all the available information. Therefore, searchers should not try to second guess the search manager or the planner, but instead concentrate on performing their assigned tasks to the best of their abilities. The number and type of resources assigned to each segment will be whatever is required to maximize the overall chances for success. A good search, therefore, is one where the search crew performed their assignment safely and precisely as instructed.

SEARCH AND RESCUE TIP

A good search is one where the search crew performed their assignment safely and precisely as instructed.

People are not good at estimating probabilities directly. It would be great if searchers could simply be asked to estimate what their POD was for a search, but experiments show that a searcher asked to estimate the POD of a recently conducted search will be wrong as often as right. In fact, in multiple experiments, POD estimates from searchers were only within 10% of the actual POD as often as if the value had been randomly chosen (Koester et al., 2004). Such an estimate can be even further biased when the severity of any negative results is more significant, such as when the searchers feel that if they do not find the subject, they will die (Harris et al., 2008). This is why search planners do not, and should not, ask field personnel to directly estimate POD or any other probability. Instead, search crews will be asked what they observed, what they did, and where they did it to provide the information necessary for POD to be computed by search planners.

As implied by the prominent role POS plays in search theory, success is important in a search, but a search that takes a long time increases the chances of turning the rescue of a live subject into the recovery of a dead body. Delays in locating a subject increase the chances of death and injury due to exposure, trauma, dehydration, and similar significant problems that can affect both the subject and searchers. Therefore, a successful search for a live, human subject must also include the element of time. If we want to save a life during a search, we must find the subject quickly. In other words, the driving concept of the application of search theory is to search in such a way as to maximize the chances of finding what you seek as fast as possible, that is, "Success Fast"—a very sensible and intuitive goal.

SEARCH AND RESCUE TIP

The driving concept of the application of search theory is to search in such a way as to maximize the chances of finding what you seek as fast as possible, that is, SUCCESS FAST.

Origins of Search Theory

Operations research (OR) is a professional, scientific discipline that provides for a systematic approach to informed decision-making, especially in uncertain situations. It involves the application of scientific and mathematical methods to the study and analysis of problems involving complex systems (Informs, 2017). *Search theory* is an applied mathematical subdiscipline of OR that uses OR principles and methods to help solve search problems. In short, search theory is a mathematical approach to determining how best to find that which is sought, and the principles of search theory apply to any situation where the objective is to find, in the most efficient manner, a person or object contained in some geographic region.

Bernard O. Koopman (1900–1981), a Harvard-educated scientist, established the basis for a rigorous study of search theory and practice with his pioneering work for the U.S. Navy during World War II. The work initially done by Koopman and colleagues was instrumental in the Allied approach to the Battle of the Atlantic and antisubmarine warfare. Although this application may seem far removed from searching for lost people on land, the basic theory of search established by Koopman applies to all types of searching, including that of inland search (Koopman, 1980; Washburn, 2002).

Search theory was applied to military SAR operations during and after World War II, but the U.S. Coast Guard provided the first comprehensive application to civil SAR in the 1950s. The methodology was incorporated into the first edition of the *U.S. National Search and Rescue Manual* in 1959, and it quickly gained acceptance by maritime SAR agencies worldwide and has remained in global use ever since. In addition, scientific research and development in search theory has progressed in fields as diverse as mining, mineral and oil exploration, and even archeology.

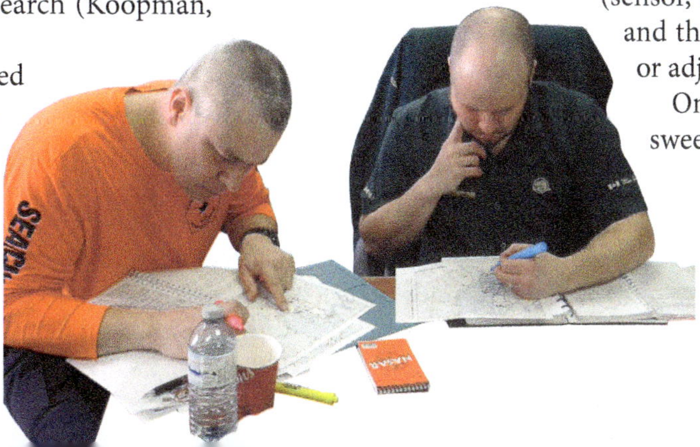

Search theory is used because it allows search planners to achieve success quicker, thus achieving three other goals of all search operations: minimizing the amount of time searchers are exposed to hazardous conditions, minimizing the costs involved (searching and supporting searchers can be expensive), and ultimately saving more lives. In short, search theory is used because it works.

Searcher's Role

One of the most significant contributions that field searchers can make is accurately and completely describing to search planners what was done and seen during a search, usually at the debriefing. This information is used by search planners to compute POD and, in turn, is used to compute POS, which ultimately guides all other search efforts.

Sweep Width

How easy or difficult a search object is to detect is measured by something called *effective sweep width* or just **sweep width**. Put simply, sweep width is a measure of detectability that represents a unique combination of the characteristics of the three detection variables (sensor, object, and environment). A specific combination of these three variables that would make detection easier suggests a larger sweep width. A specific combination of these three variables that would make detection difficult suggests a smaller sweep width. Sweep width is a key element in the determination of probability of detection (POD), which in turn is an important element in planning and evaluating a search.

Search planners can choose where and how many search resources to assign to various segments, which is the essence of the search planner's job, but they cannot control the nature of the three detection variables (sensor, object, and environment) and thus cannot directly control or adjust sweep width.

One group of authors describes sweep width this way:

> The *sweep width* concept is extremely robust and extremely practical. An important property of *sweep width* is its relative independence from the

> details of the detection processes themselves, such as the exact shape of the detection profile or exactly how the searcher's eyes and brain function to see and recognize the search object. In fact, *sweep width* integrates the effects of all the myriad factors affecting detection in a given situation into a single numeric value that is then easy for search planners to use. *Sweep width* is simply a measure (or estimate) of the average detection potential of a single specific "resource" (e.g., a person on the ground, an aircraft or vessel and its crew, etc.) while seeking a particular search object in a particular environment. Thus the concept may be applied to any sensor looking for any object under any set of conditions (Koester et al., 2004, p. 188).

One way to think about sweep width is as a variable measure of detectability that is carried around by a searcher (sensor) and applied as he or she searches. This measure (sweep width) is larger when a specific object is easier to detect by the searcher in a specific environment. Consider the previously described example of a visual human searcher looking for a green golf ball in an open field with short, green grass on a cloudy day. The unique combination of the three detection variables involved suggests a somewhat small sweep width, meaning a somewhat difficult situation for detection. Now consider the same searcher on the same cloudy day in the same open field looking for an orange, much larger, beach ball. It is easy to conclude that the sweep width in this situation would be much larger, suggesting a far easier situation for detection. In fact, changing the characteristics of any one of the three detection variables (sensor, object, or environment), like we did with the size and color of the ball in the example, could make the situation easier or harder in terms of detection.

Some important characteristics of sweep width can help clarify its meaning. It is described as a width and so is measured in feet or meters like a width would be. For a human, visual searcher, sweep width is centered on the searcher. That is, half of the sweep width extends to each side of the searcher as he or she passes through the search area.

Actual sweep width values for specific situations are determined by rigorous scientific experiments. However, reasonably accurate estimates may be made in one of two ways: (1) the use of tables of sweep width values that have been established by rigorous experiments for various typical search situations, then applying appropriate "correction factors" to accommodate other search situations; and, (2) the use of a field-expedient procedure conducted while in the segment to be searched that can be used by search planners to estimate sweep width.

TABLE 14-1 shows a table of sweep width values from the *International Aeronautical and Maritime Search and Rescue (IAMSAR) Manual* that can be used when searching for various search objects from an aircraft. For example, when searching for a person on the ground (left column) from an aircraft flying at 1,000 feet (300 meters) (second column from left), and with meteorological visibility of 10 nautical miles (19 kilometers), the sweep width is 0.5 miles (0.9 kilometers). This value is then corrected for factors that affect sweep width, such as vegetation and mountainous terrain (**TABLE 14-2**), flight speed (faster reduces sweep width), and high winds (more wind reduces sweep width). Thus, a corrected sweep width value can be computed by starting with an uncorrected sweep width value in Table 14-1 and applying correction factors such as those included in Table 14-2 (there are others).

These tables have been in use for decades around the world, but at the time of this writing, very few such sweep width tables are (yet) available for searches conducted on the ground for lost and missing people. Interestingly, the very research intended to develop sweep width values for land search revealed a relatively simple field procedure for estimating sweep width (Koester et al., 2014). This "range of detection" procedure is described in Chapter 15, *Search Operations*.

Defining sweep width precisely is difficult, and some find it helpful to visualize how sweep width is experimentally derived. Sweep width experiments start with a search segment—represented in **FIGURE 14-6** as the rectangle. In the segment, many targets are randomly placed, represented in Figure 14-6 by the dots, before a searcher (sensor) passes through. The track of the searcher is depicted in Figure 14-6 by the arrow pointing upward. As the searcher passes through the target-rich environment, some targets are detected (the white dots) and some targets are not detected (the colored dots). In this example, all targets (dots) were detected out to some distance from the sensor—a clean sweep. Although this example is not necessarily realistic (rarely does a sensor detect all there is to find), this "definite range" sensor example is often used to demonstrate perhaps the most important characteristic of sweep width: sweep width is the width of the swath where the number of objects *detected outside* the swath equals the number of objects *missed (not detected) within* the swath. In Figure 14-6, a total of 40 objects lay within the swath, and all 40 were detected. Thus, the number of the targets detected outside the swath (zero) equals the number missed within the swath (also zero), so the two values are equal, and the width of the swath is the sweep width. A clean sweep

TABLE 14-1 Sweep Widths for Visual Land Search (Searching from an Aircraft)

		Visibility (km[NM])				
Search Object	**Height in m (ft)**	**6 (3)**	**9 (5)**	**19 (10)**	**28 (15)**	**37 (20)**
Person	150 (500)	0.7 (0.4)	0.7 (0.4)	0.9 (0.5)	0.9 (0.5)	0.9 (0.5)
	300 (1000)	0.7 (0.4)	0.7 (0.4)	0.9 (0.5)	0.9 (0.5)	0.9 (0.5)
	450 (1500)	—	—	—	—	—
	600 (2000)	—	—	—	—	—
Vehicle	150 (500)	1.7 (0.9)	2.4 (1.3)	2.4 (1.3)	2.4 (1.3)	2.4 (1.3)
	300 (1000)	1.9 (1.0)	2.6 (1.4)	2.6 (1.4)	2.8 (1.5)	2.8 (1.5)
	450 (1500)	1.9 (1.0)	2.6 (1.4)	3.1 (1.7)	3.1 (1.7)	3.1 (1.7)
	600 (2000)	1.9 (1.0)	2.8 (1.5)	3.7 (2.0)	3.7 (2.0)	3.7 (2.0)
Aircraft less than 5700 kg	150 (500)	1.9 (1.0)	2.6 (1.4)	2.6 (1.4)	2.6 (1.4)	2.6 (1.4)
	300 (1000)	1.9 (1.0)	2.8 (1.5)	2.8 (1.5)	3.0 (1.6)	3.0 (1.6)
	450 (1500)	1.9 (1.0)	2.8 (1.5)	3.3 (1.8)	3.3 (1.8)	3.3 (1.8)
	600 (2000)	1.9 (1.0)	3.0 (1.6)	3.7 (2.0)	3.7 (2.0)	3.7 (2.0)
Aircraft over 5700 kg	150 (500)	2.2 (1.2)	3.7 (2.0)	4.1 (2.2)	4.1 (2.2)	4.1 (2.2)
	300 (1000)	3.3 (1.8)	5.0 (2.7)	5.6 (3.0)	5.6 (3.0)	5.6 (3.0)
	450 (1500)	3.7 (2.0)	5.2 (2.8)	5.9 (3.2)	5.9 (3.2)	5.9 (3.2)
	600 (2000)	4.1 (2.2)	5.2 (2.9)	6.5 (3.5)	6.5 (3.5)	6.5 (3.5)

Material from the IMO publications IAMSAR Manual Volumes I, II and III (2016 - II960E/IF961E/II962E and 2013 - IH960E/IE961E and IH962E) and/or the IMO website www.imo.org is reproduced with the permission of the International Maritime Organization (IMO), which does not accept responsibility for the correctness of the material as reproduced: in case of doubt, IMO's authentic text shall prevail. Readers should check with their national maritime Administration for any further amendments or latest advice. International Maritime Organization, 4 Albert Embankment, London, SE1 7SR, United Kingdom.

TABLE 14-2 Correction Factors—Vegetation and High Terrain

Search Object	15–60% Vegetation or Hilly	60–85% Vegetation or Mountainous	Over 85% Vegetation
Person	0.5	0.3	0.1
Vehicle	0.7	0.4	0.1
Aircraft less than 5700 kg	0.7	0.4	0.1
Aircraft over 5700 kg	0.8	0.4	0.1

Material from the IMO publications IAMSAR Manual Volumes I, II and III (2016 - II960E/IF961E/II962E and 2013 - IH960E/IE961E and IH962E) and/or the IMO website www.imo.org is reproduced with the permission of the International Maritime Organization (IMO), which does not accept responsibility for the correctness of the material as reproduced: in case of doubt, IMO's authentic text shall prevail. Readers should check with their national maritime Administration for any further amendments or latest advice. International Maritime Organization, 4 Albert Embankment, London, SE1 7SR, United Kingdom.

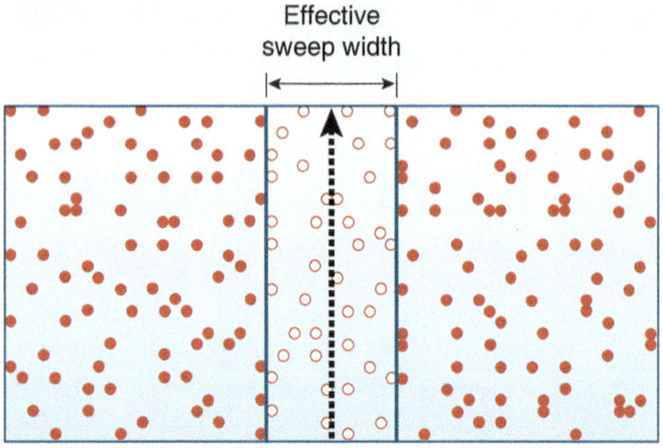

Effective sweep width

FIGURE 14-6 Illustration of an experiment from which effective sweep width is determined. The dotted line represents the searcher's track; detected objects are denoted by white dots. The number missed within the swath is zero, and the number detected outside the swath is zero (a clean sweep). Since the number of detected objects outside the swath equals the number of undetected objects within the swath (a characteristic of sweep width), the width of this swath equals the sweep width.

Effective sweep width

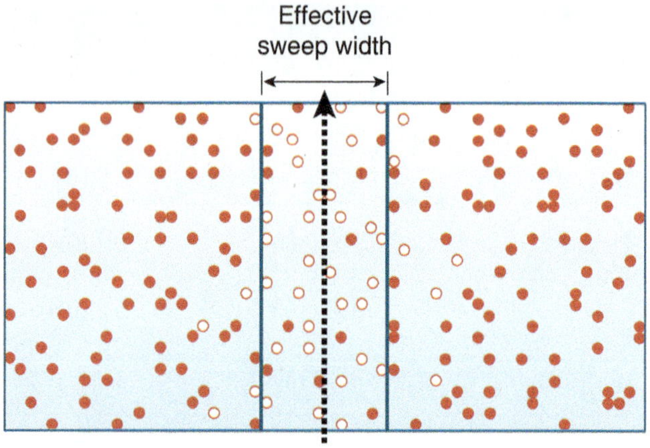

FIGURE 14-7 Illustration of an experiment from which effective sweep width is determined. The dotted line represents the searcher's track; detected objects are denoted by white dots. The number missed within the swath is 11, and the number detected outside the swath is 11. Since the number of detected objects outside the swath equals the number of undetected objects within the swath (a characteristic of sweep width), the width of this swath equals the sweep width.

where the searcher/sensor is 100% effective out to a definite range on either side of the track and completely ineffective at greater distances is unrealistic, but it serves to illustrate the sweep width principle.

FIGURE 14-7 illustrates a more realistic situation where objects are detected over a wider swath, but not all the objects within that swath are detected, and some objects outside the swath are detected. In this illustration, the number of objects detected outside the swath (11) also equals the number of objects missed within the swath (11). Instead of making a clean sweep, the detections are more widely distributed. Thus, the width of the swath where as many targets were missed within as detected beyond is the sweep width.

The concept of sweep width recognizes that some objects near the searcher may be missed, and some objects far from the searcher may be detected. Indeed, sweep width is an average measure of detectability over a wide range of detection opportunities. It is not a measure of the maximum distance at which an object might be sighted. In fact, some search objects may be detected well beyond the sweep width, and some may be missed within the sweep width. This is required by the very definition of sweep width.

If sweep width is known, the number of objects to be found can be accurately predicted, on average, for a single searcher's pass through the area. This is extraordinarily valuable information for the search planner. Knowing (or estimating) the sweep width for a given sensor, search object, and environment provides the first information needed by a search planner interested in computing POD. The next step is using the sweep width to determine the **area effectively swept**.

Field Contributions to Measuring Detection

The area effectively swept—sometimes referred to as *search effort*—is an area, described in square feet or meters, that results from multiplying the sweep width by the total **track line length (TLL)**. This value represents exactly what the term suggests: a measure of the area that can be (or was) effectively searched. Total track line length can be determined by several methods, but it must account for all searchers who are expending effort in the search segment. It can be computed by determining the track line length for each individual search resource (e.g., each member of a search crew), then summed across all searchers to compute a total track line length, or it can be computed for one representative member of a search crew and multiplied by the number in the crew to compute a total track line length.

Ideally, a GPS device can be used to store the track of one (or all) searchers, which can then be uploaded to search planners at the debriefing, but this is not always possible. If a forward speed of the searcher can be estimated, this **search speed** (in miles per hour [mph] or kilometers per hour [kph]) can be multiplied by the time spent searching to compute the track line length (speed × time = distance). For example, a person searching at 0.5 mph (0.8 kph) for 30 minutes would have a track line length of 0.25 mile or 1320 feet (0.4 kilometers or 402 meters).

This raises at least two questions: (1) what does area effectively swept have to do with searchers in the field, and (2) how can search speed be estimated? Although computing the area effectively swept is vital to search planners, it has little or no value to field personnel. However, for search planners to make this important calculation, they need information from the field, such as observations that allow an estimation of sweep width, an estimate of search speed, the exact time spent searching (minus travel time to and from the segment and breaks), and other useful observations and experiences from search crews. Without input from the field, planners are only guessing. Input from search crews is critical to effective search planning.

Search speed can be estimated in several ways and will likely be requested by search planners if another method of determining track line length is not available. It can also be useful to searchers when planning a search task.

The easiest method of determining search speed may be, like track line length, through the use of a GPS receiver. Many of these devices display speed of travel. A searcher carrying one may therefore be able to use it to directly determine search speed over a given track. Alternatively, several sources also suggest wilderness hiking speeds ranging from 2 to 4 miles per hour (Tawrell, 2007; Trailtrove.com, 2017; NSARC, 2011), which could be used as a basis for estimating search speed. The Naismith Rule, named after a 19th century Scottish mountaineer, can also be used in estimating hiking speed: For the average walker, allow 1 hour for every 3 miles (5 kilometers) forward, plus 1 hour for every 2000 feet (600 meters) of ascent; when walking in groups, calculate for the speed of the slowest person (www.mountainsafety.co.uk, 2017). Experience suggests adjustments to this rule that include subtracting 10 minutes for every 1,000 feet (300 meters) of gentle descent and adding 10 minutes for every 1,000 feet (300 meters) of steep descent. Search speeds can be derived from these suggestions, depending on the terrain (i.e., open land, on trail, off trail, heavy underbrush, heavy timber, etc.) and other environmental conditions, but they are almost always slower, by a significant margin, than hiking speeds.

Another way to determine search speed is by performing an experiment of sorts during a training session. Using terrain representative of a typical search area, determine the distance from the start of a search to some location a short but measurable distance away, say one-quarter mile (0.4 kilometer). Search the measured distance at a normal pace and note how long it takes. Then, the search speed can be computed by dividing the distance measured by the time it took to search. For example, if the distance was one-quarter mile (0.4 kilometer) and it took 15 minutes (1/4 hour), your search speed was 1 mile per hour (0.25/0.25 = 1 mph or 1.6 kph). This type of experiment can be performed in each of the typical types of terrain in which you might be called to search. With some practice and experience, a searcher can estimate his or her actual search speed by adjusting this "normal" search speed up or down to match the terrain, steepness, weather, and other factors that affect search speed. Eventually, search planners familiar with their search crews will know their normal search speed and, at the debriefing, just need to know if they went faster or slower than normal (see also Chapter 15).

With all these rough estimates of probabilities, search speed, track line length, and other variables used in the application of search theory, one might presume that mathematically combining all of these "fuzzy" numbers produces even fuzzier results. In fact, the use of estimated, less than perfect, input values may take the proper application of search theory more time to achieve success, but it will still get there. Search theory, when properly applied, is so robust and adaptable that even when imprecise or approximate values are used, it will still eventually push search planners toward the right answer. This robustness is one of the many strengths of this method. In addition, using the right process, even with less than ideal inputs, gets users in the habit of following a time-tested methodology so that when more accurate data are available—say, after we have more data from additional sweep width experiments—the results of the process will be even more useful.

Coverage and Probability of Detection

Getting back to the process of computing POD, now that search planners have computed the area effectively swept, they can use it to determine coverage, which is the last step in ultimately computing POD. Search planners compute coverage, or **coverage factor (C)**, by dividing the area effectively swept by the area of the search segment. That is, coverage is the ratio of the area effectively swept to the area of the segment searched. It is also a unitless value. That is, coverage is not described in feet, meters, square feet, square meters, or any other unit. It is simply a numerical value that describes a measure of thoroughness, effort density (searching effort per unit of area), or how well a segment was covered. The higher the coverage, the more thorough the search; the lower the coverage, the less thorough the search. A higher coverage suggests more search effort (i.e., area effectively swept) was used per unit of area of the searched segment.

While the actual coverage value may have little meaning to search crews, the general concept can be intuitive and useful. Search planners may use the term in a briefing of search crews to describe how thorough they would like the search task to be. For example, the instruction may go something like this: "please conduct a high coverage search in this small segment; you will be given plenty of time to complete the task," or, "please conduct a low coverage search in this segment and get it done quickly so you can be used in another segment; the subject is still thought to be responsive." If a search crew understands the concept of coverage and how it is derived, these types of instructions can be informative, helpful, and effective.

Probability of detection (POD) has a mathematical relationship to coverage that is represented in the curves (and their underlying mathematical functions) represented in **FIGURE 14-8**. The lower curve shows the relationship between POD and coverage as derived by Koopman (1946; 1980) for situations where searchers do not move along a set of long, perfectly straight, parallel, equally spaced tracks but instead follow more irregular paths. This curve—known as the "normal search" or "random search" curve—also works well when other random influences are present, such as uneven terrain and vegetation, even when the searcher tracks are perfectly straight, parallel, and equally spaced (Koester et al., 2004), which is why this curve is generally recommended for land search. Once the coverage is computed, search planners enter the graph at the coverage value at the bottom, move up to the normal search curve, and move horizontally to determine the POD value. The upper curve in Figure 14-8 represents ideal search conditions where there are no gaps or overlaps in search tracks, which is difficult to achieve in land search. **FIGURE 14-9** illustrates how the detection elements of search theory combine to compute POD.

When in the possession of skilled search planners, POD has powerful predictive value when planning a search. It can be used to compare the effectiveness of multiple search plans to choose the best option. POD computed after a search and based on the actual observations and experiences of field crews in the debriefing is even more powerful; it can be used to evaluate the effectiveness of the search operation. Both applications of POD are important to search planning, but the latter (retrospective POD) is more meaningful because it is based on real feedback from search crews rather than just estimates.

It seems intuitive that the total level of detection brought to bear in a segment should somehow increase overall if the segment is searched multiple times. This is indeed true and is one reason search

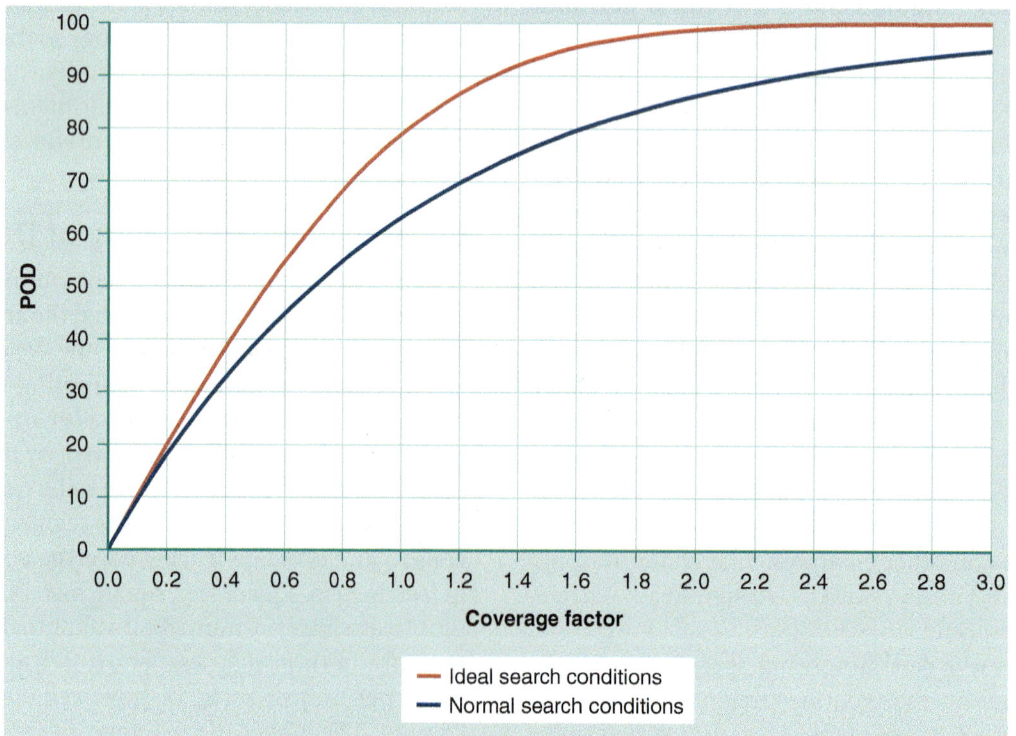

FIGURE 14-8 Average probabilities of detection (POD) over an area for visual searches using parallel sweeps. To calculate the POD, find the computed coverage across the bottom of the graph, move up to the bottom curve (the "normal search" curve is recommended for land search), and then move horizontally to the associated POD value.

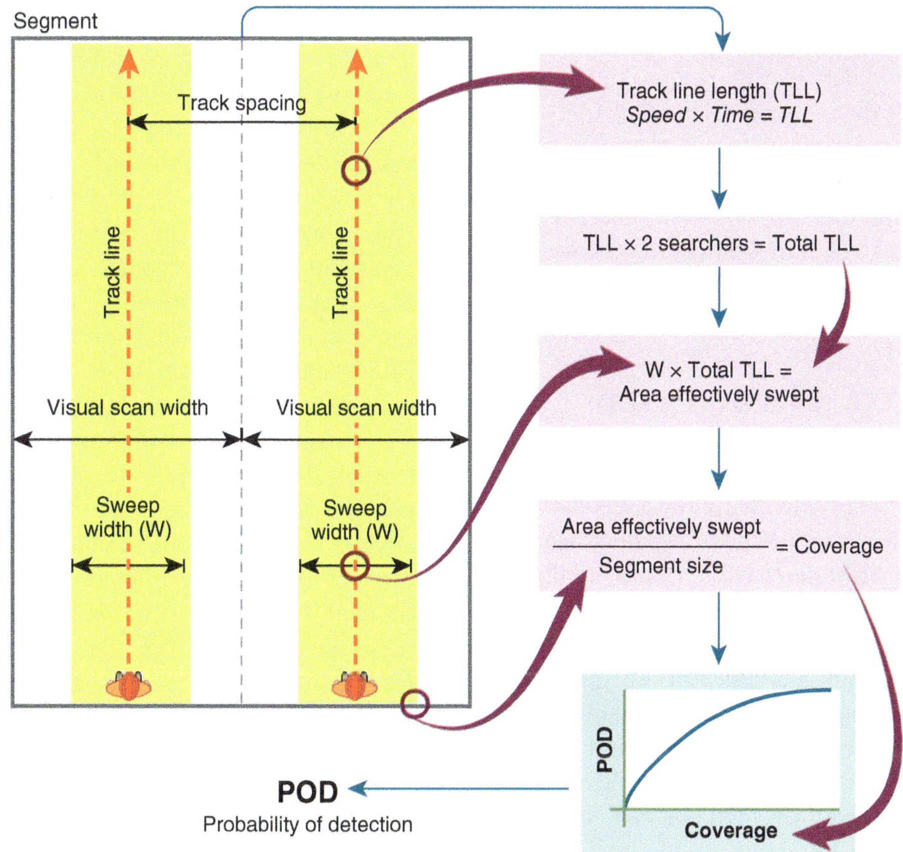

FIGURE 14-9 Detection elements of search theory. Probability of detection (POD) is computed by multiplying the sweep width (W) by the total track line length (total TLL) and dividing the result, called the "area effectively swept," by the area of the segment. The resulting value is the coverage factor from which POD can be determined by using the POD graph shown in Figure 14-8.

managers may direct search crews to search the same segment multiple times. In search theory, this is called cumulative POD. If a segment is searched the first time to a coverage of 0.5, then searched a second time to a coverage of 0.5, the cumulative POD can be computed by first summing the multiple coverage factors for each search. Then, using the sum of the multiple coverage factors as the entry point in the graph in Figure 14-8, cumulative POD can be determined. In this example, the sum of coverage factors is 1.0 (0.5 + 0.5 = 1). Then, Figure 14-8 can be used to determine that the cumulative POD for the two searches is about 63%.

Although cumulative POD is a very useful concept, recall that achieving the highest POD possible is not the goal of search crews or search planners. POD does not account for whether the search object is in the segment searched; thus, more information is needed to predict or determine the probability of success of a search. This is a good place to reiterate that the goal of search planners is to maximize the over POS, and the goal of search crews is to perform their assignments safely and precisely as instructed.

With POD computed, search planners can now combine it with POA (estimated in any number of ways) to compute POS for each segment searched and for the overall search area. While most of these calculations hold little practical value to search crews, they are used by search planners to numerically represent intangible possibilities that can be very useful for planning purposes. POS in particular can help the search planner make very important decisions that would likely be significantly more difficult without the tools search theory provides.

Specifically, search planners use search theory to help them achieve the following:

1. Allocate resources so that the maximum overall POS possible is achieved with the available resources and in the shortest possible amount of time.
2. Decide when and how to search or re-search a segment.
3. Decide when to increase or decrease the size of the search area.
4. Decide when to suspend an unsuccessful search or move the search area.

5. Rationalize actions to family, media, and authorities.
6. Justify actions to others.

Search theory cannot be applied properly by even the most skilled and experienced search planners without detailed input from searchers. Effectively communicating to search planners what is done, observed, and experienced by searchers in the field may be the most important and relevant task performed in any search operation.

Handling External Influences

When a person is reported missing and a search ensues, there is often great interest shown by news agencies (television, radio, print news, etc.), friends, family, and political entities (sometimes local but also state, federal, and international depending on the situation and individuals involved). Thus, it is likely that during a search someone who is a journalist, a friend, a member of the subject's family, or someone with interest and influence beyond the scope of the search operation will eventually confront field SAR personnel (**FIGURE 14-10**). When this happens, the potential for significant problems and/or embarrassment exists, and field personnel must have a plan to handle the situation.

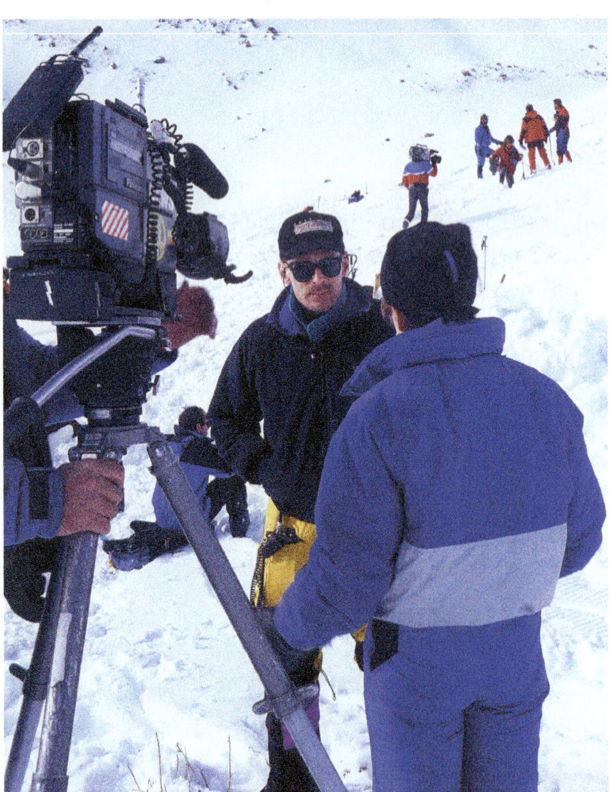

FIGURE 14-10 When media representatives inquire about search details, the potential for significant problems (and at least embarrassment) exists, and field personnel must have a plan to handle the situation. A polite referral to the incident commander or public information officer is best.

In most SAR incidents, the incident commander usually designates someone to deal with external influences. Typically in ICS, the public information officer communicates with the news media, the liaison officer deals with external organizations, and a family liaison is assigned to deal with and manage family issues. The important point is that someone (or group) is specifically assigned to these duties, and only the individuals assigned to these duties should be carrying them out. Before journalists, family members, and other interested parties are made aware of the proper channels for inquiries and information retrieval, they may approach anyone involved in the incident for information. Because of the potential for incomplete, uninformed, and/or inappropriate information to be disseminated, only those authorized by the incident commander should respond to these inquires. All others must be gently and courteously referred to the proper SAR personnel: the incident commander, public information officer, liaison officer, etc. Direct the media and other non-SAR individuals to someone who can talk to them because most likely you are not authorized to do so.

Lost or Missing Person Behavior

Understanding and predicting the behavior of a lost or missing person can greatly enhance the chances for a successful search. Search managers especially need to know what to expect from a lost or missing person, but information regarding how this person might act can also be helpful to field personnel.

In this context, subjects who have been reported missing and subjects who are believed to be lost shall both be referred to as "lost persons."

Lost Person Behavior for SAR Management

Search managers and planners, by analyzing the behavior of past lost persons, may be able to predict what the subject of the current search might do, how he or she might behave/react, where he or she might go, and where he or she might end up under similar circumstances. A skilled search manager or planner seeks answers to the following questions:

- What is the subject's state of health?
- What is his or her experience base? What has he or she experienced before?

- How does he or she handle being lost or confronting the environment in which he or she is lost?
- What could a lost subject do to affect the strategy of the search?
- What category does the subject fall into?
- How have other lost subjects behaved in similar circumstances?
- What does history indicate? Are there statistics?

Statistics compiled from past incidents indicate that members of a specific predetermined category of lost persons (e.g., children, teens, elderly folks, hunters, hikers) tend to act like others in the same category. If a search manager understands how members of the category that the lost subject fits into may act, the behavior and actions of the lost subject can be better anticipated. Koester (2008), in his landmark book on the subject, succinctly states it like this: "Knowledge of lost person behavior is a powerful tool that helps to determine where to look for the lost person" (p. 4).

Studies of thousands of past searches show that there are trends in the way most people act. These historical and statistical trends are often used to help determine how best to manage a present situation.

Lost Person Behavior in the Field

Knowledge of lost person behavior can also be advantageous to field personnel. It can help a searcher understand where to look and what to look for, even within a single assigned segment (Koester, 2008). Basically, the advantages of applying lost person behavior in the field are rooted in two concepts:

1. An understanding of the behavior of similar subjects from past SAR cases can be applied in the present situations to help predict the actions of the current subject.
2. An understanding of how the present lost subject has acted in the past might help predict his or her future actions.

What has been learned from analyzing past SAR cases and their subjects is that most categories of lost subjects tend to travel the path of least resistance. Places such as roads, paths, railroad tracks, power lines, game trails, streams, and clear cuts are much more likely to produce clues than thickets, the other side of wide rivers, deep woods, mountains, deep snow, and obvious paths of great resistance. There are some notable exceptions. For example, Alzheimer's (dementia) patients tend to "...go until they get stuck" (Koester, 2008, p. 162), and this is often in areas through which other people would not have attempted to travel.

Weather and visibility also seem to play an important role in determining actions of a lost person. For example, bad weather usually forces a person to take cover and stop; darkness tends to cause a person to rest and/or sleep; or fog and low visibility may limit a lost subject's wandering. These historical trends are based on the examination of what others have done in the past but do not always hold true.

Analyzing past situations also indicates that a subject might do certain things to affect their survivability and/or detectability. This information can be of great value to field personnel. For instance:

1. Can the subject build a fire or shelter?
   - Fire rings, shelters, fires, etc., might be clues.
   - The ability to perform these skills can suggest greater survivability.
2. What equipment is the lost subject carrying?
   - Discarded gear might be a clue and may be able to be confirmed as belonging to the subject.
   - Equipment available to the subject can directly affect survivability.
3. What is the subject's detectability?
   - Is the subject wearing brightly colored clothes or camouflage?
   - Will the subject be easy or difficult to see?
   - Is the subject likely to be responsive?
4. Can the subject respond to a searcher?
   - Does a searcher have to stumble over the subject or just get within earshot?
5. Will the subject hide or come running?
   - An evasive subject (one who does not want to be found and avoids searchers) is always more difficult to find and may be dangerous.

Where knowledge of lost person behavior is most likely to contribute to a search is in the field when a searcher simply puts himself or herself in the "shoes" of the lost subject. Trying to think like the lost subject can enhance one's understanding of where to look and what to look for.

Anticipating how a subject might act requires that SAR personnel have a thorough understanding of the subject's personality, attitudes, and other personal characteristics. This understanding should come from a complete subject profile, which is compiled from facts collected by an effective search management team. A complete profile must also be available to field personnel. The management team should not hesitate to distribute a subject profile to field personnel to ensure maximum effectiveness of the information. A complete subject profile can be invaluable to field personnel, but search managers compile the subject information.

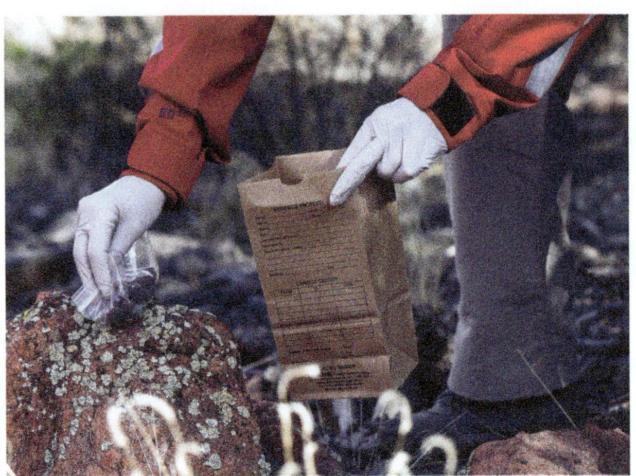

FIGURE 14-11 Evidence being collected. Whether SAR personnel find a small clue or an injured subject, how the individual or team handles the situation may have a significant effect on the outcome of the search and any potential investigation.

The ideal subject profile is comprehensive, leaves nothing to the imagination, and includes a complete list of all information related to the lost subject. The profile is compiled through systematic and thorough investigation, interrogation, and questioning by the management team and should include a complete missing person questionnaire. All available information should be included in the subject profile. Nothing should be left out. As a minimum, it should include the following:

1. Physical description of subject, clothing, and all equipment carried
2. Point last seen or last known point
3. Activities the subject is most likely to engage in (includes interests, hobbies, friends, etc.)
4. Standard practices (what they usually do, where they usually go, how they usually act, etc.)
5. Personality traits (aggressive, loner, despondent, dangerous, fearful, etc.)
6. Has this happened before, and, if so, what did they do before? (Where did they go, who did they see, etc.)
7. Physical and mental condition (whether the subject is healthy or sick, how [and how well] he or she handles stress, whether he or she is experienced in the wilderness)

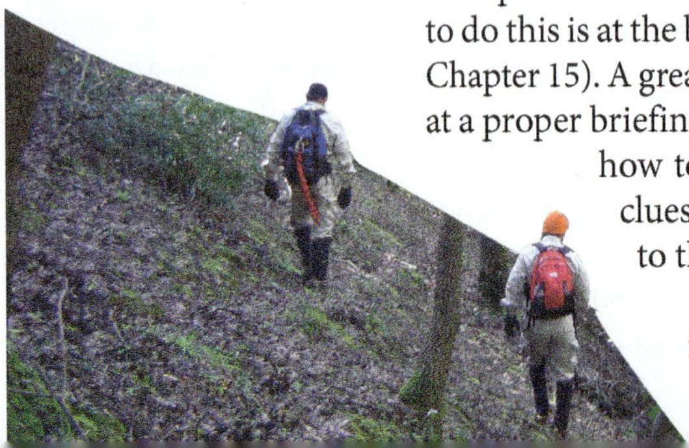

Put yourself into the lost person's shoes and allow this to influence your thoughts and ideas while acting within the constraints of the search plan. Think of how they might be feeling; imagining what they might be thinking; and ask, "What would I do if I was this lost person?"

Lost persons are much more likely to follow a route of easy travel. Consider these paths as likely areas for evidence/clues and check them thoroughly. Most, but not all, lost subjects follow paths of least resistance. Know this but be mindful of the exceptions.

Many studies regarding lost person behavior have been undertaken over past years, and studying this information enhances the knowledge of any member of the SAR community. Examining these documents, as well as others that deal with the behavior of lost people, is strongly encouraged but is beyond the scope of this book. The list of references at the end of this chapter is a good starting point for educating yourself.

Handling Evidence

SAR personnel can be the first to find a lost subject or clue. Whether SAR personnel find a small clue or an injured subject, how the individual or team handles the situation may have a significant effect on the outcome of the search and any potential investigation (**FIGURE 14-11**).

Proper processing of discovered evidence is essential for search success. As clues are discovered, they must be interpreted and acted upon. The ability to search must be combined with the knowledge of how to handle what is discovered. If a searcher expects to locate the subject or solve a mystery, clues must be handled in such a way to facilitate all search efforts and to preserve evidence for subsequent investigation.

Although scene and evidence protection are not necessarily a primary responsibility of SAR personnel, a thorough knowledge of essential guidelines serves to build better relations with all authorities, gets the most from all clues, and preserves evidence for further examination.

Briefing

The best way to handle any clue or piece of evidence is to have planned for its discovery and processing. The place to do this is at the briefing (see the Briefing Checklist in Chapter 15). A great deal of information can be conveyed at a proper briefing, but specific instructions regarding how to handle and act on any discovered clues may be among the most important to the success of the search.

Since evidence can take so many forms, instructions on how to handle it should cover all the possibilities, leaving very little to chance. Handling clues and evidence can be the single most important part of the investigation and, therefore, may weigh heavily on its outcome. Searchers are often confronted with situations not common to many other field personnel. Therefore, searchers need to ask all the standard questions at a briefing with some search-specific additions. If not told, searchers should ask, and get answers to, the following questions regarding the handling of evidence:

1. Exactly how should the evidence be recorded (sketch, photograph, narrative description in writing, all the above)?
2. Exactly how, if at all, should a print or sign be protected (cordoned off, covered, plaster cast, guarded)? Should someone else be called to handle this?
3. Should I act upon my interpretation of a specific piece of evidence, or should I report my findings and wait for further instructions? To what extent can I act on what is found?
4. What should I do as a searcher if I am confronted with two trails? Should I act as I see fit, or report it and wait for instructions? Is splitting up the team a viable alternative?
5. If the clue is an item that may have been discarded by the subject, do I note the location, mark the location in an obvious way, and leave the item in place? Do I do all the above except recover the item and bring the information to the command post (immediately or at the end of the search assignment)?
6. If the clue is to be retrieved, exactly how should this be done? Does this require carrying additional equipment?

Often, experienced search teams suggest to the person briefing them how they may handle certain situations. This may be the best course of action, especially if those charged with managing the incident are not fully familiar with the capabilities of the search team.

Specific Situations

SAR personnel may encounter four primary SAR situations involving evidence and clues:

1. *Evidence.* Clues that are discovered and must be processed.
2. *Crash scene.* Usually a vehicle, occasionally an aircraft, often involves injury and death, and always involves important evidence.
3. *Human remains.* May involve any number of situations that might have caused harm to an individual or group. Bodies often involve injury and always involve important clues.
4. *Injury.* Scenarios that may require the treatment of injuries and where death may be encountered. These situations may involve evidence as well.

At any one of these situations, SAR personnel may be confronted with evidence that might be critical to the success of a SAR mission. Therefore, all evidence, no matter how seemingly insignificant, should be handled as if it were of extreme value.

Evidence

Generally, evidence can be categorized as either *physical* or *incorporeal.* Physical evidence is something that can be touched and held. Tangible objects such as shoes or gum wrappers are examples, but foot prints and sign also fall into this category. **Incorporeal evidence**, on the other hand, is nonphysical information or knowledge; these are intangible items, meaning that they cannot be touched or held. Examples include the subject's age, a whistle blowing, a flashing light, or a report from a witness. The effectiveness of this type of evidence ultimately depends on how well it was recorded. In fact, this type of evidence is usually converted to physical evidence by field personnel. Photos of an event and written records of what happened, for example, were all once incorporeal items turned into reproducible evidence by field personnel.

Physical evidence is far more desirable in the long run because it is usually relatively easy to preserve and reproduce later. Incorporeal evidence, however, can also be important. It just may not be as persuasive when its credibility rests solely on how well it was recorded. After all, which would you find more persuasive: a fisherman with a tale of the "big one" that got away, a fisherman with a photo of the fish, or a fisherman with a big fish in hand? Physical evidence is always preferred.

Ideally, the recording and documentation of a clue and its surroundings should be of such quality, accuracy, and completeness that the entire scene could be reenacted or reproduced. The scene should be recorded so well that what went on before, during, and after the discovery of a particular piece of evidence can be accurately relived. This can be difficult when evidence is intangible and difficult to preserve. The recording of the event (photo, notes, sketches, etc.) becomes the physical evidence, so the more thorough the recording of the evidence, the better the evidence.

The following actions taken by the searcher can help turn intangible clues into physical evidence (Taylor and Cooper, 2014):

1. *Take notes.* Document placement of clues, position of people or bodies, and pertinent facts surrounding the scene. Leave nothing to the

imagination, but do not expound. Stick to the facts and be able to corroborate them, if possible. Basically, describe in prose everything that you know regarding the scene and the situation.

2. *Sketch the scene.* Draw diagrams and pictures of pertinent objects involved at the scene and their position relative to each other. Not everyone is an artist, but simple line drawings showing the relationship between items can be invaluable.
3. *Photograph.* Take photos, if possible. This is an excellent way to document a scene, but it relies heavily on light and equipment availability. Make sure to include something in the photo that indicates scale, time, and date, if possible (a ruler, coin, newspaper, etc.). Attempt to photograph at least three sides (four is better) of any one object, and back off for a larger view of the location of the object or person in relation to the surrounding landscape. Note that the camera may itself be taken to retain the chain of custody.
4. *Corroborating witnesses.* Get information from any witnesses who saw what you saw or who saw anything at all. Write down at least their names, addresses, and phone numbers so that they can be contacted later, if necessary. Also, note what they saw and/or did at the scene.
5. *Retrieve and preserve.* Collect clues, if doing so is within the scope of the briefing and if it can be done properly. Evidence and clues should be the focus of all sketches, photographs, and documentation, but retrieving and preserving the evidence itself is the ultimate objective. Be mindful of the fact that notes, sketches, photographs, and camera may themselves become evidence.

In tracking, evidence usually takes the form of a print or sign that, of course, cannot be directly retrieved. More importantly, both sign and prints are usually time sensitive. Because they tend to disappear with time, the sooner prints are discovered and recorded, the more valuable they are to an investigation. Tracks tend to disappear quickly. This means that photographs, sketches, and other documentation may need to be produced immediately upon discovery of such evidence. The tracker or searcher who finds tracks needs to record a print right away to maximize its usefulness (Taylor and Cooper, 2014).

Evidence should not be allowed out of your possession or protection until it can be conveyed to an equally responsible person. When evidence is considered for use in a case, opportunities for alteration of the evidence, by natural or human-made causes, can reduce its credibility and reliability. That is, the better the chances that a piece of evidence could have been changed or altered, the less its significance, particularly in court. This is referred to as *maintaining the chain of evidence* and may weigh heavily on a clue's acceptability in court, where it counts. The "chain" is most relevant to law enforcement personnel and investigators, but SAR personnel must also understand and appreciate its existence and purpose (Taylor and Cooper, 2014).

Any SAR operation where evidence is found should be considered the scene of a crime until proven otherwise. Just as in emergency medical care where, to be safe, patients are treated for the worst possible injury or illness, any situation where evidence is collected should be considered a crime scene until a responsible authority establishes otherwise. This allows everything to be considered evidence until you have reason to believe otherwise, thereby preserving any possibilities.

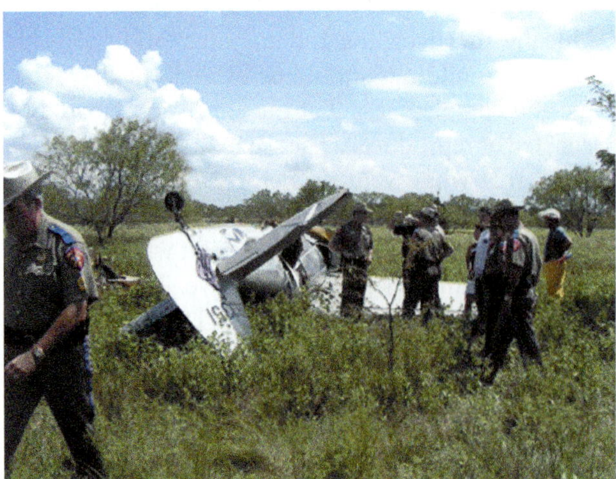

FIGURE 14-12 At a crash scene, there are many things that SAR personnel can do to help victims of the incident as well as the subsequent investigation.

Crash Scene

A crash scene may involve an aircraft, automobile, or other vehicle or machinery. Crash scenes may include injury and death but almost always involve evidence. Often the only way to find out exactly what happened is to piece together the clues. How these clues are handled and processed initially may mean the difference between determining exactly what occurred and only guessing.

At a crash scene, there are many things that SAR personnel can do to help victims of the incident as well as the subsequent investigation (**FIGURE 14-12**). However, there are also actions that could hamper an investigation, further complicate the victim's situation, and even result in personal injury to SAR personnel.

In the United States, the National Transportation Safety Board (NTSB), the Federal Aviation Administration (FAA), and the military all have a responsibility to investigate aircraft accidents within their respective jurisdictions that involve serious injury or death (U.S. DOT FAA, 2010). In general, civil aircraft accidents are investigated by the NTSB. Some nonfatal accidents may be looked at by the FAA, and all military crashes are handled by a respective branch's investigating team. All these agencies would like to see the site disturbed as little as possible. Notes, sketches, photographs, and relevant comments such as body positions, locations of aircraft parts or pieces, and other pertinent observations are all appreciated when retrieved with permission to do so. The default for SAR personnel, after treating any injuries, should always be protecting the scene from disturbance and contamination until authorized investigators arrive to take charge.

The NTSB may also get involved with local and state agencies when modes of land-based mass transportation are involved in a crash. Some examples include crashes involving trains, buses, and subways. The U.S. Coast Guard (USCG) might get involved in any crash that involves U.S. waterways, and state and local agencies may get involved when a crash involves a vessel (or vehicle) on state or locally governed waterways.

The most common crashes in the world involve motor vehicles on roadways. When this type of incident occurs, local law enforcement, fire service, and emergency medical services (EMS) will likely be involved, but each of these agencies usually has responsibility for different aspects of the scene. Most often at a crash scene in the United States, law enforcement generally has responsibility for maintaining/returning traffic flow, crash investigation, and criminal investigation; the fire service has responsibility for scene safety, fire protection, vehicle extrication, and assisting with medical care; and EMS personnel have responsibility for treating injuries and transporting patients. Since SAR personnel may be members of any of these agencies, everyone involved should have a basic understanding of his or her role in this type of scenario.

In situations involving remote incident sites, SAR personnel may be asked to assist investigators in getting to the site. In these cases, pointing out observations and subtle clues not readily apparent to the investigator could be very helpful. At sites that would be inaccessible to all but trained SAR personnel, team members may even be asked to conduct the entire on-scene investigation.

If wreckage must be disturbed to remove bodies, the coroner or medical examiner needs to coordinate with the responsible agency. If the investigator is not readily available, some other agencies can allow removal of bodies by the authority of the coroner. Any activity concerning the dead should strictly follow guidelines established by the authority having jurisdiction over the situation.

A final step in the resolution of a crash site investigation is the disposition of the wreckage. In some cases, salvage may be by an insurance company or even private individuals. The removal of any wreckage must be coordinated with the investigating agencies and is usually performed in a specifically prescribed manner. If the wreckage of an aircraft is to be left at the site and it is visible from the air, it must be marked in an appropriate manner prescribed in that state. This is to preclude mistaking the site for a recent crash should another search be initiated in the same area.

Guidelines for handling crash scenes include the following:

1. Proceed with caution! Safety of SAR personnel is paramount. If the smell of spilled fuel is strong, approach from uphill and upwind, or do not approach at all.
   - With the presence of any fuel in the area, extreme caution should be used during any activities. Absolutely no smoking or use of fire- or spark-producing devices is allowed, which may include portable radios.
   - Absolutely ensure the safety of personnel. Do whatever is necessary to see that everyone is prudently safe. This may include leaving the scene altogether.
2. Prevent further injury to the patient or patients by stabilizing the scene. This step usually involves minimizing hazards and should not be neglected.
3. Determine whether any subjects are alive or dead. If alive, begin emergency care to the best of your ability and training. If dead, secure the scene and notify a higher authority.
4. Establish a security perimeter for the site, but remember that SAR personnel, including trackers, usually have no legal authority to perform law enforcement functions and may not be able to forcibly prevent people from accessing the scene. If the scene is breached, note the circumstances and document what was done and when.
5. Handle any evidence such as baggage, personal effects, cargo, mail, tracks, etc., as specified in the briefing. If no such determinations have been made, protect and leave any evidence where it was found, unless it is in danger of obliteration or alteration by weather or environmental hazards.
6. Document, photograph, and/or sketch all pertinent evidence, especially if investigators will rely heavily on your observations (i.e., if investigators cannot access the scene or if evidence is affected by weather or time).

Handling the Deceased at a SAR Scene

The discovery and investigation of serious injuries and accidental death can be one of the least enjoyable but most important aspects of SAR. As with most investigative cases, someone is tasked with collecting clues, finding cause, and explaining a set of circumstances. The detailed study of the event and evidence of the situation is the legal responsibility of trained public officials such as coroners, medical examiners, and law enforcement officers, depending on the nature and location of the mishap. Frequently, however, evidence is produced or discovered by searchers, who are obliged to help the responsible authorities as best they can.

While at times the circumstances or the facts that lead up to a death may seem rather obvious, SAR personnel should understand that there are certain requirements and obligations, both to the state and to family or friends. The inquiry process varies from jurisdiction to jurisdiction and state to state, but basic guidelines that apply to SAR team members have been established.

The first responsibility of someone arriving on the scene is to determine whether the subject is dead, alive, or critically injured. If this means moving or touching the individual, then go ahead and do whatever is necessary. Proper emergency care supersedes investigation at this point, and medical treatment is never interrupted, just supplemented, by evidence considerations. At the point that responders determine the subject is dead and medical treatment is deemed unnecessary (by whatever means is generally accepted), every attempt should be made to preserve the surroundings and the exact position of the deceased and associated evidence.

Observe the scene and look for clues, evidence, or indications of what might have happened. If anything in the way of tracks, imprints, scuff marks, or possessions is in danger of being lost, preserve the information or scene description by writing it down or photographing objects before recovering them. Whichever approach to evidence handling is followed, it should correspond with the guidelines indicated in the briefing.

The area immediately surrounding a body or bodies should be secured with a rope, string, or tape after a subject(s) is (are) determined to be dead. This physical barrier not only ensures that officials do not casually walk in and out of the area, but it should keep other curious onlookers out as well. Again, pay attention to any item within the cordoned area. In writing down whatever was observed, make sure that plenty of emphasis is placed on disturbances or movements made within the scene by SAR personnel, intentional or not. Failure to do this could result in being suspected of acting beyond one's authority or even destroying evidence. If possible, even if alone, remain at the scene until official help arrives. This could involve sending a passerby or another team member for help, if a radio is not available. Remember the chain of evidence. Finding a clue and then abandoning it, for any length of time, could mean the difference between accepting and refuting certain evidence in court.

You or someone in your team may be required to make a written statement. This must be as accurate and detailed as possible and involve only the facts, not conjecture. Ask for the advice of a knowledgeable person when considering what to include in an official statement. The advice of an attorney may also be prudent.

Unless specific instructions have been given to do so, do not search a deceased person for identification. That is an official function that must be carried out by responsible authorities. Depending on the state and local jurisdiction, a body may be moved or pronounced dead only by a coroner, deputy coroner, or medical examiner. Essentially, one of these people is in total command of the site. Often, however, SAR personnel are called upon to assist in the investigation under the specific direction of one or more of these officials.

Always try to have a witness to any activity you are involved with around the scene of a death. Everyone becomes suspect when the ultimate tragedy becomes reality and a person dies. Nothing is protected, and everything is possible. Most importantly, protect your own interests, have a reason for all that you do, and document everything well.

Handling Injuries at a SAR Scene

Considerations for handling injuries are similar to those for handling deaths. Protecting evidence is important, but it falls second to proper emergency care. Treatment of injuries and alleviation of pain are major goals in SAR and should not be precluded by the collection of evidence. However, when medical treatment is being addressed or complete, the entire investigation may still hinge on any clues, observations, and recollections of those involved. Therefore, be mindful of investigative considerations while treating a patient, and try to protect evidence while doing your best for the patient.

In summary, handle any clue as if it were the only piece of evidence, consider each and every discovery to be absolutely important until proven otherwise, and follow these simple guidelines:

1. Plan for the handling of evidence, including search-specific considerations, in the briefing. Do not wait until something is found.

2. Generate an accurate record of the evidence and its environment by taking notes, making sketches, photographing, or retrieving the evidence.
3. Understand and maintain the chain of evidence.
4. Treat injuries or assist the injured first, but be mindful of any evidence.

Wrap-Up

READY FOR REVIEW

- It is important that the motivation of the search and rescue (SAR) personnel be consistent with the search and rescue community's motto—". . .these things we do, that others may live"—if satisfaction and any level of success is expected.
- The fundamentals of land search are based on principles that have long been accepted by search managers and planners but are also important to field searchers. The principles of land search, collectively termed *crucials*, are:
  - Search is an emergency.
  - Search is a classic mystery.
  - Search for clues and the subject.
  - Focus on aspects important to success.
  - Know if the subject leaves the area.
  - Grid search as a last resort.
- There are more clues than subjects, the detection of clues reduces the search area, and the value gained from the detection of certain clues approaches that of the lost subject.
- To keep the search area as small as possible, and thus keep the search as easy as possible, steps must be taken to ensure that the subject does not leave the search area and that all possible search subject/object locations are included in the search area.
- The likelihood that a search will be successful depends on two related probabilities: the probability that the search object is in the area searched and the probability of detecting the search object, presuming it is in the area being searched.
- In most SAR incidents, the incident commander designates someone to deal with external influences. Typically in ICS, the public information officer communicates with the news media, the liaison officer deals with external organizations, and a family liaison is assigned to deal with and manage family issues.
- By analyzing the behavior of past lost persons, search managers and planners may be able to predict what the subject of the current search might do, how he or she might behave or react, where he or she might go, and where he or she might end up.
- Although scene and evidence protection are not necessarily a primary responsibility of SAR personnel, a thorough knowledge of essential guidelines serves to build better relations with all authorities, gets the most from all clues, and preserves evidence for further examination.

SEARCH AND RESCUE TERMS

Area effectively swept Also called *search effort*, a measure of the area that can be (or was) effectively searched by searchers within the limits of search speed, endurance, and effective sweep width. This area (Z) is computed as the product of the effective sweep width (W) times search speed (V) times hours spent in the search area (T). That is, $Z = W \times V \times T$ for one searcher or one resource (such as a ground searcher, dog team, boat, or aircraft and its crew) (NSARC, 2011; Cooper and Frost, 1999). "Search effort is computed as the product of search speed (V), search endurance (T), and sweep width (W), or $Z = V \times T \times W$" (NSARC, 2011, p. xxiii).

Briefing Exchange of information, usually at the onset of a situation, that conveys important knowledge from the upper levels of a hierarchy to the lower, for example information from the Incident Commander conveyed to a field team before they begin their assignment (Taylor and Cooper, 2014). A summary of the situation, past and present, conveyed by those who know to those who need to know and that provides information that will help orient personnel to all facets of the problem.

Containment Steps taken to ensure that the subject does not leave the search area; also called *confinement*.

Coverage factor (C) The ratio of the search effort (Z) to the area searched (A); C = Z/A. For parallel sweep searches, it may be computed as the ratio of sweep width (W) to track spacing (S), or C = W/S (NSARC, 2011). Coverage may be thought of as a measure of thoroughness. The probability of detection (POD) of a search is a function of coverage.

Debriefing Exchange of information, usually at the close of a situation, that conveys important knowledge and experience from the lower levels of a hierarchy to the upper; that is, information conveyed to the incident commander from a field team after completing an assignment (Taylor and Cooper, 2014).

Incorporeal evidence Nonphysical information or knowledge; intangible evidence that cannot be touched or held (Taylor and Cooper, 2014). Examples include the subject's age, a whistle blowing, a flashing light, or a report from a witness.

Last known position (LKP) (1) The last substantiated position based on clues or evidence belonging to the missing subject and indicating that the missing subject was known to be at that location. (2) Last witnessed, reported, or computed position of a distressed person or craft (NSARC, 2011).

Point last seen (PLS) The point where the search object was last seen by a witness or captured on video at a specific time and location (NSARC, 2011).

Possibility area (1) The smallest area containing all possible survivor or search object locations. (2) For a scenario, the smallest area containing all possible survivor or search object locations that are consistent with the facts and assumptions used to form the scenario (IMO/ICAO, 2016).

Probability density (Pden) Probability of containment per unit area; often POC or POA/mi^2. Pden is constant throughout any given region (NSARC, 2016).

Probability of area (POA) The probability that the search object (or subject) is contained within the boundaries of an area, subarea, or grid cell; also called *probability of containment (POC)* (NSARC, 2011).

Probability of detection (POD) The probability of the search object being detected, assuming it was in the areas that were searched. POD is a function of coverage factor, sensor, search conditions, and the accuracy with which the search unit navigates its assigned search pattern. Measures sensor effectiveness under the prevailing search conditions (IMO/ICAO, 2016).

Probability of success (POS) The probability of finding the search object with a particular search. For each subarea searched, POS = POA × POD. Measures overall search effectiveness (NSARC, 2011). The accumulated probability of finding the search object with all the search effort expended over all searches to date is called *cumulative POS (POScum)*.

Probability theory A branch of mathematics used to systematically deal with uncertain events.

Region "A delineated portion or subset of the search area within which there is a nearly uniform distribution of likelihood for containing the search subject or object." (NSARC, 2011, p. xxii).

Scenario A consistent set of known facts and assumptions describing what may have happened to the survivor(s) (search subject) (NSARC, 2011).

Search area The area, determined by the search planner, that is to be searched. This area may be subdivided into search subareas for the purpose of assigning specific responsibilities to the available search facilities (IMO/ICAO, 2016). It includes the smallest area, consistent with all available information, which contains all possible search object locations and, therefore, includes all regions and segments that are consistent with a particular scenario. This area may be divided into regions based on the probable scenarios and into segments for assigning specific tasks to the available search resources.

Search object A ship, aircraft, or other craft missing or in distress, or survivors or related evidence for which a search is being conducted (IMO/ICAO, 2016). A generic term used to indicate the lost subject or evidence (clues) related to a lost subject.

Search speed (v) The average rate of travel (speed over the ground) of searchers while engaged in search operations within a segment (Cooper and Frost, 1999).

Search subarea A designated area to be searched by a specific assigned search facility, or possibly two facilities working together in close coordination (IMO/ICAO, 2016).

Search subject The person being searched for, commonly referred to as the *subject*.

Segment "A delineated portion or subset of the search area bounded and sized to be searchable by assigned facilities" (NSARC, 2011, p. xxiii). Segments and their boundaries are based on factors that affect the searchers. The search planner determines the size of a segment. The boundaries of a segment are identifiable both in the field and on a map and are based on suitability for assigning search resources, not probability of the search object's location.

Sensor Human senses (sight, hearing, touch, etc.), those of specially trained animals (such as dogs), or electronic devices used to detect the object of a search (IMO/ICAO, 2016). A human, multisensor platform is often referred to as a *searcher*.

Sweep width A measure of the effectiveness with which a particular sensor can detect a particular object under specific environmental conditions (IMO/ICAO, 2016); a measure of detectability. Sweep width depends on the characteristics of the search object, the sensor, and the environmental conditions prevailing at the time and place of the search. Also called *effective sweep width*.

Track line length (TLL) Also called *effort*, the total distance traveled by a sensor while searching in the assigned segment (Cooper and Frost, 1999).

REFERENCES AND SUGGESTED READING

ASTM International. 2017. Search and rescue operations standards: List of search and rescue standards developed by ASTM. https://www.astm.org/Standards/search-and-rescue-operations-standards.html.

Benkoski, Stanley J., Michael G. Monticino, and James R. Weisinger. 1991. A survey of the search theory literature. *Naval Research Logistics*, 38, no. 4: 469–494.

Cooper, Donald C., and John R. Frost. 1999. *Selected Inland Search Definitions*. Cuyahoga Falls, OH: Private publication.

Cooper, Donald C., John R. Frost, and R. Quincy Robe. 2003. *Compatibility of Land SAR Procedures with Search Theory*. Washington, DC: U.S. Department of Homeland Security, U.S. Coast Guard, Operations (G-OPR).

Cornell, Edward H., and C. Donald Heth. 1996. Distances traveled during urban and suburban walks led by 3- to 12-year-olds: Tables for search managers. *Response*, 15: 6–9.

Doyle, Arthur C. 1903. The Adventure of the Dancing Men. http://www.eastoftheweb.com/short-stories/UBooks/AdveDanc.shtml.

Frost, John R. 1998. *The Theory of Search: A simplified Explanation*. Revised edition. Fairfax, VA: Soza and Company, Ltd. and U.S. Coast Guard.

Frost, John R. 1999a. Principles of search theory, part I: Detection. *Response*, 17 no. 2: 1–7.

Frost, John R. 1999b. Principles of search theory, part II: Effort, coverage, and POD. *Response*, 17 no. 2: 8–15.

Frost, John R. 1999c. Principles of search theory, part III: Probability density distributions. *Response*, 17no. 3:1–10.

Frost, John R. 1999d. Principles of search theory, part IV: Optimal effort allocation. *Response*, 17 no. 3:11–23.

Harris, Adam J.L/, Adam Corner, and Ulrike Hahn. 2009. Estimating the probability of negative events. *Cognition*, 110 no. 1: 51-64.

Heth, C. Donald, and Edward H. Cornell. 1997. Characteristics of travel by persons lost in Albertan wilderness areas. *Journal of Environmental Psychology*, 18: 223–235.

Hill, Kenneth. 1997. *Managing Lost Person Incidents*. Chantilly, VA: National Association for Search and Rescue.

Hill, Kenneth. 1999. *Lost Person Behavior*. Ottawa, Ontario, Canada: The National Search and Rescue Secretariat.

Hill, Kenneth. 2001. *Distances Traveled and Probability Zones for Lost Persons in Nova Scotia*. Unpublished data.

IMO/ICAO. 2016. *International Aeronautical and Maritime Search and Rescue Manual: Volume II, Mission Co-ordination*. London/Montreal: International Maritime Organization and International Civil Aviation Organization.

Institute for Operations Research and the Management Sciences. 2017. Operations Research and Analytics. https://www.informs.org/Explore/Operations-Research-Analytics.

Koester, Robert J., 2008. *Lost Person Behavior: A Search and Rescue Guide on Where to Look – For Land, Air and Water*. Charlottesville, VA: dbS Production LLC.

Koester, Robert J., Kenneth B. Chiacchia, Charles R. Twardy, Donald C. Cooper, John R. Frost, and R. Quincy Robe. 2014. Use of the visual range of detection to estimate effective sweep width for land search and rescue based on 10 detections experiments in North America. *Wilderness & Environmental Medicine*, 25, no. 2: 132–142.

Koester, Robert J., Donald C. Cooper, J. R. Frost, and R. Q. Robe. 2004. *Sweep Width Estimation for Ground Search and Rescue*. Washington, DC: U.S. Department of Homeland Security, U.S. Coast Guard, Operations (G-OPR).

Koopman, Bernard O. 1946. *Search and Screening*. In: OEG Report No. 56, The Summary Reports Group of the Columbia University Division of War Research. Alexandria, VA: Center for Naval Analyses.

Koopman, Bernard O. 1980. *Search and Screening: General Principles with Historical Applications*, revised ed. New York: Pergamon Press.

Mattson, Robert J. 1975. *Establishing Search Priorities*. Private publication.

Mitchell, B.L. 1985. *A Summary of the National Association for Search and Rescue Data Collection and Analysis Program for 1980–1985*. Washington, DC: National Association for Search and Rescue.

National Fire Protection Association. 2017a. NFPA 1670, *Standard on Operations and Training for Technical Search and Rescue Incidents*. Batterymarch, MA: NFPA.

National Fire Protection Association. 2017b. NFPA 1006, *Standard for Technical Rescue Personnel Professional Qualifications*. Batterymarch, MA: NFPA.

National Search and Rescue Committee. 2000. *United States National Search and Rescue Supplement to the International Aeronautical and Maritime Search and Rescue Manual*. Washington, DC: U.S. Superintendent of Documents.

National Search and Rescue Committee. 2011. Land search and rescue addendum to the National Search and Rescue Supplement to the International Aeronautical and Maritime

Search and Rescue Manual, Version 1.0. https://www.hsdl.org/?abstract&did=715465.

Robe, R. Quincy, and J. R. Frost. 2002. *A Method for Determining Effective Sweep Widths for Land Searches: Procedures for Conducting Detection Experiments*. Washington, DC: The National Search and Rescue Committee, USCG Contract Number DTCG39-00-D-R00009.

Stone, L.D. 1989. *Theory of Optimal Search*, 2nd edition. Military Applications Section, Operations Research Society of America. Arlington, VA: ORSA Books.

Syrotuck, William G., ed. 1976. *Analysis of Lost Person Behavior: An Aid to Search Planning*. Westmoreland, NY: Arner Publications.

Tawrell, Paul. 2007. Wilderness Camping & Hiking, 1st edition. Lebanon, NH: EXXA LLC.

Taylor, Albert, and Donald C. Cooper. 2014. *Fundamentals of Mantracking: The Step-by-Step Method*. 3rd edition, New York: Skyhorse Publishers. Available at www.NASAR.org.

Trailtrove.com. 2017. Hiking speed: What is average? http://trailtrove.com/hiking-speed.

U.S. Department of Transportation, Federal Aviation Administration. 2010. "National Policy: Aircraft Accident and Incident Notification, Investigation, and Reporting. Order 8020.11C." https://www.faa.gov/documentLibrary/media/Order/8020.11C_.pdf.

Washburn, Alan R. 2002. *Search and Detection*, 4th edition. Linthicum, MD: Institute for Operations Research and the Management Sciences.

www.mountainsafety.co.uk. 2017. Advice & info: Route planning. http://www.mountainsafety.co.uk/Route-Detailed-Planning.aspx.

CHAPTER 15

Search Operations

OBJECTIVES

Upon completion of this chapter and the related course activities, the student will be able to meet the following objectives:

- Explain the difference between direct and indirect tactics.
- Explain the difference between the search area and a search segment.
- Explain the difference between an assignment briefing and an assignment debriefing.
- Define each of the following search and rescue (SAR) terms:
  - Search area
  - Back stop
  - Decision points
  - Guide line
  - Search lane
  - Search track
- Describe at least three characteristics of a low-coverage area search.
- Describe at least three characteristics of a high-coverage area search.
- Describe at least one possible use of trail tape, ribbons, or string line during an area search.
- Explain the "searcher cube" and its use during a search.
- Describe at least four important pieces of information that should be conveyed by field personnel at the assignment debriefing after an area search.
- Explain how to conduct a range of detection (Rd) measurement.
- Describe at least two immediate actions that should be taken when illegal activities are encountered during a search.
- Describe at least three signs and symptoms of fatigue in SAR personnel.
- Discuss three of the safest uses of search resources at night.
- Discuss at least three points to consider regarding returning to service after checking out at an incident.

Tactics

Tactics are all techniques employed to find a lost subject or clues and are usually applied by the search manager or planner immediately following first notice. Tactics are important to field personnel because they are the methods by which search and rescue (SAR) team members get physically involved with the search function. Tactics usually involve a definite progression of techniques and generally fall into one of two classes—indirect or direct—although there may be some overlap between the two. Formerly, the terms *active* and *passive* have been used to describe tactics, but these terms have fallen out of favor due to how they are used by specific search resources such as radar and aviation, which uses these terms in different and potentially conflicting ways.

Indirect tactics are almost always the first to be employed, particularly with regard to fact finding or information gathering. It is through these types of tactics that the nature and the seriousness of the incident are ascertained, and a **search area** is established based on potential **scenarios**. Often, indirect tactics themselves locate the **search subject**, or the subject is discovered by other means before **direct tactics** can get underway.

Although the use of indirect tactics should continue until the subject is located or field search activities are suspended, there usually comes a point when direct tactics should be employed, and searchers are sent into the search area to locate clues and the subject. Once started, direct tactics usually continue until the subject is located or search activities are suspended pending further developments.

SEARCH AND RESCUE TIP

In the past, indirect and direct tactics were referred to as *passive* and *active*. This nomenclature was changed because the land SAR definitions of the old terms conflicted with how they were used by military and some government SAR organizations.

Indirect Tactics

Indirect tactics do not involve physically entering and moving through the search area to look for the subject or clues. Specific tactics most often used in this type of searching include fact finding (investigation), attraction, and containment. Fact finding is a process that continues from the first notice through the suspension of the search and even beyond if search success is not achieved. Attraction and containment can and should be used effectively together throughout the search, but their usefulness correspondingly declines as the chances of the subject being responsive diminish over time.

Fact Finding

Fact finding is performed by the search management team, often with the aid of other resources such as law enforcement entities. It includes collecting any information that can help focus or resolve the search. A missing person questionnaire (see Appendix A) is helpful in collecting specific data, but any information relevant to the search contributes to the available collection of facts. As in any investigation, all leads must be followed until they provide no new evidence or possibilities, the subject is found, there is sufficient evidence that the incident is not of the type for which SAR resources and methods are appropriate, or search activities are suspended pending further developments.

A version of this type of indirect technique is the **continuous limited search (CLS)**. This approach may be taken when direct search techniques achieving high levels of coverage have not turned up clues or the subject, and the incident management team has decided to continue the search on a limited basis only (e.g., no field deployment). CLS can be the best course of action when the search area has been thoroughly searched (i.e., cumulative probability of success [POS] is high) without meaningful results. In a situation like this, the incident management team may opt for continuing the investigation and/or using the area for regular training purposes, but they suspend the use of any direct tactics in the search area, which is why continuous limited search is considered an indirect search technique, often of last resort.

Attraction

Attraction techniques are efforts taken to cause the subject to be attracted to, and travel to, a desired location, which assume a mobile/responsive subject. Specific attraction techniques include noise (e.g., sirens, whistles, yelling, PA systems, horns), lights (e.g., beacons, flares, fires, strobes, car or patrol lights, search lights), smoke, aircraft, balloons, skywriting, etc. When using noise, do not forget to have silent periods in which to listen for a response from the subject, and be aware that you might be hearing other teams or echoes. It is best if all teams agree to, or are assigned, the same specific silent periods, synchronize their watches, and strictly observe these periods.

SEARCH AND RESCUE TIP

Attraction techniques are efforts taken to cause the subject to be attracted to, and travel to, a desired location. These techniques assume a mobile/responsive subject.

Sound has long been used as an attraction method. Yelling the subject's name or blowing a whistle in an attempt to get a response is used often as an indirect technique. Colwell (1992) and Manson (2009) conducted experiments using sound in SAR and concluded that, in the environments they tested, sound can be heard and recognized farther than an object can be seen and recognized. Manson (2009) also concluded that sound does not radiate with equal loudness in all directions from its source (it is directional), that sound carries farther in summer than in spring and winter, and that searchers should make sure to spend sufficient time listening for a response from the subject. Although none of this is a surprise, it does provide an important reminder that sound can be a valuable part of all field searching.

Koester (2009) described an imaginative technique used in New Zealand that combines the use of sound in the form of whistle blows and light from headlamps to attract disoriented but uninjured subjects. The unique, densely vegetated environment in which this experiment was conducted made it easy for individuals—often hunters—to become disoriented even though they were relatively close to but could not see the road where they parked their cars. While walking after dusk on the road to which they wanted to attract the lost subjects, SAR personnel in three-person teams used whistles blown at regular intervals, interspersed with periods of quiet listening, and headlamps that they "waggled" across the face of the dense vegetation to attract attention. This was often all it took to attract lost subjects to the road and self-rescue.

Another innovative variation on the attraction theme is the "passive SAR box." A passive SAR box is a durable, portable, very brightly painted, weather-proof, animal-proof, self-contained box that contains items that would be useful to a person or group finding themselves in need of assistance in an isolated, rugged area where SAR resources might not be immediately available. The box can be deployed by a SAR team in at least two ways. The first is placing it in a carefully selected location where people often need help and visiting it when someone in distress is believed to be in the area. The second is strategically placing the box after first notice of an incident along known or suspected routes of travel. In both cases, trained SAR personnel visit each box periodically to see if anyone in distress has been attracted to it. The box is brightly colored, is well labeled, and has plenty of signage on it that tells a lost subject to stay put and follow the instructions provided. Ideally, the box should have reflective material attached to the outside so it can be found at night with a light, and it can include anything the local SAR team thinks might be needed by the subject, ranging from a radio or a phone to survival gear (e.g., fire starter, shelter material, flashlight, strobe, first aid kit, nonperishable food). No navigation device should be included so the subject is not tempted to leave the box. The attached instructions might look something like this:

1. This box is the property of the Generic Search and Rescue Team. Stay with this box; do NOT leave. We will check this location often for you. If you leave, we may not find you. Stay here.
2. Use the contents of this box as needed to eat, drink, build shelter and fire for warmth, and treat injuries or wounds as best you are able.
3. Finding this box means there is an organized search for you. Trained teams with medical and other specialized training will come back here to assist you. Stay here.
4. Do not build a fire if conditions are dry and unsafe. If conditions are wet, road flare may help start a fire of wet wood and grasses.
5. In wet conditions, use large trash bags for a rain poncho by making a face hole in a bag, pulling it overhead, and covering your body with it. Other bags can be used to protect you from the damp ground. Stuff ground bags with leaves and grass to make a pad and insulate you from the cold ground.

Containment

Containment (also known as *confinement*) techniques involve efforts taken to confine the movement of a lost subject to minimize the size of the search area. Containment is an attempt to encircle the search area with resources that will immediately recognize and report if the subject leaves the search area. This type of approach is usually initiated by the search management team, often carried out by field personnel, and is implemented as early as possible in a search.

Minimally trained personnel can sometimes help achieve containment, so this may be a place where a community emergency response team (CERT) or other volunteers who may not be fully trained in field operations can help.

Some specific types of containment techniques include the following:

- *Trail blocks.* Search personnel can be placed at choke points (paths that narrow between locations) or trail junctions. If trail travelers are questioned, the subject might be located, or others can be asked if they did or did not see the subject.
- *Road blocks.* Law enforcement usually manages road blocks, which stop all traffic going into and out of the search area. This can prevent a subject who does not know he or she is the subject of a search from passing without notice and can be used to inform travelers about the search.
- *Road patrols.* One or two people in a vehicle can drive back and forth between two locations, searching for the subject while also serving as a containment resource.

- *Track traps.* As described in Chapter 13, *Tracking*, a track trap is an area particularly good for detecting sign (e.g., sand, mud, snow) that is checked for evidence periodically. It can also be human-made by clearing off an area so that sign would be more easily detected if a subject subsequently passed through.
- *Lookouts.* A lookout consists of a searcher, usually in a location selected for its wide view of the search area, set in a stationary position used for observing. From this location, a searcher could see if the subject traveled past or moved within the view of the observer.
- *Camp-ins.* A camp-in is a location where searchers are located somewhat permanently so that they can maintain an observation point for long periods of time. This type of assignment is usually longer term (multiple days) and may require logistical support.
- *String lines.* A string line is simply a continuous string deployed from a large spool carried in the pack of a searcher. It can be used in densely wooded areas or in areas where a mobile subject is likely to travel. Tags are places on the string at intervals frequent enough to be visible to a subject who may run into it. The tags may include instructions or an arrow indicating the direction the subject should travel to safety. String lines are periodically checked and are rarely used due to the time and equipment needed to deploy.
- *Other containment methods.* Containment can be supplemented through a number of imaginative methods such as placing signs or posters at locations where the subject or someone who might have seen the subject might travel, leaving notes for the subject at strategic locations such as their car and home, informing the media of the search in progress, and informing transportation providers to keep any eye out for the subject.

SAR personnel assigned to containment positions may have to remain at their posts for long periods of time. This may require additional logistical support (i.e., food, water, and other support materials), and searchers assigned to such posts should not hesitate to request it.

Direct Tactics

Direct tactics include all organized methods used to move through the search area to detect a lost subject or clues. Generally, there are three primary types of searches that can be employed by SAR personnel to find a lost subject: rapid (hasty) searches and two types of area searches, **high-coverage search** and **low-coverage search**. SAR personnel are also sometimes called upon for a fourth type of search—the evidence search—which is a special case of the high-coverage search.

Rapid (Hasty) Search

In general, a **rapid (hasty) search** is a fast, initial response of well-trained, self-sufficient, and very mobile searchers who check those places most likely to produce clues or the subject quickly. A rapid (hasty) search also could be called a search of "points and lines." In geometry, points and lines have no area. Similarly, these types of search assignments do not have definable boundaries and, therefore, involve no measurable area. Searching some place in a rapid fashion usually means that a defined search **segment** is not involved. Rather, rapid (hasty) searches are meant as a means of discovering evidence and/or the subject quickly by visiting general locations where they are likely to be found.

Rapid (hasty) search assignments might include points of interest (e.g., camps, abandoned vehicles, cabins, homes, park bathrooms, scenic overlooks, playgrounds, swimming pools, bodies of water), or linear features such as trails, tracks, paths, and roads. Searching linear features, also called *route searches*, can be searched in a parallel or serial fashion, depending on the objective of the search (**FIGURE 15-1** and **FIGURE 15-2**). A variation of the serial route search is sometimes used in night searching (see *Night Searching*, later in this chapter). When searching linear features, pay particular attention to **decision points** where the subject had to decide which path or road to take. Discovering clues or evidence indicating which path the subject took can significantly reduce search time. During these searches, some thought should also be put into transporting searchers to the tops of hilly terrain so they can walk downhill while searching (NSARC, 2011).

The criterion for a rapid (hasty) search is speed, as opposed to trying to achieve a certain level of coverage. The primary objective of rapid (hasty) searches is to check specific places where the subject or evidence is likely to be discovered quickly (success fast) and to obtain information about the search area (reconnaissance).

Features and benefits of rapid (hasty) searches include:

- An immediate show of effort
- Requiring few resources
- Fast success
- Better defined search area by gathering information or locating clues
- Clue consciousness, which is critical because teams used for rapid searches need to be track and sign aware (should have tracking skills) with a familiarity of the terrain being checked and its dangers
- A likely responsive subject
- Fast determination of where not to search further

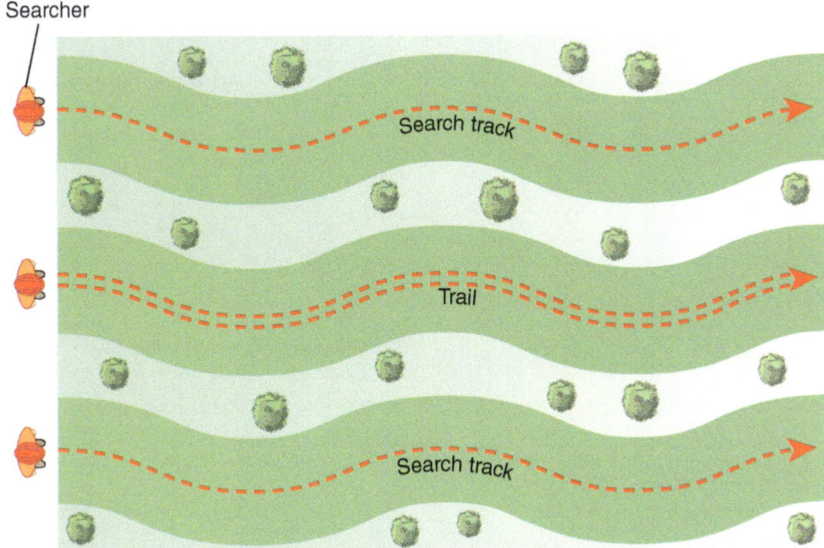

FIGURE 15-1 Example of a parallel route search. One searcher searches the trail, and two others search adjacent to the trail, scanning for evidence of the subject leaving the trail.

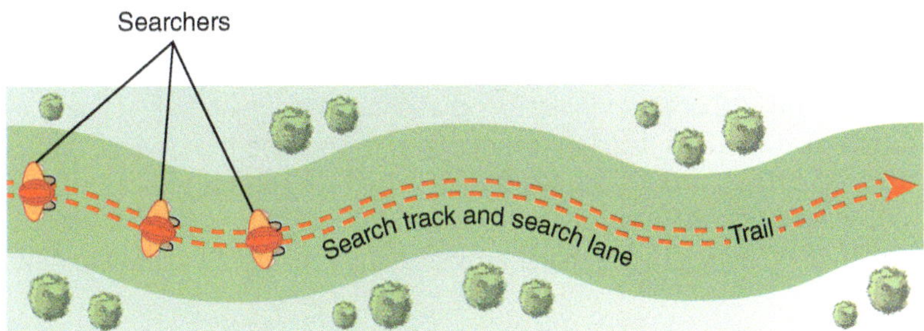

FIGURE 15-2 Example of a serial route search. Three searchers walk one after another on the trail, the leader usually scanning ahead and calling out hazards, while each of the other searchers scans different sides of the trail. This technique can also be effective at night using search lights.

- Preplanning, which is crucial for the immediate availability and effective application of this type of resource

Techniques used to accomplish rapid (hasty) searches include the following:

- Thoroughly check the last known point (LKP) or point last seen (PLS) for clues, track, direction of travel, etc.
- Following one or more known or suspected routes.
- Conduct a perimeter check, checking around the area where the subject was known to have been. This is best used in concert with containment.
- Conduct sign cutting (looking for sign) all around a piece of evidence, abandoned vehicle, PLS, or LKP. An expanding circle pattern may work well for this (**FIGURE 15-3**).
- Check all hazards, attractions, drainages, buildings, trails, roads, and any other places where the subject or evidence is likely to be discovered quickly if the subject is or has been there.

A team that performs rapid (hasty) searches usually comprises two to four searchers who are immediately available, very mobile, clue conscious, and highly skilled. The team may spread out to look for clues around a point of interest, but organized line/area searching is not usually involved. Literally running a trail, path, or road is a valid rapid (hasty) search technique. This can be a fast way to determine that the subject is not currently on a trail, path, or road.

Rapid (hasty) teams also must be prepared to conduct effective area searches if the situation requires. For example, a hasty team locating a series of clues (e.g., discarded clothing, possibly indicating a severely

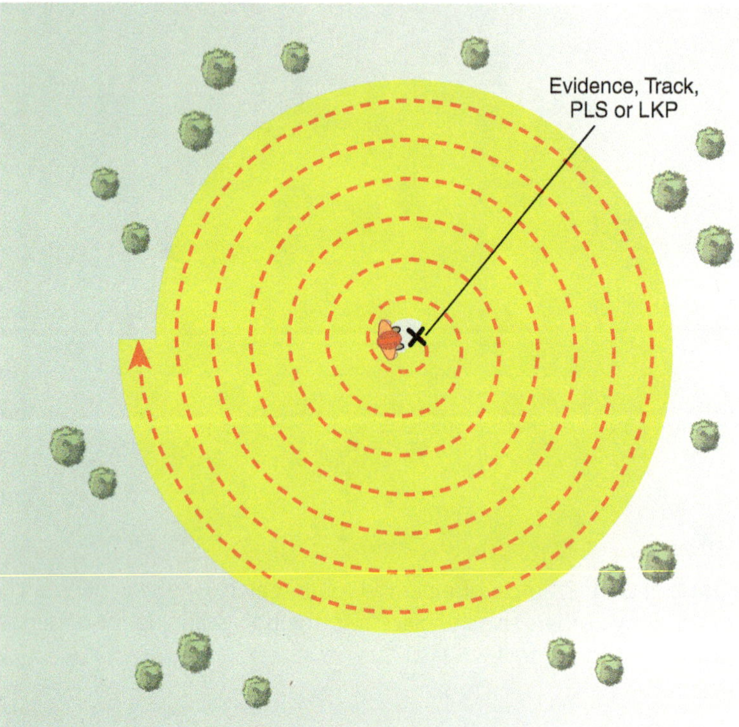

FIGURE 15-3 An expanding circle search can be used to discover tracks (sign cut) or other indicators that show the subject's direction of travel. It can also be useful when starting from the top of a hill and following the contour downward. The search starts close to a specific point—the LKP, PLS, vehicle, or track—and slowly expands outward. When done correctly, the searcher or tracker is constantly scanning new ground.

hypothermic subject) must have the training and experience to recognize the meaning of these clues, determine the area into which the subject may have traveled, and quickly conduct an effective area or route search.

Rapid (hasty) search techniques are often used in the early stages of a search but can be used anytime to check an unconfirmed sighting or to recheck specific, likely locations. The most effective rapid (hasty) search resources include trained, clue-conscious, rapidly deployable teams; trackers; dog teams; aircraft; and any very mobile, highly trained, clue-conscious resource.

In the past, other terms have been used to describe rapid (hasty) searches, including *scratch*, *eyeball*, *quick-look*, *360s*, *sign-cutting*, *ridge running*, *road/trail patrolling*, and *trail running*. A rapid (hasty) search has also been referred to as a Type I search, but this now conflicts with the National Incident Management System (NIMS) resource typing system and is no longer used.

Area Searches

Although rapid (hasty) searches alone often lead to search success, the use of area searches may be required. In an **area search**, a segment of the search area is searched in an organized manner by a specific resource. A searcher moving through a segment—a bounded, appropriately sized subset of the search area—follows a **search track**, which is the actual line of travel taken through the segment by a searcher during a search (**FIGURE 15-4**). The length of this search track—not surprisingly referred to as the **track line length (TLL)**—is an important consideration for search planners in an area search (discussed in Chapter 14, *Principles of Search and Related Issues*). The area scanned by the searcher as he or she moves through the segment is called the **search lane** (**FIGURE 15-5**). The distance between the centers of each adjacent search lane is the **track spacing**.

Be careful not to confuse the search lane with **sweep width**. The search lane is the entire area that an individual searcher can scan during a search. It includes all the area searched out as far as the searcher can see. The sweep width, on the other hand, is an estimated or experimentally derived lateral range that extends only part of the searcher's full visual scan distance. A searcher MUST scan well beyond the sweep width distance. In fact, recall from Chapter 14 that sweep width,

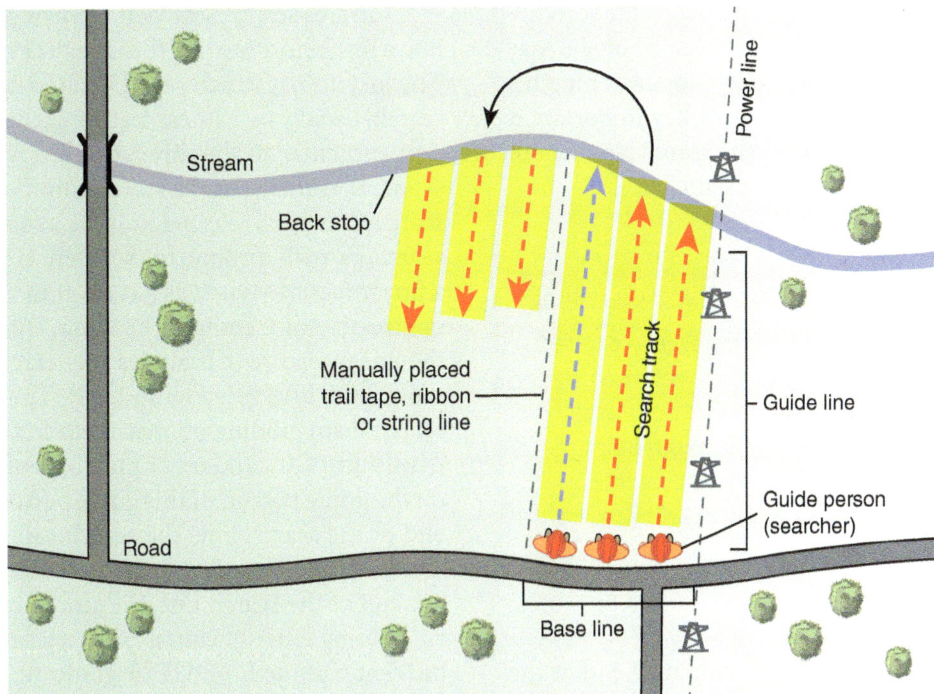

FIGURE 15-4 Example of a three-person search crew guiding (right) on a power line during an area search. Note that when the crew reaches the backstop, it moves laterally and guides (left) on the trail tape (or ribbon or string line) installed during the first pass.

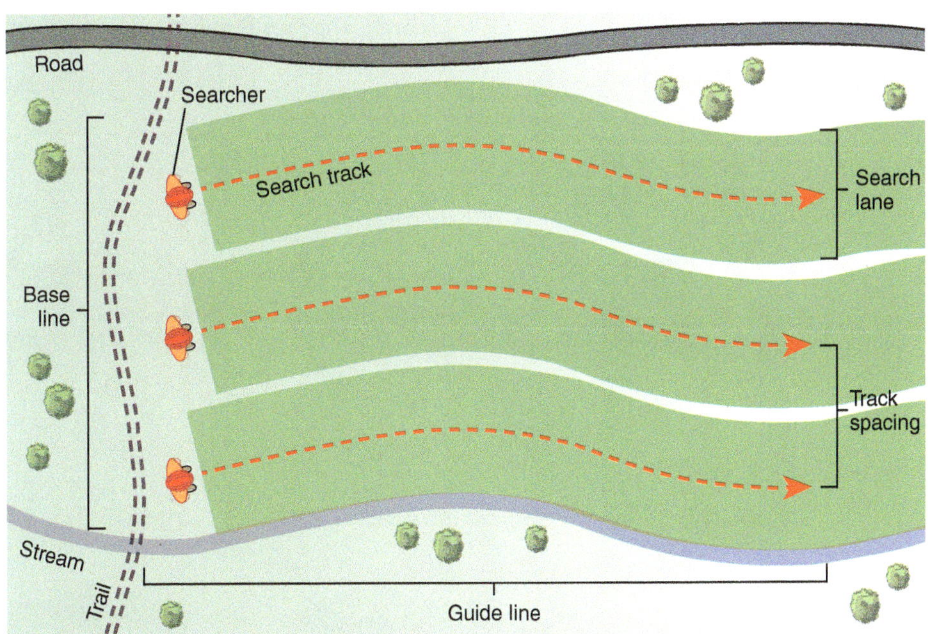

FIGURE 15-5 Example of an area search, guiding right on the stream. Depending on the gaps and overlap caused by the track spacing, this pattern could be used to achieve either a low or a high level of coverage.

by definition, is the distance beyond which the searcher can see as many objects as within which he or she may miss. A searcher is fully responsible for searching his or her entire search lane, which is of key importance. The sweep width is used only by the search planner but is based on information from the searcher.

SEARCH AND RESCUE TIP

Be careful not to confuse the search lane with sweep width. The search lane is the entire area that an individual searcher can scan during a search. It includes all the area searched out as far as the searcher can see. Sweep width is an estimated or experimentally derived lateral range that extends only part of the searcher's full visual scan distance. A searcher MUST scan well beyond the sweep width distance.

In a search segment, a search lane may end at the far side of the segment, often at a linear feature, and require the search crew to move laterally, establish their search line again, and return across the segment to continue their search (see Figure 15-4). The linear feature bounding the far side of the segment may also be referred to as a **backstop** in that it defines the end-point of one search pass and serves as the base line of the return search lanes.

In an area search, searchers often organize themselves into a line before moving through the assigned segment. The location at which searchers line up to begin their search, usually on a linear feature such as a road or trail perpendicular to the direction of travel, is called the search **baseline**. As the search commences, the line of searchers is often referred to as the **search line**, and the searchers' path through the segment is guided by either a linear feature—such as a road, trail, fence, ridgeline, or stream—or a compass heading. During the search, the linear feature that guides the search team is called the **guide line** (see Figure 15-4). The member of the search team guiding on this linear feature is called the **guide person**, and other members of the team guide on the guide person. If this guide person is on the right end of the search line, the search can be described as "guiding right" (see Figure 15-4). If this person is on the left end of the search line, the search can be described as "guiding left." Of course, such a search line can also be "center guided," and if the guide person is following a compass heading, the search can be described as "compass guided" (**FIGURE 15-6**).

If no terrain feature or compass bearing will be useful for guiding the search pattern on the return pass, during the first pass, it may be necessary for the searcher farthest from the guide line to install a **trail tape, ribbon, or string line** along the furthest boundary of his or her search lane (see Figure 15-4). On the return pass, these

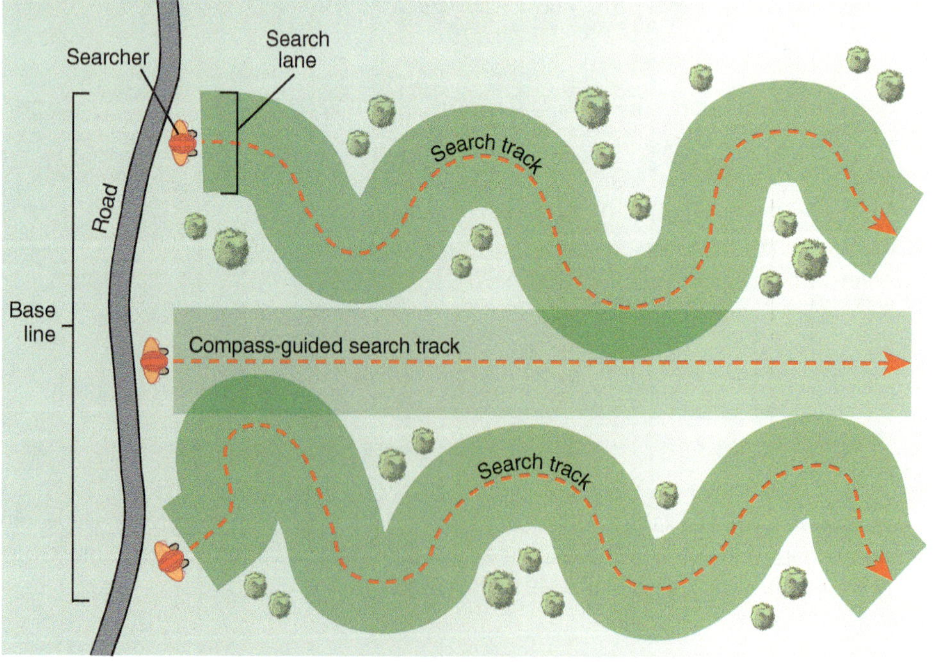

FIGURE 15-6 Example of a compass/center guided search pattern. Due to the gaps, limited purposeful wandering, and minor overlapping of search lanes, this technique could be used to achieve a low level of coverage.

temporary search lane markers can be used as guides when no other visible guide line exists. The markers can be made of toilet paper, surveyor's tape, survey markers, evidence markers, string, or other highly visible material, and they must be placed either on the ground or near eye level so that it is easily seen. When standing at one marker, one must be able to easily see at least the next marker, and perhaps two, so that a guide line is discernable. Double markers can be placed to indicate the end or a turn in the guide line. How close together the markers are placed is dependent on the terrain; obstructions to vision, such as topography and density; and type of foliage. On the return pass in the segment, the searcher guiding on the markers can recover them as time allows and necessity requires.

Searchers do not have to form a line to area search a segment. Although it might be considered less safe, searchers can operate independently, out of sight and even out of hearing distance from each other, and still achieve a measurable level of coverage in their segment. Coverage can be measured by search planners regardless of how organized, or not, a group of searchers operates during a search, but the more organized they are—that is, the less overlap and fewer gaps in their searching within a segment—the higher their coverage and resulting POD will be. Do not think that line searching is the only way to search a segment. A skillful search planner can compute coverage, and therefore probability of detection (POD), after virtually any search pattern is used in a bounded segment. The key is for search crews to completely and accurately describe what they did and where they did it during the debriefing.

Unlike a rapid (hasty) search, an area search requires that the segment being searched have established, readily discernable boundaries that are identifiable on a map as well as in the field. Each resource conducting an area search should seek to cover its assigned segment as uniformly as possible and in accordance with their briefing instructions. Search theory requires that search effort be distributed as evenly as possible across a segment, without *significant* gaps and overlaps. Search theory does well to account for small gaps and overlaps that are common to field searching, but if a significant portion of the segment was not searched at all—which search planners would learn about in the debriefing—search planners would account for it by computing coverage only for the searched portion. The unsearched part would be cut out and made into a separate segment. Thus, search teams and other resources should endeavor to spread their searching effort as evenly as possible over their assigned segments. The best way to do this is to organize the searchers in some type of line or grid search where individual searchers cover parallel search lanes.

SEARCH AND RESCUE TIP

An area search requires that the segment being searched have established, readily discernable boundaries that are identifiable on a map as well as in the field.

If unlimited resources are available, they could and should be deployed to search everywhere there is some likelihood of the subject being located. Unfortunately, resources are always limited, and search planners must determine how best to use what is available to them. In the language of search theory, this is called *optimal effort allocation*. The number and type of resources available, as well as the type of object being sought, make a difference in the type of area search chosen for the situation at hand.

Low-Coverage Area Search

In this type of area search, search teams may consist of three to seven persons but usually closer to three because coordination with fewer people is easier. The goal of this technique is to cover larger geographic areas quickly and with fewer resources, often seeking a subject that is thought to be responsive. Fewer searchers usually equates to a lower coverage (less thoroughness), but the benefit is that it allows some minimal level of coverage to be spread over a large area in a relatively short time. When a life depends on searching a very large area and there is no evidence strongly favoring one region over another, lower coverage in all segments may be better than no coverage in some to achieve higher coverage in others. This type of area search is usually associated with searching faster, which tends to produce lower coverage, and for a responsive subject that might be able to hear and respond to searchers moving through the segment.

A team conducting a low-coverage search would organize on a base line, usually at wide track (between searcher) spacing, and proceed searching on some guide line. Track spacing may be dependent on terrain and visibility and be such that adjacent searchers cannot see each other, which requires additional attention to the safety of individual searchers. Generally, with low-coverage searches, the amount of overlapping area scanned by both searchers in adjacent search lanes should be minimal, but the amount of area between adjacent search lanes that is scanned by neither searcher (gaps) may be more than with higher coverage searches.

It is best if the members of the search crew can maintain an occasional visual and voice contact with one another, but this is not mandatory. Effective searching, and measuring its resulting coverage, does not require all searchers to remain in line or contact with each other. However, organizing the search pattern does help avoid gaps and overlaps in the coverage, which improves POD.

Once the baseline and guide for the search is established, the segment is divided into an appropriate number of search lanes based on (a) the number of searchers, (b) **search speed** (affected by terrain and vegetation), (c) the amount of time assigned to the task (usually less than 6 hours), and (d) the size of the segment. One goal of the search crew should be to safely finish their assigned task in the time allotted. If a low-coverage search is assigned, it usually means that the team will have to move quickly through the segment and may have to use wide track spacing to cover the segment in the allotted time. In carrying out a low-coverage search, the goal is not to spend a great deal of time conducting a very thorough search. Thoroughness is not a characteristic of a low-coverage search.

Once the search lanes are established and their width (track spacing) determined, each searcher proceeds to search his or her assigned lane. During the search, searchers are encouraged to weave or roam in a purposeful manner while moving forward through the segment. That is, while covering their assigned search lanes as well as time permits, they should also roam laterally to look behind obstructions and investigate likely spots based on the terrain and the subject profile. Historically, this has been referred to as *purposeful wandering* (Perkins and Roberts, 2009).

The compass-guided search pattern illustrated in Figure 15-6 can be used as a low-coverage technique, but with very wide track spacing, the lateral searchers may not be able to visually guide on the compass-guided searcher in the center. The search pattern in **FIGURE 15-7** may be a better option for a low-coverage search where wide track spacing does not allow adjacent searchers to guide on each other. If each searcher is able to generally follow a compass bearing to keep overlaps and significant gaps to a minimum, this would work. Both techniques can also be used to achieve a higher level of coverage, which is discussed below.

Low-coverage searching, like area searching in general, requires skill in navigation, clue detection, and "thinking like the subject," and it has several important characteristics:

- It is more flexible and requires much less coordination of individual searcher efforts than high-coverage searching, which uses more searchers.
- Search lanes are relatively wide, often much wider than the measured range of detection.
- Searchers can adjust and tailor their movements to the environment and use "purposeful wandering," thereby making more efficient use of their time and effort.

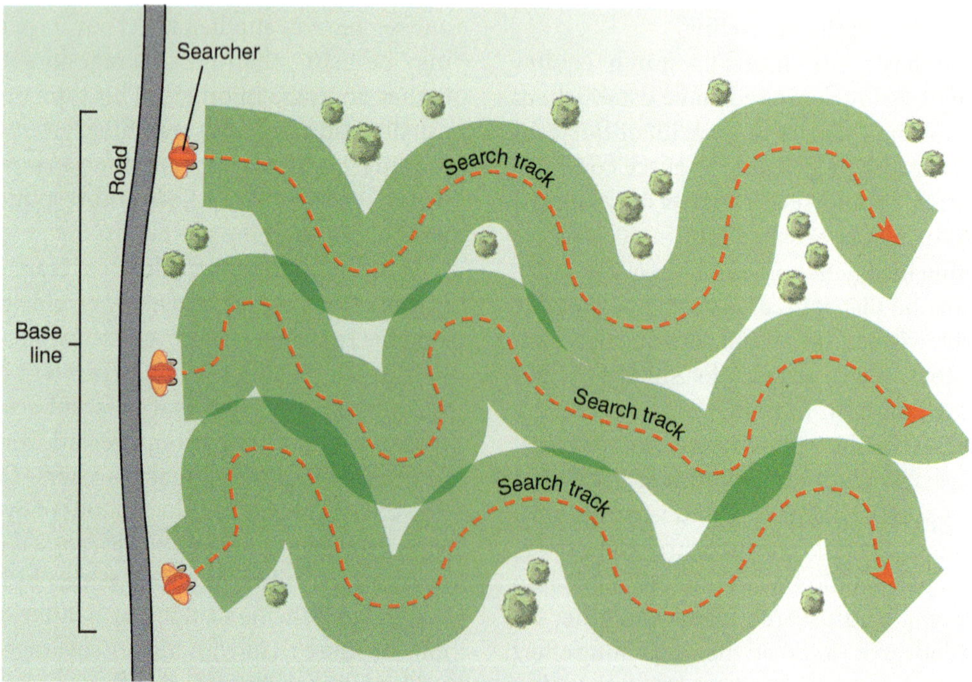

FIGURE 15-7 Example of a low-coverage search where wide track spacing does not allow adjacent searchers to guide on each other. If each searcher is able to generally follow a compass bearing to keep overlaps and significant gaps to a minimum, this would work.

- It can be used in situations where more thorough search methods are difficult or impractical.
- Because fewer searchers are often used, low-coverage searches are generally less damaging to the environment.
- Low-coverage searches are often employed after rapid (hasty) searches, especially if rapid searches found clues.
- This type of search is best used when subject responsiveness is assumed to be high.
- With appropriately skilled and alert searchers, this type of search may also locate clues.

Low-coverage searching is the preferred method for achieving low to moderate (as opposed to very high) levels of coverage in reasonable amounts of time. Techniques used to accomplish low-coverage searches include the following:

- Relatively wide spacing between the centers of adjacent search lanes. The spacing itself does not cause low coverage. The larger area being covered by the same number of searchers is what causes a reduction in coverage.
- Compass bearings or specific guides are often used to control the direction of searchers in the segment. Searchers can use purposeful wandering to quickly move back and forth laterally while maintaining a general direction of movement across the segment.
- This approach can be applied in a segment where the finding of a clue suggests an increased probability of the segment containing the subject, such as a clue that established a direction of travel.

Low-coverage searches are often used in the early stages of a search operation, such as when rapid (hasty) searches have found clues, and the time frame for subject survival is short, or when search resources are few, and the search area is large. In some segments, particularly the heavily vegetated ones, low-coverage searches may be the initial search tactic used. Low-coverage searches may also be valuable in those situations where no particularly likely regions can be identified in a large search area, and/or there are insufficient resources to achieve higher levels of coverage in all segments.

A typical low-coverage search usually achieves a coverage level of less than 0.5, and thus a POD of less than 39% (see Figure 14-8). The most effective resources for this type of search include well-trained, clue-conscious ground teams, dogs, sign cutters (trackers), and aircraft.

Many have experimented with, and taught, searchers to use sound, usually by yelling or the uncoordinated use of a whistle, to attract lost subjects. Colwell (1992) described a low-coverage approach to using sound, whistles, and portable radios in a coordinated effort to attract a responsive subject. He called this technique "sound sweeping" and "sound saturation." He found it particularly effective in the mountainous, heavily timbered, frequently snowy, Pacific West Coast coniferous forest in which he often searched.

In practical use, **sound sweep** searchers are lined up at very wide spacing along the baseline of the area to be searched. It is not necessary to coordinate a single start time for all searchers. Searchers simply walk into their search segment, usually guided by compass bearings or terrain (e.g., downhill), when they reach their starting locations. As they begin, a base or control station broadcasts over the radio a countdown call to all searchers at 1- to 2-minute intervals. For example, the base transmits, "*Whistle blast, 5-4-3-2-1 BLAST*." On this command, all searchers stop, blow their whistles (ideally this would occur simultaneously) while covering their ears to maintain their hearing sensitivity, and then listen for a predetermined period of time for an audible response. If no response is heard, the searchers continue with their sweep. This technique has the effect of saturating a large area with a sound that is easily recognized as an emergency signal (whistle). Coordinating the whistle sounds allows the sound to be sent out simultaneously then followed up with silence so that any response subject signaling a response would be able to be heard. However, the use of this technique requires a responsive subject, which is why the author suggests that it be used as soon as possible after the subject is reported missing.

High-Coverage Area Search

High-coverage area search is a slow, highly systematic area search that uses more resources and takes more time than its low-coverage counterpart. It is used when a very thorough search of a segment is desired, and the subject is thought to be unresponsive.

A high-coverage search is accomplished by searchers lining up on a baseline, usually at a closer track spacing than for a low-coverage search. They then proceed along relatively straight, parallel, equally spaced tracks—to the extent the terrain and vegetation allow—scanning a swath that extends from themselves out to their maximum range of detection. More overlap and fewer gaps in the search pattern, as well as more time spent in the segment (more searcher hours), cause higher coverage and thus higher POD. **FIGURE 15-8** illustrates an example of a search pattern that would likely produce a high coverage (shaded areas are scanned search lanes). Note the overlapping of the scanned areas and the lack of gaps, unlike in the examples used for low-coverage searching (see Figure 15-6 and Figure 15-7). **FIGURE 15-9** illustrates how more time spent in the segment—more purposeful wandering takes more time—means more

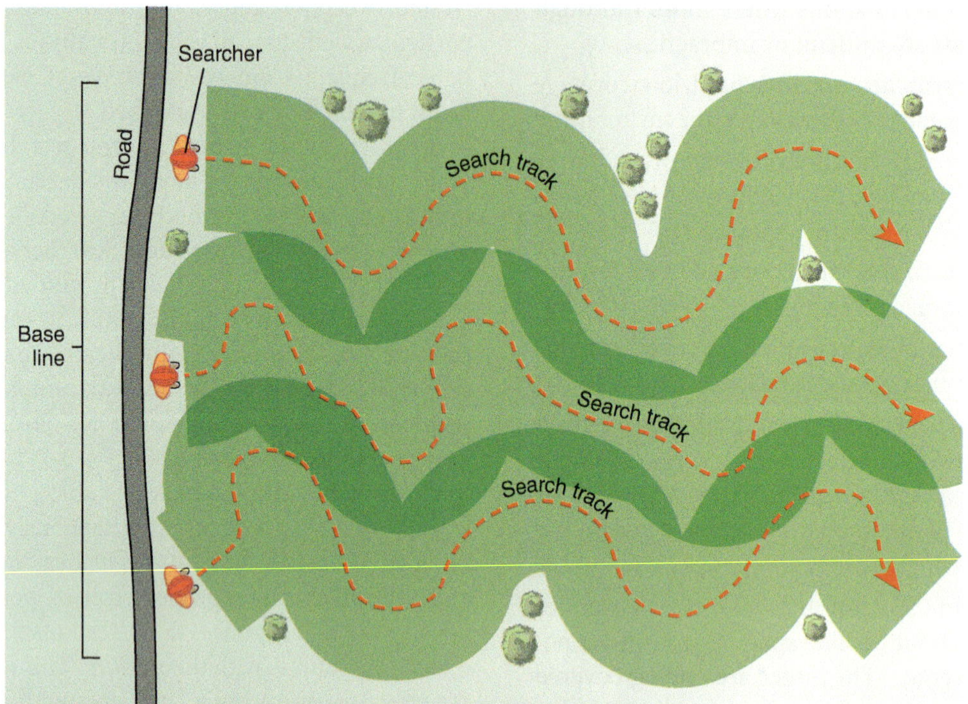

FIGURE 15-8 An example of a high-coverage search with a three-person crew. Searchers may guide on one end (guide right, or guide left) or the center, and the guide person may guide on a compass bearing or terrain feature. Note that the track spacing selected results in significant overlap and few gaps in the search lanes, which results in higher coverage.

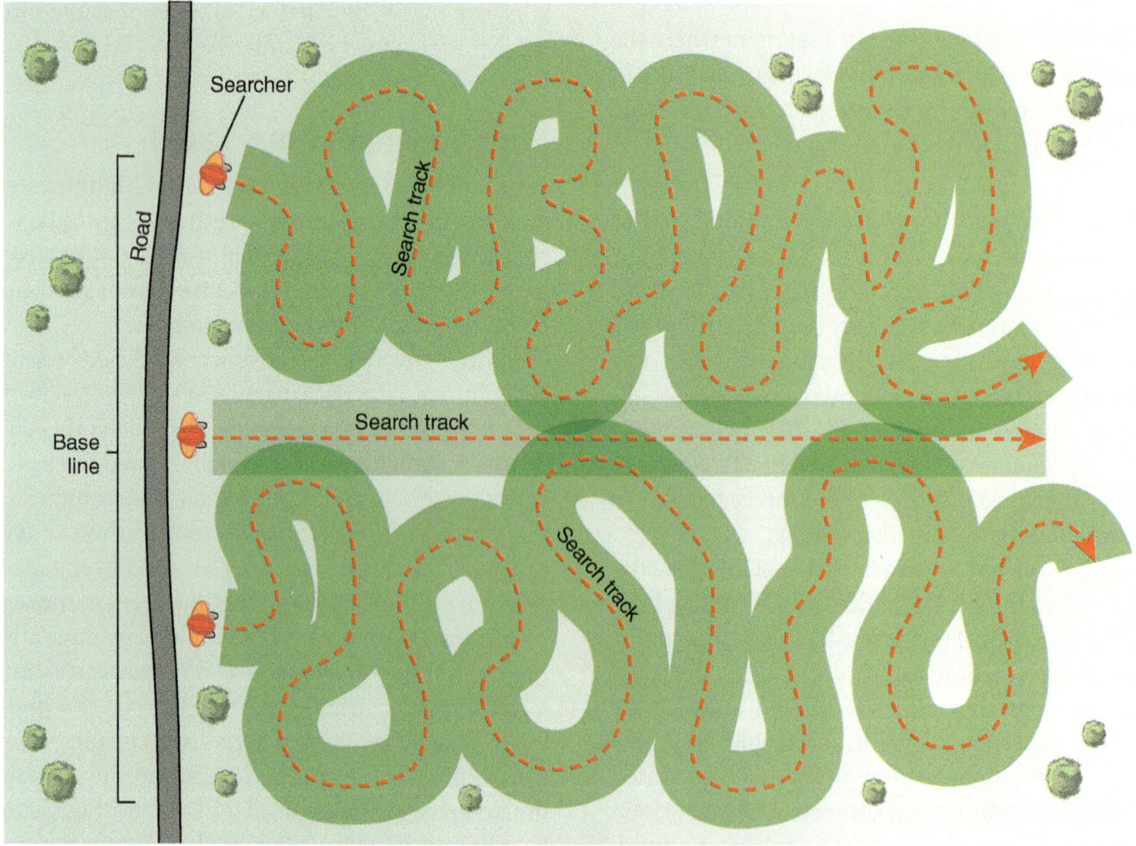

FIGURE 15-9 An example of a compass-guided search pattern with a great deal of purposeful wandering, which takes more time. More time spent searching translates to higher coverage.

search effort expended, which results in higher coverage. The more overlap in the scanned swath (search lanes), and the more time spent in the segment searching, the higher the resulting coverage.

A typical high-coverage search might achieve a coverage level of 0.5 or greater, and thus a POD of 39% or higher. Higher coverage levels may often be necessary. However, the amount of additional search effort required to significantly improve the POD diminishes as the coverage level increases—a type of diminishing return for the investment of effort. Search planners must take this into consideration when assigning resources.

The criterion for high-coverage searching is not speed but thoroughness, which can be achieved by increasing the search effort put into a segment. There are two ways to increase search effort: put more searchers into the segment, or spend more time searching in the segment. Increasing the number of resources (searchers) in a segment or the amount of time searchers spend in a segment increases coverage and thus POD. The inverse is also true: fewer resources searching in a segment or spending less time searching a segment results in less search effort being applied and, thus, less coverage.

Factors to consider in high-coverage searching include the following:

- Because it takes more searchers and/or more time spent searching, this type of searching can be extremely destructive to clues that are not detected, thereby often ensuring clues will *never* be found. Therefore, this type of search should be used *only as a last resort.*
- High-coverage searching is slow and may take a long time to cover the segment to an acceptable level. If used in the early stages of a search, especially when resources are still scarce, the overall POS generally grows very slowly, which is most often not the goal of search planners.
- A great deal of effort is needed in this type of searching to coordinate searcher movement, maintain a line abreast formation, maintain searcher spacing, and keep all searchers on parallel tracks. This "overhead" represents time and effort that cannot be expended on searching.
- Higher coverage is achieved by either (a) putting more resources (searchers) into the segment or (b) spending more time searching in the segment. The same search crew searching a segment multiple times achieves the same goal (higher coverage).
- Since keeping gaps to a minimum in search lanes is important to thoroughness, marking the searched lanes with trail tape, ribbons, string lines, or some similar method may be necessary to maintain control.
- Overlapping the scanning of search lanes by adjacent searchers increases thoroughness but reduces the overall size of the area covered.

A team that performs high-coverage searches usually consists of four to seven persons, rarely more, and with good reason. More than seven searchers is difficult to coordinate and gets cumbersome. Unskilled searchers can be mixed with skilled searchers, but unskilled searchers should never attempt this type of search without skilled help. Overlap of search lanes is permissible and may be encouraged, but it also reduces the overall size of the area being searched, which takes longer (or more searchers) to completely cover the segment. This must be taken into consideration when planning the search of a segment.

High-coverage searches should be used when lower coverage searches have been tried with a low resulting POD, or when a thorough search of a segment is desired at the onset and the appropriate resources are plentiful. In land SAR, the most effective and thorough type of search resource is almost always trained ground search teams.

Evidence Search

SAR search teams are sometimes called upon to perform evidence searches (**FIGURE 15-10**). This type of search is usually just a very high coverage search for what is usually a relatively small item, but there are at least four potential differences between a search for a human subject and an evidence search:

1. An evidence search does not usually involve a live subject, and, thus, speed and urgency are often less relevant.
2. Evidence searches often involve looking for small objects in limited areas.
3. Inanimate objects do not usually move once they are lost.
4. The rules of evidence (e.g., maintaining the chain of evidence, protection of the evidence from contamination, and recording the evidence as it is found) are strictly enforced on evidence searches. Nevertheless, the same techniques for organizing and employing searchers in a high-coverage search apply.

Because a high level of coverage is often needed in an evidence search (i.e., a high level of confidence that nothing was missed), more search effort is usually required. Because there is a direct correlation between search effort and coverage, doubling the search effort (area effectively swept) also doubles the coverage (but not the POD). In an evidence search, the amount of search effort employed, and the resulting coverage, is usually increased by searchers simply spending more time searching and taking their time to be very thorough.

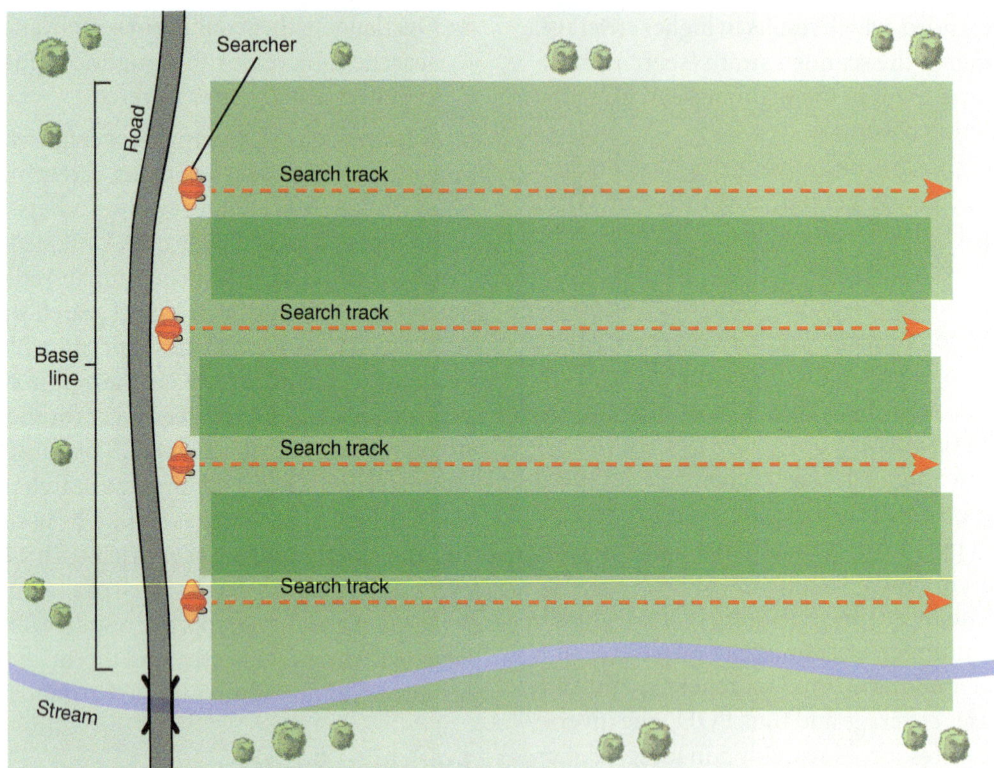

FIGURE 15-10 An example of an evidence search with four searchers. Their small track spacing allows for their search lanes to overlap significantly, increasing coverage in the area they are searching.

Spending twice the time searching should roughly translate to twice the coverage. As mentioned previously, search effort can also be increased by increasing the number of searchers; that is, twice the number of the same type of searchers at the same search speed in the same segment translates to twice the coverage. Both approaches are usually needed in an evidence search.

SEARCH AND RESCUE TIP

Because there is a direct correlation between search effort and coverage, doubling the search effort, or doubling the amount of time spent searching, doubles the coverage.

Important characteristics of evidence searches include the following:

- Time is not usually as important a factor as it is in searches for human subjects, but this does not mean the search is unimportant or not urgent.
- In this type of search, there is often no second chance. Evidence not discovered on the first pass may be destroyed, damaged, or modified by the search activity itself to the point where it is no longer useful.
- Large amounts of effort are required to achieve high levels of coverage for what are often small search objects. Searching on hands and knees and shoulder-to-shoulder in closely spaced parallel tracks is often necessary.

It is important that each object found in an evidence search be left in place untouched and undisturbed by the searcher, unless specifically instructed to do otherwise in the briefing. When possible evidence is found, the searcher should immediately stop, announce the find so all other searchers stop as well, and call the object to the attention of a law enforcement official who then decides what action to take. Often the actions taken will be to photograph the item in place; note exactly where, when, and by whom it was found; retrieve, mark, and bag the item; and start a chain-of-custody record. Searchers may resume searching only when directed to do so by an authorized official.

Information to Report to Planners after a Search

As a minimum, field personnel should convey several important pieces of information at the debriefing after an area search is conducted:

- Estimated forward search speed of the individual or team while searching (e.g., slow, normal, or fast)
- How long the individual or team searched, in minutes (excluding breaks and travel time to and from the segment)
- Field measurements of range of detection (Rd)
- Other field-observable measures identified and requested by search planners prior to the assignment

- A qualitative description of how well the team did with the search (e.g., excellent, good, fair, or poor)
- A qualitative description of the search conditions (e.g., rough terrain that slowed and fatigued searchers, numerous thickets that could not be thoroughly investigated and still finish the assignment on time)

Forward Search Speed

In the absence of a GPS receiver or other means of directly measuring average search speed, an estimate of the search speed is needed so that effort, or total distance traveled while searching, can be computed by search planners. As mentioned in Chapter 14, effort is needed to eventually compute POD. In addition, the search speed itself may affect the sweep width. If searchers move very quickly or run, they may devote more of their attention to navigating the terrain and less to searching. In short, faster travel could reduce the effective sweep width and thus coverage and POD. The opposite is true for much slower than normal search speeds. Spending more time in a segment due to very slow forward speed has the effect of increasing sweep width and thus coverage and POD. Therefore, it is essential that searchers provide an estimate of their average speed while searching because it will affect the search planner's estimate of the POD and POS that were achieved.

As mentioned in Chapter 14, one way to estimate forward search speed is to first measure search speeds during SAR exercises or on actual searches to determine the "normal" speed for you and your team. Using this measure as a reference, searchers can then describe their forward speed in comparison as either slow, normal, or fast. Values could then be assigned to each of these speed categories and used by search planners (e.g., slow = 0.5 × normal search speed; normal = 1 × normal search speed; and fast = 1.5 × normal search speed). Since differences of these magnitudes are not likely to have a big effect on sweep width for ground searches, such general estimates are usually sufficiently accurate. However, to more accurately estimate forward speed during a search, experiments could be conducted by field searchers (see also Chapter 14 under *Field Contributions to Measuring Detection*). For example:

- It takes 30 minutes (0.5 hour) to search from Point A to Point B.
- The distance between Point A and Point B is 0.5 mile (0.8 kilometer).
- Searchers describe their speed in this segment as "normal."
- 0.5 mile (0.8 kilometer) divided by 0.5 hours = 1 mile per hour (1.6 kph).
- Thus, normal speed = 1 mile per hour.

Similar experiments could be conducted in other environments to determine normal search speeds for that environment. Search planners could then use these experimentally derived speeds when field personnel report their search speed as slow, normal, or fast.

Time Spent Searching

If search planners have an estimate of how fast searchers are traveling (v) and exactly how long they have been searching (t), the track line length (TLL) can be computed by multiplying the two values:

$$v \times t = \text{TLL}$$

This value (TLL) is very important to search planners because they can use it as part of their computation of POD, thus searchers providing an estimated search speed and an accurate description of how long they have been searching is also important. Therefore, at least one of the searchers on a crew (the time keeper) should keep track of exactly how long the team has been searching, which should exclude rest and meal breaks, traveling to and from the search segment, and any time the group was not actually searching.

If there is a direct means of measuring TLL, such as with a GPS device, estimating search speed and search time becomes less important—until the GPS device stops working. Field personnel should become accustomed to estimating their search speed and recording their search time so both can be reported at debriefing.

Field Estimation of Sweep Width

The concept of sweep width (see Chapter 14) as a key element of search theory has been in use in SAR since just after World War II. Since then, perhaps hundreds of experiments to determine sweep width values under various environmental conditions have been conducted for the maritime and aeronautical search environments, including for searches from aircraft over land (see Table 14-1). Federal government and military objectives were the primary impetus for these efforts, and, thus, funding was available. Tables of sweep width values for both types of searches are available in the *International Aeronautical and Maritime Search and Rescue Manual* published jointly by the International Maritime Organization and the International Civil Aviation Organization (IMO/ICO, 2016). This three-volume document is recognized globally as the standard text on aeronautical and maritime SAR operations and methods.

Unfortunately, prior to 2002, no sweep width experiments had been conducted for land-based ground searches. Recognizing this fact, between 2002 and 2004, the National Search and Rescue Committee (NSARC), a consortium of U.S. federal agencies, funded the development of an experimental model that could be used by inland search teams to develop their own sweep width data (Frost and Robe, 2002; Koester et al., 2004). This seminal work served as a precursor to several other land-based sweep width experiments that followed over the subsequent decade and led to a method of estimating sweep width in the field (Koester et al., 2014).

Until experimentally determined sweep width data becomes widely available for land search, some method for estimating sweep width is necessary if the full benefit of search theory is to be realized. Using a method supported by research and widely thought to be reliable, search planners can use certain measurements reported from the field by search crews as the basis for an estimate of sweep width in a particular segment. This field measurement, referred to as a **range of detection (Rd)** measurement, is helpful because it depends on the same variables as sweep width (i.e., the unique combination of the characteristics of the search environment, **search object**, and search **sensors**). Field personnel should be prepared to report Rd and related field-observable measurements after a search in the debriefing.

The range of detection should be measured in the segment in which the search will be conducted, using a search object representative of that which is being sought. For example, if a human subject is the target of the search, a backpack (or two) or sleeping bag could be used. Range of detection can be quickly measured and documented in the search segment and then reported to search planners.

In the past, other authors have referred to similar measurements as the "Northumbrian rain dance" (Perkins, 1989), the "visibility petal" (Colwell, 1992), and "average maximum detection range" (Robe and Frost, 2002). We have learned a great deal in the intervening years since these innovative authors described their ideas. We now know that the difference between previous methods and the range of detection measurement is significant enough to completely replace any other similar sweep width estimation methods previously used. Because a full explanation of this significance is beyond the scope of this book, the focus here is on determining range of detection in the field, which is done by searchers in their assigned search segment.

To measure the Rd in the segment to be searched, place an object on the ground that serves as a suitable proxy for the primary object being sought (**FIGURE 15-11**). A backpack with coloration and contrast with the environment similar to that expected on the lost subject works well. Note and record whether the object might be considered low visibility (camouflage or low contrast with the environment), medium visibility (blue or only moderately contrasting with the environment), or high visibility (florescent orange or highly contrasting with the environment). This becomes important to the search planner later. Place this object at a location judged to be

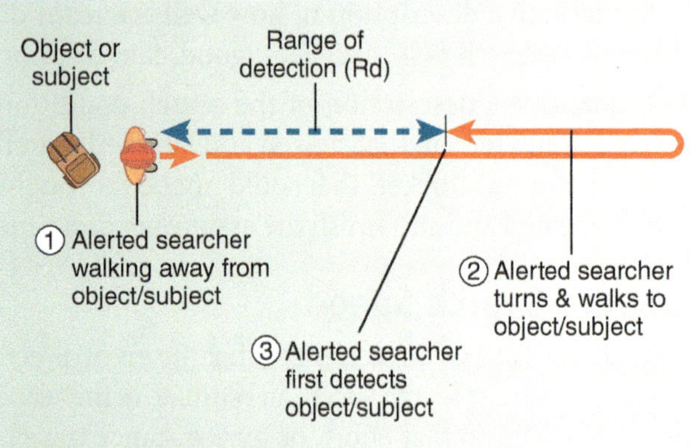

FIGURE 15-11 Range of detection (Rd) exercise done in the segment to be searched.

representative of the conditions in the search segment. Beginning at the object, establish a random compass bearing (say, 10 degrees) and walk away from the object until it is no longer visible. Continue walking away from the object for another 30–50 feet (9–15 meters), or until you are sure you can no longer see the object, then reverse your compass heading (back azimuth; 190 degrees) and walk toward the object, visually scanning for it as you walk. At the point you reverse your heading, you should not be able to see the object. Continue to move toward the object until it is sighted, then stop. The straight-line distance from this point to the object is the Rd. Measure and record this distance as accurately as possible. A laser range finder is ideal, but for those without one, the distance can be easily estimated by having calibrated the length of one's pace, walking to the object, and counting the number of paces. Repeat this exercise at least four times, each time adding 90 degrees, or so, to the bearing previously used (**FIGURE 15-12**). Repeating the exercise eight times is better, each time adding 45 degrees to the initial bearing (**FIGURE 15-13**). Having each teammate make an Rd measurement at random compass bearings is better and faster than one person repeating the exercise multiple times.

Experience has shown that searchers should carry their SAR packs and communication devices while making Rd measurements. More than one searcher has become disoriented after walking away from the search object, only to turn to walk in a direction that took him or her farther from the group. Safety and accountability must be a priority, even during the Rd measurement.

Terrain and obstacles such as trees, rocks, and vegetation may cause significant variation in the Rd of each measurement, which is to be expected. Record all Rd measurements for reporting in the debriefing. Search planners will likely combine the values to establish an "average range of detection." This average Rd is multiplied by a correction factor, which is dependent on the

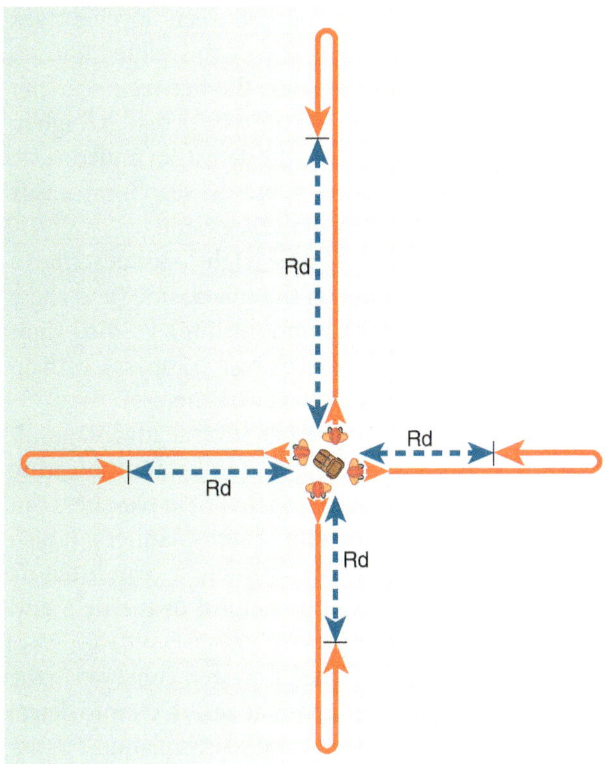

FIGURE 15-12 Four field measurements for range of detection (Rd) is minimally adequate, but more is better.

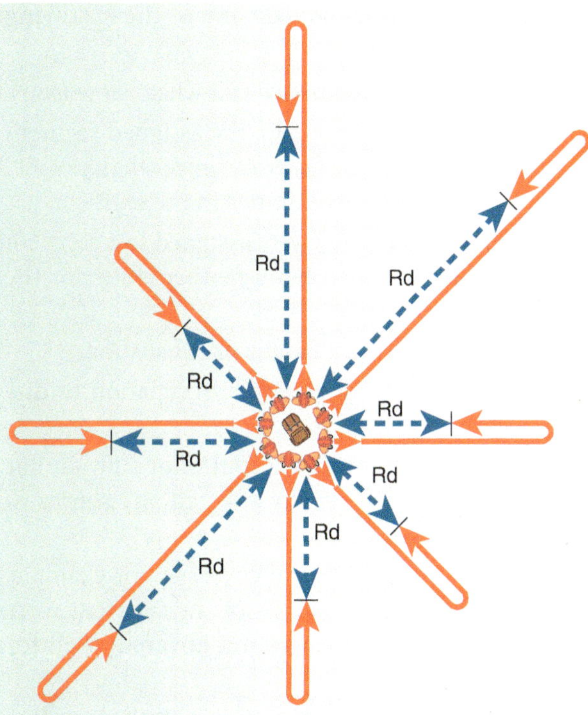

FIGURE 15-13 Eight measurements for range of detection (Rd) is best, although fewer can be adequate.

level of contrast the object has with the environment (i.e., high, medium, or low visibility), resulting in a value that can be used as an estimate for sweep width. In mathematical terms, it might look like this:

Average Range of Detection × Correction Factor
= Sweep Width Estimate

The Rd measurement process performs several important functions:

- It gives searchers the experience of seeing how an object like the search object appears in the environment where the search is to take place. (However, searchers must avoid becoming so fixated on this image that they overlook other items of importance that look different, such as clues or even the subject.)
- Although Rd, strictly speaking, is not itself a measure of detectability, providing it does give the search planner a basis for estimating sweep width.
- Having had the experience of performing an Rd measurement, searchers will be in a better position to make other observations about their environment and search conditions.

If a segment includes two or more significantly different environments (e.g., both open field and timbered forest)—something search planners try to avoid—an Rd measurement should be made in each of the representative environments and reported accordingly in the debriefing. Search planners can then use these measurements to help compute coverage in each portion of the segment searched.

Qualitative Description of a Search

Fatigue is believed to decrease sweep width by 10% (IMO/ICAO, 2016; Koester et al., 2014), and there is evidence that at least some search distractions—such as precipitation and wearing a hat while searching—reduce sweep width by some amount (Koester et al., 2004). However, there are likely many situations, conditions, and influences on the effectiveness of a search that are not yet recognized or understood. Additional experiments in inland environments using land search resources are needed to provide more insight. Until this is accomplished, some method of subjectively estimating the overall quality of the search may be helpful. This can be as easy as subjectively reporting, during the debriefing, an assessment of how well the search went and how searchers feel about their efforts. Offering four options should be adequate: excellent, good, fair, or poor. Reporting, for example, that "the search seemed to go fine" might not be that meaningful. However, given the four choices and a search crew choosing to rate the overall search as poor should at least trigger some relevant questioning by the person conducting the debriefing.

A detailed description of the conduct and effectiveness of the search should be provided during the debriefing, which may include any of the following (**FIGURE 15-14**):

- The crew felt rushed/hurried (for whatever reason).
- The size of, or the terrain in, the assigned segment caused the crew to go faster or slower than normal search speed for the conditions in the segment.
- Searchers thought they were assigned to a segment they thought would contain neither clues nor the subject (bias).
- The crew experienced fatigue or exhaustion.
- Searcher boredom or other preoccupation or distractions affected the search.
- Loud noises, bright lights, foul odors, or similar distractions detrimentally affected any senses of the searchers.
- Coverage was not uniform coverage; for example, difficult-to-search portions of the segment were avoided, or a portion was not covered at all for whatever reason.
- Conditions (terrain, vegetation, weather, and/or lighting) were different from those described in the pre-search briefing.

The importance of accurately and completely reporting all observations made during a search cannot be overemphasized. When observations are reported by experienced search crews, search managers and planners take them very seriously. Erroneous, inaccurate, or vague information from field SAR personnel can be devastating to an otherwise reasonable search plan.

Grid Naming System

A grid naming system was developed by the Boy Scouts of America-affiliated Explorer Search and Rescue teams (now called *Venturing*) in the Pacific Northwest. This scheme can be used to describe any specific line (area) search pattern (WESAR, 1999). The system consists of a *number-word-number* sequence that serves as the name of the pattern.

For example, "6–guide [right]–30," where the first number (on the left) describes the number of searchers on the search line (6 searchers). The team leader is not included in this number if he or she is working behind the baseline, which might be done if the number of searchers on the search line is large (closer to the limit of seven), like in this example. The word is either "compass" or "guide" and indicates what the team is using as the guide. The word is "compass" if the team is using a compass bearing for directional control and "guide" if the team is guiding on a linear feature such as a stream, road, ridgeline, or virtually anything other than a compass. "Left" or "right" can be added to the word "guide" to indicate which direction the search line should guide. The second number in the system describes the average between searcher track spacing in feet or meters. Note that this value indicates the *average* track spacing. Since the between-searcher distance may be dependent on the type of search (high or low coverage), the terrain, and the density of underbrush, the track spacing estimated before the search can easily vary once the team arrives in the segment.

The above example (6–guide [right]–30) describes a search with six searchers on the search line (and there may be one team leader behind the line), guiding right on something (as opposed to using a compass), with an average track spacing of 30 feet (9.1 meters).

This grid naming system has several advantages. It offers an easily recognized method of communicating the details of a search pattern so that field searchers can effectively communicate with search planners. It also provides an opportunity to estimate a search team's baseline width, which can be helpful in the field and in the command post.

This level of operational detail is rarely conveyed in the briefing and is usually left up to the search crew to determine, given the instructions from search planners in the briefing. For example, the search crew may be instructed only to conduct a high-coverage search, leaving the details of the specific search operation up to the search crew to determine. The search crew can then use this terminology to communicate accurately in the debriefing exactly how the segment was searched. Alternately, if the search planners wanted a specific type of search conducted, they could use this terminology to accurately communicate it to the field search crews in the briefing.

Skillful Searching

Experienced SAR personnel have developed certain practical techniques and guidelines for searching that have been found to be useful over the years.

Proper Attitude

It is essential that searchers stay alert and maintain the proper attitude for effective searching. Searching is hard work and can be boring, tedious, and fatiguing. You must be able to stay alert and maintain your usefulness during a search if you expect to be of any help at all. The only thing worse than not keeping alert is not keeping alert and doing nothing about it. Many find it useful to mentally talk to themselves, "telling" themselves what to do, as an effective way to maintain focus and alertness. ("Look behind that log. What's in that creek bed?") This also helps preclude the, "I'm cold; it's wet; how much longer?" type of thought patterns. You must be able to recognize at what point you stop being an effective searcher. Furthermore, you must assert yourself when this occurs,

BRIEFING AND DEBRIEFING CHECKLISTS

Briefing

1. Incident Action Plan - what is it and how I fit in
   - Organizational overview
2. Situation status, objectives, strategies, and predictions
3. Subject information/profile
   - Physical description and clothing worn and carried
   - Sole pattern of footwear, procure sketch/photo
   - Items/equipment carried
   - Trip plans, intended routes, favorite spots
   - Mental condition, behavioral traits
   - Circumstances surrounding search
4. Tactical assignments with explicit instructions
   - Procure briefing form, if possible
   - If area search, general level of coverage desired
5. Weather - present and forecast
6. Specific equipment needs
   - How long will you be in the field?
7. Communications details:
   - Frequencies/Talk Groups to be used
   - Phone numbers to call (provide yours, too)
   - Designators and codes
   - Contact persons and times
   - What to do if communications problems arise
   - Emergency communications (whistle?)
8. Transportation details (if needed)
9. Reporting locations and times
   - For transportation, debriefing, etc.
10. How to deal with media/family - where to refer
    - Identify who is family, friends, media
11. General terrain description and map of segment
12. How to handle discovered evidence/clues
    - Log, retrieve, photograph, mark, etc.
13. General hazards and safety instructions
    - Natural and manmade hazards, plants, animals, chemicals, illegal activity, aircraft, mines, caves, water features
    - What to do if someone becomes injured
    - Emergency signal?
    - What to watch out for
    - What to do if you discover illegal activity
14. Debriefing procedures:
    - Where, when, and with whom to debrief
    - Can GPS track be uploaded?
    - What info will be expected, needed, or required, and in what format (oral, written, sketches, maps, etc.)?
    - If a debriefing form is used, procure an example

Briefing should last less than 30 minutes and should be held before, not during, shift (operational period). A combination of written and oral briefings is most successful. *Take notes, ask questions, and get a map, if possible.*

Debriefing

1. Explicit description of search area covered (and not covered) and activities carried out during search
2. Range of detection measurements (Rd) or other estimate of sweep width for each subarea of the assigned segment
3. Report other field-observable measures identified and requested by search planners in briefing.
   - Upload GPS track, if available
4. Describe any hats or hoods worn during search. Explain.
5. Describe any precipitation, fog, or darkness encountered, and when.
6. Qualitative description of search (excellent, good, fair, poor). Explain.
7. Was team fatigued during search? Explain.
8. Estimate of forward speed of search unit (fast, normal, slow).
9. Exact amount of time in minutes spent searching
10. Location of any clues found, regardless of how insignificant they may seem
    - Show on map
    - Show photograph
    - GPS waypoint
11. Specific difficulties encountered in segment or any problems with the search at all. Explain.
    - Gaps in coverage
    - Severe weather; excessive heat or cold?
    - Fitness problems?
    - Illness or injuries?
    - Communications problems?
    - Caves, mines, water features, or cliffs discovered?
    - Inaccessible or impassable terrain or obstacles such as dense vegetation, fences, walls, etc.?
12. Hazards in the area? Be specific with respect to location and description.
13. Suggestions, recommendations, and ideas for further search activity in the segment?
14. Complete and submit any debriefing and ICS 214 forms.

Proper info conveyed in the debriefing is absolutely essential for an effective search. Use any means to convey what you want to say about the area searched. (sketches, maps, notes, photos, videos, GPS tracks, etc.)

Debriefing should be done in writing, if possible, perhaps using an open-ended questionnaire for personnel coming out of the field. All debriefings should be performed one-at-a-time, on an individual basis, if possible. However, team leaders could debrief their team members and someone in turn debrief the team leader.

The above list is a minimum.
Please feel free to copy this page (shrink it if necessary), laminate it, and carry it with you during a search.

FIGURE 15-14 Briefing/debriefing checklist.
Courtesy of Donald Cooper.

so that you can be replaced and given a chance to correct the problem. If you cannot discipline yourself to search effectively in less than ideal conditions (bad weather, cold, hot, tired, lack of success, etc.), then you should not participate in the search at all or at least reconsider your position.

Searcher Safety

The safety of the searchers is more important than the mission itself. You are more important than your partners, your partners are more important than the subject, and the subject is the reason why the search is underway. The subject is not the last priority; the subject is third in a long list of priorities. It may seem arrogant, but the above is always true. However, the searchers should be so confident and capable in their own skills and those of their partners that they can concentrate on the subject. When this confidence is lacking, searchers may have to move their focus away from the subject and back to themselves, which is never desirable.

SAFETY TIP

The safety of the searchers is more important than the mission itself.

Personnel Accountability Report

The term **personnel accountability report (PAR)** is borrowed from the fire service but is applicable to all emergency services. It is a roll call procedure usually initiated by a supervisor or an incident commander to confirm that all personnel are accounted for and safe. An important requirement for the procedure to work is that all personnel working at an incident must have checked in and are being tracked within their respective crews and assignments at the incident.

In practical use, using a radio or a mobile phone, a supervisor or incident commander would ask a crew leader for a PAR with a question such as, "Do you have PAR?" If the crew leader can immediately account for all assigned personnel, the appropriate response would be "I have PAR." If the crew leader must take a minute or two to account for his or her personnel, the response would be "stand by" as all personnel are accounted for, followed soon thereafter by the appropriate response. "Stand by" serves as a code word indicating a crew leader, or other supervisor, is requesting a couple more minutes to account for his or her personnel. A PAR request can also be effectively communicated via texting with a simple "PAR?" when asking for PAR, and a response of "PAR" when all personnel are accounted for. Some automatically text "PAR" to their supervisor once they arrive home safe after an operation. The supervisor then, in turn, notifies his or her supervisor in a similar fashion once all personnel under their supervision have sent a PAR text.

Two other related practices can also be useful in SAR operations. The term *Mayday* is used by pilots, as well as emergency service personnel, to indicate that the aircraft/individual is in distress. Typically, it is repeated three times, which is the universal radio distress signal (FAA, 2015). SAR personnel can also use this term to indicate an emergency, especially when communicating over the radio, but it must be established in team policy.

Another helpful practice for SAR personnel is the use of the phrase "emergency traffic," which is also borrowed from emergency services. When this phrase is announced over the radio, it indicates that the user has a critical, life safety-related message to convey. Upon hearing this phrase, every listener should immediately stop talking and yield the radio talk group or frequency to the person making the announcement. The response from the incident commander, or a designee, to hearing "emergency traffic" should be "emergency traffic, go ahead" followed by radio silence so the speaker can announce the urgent message. No other communications are authorized on that talk group/frequency until it is released by the incident commander.

Procedures vary from team to team and region to region. SAR personnel must be familiar with their local radio protocols, especially as they relate to emergency and urgent communications. None of these procedures will be useful if they are not integrated into operational policies and protocols at all levels. If they do not already exist, speak to your team leader(s) about developing these or similar protocols.

Be Prepared

Always take the Boy Scout motto to heart and "be prepared." Have the proper equipment and clothing with you so that you can be an asset rather than a detriment. Have a ready pack, know what is in it, and know how to use what it contains.

Searcher "Cube"

Scan the "searcher cube" while searching and while approaching the search segment. That is, look up and down, look left and right, and look forward and behind. This technique allows you to see things that might not be visible when merely looking forward. While approaching a segment, searching the searcher cube also allows the searcher to become familiar with the surrounding terrain so the return journey is easier.

SEARCH AND RESCUE TIP

Scan the "searcher cube" while searching and while approaching the search segment. That is, look up and down, look left and right, and look forward and behind.

Use All Senses

Use all sense organs for searching: your eyes, your nose, your ears, and most importantly, your head. Although human searchers are primarily visual searchers, they also possess several other senses that can be useful during a search. Sound has already been mentioned as an important element in searching, but the sense of smell is often overlooked in its potential for contributing to overall search efforts. Have you ever discovered something by smell, such as a decaying animal carcass or a freshly dropped pile of bear feces? Smell is a powerful and memorable resource that should not be overlooked while searching.

More important than any of the senses is one's ability to think and reason. The brain is what is used to recognize something that is relevant and important. The brain is also what is used to interpret the meaning of a clue and to recognize that something is out of place. Do not underestimate the power of thinking hard about what you see as a searcher.

Search for Clues and the Subject

Search for clues as well as the subject. There are many more clues than subjects. Clues can substantially decrease the search area and indicate where not to search further. A lack of clues can be just as important as a great number of them. Do not be discouraged if you know you are searching effectively, yet you have turned up nothing. This negative information is very important to search planning.

Use Sound and Listen

Yell and make noise occasionally, but intermix regular moments of silence so you can listen. Noise may attract or cause a response from a lost subject, and the silence permits you to hear the response and respond to it. This can be particularly effective when the subject is thought to be lost but responsive, which is often the case early in a search.

Know Your Surroundings

Constantly scan your surroundings. Know what is behind you and from where you came. Study what is ahead and how it may affect your search. Be constantly mindful of your location; within your segment, within the search crew, and on the map. Within the search organization, know to whom you answer and who answers to you. Know your responsibilities within the search crew and the responsibilities of those working with you.

Learn the names of the searchers on either side of you in a line search, and remember what color and type of clothing they are wearing. Know if those people change their outer layer of clothing, and inform them if you change yours. Searchers wearing brightly colored clothing are important during searches. Camouflage is unacceptable to wear during a search.

Always Check the Obvious

Use common sense and talk to hikers you run into, check buildings and caves, and ask people in the area if they have seen anything. More than one search has ended when the subject was found helping in the search.

Dealing with the Media

A field searcher has no reason to be talking with the subject's family or the media unless he or she has been assigned to do so. The proper way to handle the inquiry is to refer the individual to the incident commander or the appropriate responsible personnel. For the same reasons, there should be no loose talk in or around the incident site. Think what you want, but speak only after thinking. Complaints about the mission should be made in private to one's supervisor or saved for the post-mission critique.

Scanning

Experience and experiments have taught us the errors in search technique that can reduce the effectiveness of searching (Koester et al., 2004).

The most successful searchers walk a short distance, stop, and then perform a thorough scan in all directions (the searcher cube). Research shows that a searcher's ability to make detections appears to be higher when stopped than when in motion. Searchers should therefore use this "stop and scan" technique, which should include looking behind frequently, as much as possible.

Visual scanning should be done out to the farthest distance possible, regardless of distractions and obstacles.

Research shows that many searchers limit their scanning due to foliage that screens their view and distractions that focus their attention on one or two places rather than the entire search lane. To avoid these mistakes, searchers should:

1. Try to scan past and through the first trees and foliage encountered. Do not let foliage prevent you from looking through gaps between trees and past screens that only partially obscure what is beyond them.
2. Regroup and scan after a distraction such as crossing a log, jumping over a creek, or crawling over a fence. Recognize when a distraction occurs, then stop and scan before continuing.
3. Get low, if needed, and look under close-in obstacles or screens. Do whatever you can to scan into the furthest reaches of the search lane.
4. While searching, treat talking—on the radio, with other searchers, etc.—as any other distraction. When recognized as a distraction, stop and scan. Avoid unnecessary talking while searching.
5. Use corrected vision. If corrective lenses are needed to better focus on close and/or distant objects, wear them when searching.

Some people see color differently than what most people see, and the most severe of these deficiencies are referred to as color blindness. Color blindness causes those affected by it not to see differences in color, and many are not aware they have it. This can have a significant effect on search effectiveness in that a color-blind searcher may not be able to tell the difference between a fluorescent orange jacket and the green foliage around it. There are three different kinds of color blindness, but the red-green deficiency type (deuteranope) is the most common. Men are most often affected by it—about 8% of the population—but 0.5% of women are also afflicted (NIH NEI, 2017). Searchers with color blindness should inform their supervisors and teammates.

Encountering Illegal Activities

During SAR field operations, personnel may encounter suspicious or illegal activities such as drug smuggling, human trafficking, illegal marijuana growing operations, alcohol stills, methamphetamine labs, and chemical dumping sites. Each of these situations is accompanied by unique hazards, and many may involve armed individuals or booby traps. Some involve hazardous chemicals that can be caustic, poisonous, flammable, or have the potential to explode.

Field personnel should be constantly vigilant regarding the potential for this type of threat, and if these or similar threats are recognized, they should immediately stop their task and retreat to a position of safety, inform their teammates, report it to the incident commander, and follow local policies and procedures.

Searcher Fatigue

Fatigue is a natural physiological reaction to prolonged physical and/or mental stress. It can be caused from long periods of work, any amount of hard work, lack of sleep, disrupted sleep, environmental stress (e.g., heat, cold), poor fitness level, age, and physiological causes such as dehydration. Fatigue may be the number one contributor to human error (Dupont, 2009).

SAFETY TIP

Fatigue may be the number one contributor to human error and can affect the human body much the same as being intoxicated.

In SAR, fatigue may have numerous and significant effects on personnel. It can impair and reduce judgment, decision-making, reaction time, ability to communicate, physical capabilities, memory, focus, and attention span. In short, it can affect the human body much the same as being intoxicated. For searchers, fatigue can reduce clue awareness and dramatically affect muscular coordination, which can make traveling across difficult terrain dangerous. Thus, searching while fatigued may do more harm than good.

It is important that personnel are aware of the signs and symptoms of fatigue—in themselves and others. The prevention and mitigation of fatigue requires regular sleep, healthy diet (including reduced use of alcohol and other drugs), and regular exercise. Searchers must never arrive on the scene already fatigued. Fatigued individuals must recognize and acknowledge fatigue in themselves and decline to participate in a search, if invited. Doing otherwise endangers everyone, including the subject and other searchers who may be further endangered should they have to rescue you.

Circadian rhythms are physical, mental, and behavioral changes that follow a roughly 24-hour cycle, usually related to exposure of humans to light and dark (NIH NIGMS, 2017). Some scientists suggest that work of a critical and complex nature is not recommended during the low point on the body's circadian rhythm (usually 3:00–5:00 a.m.), and work performed while fatigued should always be checked by another (Dupont, 2009).

As a final thought on the subject, consider the tragic line-of-duty death of 24-year old Lisa Hannon on May 3, 1994. In college at the University of Virginia,

Lisa joined the Blue Ridge Mountain Rescue Group, a member group of the Appalachian Search and Rescue Conference (ASRC), where she worked through the ranks until becoming an ASRC and Virginia State certified incident commander. On May 2, 1994, Lisa was requested by the Virginia Department of Emergency Services to help with a search for a 5-year-old boy that had been underway for three days in the mountains of Hampshire County, near the town of Kirby, West Virginia. Lisa worked throughout the day and night to build a well-run incident organization that coordinated all Virginia SAR resources and eventually included over 1,000 personnel. At 8:00 a.m. on May 3, 1994, after 23 hours without sleep, Lisa left the base on her way to her afternoon job near Washington, DC. Twenty minutes later, while driving on Route 50, her truck hit a tree, and she was killed instantly. She is believed to have fallen asleep (ASRC, 2017). Please use this unfortunate incident as a poignant reminder of the importance of the recognition and mitigation of fatigue and its potential, and of a young life well lived in the service of others.

Night Searching

Night searching can be effective and done safely with the proper equipment, but the benefits of searching at night must be balanced with the safety of searchers. In bad weather and difficult or unfamiliar terrain, search planners may emphasize indirect tactics that are effective at night over direct area searches. Night searching can have advantages, however:

- It is quieter at night and sound carries better.
- The subject is likely stationary at night.
- The light source and angle of light can be controlled at night, which for visual searchers has advantages when looking for small items on the ground such as tracks and small evidence.
- Some search resources may be more effective at night, for example, searchers using night vision goggles (NVGs), infrared devices such as forward-looking infrared (FLIR) and thermal imagers, and dog teams. Human eyes do adapt to low light, but it may take 30 minutes or so for full night vision.
- Subjects are often located at night by searchers who first detect the subject's flashlight, light from a fire/stove, or light from an illuminated cell phone. Searchers should recognize this possibility and search beyond the light of their search light.

Due to the anatomy of the eyes and how they work, it is best to view an object at night through peripheral vision and by moving your eyes in short, abrupt, irregular movements over and around the target without actually looking directly at it (Perkins and Roberts, 2009). Because human searchers are primarily visual searchers, lighting is important for night searches. Two types of lights are needed: one for personal use (usually a headlamp), and one for searching (usually a handheld light with a powerful beam). Searcher discipline is important because one moment of shining a light in a searcher's eyes can significantly impair night vision. Thus, lights should be used sparingly, which also extends the life of batteries.

At night, never shine your flashlight or headlamp into your eyes or those of other searchers. It takes quite a while to adjust one's eyes to the dark again. Sometimes not using lights at all is preferred if safety and effectiveness can be maintained.

Difficulties of traveling across terrain are worsened by darkness, so night searching requires more attention to travel safety than during daylight. This means that night searching is generally more difficult, less searching may be accomplished in the same amount of time, and searcher fatigue occurs at a faster rate.

Due to the challenges presented by area searching at night, the safest use of search resources at night may be:

- In and directly around buildings, shelters, vehicles, and specific points of interest that can be well lit
- On trails, paths, and roads where foot travel is unobstructed
- On boundaries, fences, garden walls, breaks in vegetation, and edges of vegetation transitions
- On roadside ditches where safe travel on the adjacent road is possible.

Perkins and Roberts (2009) from the United Kingdom suggest a method of night searching on trails that has been found effective and is similar to that which is used in Koester (2009) in New Zealand. The authors suggest lining up a group of five searchers on a trail using search lights as follows:

- The lead searcher navigates for the group and illuminates the path ahead while announcing information about the terrain and hazards.
- The second and third searchers illuminate the ground close to the trail, each on a different side.
- The last two searchers illuminate the ground at a distance from the trail, each on a different side.

With some practice, and perhaps some experimentation, the distance at which one's search light can be used to detect a subject can be determined. This distance effectively establishes the width of one's search lane, can be used to help establish track spacing during the search, and should be communicated at the debriefing.

The following standards include requirements for search operations and are recommended reading for SAR personnel who may be involved in search operations:

- ASTM F1633, Standard Guide for Techniques in Land Search (ASTM, 2017)
- NFPA 1670, Standard on Operations and Training for Technical Search and Rescue Incidents (NFPA, 2017a)
- NFPA 1006, Standard for Technical Rescue Personnel Professional Qualifications (NFPA, 2017b)

Anatomy of a SAR Incident

The elements of the SAR Incident Cycle (preplanning/preparation, notification [first notice], check-in, briefing, tactics/operations [assignments], debriefing, check out, and critique) are used to illustrate what SAR personnel should be doing at these various benchmarks. The details of this process are extremely important to the searcher because the process may not be explained at the scene of a SAR incident. Arriving with an understanding of how the overall process works, from before the call-out to the post-mission critique, is a distinct advantage for everyone involved.

Preplanning and Preparation

Preplanning to a searcher means having the skills, knowledge, and equipment ready to perform in a SAR incident, as well as being physically and mentally prepared. SAR personnel must know before an incident what may be expected of them. They must understand the standards by which they will be measured.

Equipment

Proper equipment must be ready for use at the first notice of an incident. Different areas and environments require different equipment. Knowledge of what is needed—both generally and specifically—is imperative. Equipment must be ready for use and not require collection or repair at the time of call-out.

Self

Through study and experience, SAR personnel must possess an understanding of the fundamental information that is necessary to perform safely, efficiently, and effectively at an incident. Everyone must be fully prepared educationally, emotionally, physically, and mentally for the rigors of a SAR incident. One's attitude is the capstone on the well-rounded field operator.

The searcher must be physically up to the challenges presented by most SAR incidents. Anything else shows a lack of planning and preparedness. The searcher must be mentally prepared to endure the strain of boredom, fatigue, and discomfort while maintaining an attitude of urgency and optimism for the cause. A searcher who responds to an incident in which he or she does not want to be involved should stay home. A searcher must want to search and be ready to do so at any time. The credo for SAR personnel should be, "be prepared," before a call-out occurs.

First Notice

First notice is the initial notification of responders to a SAR incident. First notice should really be broken into two distinct parts:

1. First notice of incident
2. First personnel notice (call-out)

First notice of incident usually involves an individual in some official capacity (but not necessarily) to whom a lost or missing person(s) is reported. The report could be from relatives or friends, from a member of a party that recognizes a person is missing, by the discovery of evidence or clues (e.g., abandoned vehicle, registration system, deserted camp or equipment), distress signals, emergency locator transmitter, and the like. This type of notification usually involves some organization that the public believes has the authority and/or responsibility for SAR by way of an individual who represents that authority.

First personnel notice involves calling SAR resources to initiate a search and/or rescue. If further assistance is required, the one who takes the initial report must contact the appropriate personnel to effect further action. An individual SAR resource (searcher, rescuer, etc.) will be notified if he or she is needed, and this is termed *call-out*.

Both types of first notice are important to SAR personnel because any one person might be called upon to take the initial report or to respond to help. When an initial report of a problem is received, a chain of events begins that can determine the entire course of the SAR event.

Notice of Incident

Initial contact (whether by phone, radio, or in person) is made by the person or persons reporting a problem. The impression that the report taker gives the reporting party and the initial actions that are taken often set the tone for the rest of the mission. If the report comes into an agency (such as a sheriff's office, park service, or fire service), the degree of professionalism and responsiveness may affect future missions as well. The most important initial considerations by the initial report taker should include the following:

- *The attitude of the report taker/interviewer.* The report taker should remain calm and professional, be inquisitive, have a tone of concern, and express a willingness to help.
- *The name and call-back telephone number and location of the reporting party.* The reporting party should be told to remain there until told to do otherwise.
- *Urgency.* This is not disorganized haste but directed, efficient, planned, and coordinated action.

The report taker/interviewer must sort out the initial information offered by the reporting party for importance and relevance while also attempting to acquire specific information that must be collected immediately for effective decision making. Formats for the specific information required can be found in sections A through E of the missing person questionnaire (Appendix A, first notice information). Once this information is collected, a search planner/manager can enter it into an urgency determination form, and the relative urgency can be determined.

The initial report taker/interviewer must now evaluate the information received in a calm, intelligent manner for subsequent action. This is also the time when a trained search manager should be involved. A trained search manager will want to interview the reporting party in person, evaluate the initial information, determine the reliability of the sources, consider the facts, consider the probabilities, consider the possibilities, and then combine the information objectively before acting further. This might also be where a search manager begins to call-out initial resources.

One of the first actions of a trained search manager in an interview is to request more information about the lost subject(s), and this is where the initial report taker (management trained or not) can begin filling out the missing person questionnaire (MPQ; see Appendix A). All questions on the MPQ should be filled in, if possible, leaving no blank spots for someone later to have to guess whether the question was ever asked.

The following is a general summary of what should be determined during the initial reporting of an incident:

1. Is there a problem?
2. How serious is it or could it get?
3. Where is the problem?
4. Who and how many is/are involved?
5. How did it happen?
6. When did it happen?

Information should be compiled so it can be used to make decisions about what is to be done.

If a trained search manager is not available, the report taker may have to interview the reporting party directly to collect enough information to initiate the search. Physical evidence may also be brought to the attention of the interviewer, which requires that it be properly collected or protected, interpreted, and documented so that the chain of custody is maintained (see *Handling Evidence* in Chapter 14). Using at least sections A through E of the missing person questionnaire (Appendix A) as a guide is helpful and is the perfect place to document responses to questions. As the missing person questionnaire is completed, it can serve as the basis of a subject profile.

Personnel Call-Out

For searchers, the initial call-out is the process by which they are notified that their services are needed. Certain information must be acquired from the notifying source so that the individual whose services have been requested can make an efficient and effective response. This checklist identifies what minimum information should be available to the resource being requested:

- Description of the situation (abbreviated), who is in charge (individual or organization), and who is making the call-out (name of person you are talking to and call-back number)
- Description of terrain, weather, weather forecast, and elevation range where you will be involved
- Length of time needed (best guess will do) and length of time available
- Special equipment (personal or team) needed
- Map? Of where? What type, scale, etc.?
- Meeting place (check-in) as well as detailed directions (signs, suggested route, markers, how long should it take, etc.)
- The name of the person to whom searchers should report upon arrival
- Any other pertinent information

Certain information must be offered to the notifying source so that they know what advantages or limitations an individual's (or organization's) involvement may carry. For example:

- How long are you available (minutes, hours, days, or months)?
- What equipment do you (or don't you) have?
- What are your physical limitations (handicaps, conditioning, injuries, etc.)?

- Do you need transportation, or can you supply it?
- Describe training limitations (especially if your training differs from what is expected).
- Any other pertinent information that is requested of you.

Check-In

Once the call-out procedures have taken place, all SAR personnel must travel to the reporting location and check in. The type of check-in required (formal versus informal) varies depending on the complexity and size of the incident; it may be verbal or may require checking-in on a form such as an ICS 211, which is highly recommended. Regardless of the method, check-in is an essential accountability element that is necessary to maintain a safe working environment. Insist that your presence be documented and tracked, even if that service does not appear to be offered.

Briefing

After check-in and general assignments have been made, briefing takes place so that specific task assignments can be made (**FIGURE 15-15**). The **briefing** is a summary of the situation, past and present, conveyed by those who know to those who need to know. It provides information that helps orient personnel to all facets of the problem (safety, strategic, environmental, and tactical). A general briefing usually occurs initially when an individual is first indoctrinated at an incident and may be repeated when the incident management team changes shift. The purpose of a briefing is simply to convey necessary information to the personnel who need it.

Another type of briefing is assignment specific; that is, it involves the description of a particular task assignment. This assignment briefing takes place prior to every assignment that is made.

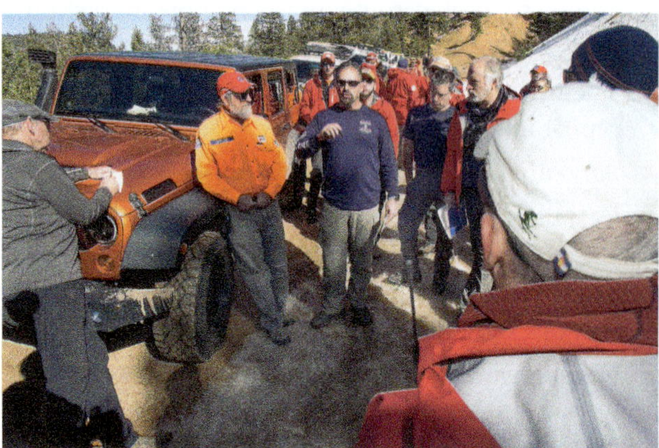

FIGURE 15-15 Before field deployment, briefing is necessary to convey to searchers what they need to know before going into the field.

The term *briefing* is used whenever information is conveyed from the top of a hierarchy down to the ranks. Getting "briefed" basically means learning from superiors the details of the tasks you are expected to do. Briefing is just the information that searchers need to know.

The planning section chief (ICS function) or a member of his/her staff is usually responsible for briefing. Team leaders are usually briefed, but entire teams may be briefed together in certain situations. Where team leaders are briefed, they in turn brief their teams. In larger incidents, the planning section chief may delegate briefing to a subordinate.

All SAR personnel should be aware of certain characteristics of a briefing:

- A briefing should be performed prior to a search shift (operational period) rather than during it.
- A briefing should last less than 30 minutes—far less is better—and should be in both oral and written formats, if possible.
- Short, as opposed to lengthy, briefings maintain a high morale and the credibility of SAR personnel and ensure a timely response to the field.
- Notes should be taken, and instructions should be repeated back to the briefer to ensure accuracy. It is important to ensure that the information is conveyed and understood.
- Briefings should take place in a designated area, with plenty of room. That is, the area should be sheltered, quiet, and free from interruptions and distractions.

Ideally, much of the specific information needed in a briefing is included on an assignment list form (ICS 204) or a task assignment form, and it is provided to search crew leaders. It can also be helpful for an individual or team to design or procure a briefing checklist (see Figure 15-14) to ensure that at least the most important issues are covered in a briefing. As a minimum, such a checklist should be based on the following information:

- *Incident action plan.* Procure a copy, if possible, including an organizational overview showing where you fit into the organization, who answers to you (if anyone), and to whom you answer.
- *Situation status, objectives, strategies, and predictions.* This includes what is happening now, what may happen later, and what we want to happen.
- *Subject information.* This includes a complete physical description, sole pattern of footwear (photo or sketch is helpful), clothing and items/equipment description (carried and worn), physical and mental condition, behavioral traits, circumstances surrounding the search, medical/health problems of the subject, trip

plans, intended routes, favorite spots, etc. Photos are helpful.

- *Tactical assignments with explicit instructions.* Know exactly where and how to search.
  - Specific area, where to start, and how to get there (copy of map).
  - Team configuration.
  - Procedures for handling discovered clues or evidence.
  - Adjacent teams and their location(s).
  - Have other teams searched the area?
  - When to start and stop, and what to do if an area is not finished when you are supposed to return.
  - Instructions for subject contact: what to do if the subject(s) is found dead, injured, or well. Make sure the rescue/evacuation plan is understood.
  - Instructions for protecting the scene, if necessary.
- *Current and forecast weather in the assigned search segment.*
- *Equipment needed by searchers.* Examples include specific clothing, safety equipment, food and water, camera, medical gear, climbing gear, and radios.
  - How long will you be in the field?
- *Communication details.* These include frequencies/talk groups to be used, phone numbers to call (provide yours to the briefer), designators and codes, contact person and times, communications failure procedures, emergency communications procedures (whistle?).
- *Transportation details.* How do you get where you are supposed to be: who will take you, and how?
- *Reporting detail.* These include reporting locations; times; and where, when, and to whom to report.
- *How to handle external influences such as the media and the subject's family and friends, should they be encountered.* Identify who is family, friends, and media, as well as where to refer them.
- *General terrain description and map of the assigned segment.*
- *Precisely how to handle and report discovered evidence or clues* (e.g., log, retrieve, mark, photograph).
- *Description of general hazards in the segment, ideally marked on map, with safety instructions.* These include dealing with human-made hazards (helo, aircraft, fuels, etc.), terrain hazards, and natural hazards (snakes, dogs, poisonous plants, other animals, etc.).
  - What do you do if someone becomes injured? Stay with them, go get help, or use the radio?
  - What should you watch out for?
  - What should you do if . . .?
  - Illegal activity?
  - Precise debriefing procedures.
  - Where, when, and with whom to debrief.
- *What information is required and in what format* (oral, written, sketches, maps, etc.)?
- *If a debriefing form is used, procure an example.*

Assignment

Once the briefing has been completed, it is time to carry out the assignment described in the briefing.

Individual Responsibilities

While on assignment, an individual has certain responsibilities that bear directly on the effectiveness and safety of him/herself and his/her crew. Search crews can vary in size but should meet ICS doctrine for span of control, which dictates that five be the rule of thumb for maximum unit size, but up to seven is permitted. Within that unit, certain obligations must be met, and it should be the job of all crew members to see that their responsibilities are carried out.

- All members of the search crew must have their own personal gear and should not be dependent on anyone else for equipment. "Have your own and carry your own" should be the credo.
- All crew members should be dressed properly for the terrain and environment in which they will be involved. Everyone should have appropriate back-up clothing where necessary.
- All crew members should be physically and mentally prepared to perform difficult search and rescue operations and not depend on it being an easy day.
- Skills and skill limitations should be immediately relayed to the crew leader. Nothing should be assumed.

Team Responsibilities

Every crew should immediately assign, before deployment into the field, at least one member to the following responsibilities: navigator, tally, time keeper, and crew leader. A crew leader may be assigned before the group is put together because every crew must have a leader.

Even though every member of a crew should always know where they are (geographically and with respect to the search area), one member should be assigned as navigator so that everyone can check his or her accuracy.

A "tally" (distance measurer) is one who, by some method (usually stride), keeps track of distance traveled with relationship to the baseline and segment boundaries.

The time keeper maintains a chronology, in writing, of what goes on and the time it happens during the operational period. Documenting everything is always a good idea. A team may assign one individual to do all the writing, especially if someone takes shorthand or finds it easier than others to write while on the move.

Any job that the crew leader deems necessary should be assigned before going into the field because an individual may need time to prepare. Remember that, in addition to everything else, a searcher must search and search well. If you have a problem with anything to which you have been assigned, speak up. Perhaps you can be reassigned.

Debriefing

After a field assignment is completed, debriefing is necessary for the extraction of pertinent information from field SAR personnel (**FIGURE 15-16**). **Debriefing** is the transfer of information from field personnel to the search management team after an assignment has been completed. The purpose of debriefing is to convey as much of the relevant information as possible to the search management team. Management's purpose is to extract the information from the field personnel. Without thorough information, subsequent planning can be misdirected, improper, inadequate, and incomplete. The term *debriefing* is used whenever information is conveyed from subordinates to supervisors in a hierarchy. Simply put, debriefing is the acquisition of information that management needs from field personnel.

The following are general guidelines regarding debriefing:

- The planning section chief (ICS function), or his/her equivalent, is responsible for seeing that an adequate debriefing is performed, but coordination of the debriefing is usually handled by a member of the planning section.
- The team leader may debrief his/her team and then, in turn, be debriefed; eventually, all field personnel should be debriefed.

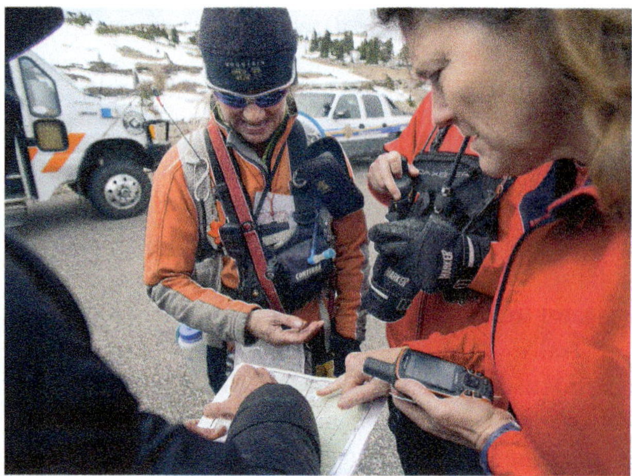

FIGURE 15-16 After a field search assignment is completed, debriefing is necessary for the collection of relevant information by search planners from field SAR personnel.

- The debriefing of field personnel should be done on an individual basis, rather than two or three at a time, and it should take place as soon as possible after an individual (or team) exits the field.
- Debriefing should be done in writing, if possible. Written information reduces confusion and misunderstanding and can easily become part of the final documentation of the incident.

All pertinent information should be solicited and conveyed during a debriefing, including the following list. Refer also to the briefing and debriefing checklists found in Figure 15-14.

- Include explicit and complete descriptions of the search areas covered (and not covered) and activities carried out during search.
- Note range of detection measurements (Rd) for each segment and, if needed, the specific subarea of the assigned segment (see Figure 15-13).
- Report any other field observations identified and requested by search planners in the briefing.
- Describe any hats or hoods worn during the search. Explain.
- Describe any precipitation, fog, or darkness encountered during the search and when.
- Include a qualitative description of the search (excellent, good, fair, or poor). Explain.
- Note whether any members of the search crew were fatigued during the search. Explain.
- Estimate the forward speed of the search unit (fast, normal, or slow).
- Note the exact amount of time spent searching, excluding rest breaks and traveling to and from the segment.
- Note the exact location of any clues located, regardless of how insignificant they may seem (use maps, sketches, etc., to convey location).
  - Show on map and describe GPS waypoint, if possible
- Note specific difficulties encountered, such as gaps in coverage, terrain problems, communication problems, weather difficulties, physical fitness or illness, or injuries.
- If there were hazards encountered in the area, be specific with respect to the location and description.
- Include suggestions, recommendations, and ideas for further activity in the segment.
- Complete and submit any debriefing and ICS 214 (Unit Log) forms at the debriefing.

SAR personnel should use any and every method of conveying information. Sketches, maps, photos, briefing reports (assignment forms), notes, etc., may all be of value. Proper information conveyed in the debriefing is essential for an effective search and can be the most important part of an operation.

SEARCH AND RESCUE TIP

Proper information conveyed in the debriefing is absolutely essential for an effective search and can be the most important part of an operation.

Check-Out

Once SAR personnel have performed their duties, they are released from the incident and allowed to "check out." This is an important step that includes at least two parts:

1. An evaluation of the individual to confirm that he or she is healthy, rested, and has appropriate transportation
2. An accounting for the individual that documents his or her departure

The level of formality varies depending on the complexity and size of the incident, but precise check-out and demobilization details should be acquired at the incident briefing or debriefing. At check-out, a final accounting is made of all field personnel. If a formal critique is planned, details (such as when and where) can be relayed at this time.

The responsibility for the safety of SAR personnel does not end at check-out. It ends when all SAR personnel have safely arrived at their intended destinations. SAR personnel should not hesitate to request assistance or transportation if they are too tired to drive home on their own. Tragedies have occurred when fatigued SAR personnel have attempted to return home on their own after many hours of rigorous operations (ASRC, 2017).

Return to Service

It is useful to begin mentally preparing for returning to response-ready status even before checking out of the current incident. This usually involves two steps: finishing up current involvement with the incident, and returning everything to full mission-ready status.

First, make sure all paperwork and physical work is done for the present mission. Consider the following:

- Debriefing forms finished?
- Checked-out?
- Injury claim forms filled out?
- Expendable supplies used?
- Personal supplies that need to be reimbursed?
- Can you do anything to help others get back into service?
- Does the incident management team need any help demobilizing?
- Can you help in any way at all?
- What expendable gear needs to be replaced? Replace, replenish, and clean all gear and equipment so it is ready for its next use, which could be at any time).
- What food and/or water must be replaced?
- Batteries?
- Medical supplies?
- Does gear need to be cleaned?
- Does clothing need to be cleaned?
- Did you lose anything?
- Did you break anything?
- Did anyone borrow anything from you?
- Did you borrow anything that needs to be returned?

Rest, eat, drink, and return your body to full mission-ready status.

Maintaining a Personal Search Mission Log

SAR personnel should maintain a personal "search mission log" (see Appendix C for an example). This log should, as a minimum, contain the date and time of your involvement in a SAR mission and a description of the details of your involvement (functions performed, positions held, etc.). It is also a good idea to have your mission supervisor sign the log to validate your documented actions during the mission. Not only can such a log help track your experience, it can also help document your actions should questions arise later.

Some SAR organizations require the maintenance of such logs. For example, The SAR Program of the Commonwealth of Virginia Department of Emergency Services requires documentation of a certain amount of experience before becoming certified as a ground SAR incident commander. A mission log validated by your team leader is permitted to satisfy this requirement.

Mission Critique

Participating in the mission critique, also called the incident debriefing or after-action review, is an opportunity to help ensure that mistakes made are not repeated and that things that were done right are noted. Make sure that you have made your ideas and problems known before you leave, and offer a constructive critique rather than a destructive one. Be aware that some management teams include a brief critique at the end of each assignment. In these cases, no incident critique may be performed.

A formal critique of any SAR incident, no matter how large or small, should always be attempted as soon as possible after the incident. Although trying to accomplish this before everyone goes home may not be possible, some information can be gleaned by performing a "hot wash." A hot wash is an after-action discussion and evaluation of one or more organization's performance immediately following an operation, exercise, or training session. A more formal incident debriefing and critique may follow, but a hot wash allows information to be collected while it is fresh in the minds of those who participated. Whether a formal debriefing or a hot wash, the exercise is intended to identify the lessons learned and is not for placing blame, pointing fingers, or allowing adversaries to embarrass each other. The participation of all involved SAR personnel is encouraged and may be required.

It is the responsibility of the SAR manager to provide for an effective critique of the entire search operation, but often an individual must make the right noises to provoke action. It is especially important to hold a critique when a subject was not found. For a team or an organization, a critique can help to review, revise, and improve the preplan. For the individual, it can help identify opportunities for improvement on a personal level.

An individual's critique of himself or herself should include at least the following:

- What gear did I need that I did not have (personal, team)?
- How long did it take for me to mobilize? Could it be done better next time?
- What particular skills do I need to work on (navigation, search technique, wilderness travel, physical condition, etc.)?
- How can I improve myself?

The purpose of a mission critique should be to identify why and how the search occurred and how it could have been prevented, and to assess the effectiveness and efficiency of one's involvement in the operation. The questions are: what went right, what went wrong, and why? What can you, as an individual resource involved in the operation, do to improve not only your response and actions but also those of your team and the entire operation? If you see something that would have made the operation run better, do something about it and mention it to someone who can effect change.

Wrap-Up

READY FOR REVIEW

- Tactics are important to field personnel because they are the methods by which search and rescue (SAR) team members get physically involved with the search function.
- Indirect tactics do not involve physically entering and moving through the search area to look for the subject or clues. Specific tactics include fact finding (investigation), attraction, and containment.
- Direct tactics include all organized methods used to move through the search area to detect a lost subject or clues. Generally, there are three primary types: rapid (hasty) searches and two types of area searches, high-coverage search and low-coverage search.
- It is essential that searchers stay alert and maintain the proper attitude for effective searching.
- The safety of the searchers is more important than the mission itself. You are more important than your partners, your partners are more important than the subject, and the subject is the reason why the search is happening.
- A personnel accountability report (PAR) is a roll call procedure usually initiated by a supervisor or incident commander to confirm that all personnel are accounted for and safe.
- Use all sense organs for searching: your eyes, your nose, your ears, and most importantly, your head. Although human searchers are primarily visual searchers, they also possess several other senses that can be useful during a search.
- Know what is behind you and from where you came. Study what is ahead and how it may affect your search. Be constantly mindful of your location; within your segment, within the search crew, and on the map. Know your responsibilities within the search crew and the responsibilities of those working with you.
- The proper way to handle inquiries from the subject's friends or family or the media is to refer the individual to the incident commander or the appropriate responsible personnel.

- The most successful searchers walk a short distance, stop, and then perform a thorough scan in all directions (the searcher cube).
- Night searching can be effective and done safely with the proper equipment, but the benefits of searching at night must be balanced with the safety of searchers.
- The details of the SAR incident cycle process are extremely important to the searcher because the process may not be explained at the scene of a SAR incident.
  - Preplanning/preparation
  - Notification (first notice)
  - Check-in
  - Briefing
  - Tactics/operations (assignments)
  - Debriefing
  - Check-out
  - Critique

SEARCH AND RESCUE TERMS

Area search When a bounded segment of the search area is searched in an organized manner by a specific resource.

Back stop The linear feature bounding the far side of the segment that defines the endpoint of one search pass and serves as the baseline of the return search lanes.

Baseline A line, perpendicular to the direction of travel, on which searchers line up to begin their search.

Briefing Exchange of information, usually at the onset of a situation, that conveys important knowledge from the upper levels of a hierarchy to the lower, that is, information from the incident commander conveyed to a field team before they begin their assignment (Taylor and Cooper, 2014). A summary of the situation, past and present, conveyed by those who know to those who need to know and that provides information that helps orient personnel to all facets of the problem.

Confinement see *Containment*.

Containment Steps taken to ensure that the subject does not leave the search area; also called *confinement*.

Continuous limited search (CLS) An indirect, last resort search technique in which the use of any direct tactics in the search area are suspended, but the incident management team may opt to continue the investigation and/or use the area for regular training purposes.

Debriefing Exchange of information, usually at the close of a situation, that conveys important knowledge and experience from the lower levels of a hierarchy to the upper; that is, information conveyed to the incident commander from a field team after completing an assignment (Taylor and Cooper, 2014).

Decision points Locations, usually on linear features such as trails, paths, and roads, where the subject had to decide which path or road to take.

Direct tactics Tactics that include all organized methods used to move through the search area to detect a lost subject or clues.

First notice The initial notification of responders to a search and rescue incident.

Guide line A linear feature, parallel to the search track, to which a searcher refers for guidance regarding the general direction of the search track; also called *control line*.

Guide person The searcher on the search line who provides guidance regarding the general direction of the search track. On guide right situations, this person is on the right of the search line and guides on a feature to his or her right. On guide left situations, this person is on the left of the search line and guides on a feature to his or her left. On guide center situations, this person is in or near the middle of the search line.

High-coverage search A systematic area search, accomplished by searchers usually lining up on a baseline at relatively small between-searcher track spacing, with the goal of spending enough time and resources in a segment to achieve a relatively high coverage. The coverage achieved is often equal to or greater than 0.5.

Indirect tactics Tactics that do not involve physically moving through the search area to detect lost subjects or clues. Examples include fact finding (investigation), attraction, containment, and continuous limited search.

Low-coverage search A systematic area search, accomplished by searchers usually lining up on a baseline at relatively wide between-searcher track spacing, with the goal of covering larger geographic segments with fewer resources in a relatively short period of time. The coverage achieved is often less than 0.5.

Personnel accountability report (PAR) A roll call procedure usually initiated by a supervisor or incident commander to confirm that all personnel are accounted for and safe.

Range of detection (Rd) The linear distance at which a search object is first detected when moving toward it from multiple angles (Koester et al., 2014).

Rapid (hasty) search Quickly looking for the search object along likely routes of travel, along linear geographical features, or in high probability locations; also called *initial reflex search* (NSARC, 2011).

Scenarios Consistent sets of known facts and assumptions describing what may have happened to the survivors (search subjects) (NSARC, 2011).

Search area The area, determined by the search planner, that is to be searched. This area may be subdivided into search subareas for the purpose of assigning specific responsibilities to the available search facilities (IMO/ICAO, 2016). This area includes the smallest area, consistent with all available information, which contains all possible search object locations and, therefore, includes all regions and segments that are consistent with a particular scenario. The search area may be divided into regions based on the probable scenarios and into segments for the purpose of assigning specific tasks to the available search resources.

Search lane The area an individual searcher is assigned to scan during a search.

Search line A series of searchers forming a line to conduct an area search.

Search object A ship, aircraft, or other craft missing or in distress, or survivors or related search objects or evidence for which a search is being conducted (IMO/ICAO, 2016). A generic term used to indicate the lost subject or evidence (clues) related to a lost subject. A live human search object is often referred to as a search subject.

Search speed The average rate of travel (speed over the ground) of searchers while engaged in search operations within a segment (Cooper and Frost, 1999).

Search subject The person being searched for, commonly referred to as the "subject." Searches focusing primarily on the discovery of objects as opposed to persons (e.g., aircraft or vessels) commonly use the term *search object*.

Search track The general line of travel a searcher or search line takes through the search area during a search.

Segment A delineated portion or subset of the search area bounded and sized to be searchable by assigned facilities (NSARC, 2011). Segments and their boundaries are based on factors that affect the searchers, and the search planner determines the size of a segment. The boundaries of a segment are identifiable both in the field and on a map and are based on suitability for assigning search resources, not probability of the search object's location.

Sensors Human senses (sight, hearing, touch, etc.), those of specially trained animals (such as dogs), or electronic devices used to detect the object of a search (IMO/ICAO, 2016). A human, multisensor platform is often referred to as a "searcher."

Sound sweep An effective search technique that combines a sound attraction tactic with the direct tactic of wide-spaced grid searching. The use of sound, typically whistle blasts, is closely choreographed with simultaneous blasts followed by a uniform listening period for subject response. The use of this technique presumes a responsive subject and, thus, is most effectively utilized in the early stages of a search (NSARC, 2011).

Sweep width A measure of the effectiveness with which a particular sensor can detect a particular object under specific environmental conditions (IMO/ICAO, 2016); a measure of detectability. Sweep width depends on the characteristics of the search object, the sensor, and the environmental conditions prevailing at the time and place of the search.

Tactics The deployment and directing of resources on an incident to accomplish the objectives designated by strategy.

Track line length (TLL) Total distance traveled by a sensor (i.e., searcher, boat, or aircraft) while searching in the assigned segment; also called *effort* (Cooper and Frost, 1999). It is the sum of all track lines lengths used on a search. For example, four searchers each with a track line length of 500 feet (152 meters) would have a total track line length of 2,000 feet (608 meters).

Track spacing The distance between the centers of each adjacent search lane.

Trail tape, ribbon, or string line The use of markers to install a guide line where no visible guide line exists. Toilet paper, surveyor's tape, survey markers, evidence markers, string, and other similar material can be tied, placed, or anchored to indicate a line or boundary of a search lane.

REFERENCES AND SUGGESTED READING

Appalachian Search and Rescue Conference. 2017. In memory: Lisa Hannon. http://www.asrc.net/in-memory/.

ASTM International. 2017. Search and rescue operations standards: List of search and rescue standards developed by ASTM. https://www.astm.org/Standards/search-and-rescue-operations-standards.html.

Colwell, Martin. 1992. New concepts for grid searching. *Search and Rescue Technical Publications Series*, 1 no.1,

Olympia, WA: International Search and Rescue Trade Association.

Cooper, Donald C., and John R. Frost. 1999. *Selected Inland Search Definitions*. Private publication. Cuyahoga Falls, OH.

Cooper, Donald C., John R. Frost, and R. Quincy Robe. 2004. *Compatibility of Land SAR Procedures with Search Theory*. Washington, DC: U.S. Department of Homeland Security, United States Coast Guard, Operations (G-OPR).

Dupont, Gordon. 2009. Human factors: Avoid the dirty dozen with safety nets. Air Beat Magazine.

IMO/ICAO. 2016. *International Aeronautical and Maritime Search and Rescue Manual: Volume II, Mission Co-ordination*. London/Montreal: International Maritime Organization and International Civil Aviation Organization.

Koester, Robert J., Kenneth B. Chiacchia, Charles R. Twardy, Donald C. Cooper, John R. Frost, and R. Quincy Robe. 2014. Use of the visual range of detection to estimate effective sweep width for land search and rescue based on 10 detections experiments in North America. *Wilderness & Environmental Medicine*, 25, no. 2, 132–142.

Koester, Robert J. 2009. Sound-light line detection index experimental methodology for search and rescue, Search and Rescue Institute of New Zealand. Charlottesville, VA: dbS Productions LLC.

Koester, Robert J., Donald C. Cooper, J. R. Frost, and R. Q. Robe. 2004. *Sweep Width Estimation for Ground Search and Rescue*. Washington, DC: U.S. Department of Homeland Security, U.S. Coast Guard, Operations (G-OPR).

Koopman, Bernard O. 1946. *Search and Screening*. OEG Report No. 56, The Summary Reports Group of the Columbia University Division of War Research. Alexandria, VA: Center for Naval Analyses.

Koopman, Bernard O. (1980). *Search and Screening: General Principles with Historical Applications*, revised edition. New York: Pergamon Press.

Manson, B. 2009. *Using Sound in Searching for the Lost Subject: Examining Factors Affecting Optimization*. Self-published.

National Fire Protection Association. 2017a. NFPA 1670, *Standard on Operations and Training for Technical Search and Rescue Incidents*. Batterymarch, MA: NFPA.

National Fire Protection Association. 2017b. NFPA 1006, *Standard for Technical Rescue Personnel Professional Qualifications*. Batterymarch, MA: NFPA.

National Institutes of Health, National Eye Institute. 2017. Facts about color blindness. https://nei.nih.gov/health/color_blindness/facts_about.

National Institutes of Health, National Institute of General Medical Sciences. 2017. Circadian rhythms fact sheet. https://www.nigms.nih.gov/education/pages/Factsheet_CircadianRhythms.aspx.

National Search and Rescue Committee. 2000. *United States National Search and Rescue Supplement to the International Aeronautical and Maritime Search and Rescue Manual*. Washington, DC: U.S. Superintendent of Documents. http://www.dco.uscg.mil/Portals/9/CG-5R/manuals/Natl_SAR_Supp.pdf.

National Search and Rescue Committee. 2011. Land search and rescue addendum to the National Search and Rescue Supplement to the International Aeronautical and Maritime Search and Rescue Manual, Version 1.0. https://www.hsdl.org/?abstract&did=715465

National Search and Rescue Committee. 2012. Catastrophic incident search and rescue addendum to the National Search and Rescue Supplement to the International Aeronautical and Maritime Search and Rescue Manual, Version 3.0. http://www.dco.uscg.mil/Portals/9/CG-5R/nsarc/CISAR%20Addendum%20-%20Version%203-0%20(062112)%20Final.pdf.

National Search and Rescue Committee. 2016. National search and rescue plan of the United States. http://www.dco.uscg.mil/Portals/9/CG-5R/manuals/National_SAR_Plan_2016.pdf.

Perkins, Dave. 1989. Critical separation: its role in search management in theory and practice. In LaValla, P. (ed.). *Probability of Detection (POD) Research, and Other Concepts for Search Management*. Olympia, WA: Emergency Response Institute (ERI), pp. 1–39.

Perkins, Dave, and Roberts, Pete. 2009. Field search skills: A practical handbook. UK edition. Ashington, UK.: The Centre for Search Research.

Robe, R. Quincy, and J. R. Frost. 2002. A method for determining effective sweep widths for land searches: Procedures for conducting detection experiments. Prepared for the National Search and Rescue Committee, USCG Contract Number DTCG39-00-D-R00009. Alexandria, VA: Potomac Management Group, Inc.

Stone, Lawrence D. 1989. *Theory of Optimal Search*, 2nd edition. Military Applications Section, Operations Research Society of America. Arlington, VA: ORSA Books.

Taylor, Albert, and Donald C. Cooper. 2014. *Fundamentals of Mantracking: The Step-by-Step Method*. 3rd edition, New York: Skyhorse Publishers. Available at www.NASAR.org.

U.S. Department of Transportation, Federal Aviation Administration. 2015. Aeronautical information manual: Official guide to basic flight information and ATC procedures. https://www.faa.gov/air_traffic/publications/media/aim.pdf.

Washburn, Alan R. 2002. *Search and Detection*, 4th edition. Linthicum, MD: Institute for Operations Research and the Management Sciences.

Washington Explorer Search and Rescue. 1999. *Washington Explorer Search and Rescue Team Member Training Manual*, 4th edition. Tacoma, WA: Washington Explorer Search and Rescue.

CHAPTER 16

Rescue

OBJECTIVES

Upon completion of this chapter and the related course activities, the student will be able to meet the following objectives:

- Explain the difference between rescue hardware and software.
- Explain the difference between a bend and a hitch.
- Explain the difference between static and dynamic kernmantle rope.
- Explain the difference between flat and tubular webbing.
- Describe at least five life safety performance characteristics that should be considered for any use of rope in rescue.
- Identify and describe at least three characteristics of the most common material used in manufacturing rescue rope.
- Identify the cardinal rule of caring for rescue software.
- Discuss at least three considerations for storing rescue software.
- List and describe at least three signs of wear on rescue rope.
- List at least three rules of rescue software care.
- Identify at least four parts of a carabiner.
- List and describe at least three different types of litter carries.

Life Safety Rope

Around the world, the use of rope and rescue equipment by search and rescue (SAR) personnel has evolved to a very high level. The intent of this chapter is to convey the most basic rescue information SAR personnel will likely encounter on a mission. This introduction is not meant to serve as a complete or comprehensive training program in rescue of any type. Interested readers should consult more detailed references and pursue technical training to advance their knowledge in this important subject area.

Even if proper equipment and techniques are used, the potential danger and harm that can occur to SAR personnel and patients cannot be overstated (**FIGURE 16-1**). Any rescue activity that requires the use of a rope to support a life is inherently dangerous. Proper and extensive training and experience should be gained from qualified sources if these skills are to be used in the field.

Rope used to support a human life (life safety rope) must be specially designed and engineered to do so. Not just any rope can serve as a life safety rope. For example, ropes sold in discount and hardware stores—commodity ropes—are not intended to be used for life safety applications. Using these non-life safety ropes inappropriately has led to many unfortunate tragedies.

Life safety rope should be certified to life safety standards, such as those promulgated by American National Standards Institute (ANSI), ASTM International (ASTM), National Fire Protection Association (NFPA), International Climbing and Mountaineering Federation (UIAA), Cordage Institute (CI), or Committee for European Normalization (CEN). SAR personnel should look for one of these certifications before using any rope in a life safety application.

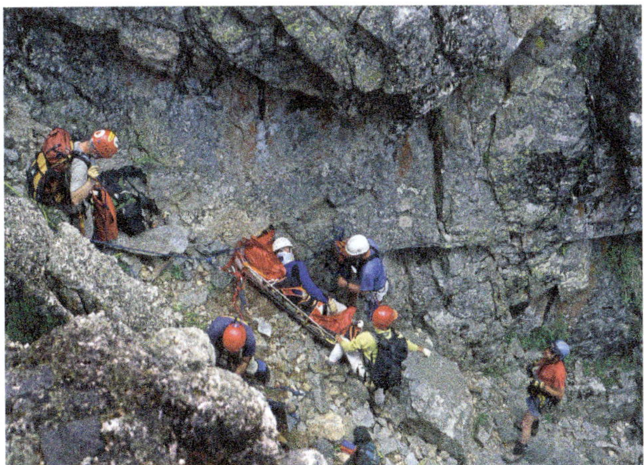

FIGURE 16-1 Any rescue activity that requires the use of a rope to support a life is inherently dangerous. Extensive training and experience should be gained from qualified sources if these skills are to be used in the field.

Life safety rope can be used in many ways—climbing, caving, recreation, rescue, rope access—and each application requires different characteristics, or combinations of characteristics, in the rope. Specific life safety performance characteristics that should be considered for any use of rope should include the following (McCurley and Evans, 2017):

- Strength
- Impact force transmitted during a fall
- Number of falls held
- Elongation
- Diameter
- Abrasion resistance
- Compatibility with other equipment
- Hand (flexibility and handling characteristics; knotability)
- Weight
- Flotation

ASTM publishes a standard that describes the inspection of life safety rope: *Standard Guide for Inspection of Nylon, Polyester, or Nylon/Polyester Blend, or Both Kernmantle Rope*, F1740-96. SAR personnel should become familiar with this and related standards (ASTM, 2012a).

Life Safety Rope Materials

Since the discovery of nylon in 1938, synthetic fibers have proved indispensable in the construction of life safety rescue rope. The most common material now used to manufacture these ropes is nylon, but some are also made with polyester. These materials do not rot and have a high strength-to-weight ratio. For several reasons, natural fibers such as sisal, hemp, and manila are not acceptable for life safety use.

TABLE 16-1 Minimum Breaking Strengths for Rope

Diameter	Minimum Breaking Strength
7 mm (0.28 inch)	2200 lbf (9.8 kN)
8 mm (0.31 inch)	2875 lbf (12.8 kN)
10 mm (0.38 inch)	4500 lbf (20.0 kN)
11 mm (0.44 inch)	6000 lbf (26.7 kN)
12.5 mm (0.5 inch)	9000 lbf (40.0 kN)
16 mm (0.63 inch)	12,500 lbf (55.6 kN)

Note: One kilonewton (kN) is equivalent to 225 pounds-force (McCurley and Evans, 2017).

Data from McCurley, L., & Evans, T. (2017). Ropes and Knot Tying. In Auerbach, P.S., ed. Wilderness Medicine, 7th ed. Volume 2. St. Louis, MO: Elsevier, Inc. pp. 2361-2375.

Nylon is approximately 10% stronger than polyester and has higher dynamic energy absorption than polyester, but nylon temporarily loses up to 15% of its strength when wet. Both materials resist most chemicals, but nylon is degraded more by acids and polyester is degraded more by alkalis.

The **breaking strength** of various size ropes is shown in **TABLE 16-1**.

Life Safety Rope Type

The type of construction or design of rope is critical to life safety rescue applications, and today the most common type of life safety rope construction is kernmantle (German for "core in sheath").

A **kernmantle rope** is constructed using an outer, woven sheath and an inner core of parallel strands (**FIGURE 16-2**). The outer sheath of kernmantle rope is a tightly woven tube that serves to support a load and protect the inner core. The inner core consists of strands of fibers that are bundled together to provide most of the strength of the rope. These ropes are strong, easy to tie knots in, and very abrasion resistant; failure of the sheath does not greatly affect the strength of the rope.

SAFETY TIP

Rope rescue is an inherently dangerous activity that requires extensive training and practice to conduct safely.

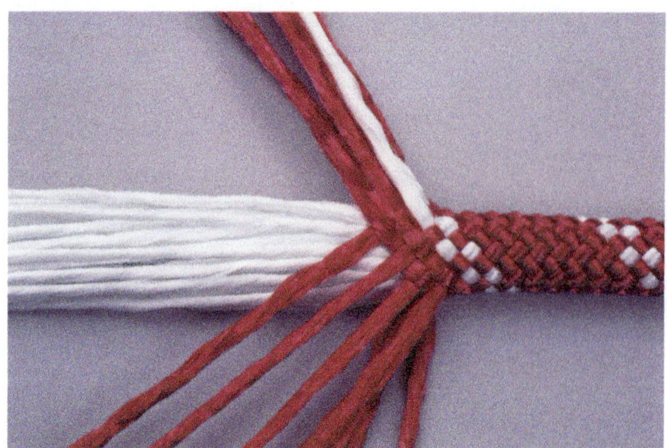

FIGURE 16-2 Kernmantle (core in sheath) rope construction.
Courtesy of Steve Hudson.

Kernmantle ropes come in three basic types: dynamic (high stretch), static (minimal stretch), and low-stretch. In a static and low-stretch kernmantle rope, the inner core is made of strands that are relatively straight and parallel to each other. When the need for energy absorption is minimal, and it is important that bouncing of the load be limited, static and low-stretch rope should be used. Static ropes may be used for rappels, lowers, traverses, and other situations where there will be no climbing above the anchor required (lower fall factor). Low-stretch rope is generally not used in situations where a rescuer may fall any distance that may shock-load a system.

SEARCH AND RESCUE TIP

When it is important that the movement and bouncing of the load be limited, static, low-stretch rope should be used.

Dynamic kernmantle rope consists of inner strands that are twisted or braided, thereby allowing them to elongate or stretch under load. This is an important consideration for any climbing activity, as the stretch of the rope acts as a shock absorber during a fall. This property benefits not only the climber but also the rope itself. High-stretch ropes tend to be more pliable and easier to knot; however, they generally are not as strong or as abrasion-resistant as their lower-stretch counterparts.

In the final analysis, most rope used on a SAR mission should be of the static or low-stretch kernmantle type, and SAR personnel should not be expected to perform rescues in a technical environment without extensive rope rescue training.

ASTM and NFPA publish standards that describe the specifications and labeling of low stretch and static kernmantle life safety rope (ASTM, 2007; NFPA 2017c), test methods for life safety rope belay systems (ASTM, 2014a), and standards on what should be included in rope rescue training (ASTM, 2012b; ASTM, 2012c; ASTM, 2014b). SAR personnel involved in the selection of life safety rope should become familiar with these and related standards.

Webbing

Another type of rescue equipment often used with ropes is webbing. Webbing is light, easy to pack, and can be used in a variety of situations. Webbing can be used to improvise a harness for a person to use when being attached to a rope, as an anchor component to attach the rope to an object, or to secure an injured victim to a litter. As with life safety rope, webbing used to support a human life must be specially designed and engineered to do so.

There are two types of webbing construction: flat and tubular. Flat webbing is a single piece of material woven into one strip of woven fibers. Tubular webbing is a continuous tube of woven material that folds flat. In cross section, it is tubular (**FIGURE 16-3**). Generally, flat webbing is stronger than tubular—although tubular webbing is still very strong—but tubular webbing is more resistant to abrasion. Webbing can be made of the same materials as rope, but it is usually made from nylon, an ultra-high-molecular weight polyethylene (UHMwPE) such as Dyneema® or Spectra®, or a combination of both nylon and a UHMwPE. The UHMwPE materials are very strong, float, have a low melting point, and a high resistance to abrasion, but they do not stretch enough to absorb dynamic energy. They are also difficult to tie into knots because of how slippery the material is, which is why sewn rather than tied slings made from these materials are preferred. Thus, for most life safety rescue applications, nylon tubular webbing, usually in 1-inch width, is the first choice.

The breaking strength of various size webbing is listed in **TABLE 16-2**.

Tubular webbing is constructed in two very different ways: spiral (shuttle loom) and chain (needle loom)

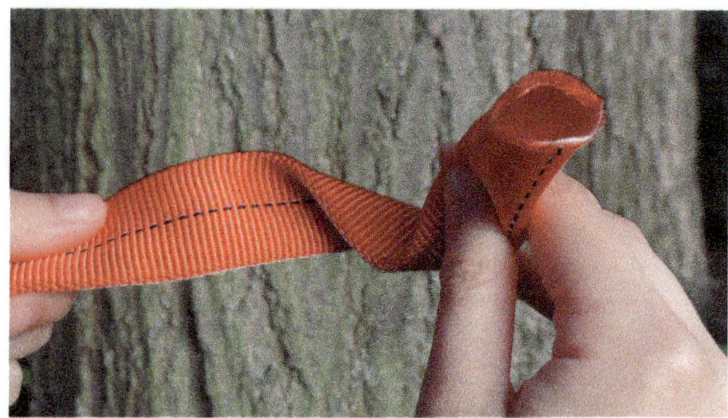

FIGURE 16-3 One-inch (25.4-mm) tubular webbing.
Courtesy of Donald Cooper.

TABLE 16-2 Minimum Breaking Strengths for Webbing

Width	Minimum Breaking Strength
9.5 mm (0.375 inch)	950 lbf (4.2 kN)
12.7 mm (0.5 inch)	1000 lbf (4.4 kN)
14 mm (0.563 inch)	1500 lbf (6.7 kN)
16 mm (0.625 inch)	2250 lbf (10.0 kN)
19 mm (0.75 inch)	2300 lbf (10.2 kN)
22 mm (0.875 inch)	3100 lbf (13.8 kN)
25 mm (1.0 inch)	4000 lbf (17.8 kN)

Note: One kilonewton (kN) is equivalent to 225 pounds-force (McCurley and Evans, 2017).

Data from McCurley, L., & Evans, T. (2017). Ropes and Knot Tying. In Auerbach, P.S., ed. Wilderness Medicine, 7th ed. Volume 2. St. Louis, MO: Elsevier, Inc. pp. 2361-2375.

structure. In the past, the spiral construction method was considered the better choice for life safety webbing due to concern that the chain structure was weaker and that abrasion could cause the lock stitch down one edge to unravel. However, improved needle loom technology and experience have helped produce better quality chain structure webbing, which today performs just as satisfactorily as spiral structure webbing for rescue work (Frank, 2013).

It is important to purchase tubular webbing intended for rescue from an appropriate and reputable source. Make sure that the vendor knows the intended use of the webbing and has worked with rescue organizations before.

Safety Factors

Rope must be stronger than the load it is intended to support. The ratio of the strength of a new rope, or any rescue component, to its intended load is called the **design factor**. If the strength of a rope is 9,000 pounds (4082 kilograms) and the load for which it is intended is 900 pounds (408 kilograms), the design factor is 10:1, but this is only for a single rescue component used in isolation. It does not consider the strength of other rescue system components, which may be weaker or stronger than the rope, or use factors that affect all equipment, such as the amount and type of use, wear, and exposure to moisture and sun over time.

Generally, component design factors tend to be high, some as high as 15:1, because one component can be built very strong. When other rescue components are factored in, however, the overall **system safety factor**—the ratio between the weakest link in a rescue system and the load to be supported—may be less than half the design factor (McCurley and Evans, 2017).

A rope used in rescue may be attached to multiple anchors using various pieces of rescue **hardware** (e.g., carabiners, ascenders, pulleys) and **software** (e.g., webbing, slings/runners, accessory cord). Thus, the strength of the entire system is only as strong as its weakest link. This is why system safety factor is so important. Ideally, the system safety factor considers system force multipliers such as the angles involved in rigging, mechanical advantage systems, and redirectional pulleys. Determination of system safety factor also requires a great deal of knowledge of rescue systems, factors that influence the strength of rescue system components, the limitations of rescue hardware and software, and experience in using all the above. The greater the chances of system failure, and the greater the consequences of such a failure, the higher an acceptable system safety factor should be. Remember, however, that only a qualified individual should determine what serves as an acceptable system safety factor.

ASTM (2015) publishes a standard guide (*Standard Guide for Determining Load Ratios for Technical Rescue Systems and Equipment, F2491-05*) that describes how to determine load ratios for technical rescue systems and equipment, which might help in determining system safety factors. SAR personnel should become familiar with this and related standards.

Software Care

Rope, webbing, harnesses, and other "soft" life safety rescue equipment are collectively referred to as "software." This easily damaged gear must be used, monitored, and maintained carefully; thus, there are several special rules that apply to its use and care.

Keep a Log

A detailed record must be kept of each piece of life safety rescue equipment, but nowhere is this more important than with life safety rope (**FIGURE 16-4**). This record should be kept on file and

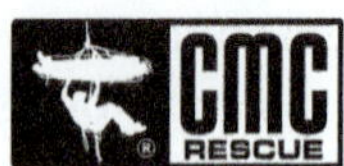

ROPE LOG

Date in service: ________________ Rope number: ________________

Length: __________ (ft) Diameter: ______ (in) Rope color: __________ Bag color: ____________

Manufacturer: ________________ Model: ________________ Tensile strength: ________________

	Date	Incident/Location [a]	How used [b]	Possible damage [c]	Inspection results	Sign in
1						
2						
3						
4						
5						
6						
7						
8						
9						
10						
11						
12						
13						
14						
15						
16						
17						
18						
19						
20						

a. Include activities such as operations, trainings, inspections, and washing.

b. Detail use of the rope such as for rappel, rappel rescue, main line, and system belay.

c. Did something happen that may have damaged the rope such as rock fall, impact load, severe abrasion, or other abuse?

A

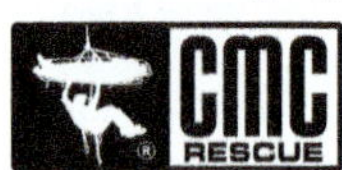

ROPE LOG

Date in service: 16 April 2015 Rope number: SCSAR 2015-006

Length: 200 (ft) Diameter: 1/2 (in) Rope color: Red (White) Bag color: Orange

Manufacturer: CMC rescue Model: Static-Pro Tensile strength: 9217 lb (41 kN)

	Date	Incident/Location [a]	How used [b]	Possible damage [c]	Inspection results	Sign in
1	4-16-15	Placed in service			OK	DC
2	4-20-15	Training/Tower	Rappel line	None	OK	JT
3	4-25-15	Gorge incident	System safety	None	OK	KC
4	5-26-15	Cuy. valley incident	Staged-Not used			TH
5	6-09-15	Miller high rise inc.	Main line	Some fraying on sheath	Check	JT
6	6-09-15	Inspection		Some wear normal	OK	DC

B

FIGURE 16-4 **A.** Example of blank rope log. **B.** Example of completed rope log.

Courtesy of CMC Rescue, Inc.

include, as a minimum, its identification marking (some unique mark or number on each component), size, type (e.g., kernmantle), manufacturer, date purchased, date in service, conditions under which equipment was used, any abuse the equipment sustained, and any actions taken (e.g., inspection, cleaning, drying, storage, and return to service) (ASTM, 2012a). Any personal, non-team, life safety equipment that might be used during a rescue should also be documented in this way.

Care and Service Life

The first and cardinal rule of caring for software is never to step on or drag it. Doing so grinds tiny, sharp particles of sand into and between the fibers of the material. In kernmantle rope, these particles can work themselves through the sheath and into the core fibers, invisibly cutting and weakening the rope. The bottom line is to never step on or drag any rescue equipment but especially rope and rescue software.

It is widely believed that with proper care, new, unused, nylon life safety rope can last up to 10 years without significant loss in strength. However, hard and improper use and storage of the same rope can quickly degrade its strength and reduce its useful life (Frank, 2013). Regardless of how well a rope has been stored, carefully maintained, and gently used, life safety rope should be discarded immediately in the following situations:

- The sheath shows significant signs of wear.
- The rope has sustained a cut.
- Damage from exposure to chemicals is suspected.
- The rope has sustained a hard shock load or has been used in any towing operation.
- Anytime there is a question about the integrity of the rope.

At least one source suggests that a static or low-stretch life safety rope that has sustained a fall factor of 0.25 or greater, or a dynamic life safety rope that has sustained a fall factor of 1.5 or greater, "...will likely cause internal invisible damage to the rope, although damage may also be caused with lower fall factors" (McCurley and Evans, 2017, p. 2363). A significant fall should also call into question all the rescue components attached to the rescue system that supported the fall.

Storage

Although many coils could be used to keep rope organized, the best way to store rope for rescue is in a rope bag. A rope bag keeps the rope ready for instant use, can be uniquely marked to identify the specific length of rope, and the color of the bag can also have meaning. Packs can be used to organize and store combinations of specialty software and hardware so they are ready for deployment. One pack might contain everything needed to build an anchor system; another might contain main line or belay line equipment. The idea is to store the equipment in such a way as to keep it compact, clean, and dry while having it ready to deploy in appropriately sized packages that are easily transported to where they are needed. Achieving this goal becomes challenging when rescue is required in isolated alpine and wilderness environments where a SAR ready pack must also be carried. This is where SAR personnel can borrow from the rock climbing community and carry some hardware and software attached to the belt, harness, or a sling draped over the shoulder (**FIGURE 16-5**).

Software must be stored out of direct sunlight. Lengthy exposure to ultraviolet radiation is known to compromise the integrity of nylon fibers and degrades its strength. This is again where the use of a rope bag can help.

Never expose rescue software to chemicals or petroleum by-products such as engine exhaust fumes and liquid fuel vapors. Avoid exposure to batteries of any type—including lead acid, "sealed," or "dry cell" batteries. The acid and chemicals they contain, and their vapors, attack and weaken most synthetic materials. Be especially cautious of this when storing software in a SAR ready pack, which may be stored in areas that are not good places to store software (such as vehicle trunks). Mildew and fungi also attack synthetic fibers, so rescue software should be dried thoroughly before being stored in a dry environment.

Keep rescue software away from high heat of any kind because it has the potential to melt and destroy synthetic materials. Also, avoid high friction and abrasion of the equipment. Do not allow nylon to run across nylon; that is, if a rope is in motion, such as in

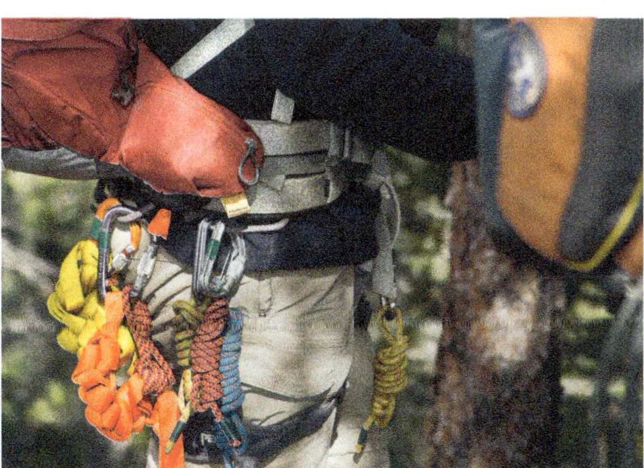

FIGURE 16-5 Example of how rescue software and hardware might be carried into isolated alpine and wilderness environments.

a haul system, it should not be allowed to contact a stationary length of rope or webbing. The heat generated from the friction can quickly melt and damage the webbing or rope.

In general, keep rescue software as clean as possible. Storing all software in a rope or gear bag can do wonders for protecting it from outside dirt, sunlight, and chemicals.

Inspections

All rescue software must be inspected before each use (ASTM, 2012a), or better yet, inspected before and after each use so it is ready for the next mission. Run the material through your hands slowly and carefully, feeling and visually checking for the following signs of wear:

- *Discoloration.* Indicates any one of many problems, including chemical damage, heat damage, or other abuses. A gray color on the exterior is not necessarily a problem, as it may be residue from an aluminum carabiner.
- *Shiny areas.* Indicates heat damage from friction, which may also show up as harder sections of the rope.
- *Fuzzy or torn sheath.* Fibers may be worn or torn; on kernmantle, this may also indicate damage to interior strands of the rope.
- *Smaller or larger diameter areas.* Indicates that the inner strands are damaged in some way, either cut or torn, or stressed and kinked upon themselves.
- *Soft spots in rope.* Places where rope is more flexible and soft also indicate interior damage.

Any significant wear and/or damage found in rescue software must be evaluated before use. Damage of the type indicated above should prompt the removal of the rope from life safety status.

If rescue software becomes dirty, it can be cleaned. For rope, there are many specially made washing devices that can be attached to a hose. In a popular version of this device, the rope is pulled through a tube in which jets of water and brush-like bristles scrub the rope as it passes (**FIGURE 16-6**). A washing machine may also be used to wash rope and rescue software. However, make sure to use a front-loading machine because the action of the agitator in top-loading machines can harm both the machine and the rope. When using a front-loading washing machine, it is best to place the rope in a mesh bag and use little or no detergent. The residual soap in a commercial machine is probably enough to clean it. If you must use soap, use the mildest type available, one that is safe for synthetic garments. Use only cold water when washing rescue software. Once washed, air dry it in a clean, dark place. NEVER dry a rope using heat or fire.

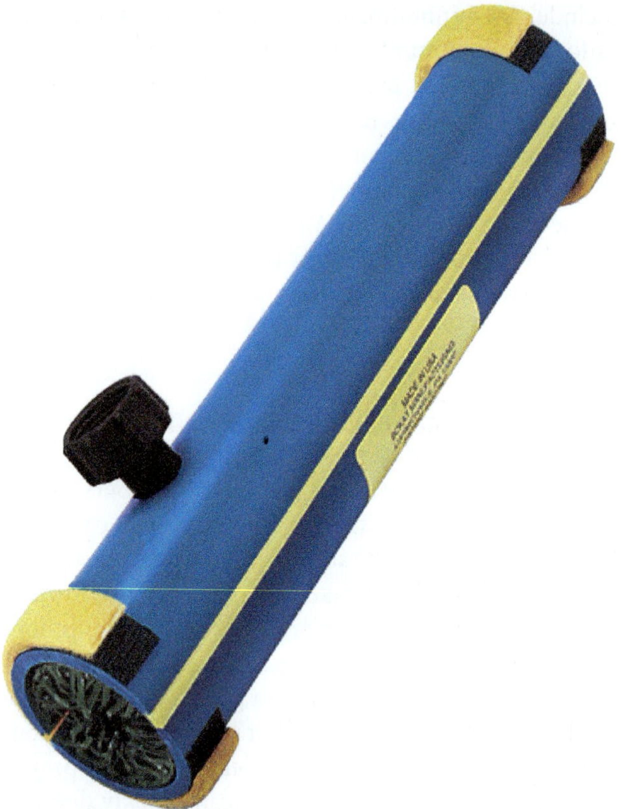

FIGURE 16-6 Rope washer.
Courtesy of Pigeon Mountain Industries.

Ten Rules of Rescue Software Care

In summary, care of rope and rescue software is important. Thus, these 10 rules should always be followed:

1. Never step on or drag a rope or rescue software.
2. Use software in a responsible manner, and keep a log of its storage and use.
3. Protect software from sharp edges and abrasion; use edge rollers and/or edge padding (**FIGURE 16-7**).
4. Do not leave rope or webbing under tension for any length of time; remove knots as soon as possible.
5. Store all software properly (i.e., cool, dry place out of direct sunlight and away from chemicals).
6. Soiled software should be gently and properly cleaned.
7. Avoid exposing software to sunlight (UV) and high temperatures.
8. Avoid nylon running across nylon (synthetic running across synthetic); the friction can cause damage.
9. Avoid exposure to chemicals.
10. Check all software for damage often, before and after each use.

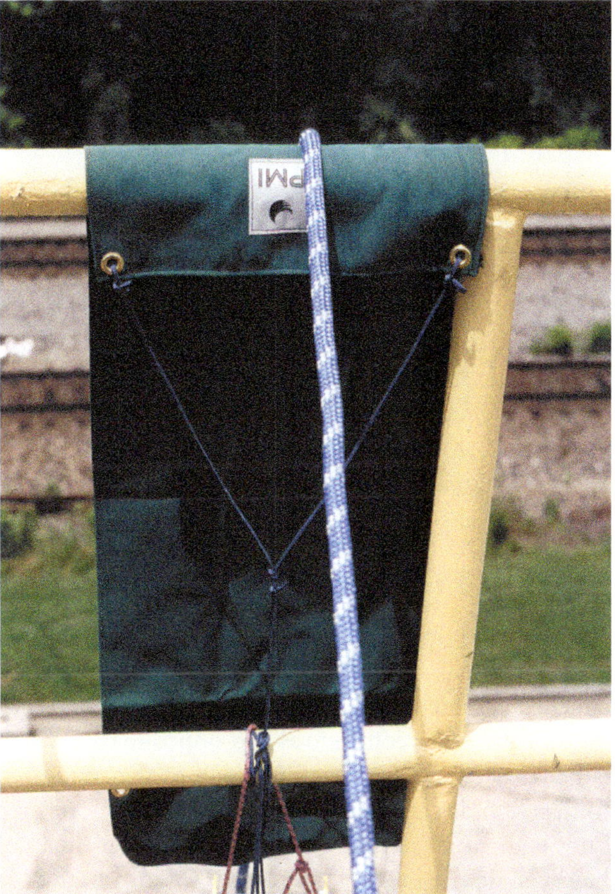

A

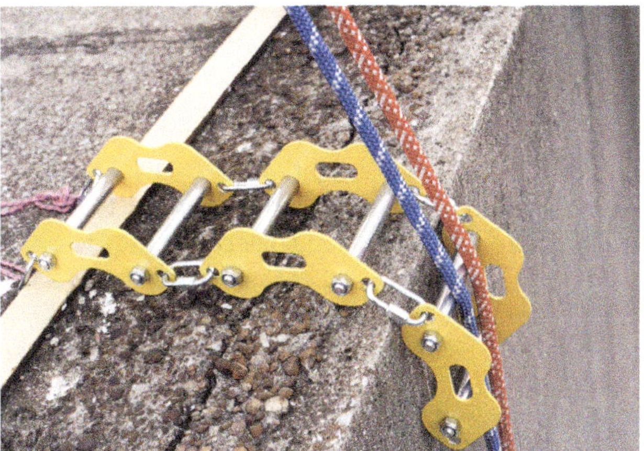

B

FIGURE 16-7 Protect software from sharp edges and abrasion. **A.** Canvas rope pad. **B.** Edge roller.

A: Courtesy of Pigeon Mountain Industries; **B:** Courtesy of Steve Hudson.

Harnesses

When choosing a harness to use, you need to determine what your function is and the type of harness that provides the necessary protection for that role. A harness can be used during a rappel, to provide protection while performing work from a height, to secure a subject in a litter or during a pick off, and when working in an exposed position. There are many situations during a SAR mission that may require personnel to be working in a harness. Therefore, SAR personnel should be familiar with harnesses that may be used in rescue. Many types of commercial rescue harnesses are available. They are typically heavier than harnesses designed for rock climbing or caving, which may or may not be appropriate for rescue.

The NFPA describes two classifications of life safety harnesses: Class II and Class III. A Class II harness is a seat harness that fits around the waist, thighs, and under the buttocks with a design load of 600 pound-force (lbf) (2.67 kN). A Class III harness is a full-body harness that fits around the waist, thighs, under the buttocks, and over the shoulders with a design load of 600 lbf (2.67 kN) (NFPA, 2017c). Although a Class III harness may be the most secure, it is also the heaviest. Thus, it may not always be the best choice for wilderness rescue.

In addition to seat harnesses and full-body harnesses, separate chest harnesses are also available. When a chest harness is combined with a seat harness, they comprise a full-body harness. However, a chest harness must never be worn alone without a seat harness. One advantage of using a chest harness with a seat harness, or a full-body harness, is to help the rescuer remain in an upright position while hanging from the rope. In some cases, attaching a chest harness improperly may be worse than not having one at all.

A climber's "swami belt," ladder belts, or Pompier belts (simple belts that only encircle the waist) are not appropriate for life-safety applications and should not be used in lieu of an appropriate rescue harness (Frank, 2013). Rappel belts that fit through the belt loops of trousers may be used in an emergency to support one's body weight, but they should not be depended upon in typical rescue scenarios.

For rescuers who (1) do not plan to be "on rope," (2) do not plan on spending long periods of time hanging from a rope, or (3) want to save weight, a commercial rescue harness may not be necessary. In these cases, an improvised harness using 1-inch (25.4-mm) tubular or flat webbing may work just fine. An improvised harness must fulfill two primary needs: it must keep the occupant securely attached to the rope, and the harness must stay securely attached to the rescuer, even when inverted or in other unusual positions. Both are easily accomplished with a "hasty harness" (i.e., "Swiss Scat" or diaper sling), which is a field-expedient, improvised harness (**FIGURE 16-8**).

Several standards are available that address rescue operations and the use of harnesses, including, but not limited to, NFPA 1670, *Standard on Operations and Training for Technical Search and Rescue Incidents*, NFPA1006, *Standard for Technical Rescue Personnel*

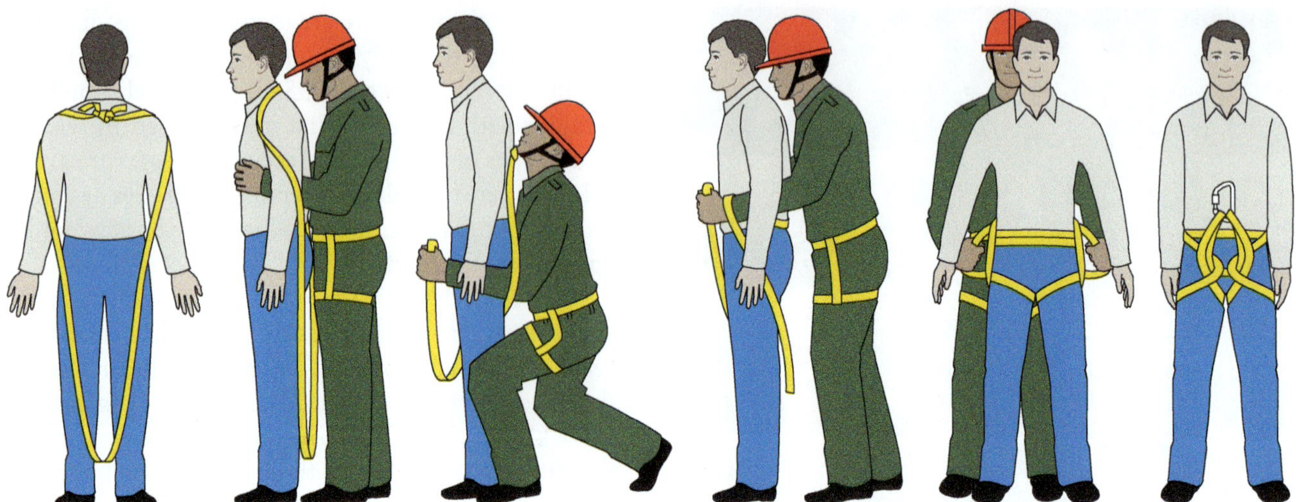

FIGURE 16-8 Tying a hasty harness.

Professional Qualifications, and several ASTM standards. Reviewing and becoming familiar with these standards is highly recommended for SAR personnel who may be required to use harnesses in or around rescue environments (NFPA, 2017a; NFPA, 2017b; NFPA, 2017c; ASTM, 2017; ASTM, 2012d).

The selection and use of a harness in rescue takes specialized knowledge and training. Such training is beyond the scope of this text. Interested readers can learn more about rescue skills and equipment by reviewing the various books and standards listed in the Reference section of this chapter and participating in training conducted by qualified instructors.

Knots, Ties, Hitches, and Bends

A variety of knots may be required in rescue, but only a few are needed in most rescue situations. The key is to learn a few useful knots and practice them often. A "knot" is a general term that refers to a broad class of rope attachments, but more specific terms also exist. For example, a **bend** is a knot used to connect the ends of two pieces of rope or webbing. A **hitch** is a knot used to attach a rope to another object or fixed rope. "Dressing a knot" is the phrase used to describe the process of neatening up a knot so that all strands in the knot are smooth and aligned.

Knowing the parts of a length of rope is also useful (**FIGURE 16-9**). A "bight" is a U-shaped curve placed in a rope that does not cross itself, and a "loop" is formed when the U-shaped end of the rope does cross itself. The "standing part" of a rope is the fixed portion attached to something, like an anchor. The "running end" of the rope is the continuous end opposite that which is being used to tie a knot. The end of the rope used to tie a knot is called the "working end." The "tail" of a knot is the unused rope that is left over after the knot has been tied. A lengthy tail can be tied into a safety or backup knot, which is a secondary knot that prevents another knot from coming untied.

Figure Eight

Possibly the most versatile family of knots is the figure-eight family. The figure eight can be used as a bend or hitch. The figure eight on a bight (**FIGURE 16-10**) is a useful knot for creating a loop that can be used to attach the rope to a carabiner or other object. **FIGURE 16-11** shows how to tie this knot.

The figure eight follow-through (**FIGURE 16-12**) is the same knot as the figure eight on a bight, but it is tied differently and used when a loop cannot be placed over an object. That is, it is used when the running end of the rope must be fed around an object like a pole or a tree. The figure-eight follow-through is a common knot used by climbers to attach their harness to the belay rope.

It is important to keep rope usage to a minimum when tying knots. For example, there is no need to tie a 1-foot-diameter loop in the end of the rope when it will be attached only to a carabiner. Also, there is no reason to leave an excessive tail (i.e., more than 6 inches [0.152 meter] after a safety knot, if used) on a knot, as it is a waste of rope and could foul the rigging.

The figure-eight knots are generally used for tying rope, and the square and water knots are generally used in webbing (backed up with safety knots). Although a

A

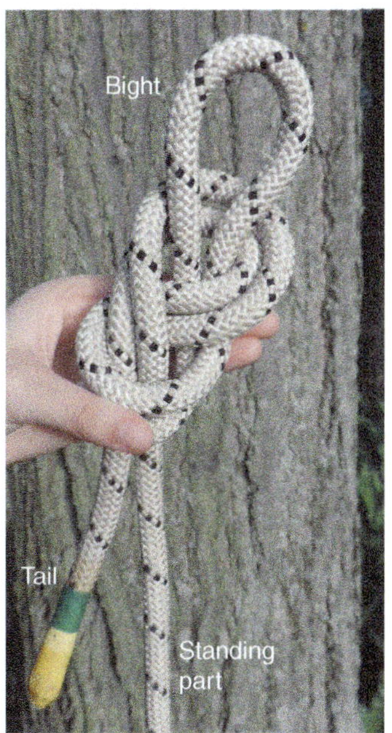

B

C

FIGURE 16-9 **A.** Rope terms. **B.** Knot terms: Figure 8 on a bight. **C.** Knot terms: Bowline with safety knot.

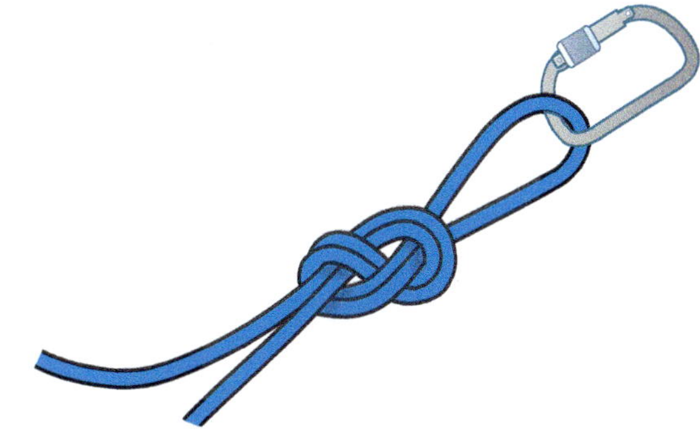

FIGURE 16-10 Figure eight on a bight attached to a carabiner.

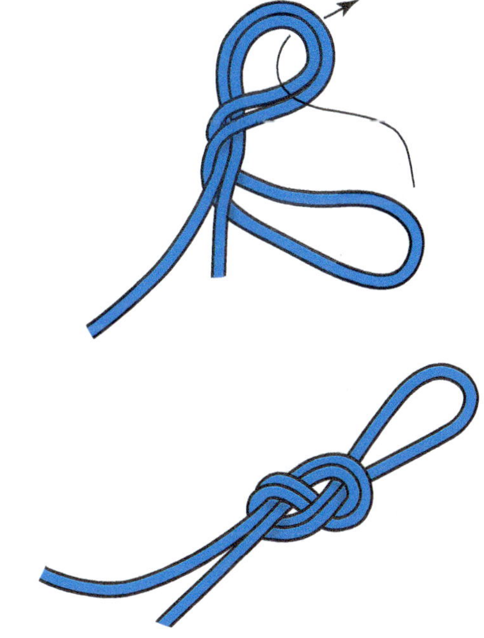

FIGURE 16-11 Tying a figure eight on a bight.

square knot can certainly be tied in rope, it is generally not considered adequate for life safety applications. The versatile figure-eight family of knots is a good choice in many situations because they are easy to tie, easy to untie, easy to teach to others, easy to inspect, easy to remember, and they hold fast—all characteristics of any good knot.

Square or Reef Knot

The square knot is useful for joining two ends of webbing together in the creation of a field-expedient seat harness (**FIGURE 16-13**). However, this knot is not appropriate for use in bending life safety rope ends together because it is easily tied incorrectly and can

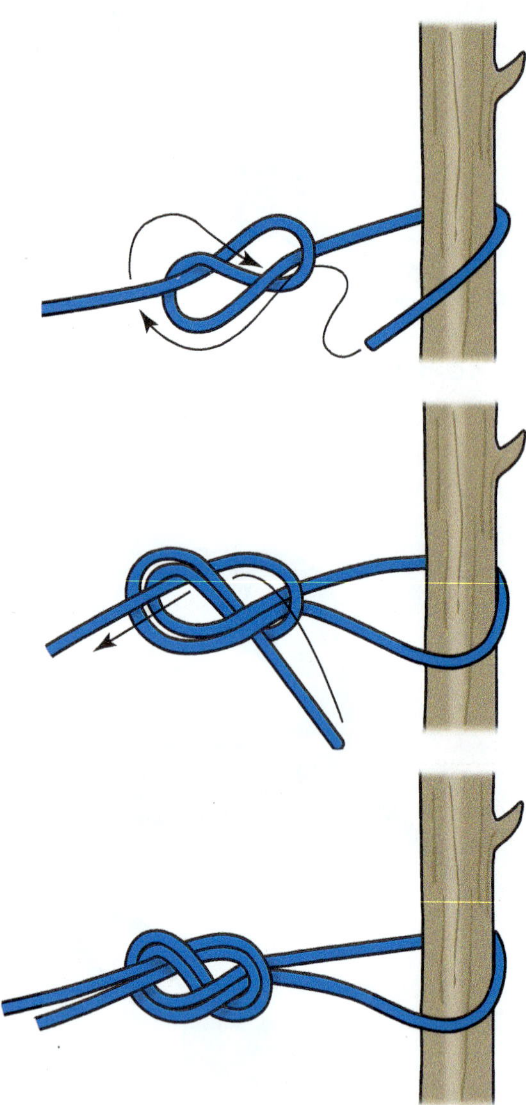

FIGURE 16-12 Figure-eight follow-through.

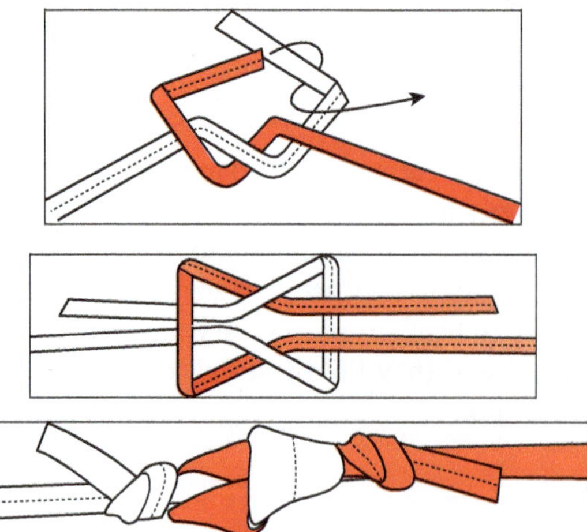

FIGURE 16-13 Tying a square knot is useful for joining two ends of webbing together in the creation of a field-expedient seat harness, but two safety overhand knots—one on each end—must be included. A square knot should not be used to bend rope ends together.

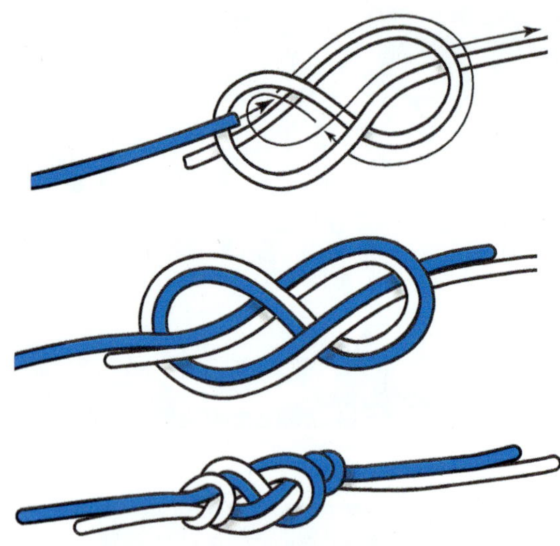

FIGURE 16-14 Tying a figure-eight bend. This type of knot is used to attach the ends of two ropes. Shown with overhand safety knots on each end.

untie itself when jostled. For tying a bend in a rope, use a figure-eight bend (**FIGURE 16-14**).

Bends

When joining two ropes, use a figure-eight bend (see Figure 16-14). Other commonly encountered bends are the ring bend and the sheet bend. The ring bend is a compact and useful knot, but it is very difficult to untie after a rope has been loaded—more difficult than the figure-eight bend, which is one reason the figure-eight bend is preferred. Again, the figure-eight family works well when bending two ropes.

Knots in Webbing

While many of the knots that work well in rope also work in webbing, webbing is a bit slicker and requires specialized knots and bends. Webbing is generally used in the construction of anchors and field-expedient seat harnesses. As such, bends are more common in webbing than knots. To bend two ends of webbing into a loop or to join two pieces of webbing, use the bend, also known as the water knot (**FIGURE 16-15**). Be aware, however, that this knot may be difficult to untie after being loaded, and it should include an overhand knot on each side of the bend as a safety.

The only place where a square knot will be encountered in rescue is in the construction of a Swiss Seat or other field-expedient seat harness. This knot can be used to join the two ends of the webbing in the last step of the construction of the seat harness (see Figures 16-3 and 16-8).

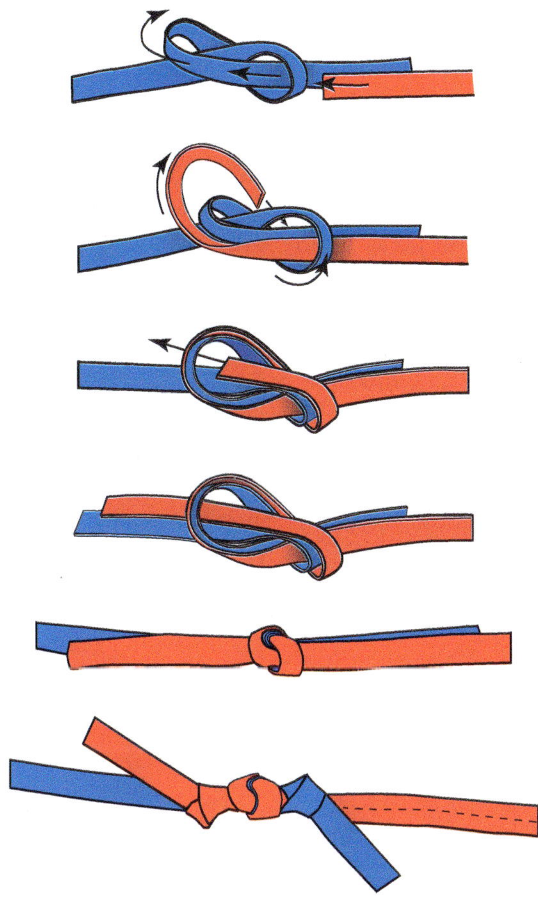

FIGURE 16-15 Tying an overhand bend, also known as a *ring bend* or *water knot*. Make sure to include an overhand knot on each side of the bend as a safety.

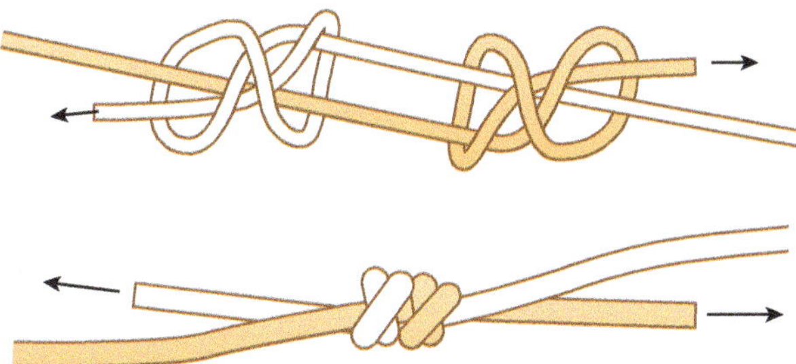

FIGURE 16-16 Tying a double fisherman's bend; used to join two ends of Prusik cord.

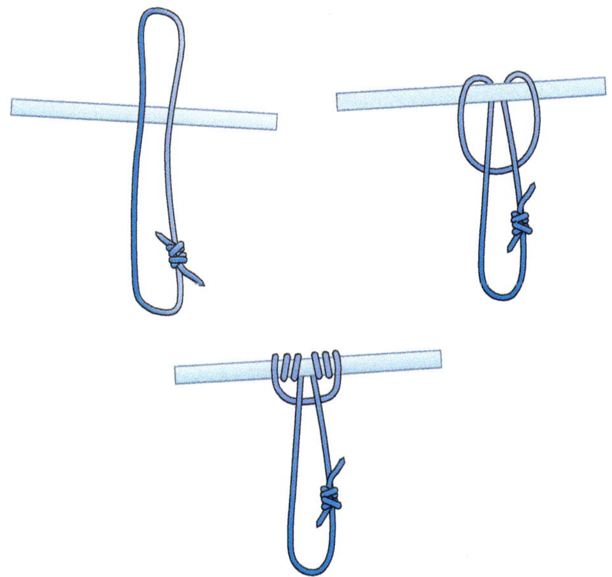

FIGURE 16-17 Tying a three-wrap Prusik to a lifeline.

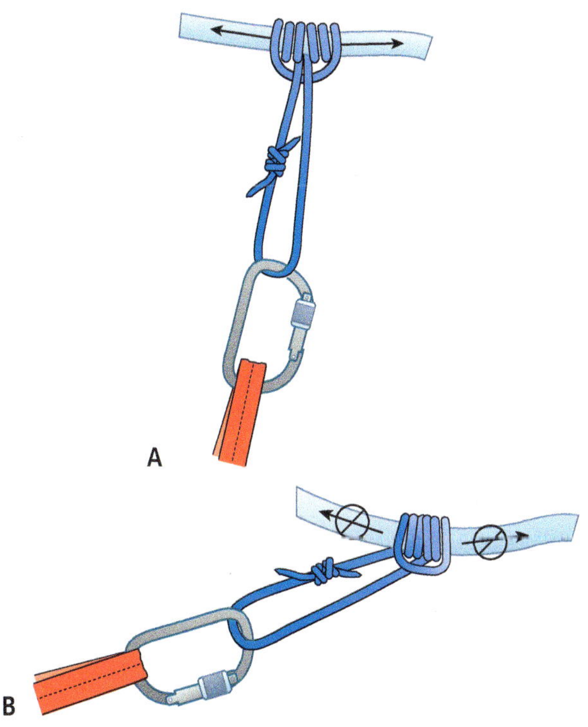

FIGURE 16-18 **A.** An unloaded Prusik attached to a lifeline. **B.** The Prusik loaded.

Prusik Slings

Another useful item to have in your SAR ready pack is a Prusik sling. This exotic-sounding item is nothing more than a piece of accessory cord tied into a loop. The Prusik sling can be used to attach a harness to a lifeline. After tying the length of cord into a sling, use a three-loop wrap to attach the sling to the lifeline. Then, use a carabiner to attach the sling to the harness. The rope for the sling should be a piece of static kernmantle cord around 4 to 5 millimeters in diameter and about 6 feet (2 meters) long. Typically, this loop is tied together with a double fisherman's (grapevine) bend. However, a figure-eight bend is also acceptable. **FIGURE 16-16** shows how the double fisherman's bend is tied, and **FIGURE 16-17** shows how to tie a Prusik to a lifeline. When it is not loaded, the Prusik moves easily along the lifeline (**FIGURE 16-18**). When loaded, the Prusik grabs the lifeline and holds fast. It is important to receive proper instruction in the use of these slings before they are used.

Carabiners

To conveniently connect webbing and rope to harnesses, litters, and anchors, and to prevent synthetic material from running across other synthetic material, a **carabiner**, which is a load-bearing, metal connector with a self-closing gate, is often used. **FIGURE 16-19** illustrates the parts of a carabiner, which come in several types, materials, and configurations.

Types of Carabiners

Carabiners come in both locking and nonlocking varieties. A nonlocking carabiner has a spring-loaded gate that closes over a pin, but there is nothing to keep the gate securely closed. Although they are not necessarily stronger, a locking carabiner has some means of preventing the gate from opening unintentionally, especially while under load. This is usually achieved by way of a screw-sliding barrel-type mechanism that slides over the gate latch. Locking carabiners are generally preferred for rescue operations.

Carabiners also come in a variety of shapes, including oval, "D," and HMS (pear-shaped) (**FIGURE 16-20**). The most common carabiner shape used in rescue is the "D." This shape focuses the load along the spine, the strongest part of the carabiner. Oval carabiners are generally not as strong by design, in that they distribute the load over the gate as well as the spine, but they may be a bit more forgiving with respect to load angles as compared to a D-shaped carabiner.

HMS is an abbreviation for the German word "Halbmastwurfsicherung," which means "Munter hitch" in English. When used in reference to a carabiner, HMS refers to the fact that the carabiner allows for the easy use of a Munter or similar hitch. Pear-shaped, or HMS, carabiners have a larger well, so that they are able to accommodate multiple ropes or other devices and fit more easily through a seat harness.

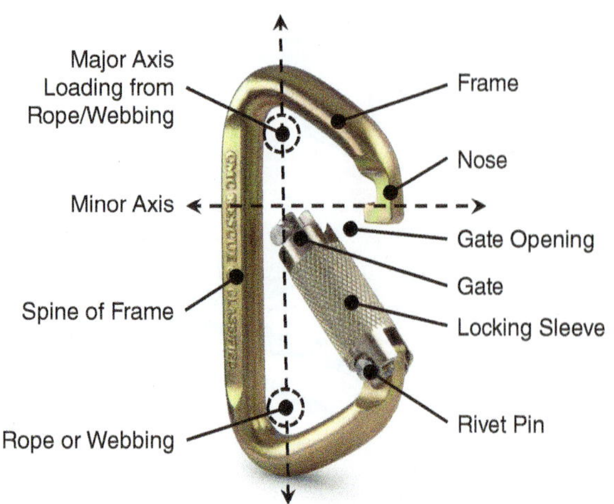

FIGURE 16-19 Carabiner terminology.
Courtesy of CMC Rescue, Inc.

Maillon Rapide Quick Links

Another type of connecting device like a carabiner is the Maillon Rapide quick link (**FIGURE 16-21**). These devices are strong and generally made of zinc-plated steel. It is important to purchase the type that has been EN 12275 (mountaineering equipment) and UIAA certified with the breaking strength stamped on the link. It is also important that these devices are only used with the gate closed. Unlike some carabiners, these devices must have a closed gate to achieve their rated breaking strength. Quick links are most useful for connections that don't require regular opening and closing. Aside from the common oval shape, quick links also come in triangular (delta or tri-link), square, and half-round configurations. These can be useful when a multidirectional load is expected.

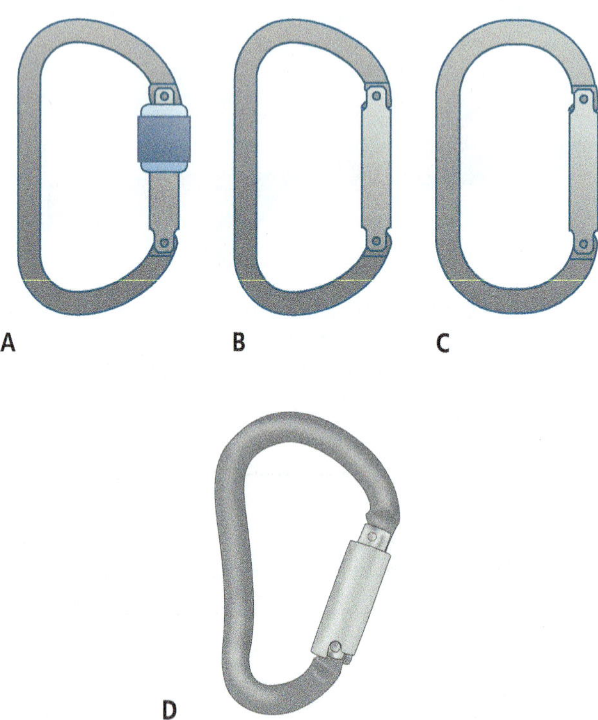

FIGURE 16-20 Types of carabiners. **A.** A "D" locking carabiner. **B.** A "D" nonlocking carabiner. **C.** An oval nonlocking carabiner. **D.** HMS carabiner.

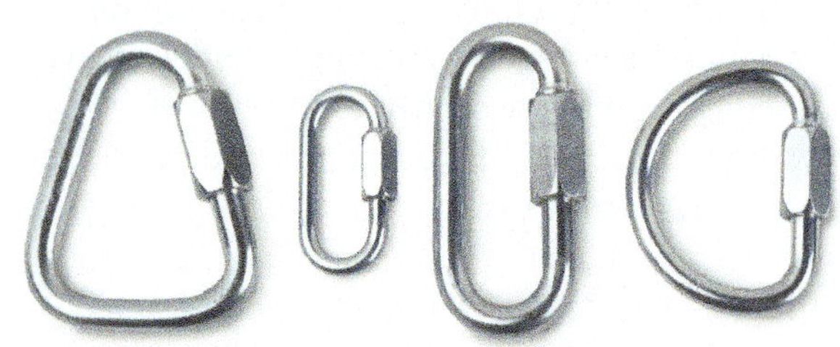

FIGURE 16-21 Maillon Rapide quick links.
Courtesy of CMC Rescue, Inc.

Which Carabiner to Use: Steel or Aluminum?

The materials used in the manufacture of carabiners are usually limited to steel and aluminum. Each has properties that are both desirable and undesirable. Steel has more strength and, to some extent, more durability; however, steel is heavy, may rust, and costs more than aluminum. Where very heavy loads are likely and gear weight is not a concern, steel is the better choice. Aluminum carabiners are lighter, do not rust (but they may oxidize), and are generally cheaper than steel. The disadvantages of aluminum include that they may be more easily damaged by dropping or shock loading, the locking device is often easier to damage, and some sizes and designs are not as strong as steel.

Loading a Carabiner

Carabiners and screw links must always be loaded axially and never across the gate (**FIGURE 16-22**). A carabiner's breaking strength is much lower when it is cross-loaded. If loading at multiple angles is required, then a tri-link or half-round screw link is a better choice.

Carabiner Care

If they are to be used in rescue, carabiners must be properly stored and maintained. Each carabiner needs to be visually inspected before it is used. The gate needs to be tested to see if it locks and examined for excessive wear or damage. The latching device and the body also should be inspected for physical damage such as deep grooves and corrosion. Carabiners should be stored in a place where they are not exposed to corrosion and/or damage.

Carabiners can be cleaned with soap and water if desired. It is not advisable to lubricate carabiners with any oil or similar lubricant, as this may collect dust and dirt. If slight lubrication is required, a small amount of dry graphite lubricant can be used.

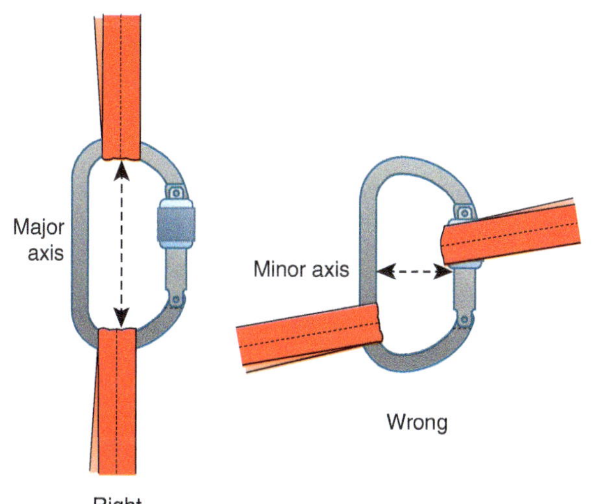

FIGURE 16-22 **A.** The right way to load a carabiner is on its major axis. **B.** The wrong way to load a carabiner is by its minor axis.

Consider removing a carabiner from service if it has been shock loaded (application of a sudden, heavy load) or has fallen from height onto a hard surface (e.g., rock or concrete). Shock loading and falls onto hard surfaces can cause small cracks to develop that can lead to weakness and premature failure. You should also remove a carabiner from service when the gate no longer closes on its own (i.e., stays in the open position).

Often the gate on a locking carabiner becomes stuck in the closed position. This can happen when a carabiner with a locked gate is loaded. The stuck gate can often be loosened by re-loading the carabiner and slightly unscrewing the gate. If this does not work, you may choose to use pliers, but be sure to be careful and inspect the carabiner for damage after opening. Remember, finger-tight is just right. Locking the gate on a carabiner does nothing for its strength. The lock only prevents the gate from opening unintentionally.

For the purposes of searcher safety in a nontechnical environment, an aluminum locking carabiner is adequate. It is recommended that SAR personnel should carry two of these in their SAR ready pack. At least one should reside on the outside of the pack, as some helicopter crews may use this link to attach your pack to the floor of the helicopter.

ASTM (2013), ANSI/ASSE (2016), OSHA (2016), and NFPA (2017c) have developed standards for industrial, climbing, mountaineering, and rescue carabiners/connectors. The European standard EN (European Norm) 12275, *Mountaineering Equipment, Connectors, Safety Requirements and Test Methods*, addresses carabiner testing protocols, rated strengths, and markings. Reviewing and becoming familiar with these and related standards is highly recommended for SAR personnel who operate in rescue environments.

Litters

A **litter** (also known as a *stretcher*) is a transfer device used to support and protect an injured subject during movement. A litter may be hand carried or transported by any number of vehicles or aircraft. Choosing a specific type of litter must be dependent on the way in which it will be used. For example, any litter that is used with a helicopter must be approved for use by the aircraft's crew. Many good litters are not acceptable for use on an aircraft.

There are a great number of litters available for use in SAR. The common types of litters that SAR personnel need to be familiar with include: improvised; basket; and flexible, wrap-around litters.

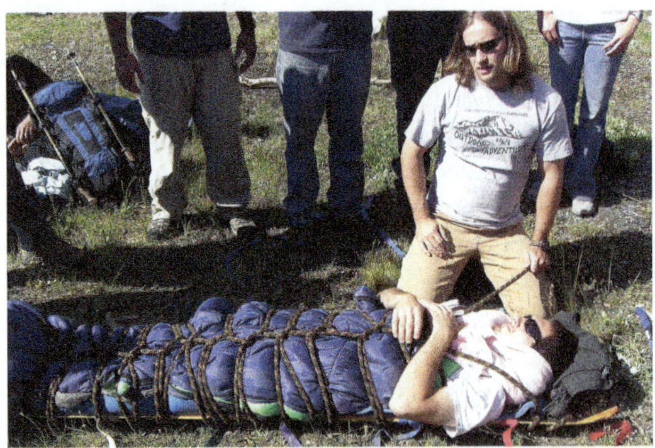

FIGURE 16-23 An improvised litter can be effective spine protection if a commercial litter is not available.
Courtesy of Jeffrey E. Isaac/Wilderness Medical Associates

Improvised Litters

In most SAR work, a litter is available when it is needed. Should such a device not be accessible and moving a patient becomes necessary, a litter can be improvised from various materials (**FIGURE 16-23**).

Although their use in organized SAR should be rare, the simplest improvised litter can be made from a heavy plastic tarpaulin, tent material, or large polyethylene bag. By wrapping the material around a rock, wadded sock, or glove and securing it with rope or twine, the rescuer can fashion handles in the corners and sides to facilitate carrying. A coil of rope can also be fashioned into a litter—called a rope litter or clove hitch stretcher—but a 150- to 200-foot (46- to 61-meter) climbing or rescue rope is required. A sturdy blanket or tarp can be used in combination with ski poles or stout tree branches to construct a litter, or a similar device can be improvised by passing the poles through the sleeves of two heavy, zipped (closed) parkas. If long distances must be traveled or if pack animals are available, a litter may also be constructed so that it can be dragged or slid along the ground like a sled. None of these methods should be first choices when a patient needs to be moved, but any of them may be necessary when the right equipment is just not available.

Basket-Style Litters

The basket-style litter derives its name from its shape. The sides curve upward to protect the victim's sides and to prevent the victim from rolling out. Most basket-style litters combine a steel frame (solid, tubular, or both) with a shell of either steel wire netting ("chicken wire") or plastic. Although the traditional materials and design (i.e., tubular and flat, welded steel with a steel chicken wire covering) are still in use today, basket-style litters are more often constructed from tubular stainless steel or aluminum because of the added corrosion resistance, increased strength, and reduced weight. Because the wire mesh of the traditional Stokes litter can be uncomfortable for the patient, nylon suspension inserts are available to suspend the patient in the basket above the wire. A sleeping pad can also be added to the bottom of the litter for added comfort and insulation.

Taking advantage of substantial improvements in polymer research, some manufacturers began producing a stretcher shell composed of rigid plastic instead of steel mesh. This has the added advantage of sliding over ice, snow, scree, and mud more easily because of the smooth bottom. As an added safety measure, when rigging this type of litter, it is important to tie into the metal rail and not just the plastic shell.

Ultraviolet (UV) light has been known to adversely affect the plastic in some of these litters. Older models in particular have been reported to become brittle upon extended exposure to UV light. Manufacturers of newer models claim this is no longer a significant problem, but it is still a good idea to protect all rescue equipment from sunlight and other elements.

SEARCH AND RESCUE TIP

Three of the common types of litters that SAR personnel need to be familiar with are: improvised; basket; and flexible, wrap-around litters.

Some of these litters are manufactured in a break-apart design that facilitates packing it into a remote site; however, the overall strength of the device often suffers a bit with this design. All older-style break-apart litters that depend on pins should be backed up with 8-mm rope or webbing, and they should be used with extreme caution in advanced technical rescue operations such as highlines (a technique where rope strung across a wide space fully supports the weight of a litter and patient). The structural weak point of many older basket-style litters, particularly aluminum varieties, is the top rail. Some rescue organizations recommend wrapping a piece of 1-inch tubular webbing around that rail for added security. Some manufacturers have no data on the strength of this rail, however, and all rescue techniques that include attachments to this rail should have a backup method of attaching to, and supporting, the device and its occupant.

Flexible, Wrap-Around Litters

Although there are others available, the Skedco SKED® litter is the classic example of a flexible, wrap-around litter. It is essentially a drag sheet made from heavy duty, polyethylene plastic (**FIGURE 16-24**). It is designed to be used with a backboard (short or long) that helps immobilize the head and neck while keeping the SKED from collapsing around the patient.

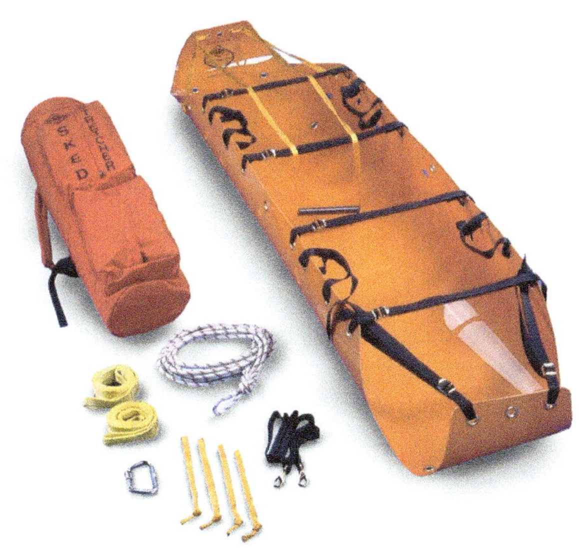

FIGURE 16-24 SKED® basic rescue system.
Courtesy of CMC Rescue, Inc.

Wrap-around litters such as the SKED have proven to be excellent choices for use in caves and other confined space situations. In fact, the SKED was primarily designed as a confined space rescue litter. The litter ends fold over the head and the feet to provide a secure, protective cocoon for the patient. There is a smaller version for children known as the Pediatric or "PED" SKED and an "HMD" (Haz-Mat/Decontaminable) version designed to be compact, easily decontaminated, and easier to drag in situations where a rescuer may be wearing a Level A protective suit (Skedco.com, 2017).

All attachments to the litter are made through built-in 3/4-inch brass grommets. The design incorporates systems for both horizontal and vertical evacuations. One of the best features of the SKED is that it rolls up into a Cordura backpack carrier, which makes the entire system extremely portable.

The SKED has some relative drawbacks. Since it is so flexible, it tends to bend at both ends. Thus, a backboard must be used to prevent the sides and the ends from squeezing the patient. An extended carry may also be difficult with the SKED due to its flexibility. While basket or wire-frame litters have a handy rail to grasp, the litter carrier on a SKED must grasp a loop of webbing.

Patient Packaging

There are a variety of ways to "package" a patient in a litter. The way the patient is packaged depends on his or her medical condition, the environment, and the manner in which he or she is to be evacuated.

Medical Condition

If the patient requires monitoring, will you be able to access the patient for taking vitals and other procedures with the method of packaging applied? Is the patient's airway clear? Will the packaging exacerbate any injuries or cause unnecessary pain?

Environment

Will the patient be warm enough? Remember, your patient is immobilized and can get very chilled even in relatively warm climates. Is there a chance of getting wet? If so, consider a vapor barrier and adequate shielding. Getting wet is not comfortable. Remember to provide shade if the weather is hot and sunny. Don't leave a patient out in the open sun for very long, especially if it is hot. Find some shade, or at least provide some sunglasses for the carry-out where shade is not available.

Evacuation

Is the patient to be evacuated vertically? If so, then take care to provide some sort of foot-loops, stirrups, or other foot supports so that the patient can bear some weight with his or her legs rather than hanging from a harness or other tie-in. Be sure to pad behind the knees (injuries permitting) and pack excess soft gear carefully around the patient. The less "slop" there is in the packaging, the more comfortable the ride. While there is some debate as to this practice, it may be a good idea to put a helmet on your patient. Some argue that a helmet is of minimal help when lying horizontal in a litter and may cause airway issues. Consult your team policies and procedures for guidance.

Litter Accessories

There are a variety of accessories that can greatly help in litter evacuation. For long, relatively flat, or trail evacuations, a litter wheel may be helpful (**FIGURE 16-25**). The litter wheel bears the load of the litter, while the litter handlers provide balance and direction. This does come with a cost, however. The litter wheel must be carried or rolled to the patient.

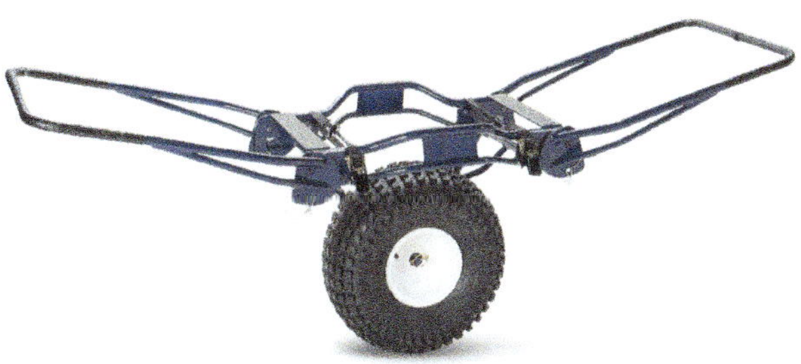

FIGURE 16-25 CMC Rescue Mule II Litter wheel with handles.
Courtesy of CMC Rescue, Inc.

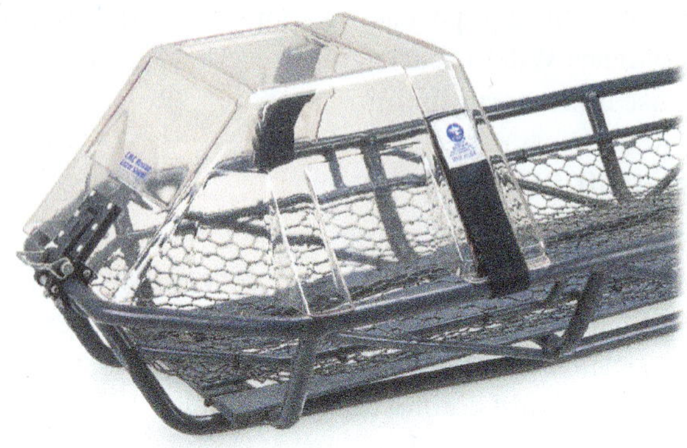

FIGURE 16-26 CMC Rescue Litter Shield.
Courtesy of CMC Rescue, Inc.

Litter shields are more effective than helmets for protecting the heads of patients (**FIGURE 16-26**). A litter shield attaches to the head of the litter and covers the head and the neck of the patient. Because nothing is on the patient's head, there is no problem with the airway, and it protects the head, the face, and the neck of the patient, rather than just the top of the head as with a helmet. Also, the shield can be covered with a pad or duct tape to provide a sunscreen.

Also available are specialized sleeping bags that are designed with a litter-packaged patient in mind. These devices open like a clamshell and have reinforced bottoms and loops on the sides to facilitate carrying. In addition, there are a variety of access openings that facilitate medical access and monitoring.

Litter Handling

Litters are used to facilitate moving patients to a place of safety, and they can be used in a variety of situations. They can be lifted by rope, carried by vehicles, or, most commonly, hand-carried by rescuers. While managing your patient, be sure to communicate and keep him or her apprised of the situation and your progress. Include them in your conversation and remember to call him or her by name. Do not refer to him or her as "the victim." Do not step over the patient if it can at all be avoided, and be careful with ends of webbing and other rescue hardware, as this can be very painful if dropped on a patient's face or body. Try not to shine a headlamp or flashlight into the patient's eyes, and be careful when using knives or scissors around the patient and the rigging.

Standard Carry

The standard litter carry involves a team of six to eight rescuers distributed around the litter, three or four to a side. Normally, one of the rescuers at the front is in charge and directs the activities of the others.

This method has the advantages of being fast, as little teamwork is required, and it usually gives the patient a comfortable ride. Its disadvantages include that it is very tiring for the handlers because it puts a constant strain on selected muscles, and view of the ground is difficult, especially at night; a handler can easily trip, stumble, and drop the litter.

If a litter handler starts to fall, he should call "Stop!" and let go of the litter. The "Stop" command is to prevent the litter team from running over the falling team member and injuring him or her needlessly.

More than one team may be needed if the distance to carry the litter is more than the team can cover in about 15 to 20 minutes. Team leapfrogging is a good method to use on long evacuations. One team takes the litter for a given distance, while the other team goes ahead to rest and pre-plan the next stretch. At the pass-off point, the first team advances to the next point for rest and planning.

SEARCH AND RESCUE TIP

Keep the patient apprised of the situation and of your progress, and remember to call him or her by name. Avoid stepping over the patient whenever possible, and try not to shine a headlamp or flashlight into his or her eyes.

This rotation can extend everyone's endurance quite a bit. Try to avoid making the distances too far. Extended rest periods can be harmful if people are allowed to cool off to the point of becoming chilled and then asked to carry a litter using cold muscles.

Caterpillar or Lap Pass

When footing is tenuous or there is an obstacle that prevents the litter team from progressing, and falling becomes a possible hazard, the caterpillar (also called "lap pass") becomes a useful option.

When the litter reaches the obstacle, the team pauses while every extra person lines up on the route at and ahead of the difficult terrain or obstacles. While remaining stationary, they form two equal length lines facing each other, about the width of the litter apart. They usually sit and try to make themselves as stable as possible. When everyone is set, the litter is passed down between the two lines of rescuers. As the litter passes each person, he or she gets up and carefully but quickly moves around the line in the direction of travel and gets set to pass the litter again. Done correctly, this provides a very stable and secure passage.

Turtle Carry

The turtle carry is most useful for negotiating very narrow passages, such as slot canyons or long spaces between two large boulders.

To accomplish the turtle carry, one hardy rescuer with gloves, kneepads, and a sense of humor gets on his hands and knees, and the litter is balanced on his back. Two other litter handlers are positioned at the head and the foot of the litter, where they mainly balance and guide the litter. They can take some of the weight of the litter, but the majority is carried by the "turtle" underneath. This is very slow and can be painful for the rescuer in the turtle role, but it is sometimes the only option available.

Strap Carry

A strap carry is very useful to prolong one's endurance on long carries. Construct a loop from webbing approximately 6 feet (2 meters) long and girth hitch it to the litter rail. While lifting the litter with one hand (over the girth hitch), bring the loop up and over your shoulders and grip the end of the loop with your other hand. This approach helps center the load on your shoulders rather than unilaterally stressing only one arm and your back. If you start to fall, you can twist out of the loop by turning away from the litter, leaving the other to temporarily support the litter.

Tag Lines

Once in a while, you will come to a place that is too low and narrow for a standard carry, lap pass, or even a turtle carry. When this happens, you may have no option but to use tag lines (short pieces of rope or webbing) to drag the litter through.

After tying a piece of webbing or accessory rope (tag line) to the head and foot of the litter, crawl through the tight spot, dragging the free end of the tag line. When one rescuer gets to the other end, pull the litter through with the tag line. The tag line tied to the other end of the litter is to help control it in case the ground is sloped or slippery. Tag lines may also be useful during low-angle and short, steep-angle maneuvers.

Wrap-Up

READY FOR REVIEW

- Any rescue activity that requires the use of a rope to support a life is inherently dangerous. Proper and extensive training and experience should be gained from qualified sources if these skills are to be used in the field.
- Webbing is light, easy to pack, and can be used in a variety of situations.
- Rope must be stronger than the load it is intended to support. The ratio of the strength of a new rope, or any rescue component, to its intended load is called the design factor.
- Software is easily damaged and therefore must be used, monitored, and maintained carefully.
- When choosing a harness to use, you need to determine what your function is and the type of harness that provides the necessary protection for that role.
- A variety of knots may be required in rescue, but only a few are needed in most rescue situations. The key is to learn a few useful knots and practice them often.
- A carabiner can be used to connect webbing and rope to harnesses, litters, and anchors, and to prevent synthetic material from running across other synthetic material.
- There are a great number of litters available for use in SAR. The common types of litters that SAR personnel need to be familiar with include improvised; basket; and flexible, wrap-around litters.

SEARCH AND RESCUE TERMS

Bend A knot used to join two pieces, or ends, of a rope.

Breaking strength The point at which a rope fails under a load.

Carabiner A load-bearing connector with a self-closing gate used to join other elements of a rescue system.

Design factor The ratio of the strength of a rope to the intended load.

Fall factor The ratio computed by dividing the fall distance of a climber attached to an anchored rope by the length of the rope between the load and the anchor or belay. For example, a 9-foot (3-meter) fall on a 9-foot (3-meter) rope would be a fall factor of 1.

Hardware In rescue, any rescue equipment not considered software.

Hitch A knot used to attach a rope to a fixed object or fixed rope.

Kernmantle rope Rope construction with two parts: a tightly woven outer sheath that serves to support a load and protects the inner core, and an inner core consisting of strands of fibers that are bundled together to provide most of the rope's strength.

Litter Body-length transfer device used to support and protect an injured subject during movement; also called a *stretcher*.

Software In rescue, any soft, pliable material that can be tied into knots. Examples are rope, webbing, and cordage.

System safety factor The ratio between the weakest link in a rescue system and the load to be supported.

REFERENCES AND SUGGESTED READING

American National Standards Institute and American Society of Safety Engineers. 2016. ANSI/ASSE Z359.1-2016, safety requirements for personal fall arrest systems, subsystems and components. Park Ridge, IL: American Society of Safety Engineers.

ASTM International. 2017. Search and rescue operations standards: List of search and rescue standards developed by ASTM. https://www.astm.org/Standards/search-and-rescue-operations-standards.html.

ASTM, International. 2015. Standard guide for determining load ratios for technical rescue systems and equipment, F2491-05(2015). West Conshohocken, PA: ASTM, International.

ASTM, International. 2014a. Standard test method for measuring the performance of synthetic rope rescue belay systems using a drop test, F2436-14. West Conshohocken, PA: ASTM, International.

ASTM, International. 2014b. Standard guide for training for level I rope rescue (R1) rescuer endorsement, F2752-09(2014). West Conshohocken, PA: ASTM, International.

ASTM, International. 2013. Standard specification for climbing and mountaineering carabiners, F1772-13. West Conshohocken, PA: ASTM, International.

ASTM, International. 2012a. Standard guide for inspection of nylon, polyester, or nylon/polyester blend, or both kernmantle rope, F1740-96(2012). West Conshohocken, PA: ASTM, International.

ASTM, International. 2012b. Standard guide for training for level II rope rescue (R2) rescuer endorsement, F2954-12. West Conshohocken, PA: ASTM, International.

ASTM, International. 2012c. Standard guide for training for level III rope rescue (R3) rescuer endorsement, F2955-12. West Conshohocken, PA: ASTM, International.

ASTM, International. 2012d. Standard specification for harnesses for rescue, safety, and sport activities, F1772-12. West Conshohocken, PA: ASTM, International.

ASTM, International. 2007. Standard specification for low stretch and static kernmantle life safety rope, F2116-01(2007). West Conshohocken, PA: ASTM, International.

Auerbach, Paul S., ed. 2017. *Wilderness Medicine*, 7th edition. St. Louis, MO: Elsevier, Inc.

Brown, Michael G. 2000. *Engineering Practical Rope Rescue Systems*. Clifton Park, NY: Delmar Learning.

Cox, Steven, and Kris Fulsass, eds. 2003. *Mountaineering: Freedom of the Hills*, 7th edition. New York: Mountaineers Books.

Frank, James A., ed. 2013. *CMC Rope Rescue Manual*, revised 4th edition. Santa Barbara, CA: CMC Rescue.

International Association of Fire Chiefs, and National Fire Protection Association. 2011. *Fundamentals of Technical Rescue*. Sudbury, MA: Jones & Bartlett Publishers.

Linxweiler, Eric and Mike Maude, Editors. The Mountaineers. 2017. *Mountaineering: Freedom of the Hills*, 9th edition. New York: Mountaineers Books.

McCurley, Loui H., and Thomas Evans. 2017. Ropes and knot tying. In *Wilderness Medicine*, 7th edition. Volume 2, edited by Paul S. Auerbach, pp. 2361–2375. St. Louis, MO: Elsevier, Inc.

National Fire Protection Association. 2017a. NFPA 1670, standard on operations and training for technical search and rescue incidents. Batterymarch, MA: NFPA.

National Fire Protection Association. 2017b. NFPA 1006, standard for technical rescue personnel professional qualifications. Batterymarch, MA: NFPA.

National Fire Protection Association. 2017c. NFPA 1983, standard on life safety rope and equipment for emergency services. Batterymarch, MA: NFPA.

National Search and Rescue Committee. 2011. Land search and rescue addendum to the National Search and Rescue Supplement to the International Aeronautical and Maritime Search and Rescue Manual, Version 1.0. https://www.hsdl.org/?abstract&did=715465.

Occupational Safety and Health Administration. 2016. 29 CFR 1910.140, Occupational Safety and Health standards, personal protective equipment, personal fall protection systems. https://www.osha.gov/pls/oshaweb/owadisp.show_document?p_table=STANDARDS&p_id=1291.

Roop, Michael, Tom Vines, and Richard Wright. 1998. *Confined Space and Structural Rope Rescue*. St. Louis, MO: Mosby.

Skedco.com. 2017. SKED® Basic Rescue System – International Orange, product description. http://skedco.com/product/sked-basic-rescue-system-international-orange/.

Vines, Tom, and Steve Hudson. 2014. *High Angle Rescue Techniques: Levels I & II*, 4th edition. Burlington, MA: Jones & Bartlett Learning.

Washington Explorer Search and Rescue. 1999. *Washington Explorer Search and Rescue Team Member Training Manual*, 4th printing. Tacoma, WA: Washington Explorer Search and Rescue.

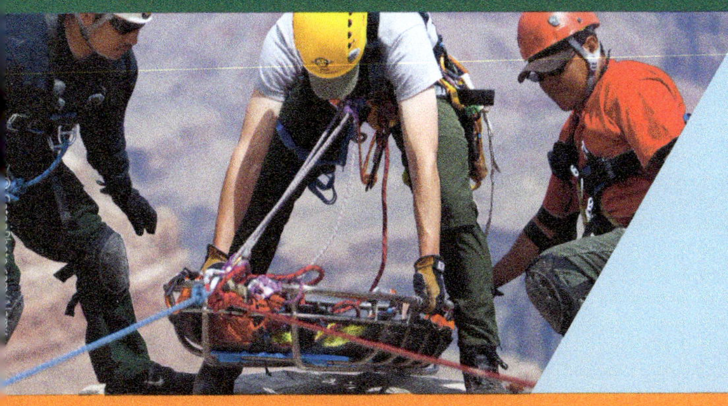

Appendix A: Missing Person Questionnaire

Incident Name: ____

____

Initial Data Capture: ______________________ Date/Time: ______________

Updated By: ______________________ Date/Time: ______________

Updated By: ______________________ Date/Time: ______________

Updated By: ______________________ Date/Time: ______________

Updated By: ______________________ Date/Time: ______________

Updated By: ______________________ Date/Time: ______________

Updated By: ______________________ Date/Time: ______________

SECTIONS

Please fill all boxes, answer all questions, and print clearly without the use of unfamiliar abbreviations and/or confusing phrases/words. (**First Notice information = sections A–E only.**)

General and Informant Information A

Case Name/Number: Agency/Org:

Date: Time: Location:

Interviewer Name: Title: Agency/Org:

Reported missing by: DOB:

Address:

Home Phone: Bus. Phone:

Mobile Phone: Other Phone(s):

Occupation: Employer:

Email(s):

Relationship to subject:

Where can be reached in next 24 hours:

What does this person think happened?

Where does this person think the subject is?

Search efforts prior to calling for SAR:

Instructions to informant:

Other persons interviewed (name, contact info, date, time, relationship, DOB):

Missing Person B

Full Name: Nickname(s):

Name to call: Alias(es):

Safe word? Y ☐ N ☐ Word: Who knows it:

Subject's primary language: Speaks English? Y ☐ N ☐

Other languages spoken: Sign Language? Y ☐ N ☐

Home address:

Home Phone: Bus. Phone:

Mobile Phone: Other Phone(s):

Occupation: Employer:

Email(s):

Category(ies) of lost subject:

General experience and familiarity with area:

General quality/quantity of equip. carried and preparedness for environment:

Police Marker:

Comments:

Physical Description C

Age: Race: Gender: Hgt: Wt: DOB:

Build:

Hair Color: Length: Style:

If balding, describe: Eye Color:

Describe all facial hair:

Glasses Regular: Sun: Contacts:

Describe glasses:

Eyesight without glasses:

Facial features, shape:

Complexion:

Distinguishing marks, scars, tattoos:

Fingerprints on file? Y ☐ N ☐ Where? Fake nails? Y ☐ N ☐

General appearance:

Clothing Worn When Last Seen D

Hat/Cap/Scarf:

Shirt/Blouse:

Trousers:

Dress:

Sweater/Pullover:

Coat/Jacket/Rain Gear:

Footwear:

Sole pattern and how known:

Hose/Socks:

Underwear:

Other:

Describe all accessories worn, such as belt, rings, watch, pins, necktie, tie clip, etc.

Details of Incident E

Location missing from:

Point last seen (PLS):

Last known point (LKP):

Day/Date last seen: Time last seen:

Last seen by whom:

Accompanied by animal(s)? (describe):

Vehicle description, if driving:

Destination(s), stated intentions:

Possible alternative destinations:

Route, possible route, how determined:

Weather at time of loss:

Use computer software to determine route(s)? What used?

Access to this computer? Where?

Other resources used to plan trip/outing (books, guides, maps, brochures):

Events of last 24 hours leading up to time of loss:

Familiar with area?

Person most familiar with area? Hazards? Contact info:

Equipment Carried F

Describe ALL items carried such as pocketbook, wallet, backpack (describe contents of each), matches, lighter, keys, pocket knife, camera, weapon, ammunition, etc. (style, color, brand, size). Use additional pages, if necessary.

Describe any food and water and/or drinks carried, including alcohol:

Describe any pets or animals: (circle pets thought to be with subject now)

Electronic Device			Battery			
Carried?	Y	Type	Status	Spare?	Type	Last Changed
Cell Phone						
GPS						
Radio						
Beacon						
Location Service						
RF Tracking Device						

Other:

Mobile Phone			
	Provider:	Number:	PIN/Password:
	Model: Smart Phone ☐	Attempt to call?	Left message?
	Text message sent?	User knows how to text?	Message sent:

GPS			
GPS	GPS Default settings:	Datum:	Able to set waypoints?
	Able to record routes?	Able to download routes?	Able to go to waypoint?
	Is the computer to which routes were downloaded available?		

Radio frequency: Radio PL/CG (used?) Check-in time/interval:

Beacon number: Beacon registered? Web password:

RF Track Freq: RFID # On subject:

Other:

Subject's Experience G

City/Township/County/
State/Country of residence: How long?

Previous residence: How long?

Birthplace:

Has the person been the subject of a search before?

If so, describe the details (date(s), circumstances, how long missing, where and when found, condition when found, actions taken by subject, lost in group (contact info for others in group, etc.)?

Additional info and comments:

Physical Health of Subject H

General physical condition:

Disabilities:

Known medical conditions:

Recent injuries/trauma: Last meal:

Recent complaints (including minor):

Pregnant? How long? Menstruating?

Physician: Phone:

Address:

Vision I

Glasses? Contacts? Type of Contacts: Time stay in:

Spare glasses/contacts: Corrected vision: Uncorrected vision:

Color blindness? Type: Night vision problems?

Other visual problems: Vision last checked:

Optometrist/Ophthalmologist contact info:

Mental/Emotional Health J

General mental health:

Known mental problems:

Suicidal? Previous attempts (explain):

Is subject dangerous to self or others? (explain)

Does subject have access to, or possibly carrying, a weapon?
(if so, describe type and size)

Are all weapons accounted for? Ammo accounted for?

Fears and phobias:

Knowledgeable person: Contact info:

Title: Address:

Physician specialist: Contact info:

Case manager: Contact info:

Therapist(s): Contact info:

Medications: Prescription and Non-prescription K

Med name, strength, dosage, etc.	Effect if not taken	Lethal dose

Identification L

Driver's License: No: Issue Date:

Passport Country: No: Issue Date:

Other ID:

Enrolled in MedicAlert®, Safe Return® or similar program? (describe)

Electronic tracking device? (describe)

Finances M

Credit & Cash Point cards: List card names and account numbers.

Checking and savings accounts: List banks and account numbers.

Does subject have credit cards or checkbook in possession? Y ☐ N ☐ Cash Carried:

Describe:

Detailed Subject History N

Single ☐ Married ☐ Divorced ☐ Widowed ☐ Adopted ☐

Spouse's name: Phone:

Address:

Siblings (name, age, residence – add page if necessary):

Father's name: Biological Father? Y ☐ N ☐ Living? Y ☐ N ☐

Contact info:

Occupation and employer:

Mother's name: Biological Mother? Y ☐ N ☐ Living? Y ☐ N ☐

Contact info:

Occupation and employer:

Other relatives/caregivers who may have info:

Occupation and Employer O

Primary occupation: Retired? Y ☐ N ☐

Employer: How long?

Contact person:

Previous/Secondary employment:

Education level (describe):

Military service branch: Reserves? Y ☐ N ☐ Currently active? Y ☐ N ☐

Contact person: Dates of service:

Religion/belief system: Active? Y N

Contact person:

Any recent contacts, changes in behavior?

Other persons who may provide info:

Hobbies, Special Interests P

Experience in outdoors, backcountry:

Survival training/experience:

First aid training/experience:

Favorite places to visit:

Athletic ability, mobility:

Swimmer, ability/non-swimmer:

Active/outgoing or quiet/withdrawn?

Attitude toward authority:

Use of social media: Facebook? Y ☐ N ☐ Twitter? Y ☐ N ☐ Other:

Online screen names/nicknames/tags:

Facebook/Twitter friends/followers:

Personal Q

Recent, current, or anticipated financial, legal, or other problems:

In whom does the subject confide and/or frequently talk to on the phone?

Who last talked to the subject at length?

When and what was the topic?

Does the subject like animals?

Reaction to dogs, horses?

Recent letter or writings (blogs, email, tweets, etc.)?

Does the subject keep a diary/journal/bible/blog?

Does the subject have access to a computer?

Describe location, user name(s), password(s)

Has Internet browser been checked?

Sites of interest?

Does subject smoke, drink, use illegal drugs, or abuse legal drugs? (describe in detail)

Additional Information and Comments R

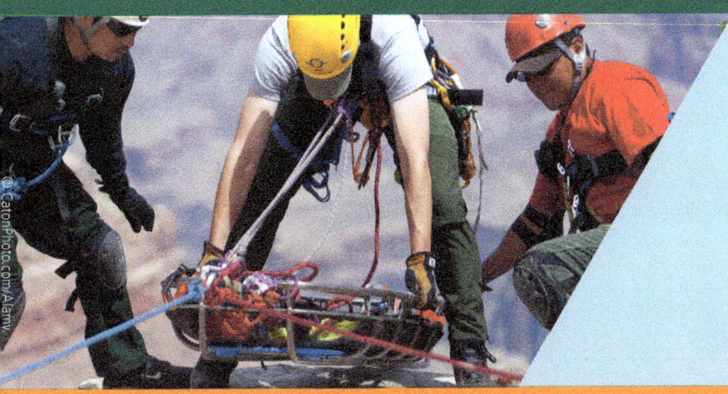

Appendix B: Cuestionario sobre Persona Desaparecida

Nombre del Incidente: ______________________

Información Inicial

Recopilada Por: ______________________ Fecha/Hora: ______________

Actualizado Por: ______________________ Fecha/Hora: ______________

Actualizado Por: ______________________ Fecha/Hora: ______________

Actualizado Por: ______________________ Fecha/Hora: ______________

Actualizado Por: ______________________ Fecha/Hora: ______________

SECCIONES

Complete todos los renglones y conteste todas las preguntas. Escriba en letra de molde, de forma clara, sin usar abreviaturas desconocidas y/o frases/palabras confusas. (informacil de Primer Aviso = secciones A–E solamente.)

Información General y del Informante A

Nombre /Número de Caso: Agencia/Org:

Fecha: Hora: Lugar:

Nombre Entrevistador: Título: Agencia/Org:

Notificado desaparecido por: Nacimiento:

Dirección:

Teléfono Hogar: Teléfono Trabajo:

Teléfono Móvil: Otros teléfonos:

Ocupación: Patrono:

Direcciones correo electrónico:

Relación con Persona Desaparecida:

¿Dónde puede ser contactado en las próximas 24 horas?:

¿Qué piensa el informante que ocurrió?

¿Dónde piensa el informante que está la persona desaparecida?

Esfuerzos de búsqueda antes de llamar a autoridades:

Instrucciones al informante:

Otras personas entrevistadas (nombre, información de contacto, fecha, hora, relación, nacimiento):

Persona Desaparecida B

Nombre completo: Apodo(s):

Nombre a llamar: Alias(es):

Palabra clave S ☐ N ☐ Palabra: ¿Quién la conoce?:

Idioma principal: ¿Habla español? S ☐ N ☐

Otros idiomas: ¿Lenguaje señas? S ☐ N ☐

Dirección hogar:

Teléfono hogar: Teléfono trabajo:

Teléfono móvil: Otros teléfonos:

Ocupación: Patrono:

Direcciones correo electrónico:

Categoría(s) de persona perdida:

Experiencia general y conocimiento del área:

Calidad general y cantidad de equipo llevado y preparación para el ambiente:

Expediente policial:

Comentarios:

Descripción Física C

Edad: Raza: Sexo: Estatura: Peso: Nacimiento:

Constitución física:

Color cabello: Largo cabello: Estilo:

Describa calvicie, si aplica: Color ojos:

Describa vello facial:

Lentes Regulares: Para el sol: De contacto:

Describa lentes:

Visión sin lentes:

Características faciales, forma:

Tez, piel facial:

Marcas distintivas, cicatrices, tatuajes:

¿Huellas digitales archivadas?: S ☐ N ☐ ¿Dónde?: ¿Uñas falsas? S ☐ N ☐

Apariencia general:

Vestimenta usada la última vez vista: D

Sombrero/Gorra/Bufanda:

Camisa/Blusa:

Pantalones:

Traje/Vestido:

Suéter/Pulóver:

Abrigo/Chaqueta/Ropa para la lluvia:

Calzado:

Patrón de la suela y porqué lo conoce:

Medias/Calcetines:

Ropa interior:

Otras:

Describa todos los accesorios usados tales como cinturón, anillos, reloj, prendedores, corbata, pines, etc.

Detalles del Incidente E

Lugar donde despareció:

Punto donde último fue vista (PUV / *PLS*):

Último punto conocido (UPC / *LKP*):

Día/Fecha vista por última vez: Hora vista por última vez:

Persona quien la vio por última vez:

¿Acompañada por algún animal? (describa):

Descripción de vehículo, si conducía alguno:

Destino(s), intenciones declaradas:

Posibles destinos alternos:

Ruta, posible ruta, ¿cómo se determinó?:

Condiciones del tiempo al desaparecer:

¿Usó algún programa de computadora para determinar ruta? ¿Cuál usó?

¿Acceso a esta computadora? ¿Dónde?

Otros recursos usados para planificar viaje/salida (libros, guías, mapas, folletos):

Eventos de últimas 24 horas conducentes a desaparición:

¿Conocedora del área?:

¿Persona más conocedora del área? ¿Peligros? Información de contacto:

Equipo Llevado F

Describa TODOS los artículos que llevaba tales como libreta de bolsillo, billetera, mochila (describa el contenido de cada una), fósforos, encendedor, navaja, camera, arma, municiones, etc. (estilo, color, marca tamaño). Use hojas adicionales, de ser necesario.

Describa cualquier alimento, agua y/o bebidas que llevaba, incluyendo alcohol: ____________________

Describa cualquier mascota o animales: (circule mascotas que se piense estén con la persona desaparecida ahora) ____________________

Aparatos Electrónicos			Carga / Baterías			
¿Llevaba?	S	Tipo	Estado	¿Repuestos?	Tipo	Última vez cambiado
Teléfono móvil						
GPS						
Radio						
Faro o baliza						
Servicio de Localización						
Aparato de Rastreo por radiofrecuencia						

Otros: ____________________

Telelos: melol	Proveedora servicio:	Número	Contraseña/número desbloqueo:
	Modelo:	¿Se ha intentado llamar?	¿Se dejó mensaje?
	¿Mensaje de texto enviado?	¿Sabe enviar mensajes de texto?	Mensaje enviado:
GPS	GPS Configuración:	Datum:	¿Capaz de marcar puntos de referencia?
	¿Capaz de grabar rutas?	¿Capaz de recibir (*download*) rutas?	¿Capaz de guiar hasta un punto de referencia?
	¿Está disponible la computadora usada para trazar o descargar las rutas?		

¿Frecuencia de Radio? ¿Radio línea privada (PL/CG) usado? Hora o intervalo para reportarse:

Número baliza (*beacon*): ¿Baliza registrada?: Contraseña para la web:

Frecuencia de rastreo: RFID # En persona desaparecida:

Otros:

Experiencia de Persona Desaparecida G

Ciudad/Distrito/Provincia/
Estado/País de residencia: ¿Por cuánto tiempo?

Residencia anterior: ¿Por cuánto tiempo?

Lugar de nacimiento:

¿Ha sido objetivo de una búsqueda anteriormente?

De ser así, describa los detalles (fechas, circunstancias, por cuánto tiempo, donde y cuándo fue encontrada, condición cuando fue encontrada, acciones realizadas por la persona, ¿perdido en grupo? [información de contacto de otros en grupo, etc.])

Información adicional y comentarios:

Salud Física H

Condición física general:

Impedimentos o discapacidades:

Condiciones médicas conocidas:

Lesiones/traumas recientes: Última comida:

Quejas recientes (incluyendo menores):

¿Embarazada? ¿Tiempo embarazo? ¿Menstruando?

Médico: Teléfono:

Dirección:

Visión I

¿Espejuelos? ¿Lentes de Contacto? Tipo de lentes: Duración lentes:

Espejuelos o lentes adicionales: Visión corregida: Visión sin corregir:

¿Daltonismo? Tipo: ¿Problemas visión nocturna?

Otros problemas visuales: Último examen visual:

Información de contacto optómetra/oftalmólogo:

Salud Mental/Emocional J

Salud mental general:

Problemas mentales conocidos:

¿Suicida? Intentos anteriores (explique):

¿La persona es peligrosa para sí misma u otros? (explicar)

¿La persona tiene acceso a, o puede estar portando, un arma? De ser así, describa tipo de arma y tamaño.

¿Falta algún arma? ¿Faltan municiones?

Miedos y fobias:

Persona conocedora: Información de contacto:

Título: Dirección:

Especialista médico: Información de contacto:

Manejador del caso: Información de contacto:

Terapista(s): Información de contacto:

Medicamentos: Prescritos y No Recetados K

Nombre, forma, dosis, etc.	Efecto si no se toma	Dosis letal

Identificación L

Licencia de conducir: Núm.: Fecha expedición:

Pasaporte/País: Núm.: Fecha expedición:

Otra identificación:

¿Registrado en *MedicAlert*®, *Safe Return*®, o en algún programa similar? (describa)

¿Aparato de rastreo electrónico? (describa)

Finanzas M

Tarjetas de crédito y débito: Enumere nombre de tarjetas y números de cuentas.

Cuentas corrientes y de ahorros: Enumere bancos y números de cuentas.

¿Tiene la persona consigo tarjetas de crédito o chequera? S ☐ N ☐ Dinero llevado:

Describa:

Historial detallado N

Soltera ☐ Casada ☐ Divorciada ☐ Viuda ☐ Adoptada ☐

Nombre de cónyuge: Teléfono:

Dirección:

Hermanos (nombre, edad, domicilio – añada página de ser necesario):

Nombre padre: ¿Padre biológico ? S ☐ N ☐ ¿Vivo? S ☐ N ☐

Información de contacto:

Ocupación y patrono:

Nombre madre: ¿Madre biológica? S ☐ N ☐ ¿Viva? S ☐ N ☐

Información de contacto:

Ocupación y patrono:

Otros familiares o cuidadores quienes puedan tener información:

Ocupación y Patrono O

Ocupación primaria: ¿Retirada? S☐ N☐

Patrono: ¿Por cuánto tiempo?

Persona de contacto:

Empleo previo/secundario:

Nivel de educación (describa):

Rama militar de servicio: ¿Reserva? S☐ N☐ ¿Activo actualmente? S☐ N☐

Persona de contacto: Fechas de servicio:

Religión/creencias: ¿Activo? S☐ N☐

Persona de contacto:

¿Contactos recientes o cambios en conducta?

Otras personas que puedan proveer información:

Pasatiempos e Intereses Especiales P

Experiencia al aire libre, campos:

Adiestramientos/experiencia en supervivencia:

Adiestramientos/experiencia en primeros auxilios:

Lugares favoritos para visitar:

Habilidad atlética, movilidad:

Nivel destrezas de natación:

¿Activa/extrovertida o callada/retraída?

Actitud hacia la autoridad:

Uso de redes sociales: ¿Facebook? S ☐ N ☐ ¿Twitter? S ☐ N ☐ Otras:

Nombres en sistemas, alias, apodos:

Amigos/seguidores en Facebook/Twitter:

Personal Q

Problemas financieros, legales, o de otro tipo, actuales, recientes o anticipados:

Personas en quien confía y/o habla frecuentemente por teléfono:

¿Quién fue el último en hablar con la persona de manera prolongada?

¿Cuándo y cuál fue el tema?

¿Le gustan los animales?

¿Reacción a perros, caballos?

¿Carta reciente o escritos recientes (blogs, correo electrónico, *tweets*, etc.)?

¿Tiene la persona un diario/bitácora/biblia/blog?

¿Tiene la persona acceso a una computadora?

Describa localización, nombre(s) de usuario(s), contraseñas

¿Se ha verificado el programa explorador de Internet?

¿Sitios de interes?

¿Fuma, consume bebidas alcohólicas, usa drogas ilegales o abusa de medicamentos legales? (describa detalladamente)

Información Adicional y Comentarios R

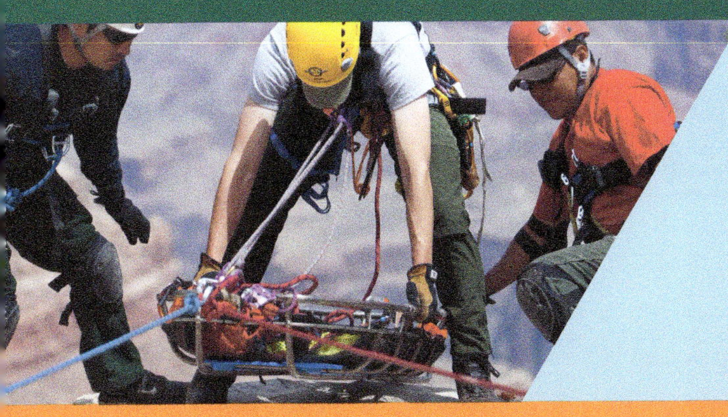

Appendix C: Search Log Book

This log book is a personal record of operational and training activity.

Entries should be made immediately following the relevant activity and counter-signed by an appropriate manager, ideally a team leader or member of the incident management team. As such, log books should be carried and completed on all operational searches and training events.

This book contains the individual record of achievement, training, and experience of the individual identified below:

Print Name: ______________________________

____

Signed: __________________________________

____

If found, please contact above at: ____________________

____

____

____

____

OPERATIONAL SEARCHES

Date	Search	Verifying Officer	Remarks - Comments

SEARCH TRAINING

Date	Search	Verifying Officer	Remarks - Comments

SEARCH TRAINING

Date	Search	Verifying Officer	Remarks - Comments

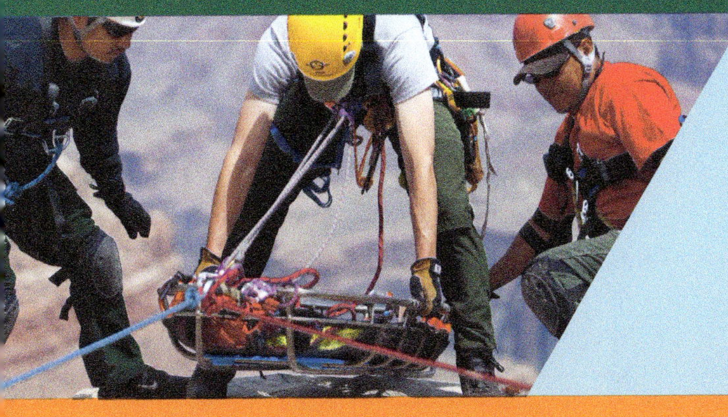

Appendix D: Search and Rescue Acronym List

AFRCC United States Air Force Rescue Coordination Center

AMBER America's Missing: Broadcast Emergency Response (AMBER Alert)

AMDR Average maximum detection range

AMS Acute mountain sickness

ARTCC Air Route Traffic Control Centers

ASTM Formerly an abbreviation for "American Society for Testing and Materials;" currently stands alone as the name of a standards writing organization (ASTM International).

ATS Air traffic services

BISC Basic Inland SAR Course (offered by the U.S. National SAR School)

BoO Base of operations (US&R)

BUBU Big, unconstricting, baggy, and ugly

CAP Civil Air Patrol

CARDA California Rescue Dog Association

CBRNE Chemical, biological, radiological, nuclear, and explosive

CE Certification evaluation (advanced US&R canine certification)

CEM Comprehensive emergency management

CERT Community Emergency Response Team

CFR Code of Federal Regulations

CISAR Catastrophic Incident Search and Rescue

CISM Critical incident stress management

CONPLAN U.S. Government Interagency Domestic Terrorism Concept of Operations Plan

COSPAS-SARSAT *Cosmicheskaya sistyema poiska avariynich sudov* (COSPAS), in English, "space system for the search of vessels in distress;" search and rescue satellite-aided tracking (SARSAT)—an international search and rescue satellite system.

CS Communications specialist (US&R)

DEET N,N-diethyl-meta-toluamide or diethyltoluamide; active chemical ingredient in popular insect repellents

DGPS Differential GPS

DHS U.S. Department of Homeland Security

DMAT Disaster Medical Assistance Team (Health and Human Services)

DOC U.S. Department of Commerce

DOD U.S. Department of Defense

DOI U.S. Department of the Interior

DOT U.S. Department of Transportation

DSCA Defense Support of Civil Authorities

EAS Emergency Alert System

ELT Emergency locator transmitter

EMAC Emergency Management Assistance Compact

EMI Emergency Management Institute

EMS Emergency medical service

EMT Emergency medical technician

EPIRB Emergency position indicating radio beacon

ESF Emergency support function

FAA Federal Aviation Administration

FCC Federal Communications Commission

FEMA Federal Emergency Management Agency (U.S. Department of Homeland Security)

FIRESCOPE Firefighting Resources of California Organized for Potential Emergencies

FLIR Forward looking infrared units

FOM Figure of measurement

FRERP Federal Radiological Emergency Response Plan

FSA Fundamental Skills Ability (basic US&R canine certification)

FSS Flight service stations

FUNSAR Fundamentals of search and rescue

GHz Gigahertz or 1000 megahertz

GN Grid north

GPS Global positioning system

GSS Ground support specialist

HACE High-altitude cerebral edema

HAPE High-altitude pulmonary edema

HELP Heat escape lessening position

HERS Heavy equipment and rigging specialist (US&R)

HHS U.S. Department of Health and Human Services

HIPAA Health Insurance Portability and Accountability Act of 1996

HMS (US&R) Hazardous materials specialist (US&R)

HMS (equipment) Abbreviation for *halbmastwurfsicherung,* which roughly translates to "half of a clove hitch." Refers to the shape of a carabiner (D or pear-shaped) intended to be used with a Munter hitch (aka, Italian hitch).

HSPD Homeland Security Presidential Directive

IAMSAR International Aeronautical and Maritime Search and Rescue

IAP Incident action plan

IC Incident commander

ICAO International Civil Aviation Organization

ICS Incident command system

IMO International Maritime Organization

ISPC Inland SAR Planning Course (offered by the U.S. National SAR School)

kN Kilonewton (1 kN = 225 lbs. or 102 kilograms)

LAST Locate, access, stabilize, transport (SAR phases acronym)

LCD Liquid crystal display

LED Light-emitting diode

LKP Last known point or last known position

LOCATER Lost Child Alert Technology Resource

LS Logistics specialist (US&R)

LSA Land SAR Addendum to the National SAR Supplement to the IAMSAR Manual

LUT Local user terminal (COSPAS-SARSAT)

MARAD Maritime Administration (U.S. Department of Transportation)

MAST Military Assistance to Safety and Traffic

MBS Minimum breaking strength

MCC Mission Control Center (COSPAS-SARSAT)

MN Magnetic north

MOU Memorandum of understanding

MRA Mountain Rescue Association

MRC Medical Reserve Corps

NASA National Aeronautics and Space Administration

NASAR The National Association For Search And Rescue

NCIC National Crime Information Center (FBI)

NCMEC National Center for Missing & Exploited Children

NCRC National Cave Rescue Commission

NFPA National Fire Protection Association

NGO Nongovernmental organization

NIMS National Incident Management System

NOAA National Oceanic and Atmospheric Administration (U.S. Department of Commerce)

NPG National preparedness goal

NPS National Park Service (U.S. Department of the Interior)

NRF National Response Framework

NSARC National Search and Rescue Committee

NSP National Search and Rescue Plan

NSS National Search and Rescue Supplement to the IAMSAR Manual

NSSL National Severe Storms Laboratory

NTSB National Transportation Safety Board

NVG Night vision goggles

NWP Neighborhood Watch Program

OFDA Office of Foreign Disaster Assistance

OPLANs Plans of operations or operations plans

OR Operations research

PFD Personal flotation device

PICAO Provisional International Civil Aviation Organization

PLB Personal locator beacon

PLS Point last seen

PMA Positive mental attitude

POA Probability of area (aka—probability of containment, POC)

POC Probability of containment (aka—probability of area, POA)

POD Probability of detection

POS Probability of success

PPD Presidential Policy Directive

PTM Planning team manager (US&R)

RCC Rescue coordination center

RCMP Royal Canadian Mounted Police

Rd Range of detection

RF Radio frequency

SA Selective availability

SAR Search and rescue

SARA Superfund Amendments and Reauthorization Act of 1986 (amended through P.L. 107-377, December 31, 2002), which amended the Comprehensive Environmental Response, Compensation, and Liability Act of 1980 (CERCLA)

SARTECH I NASAR search and rescue technician Level I
SARTECH II NASAR search and rescue technician Level II
SARTECH III NASAR search and rescue technician Level III
SCBA Self-contained breathing apparatus
SCUBA Self-contained underwater breathing apparatus
SEND Satellite emergency notification devices
SOLAS Safety of Life at Sea (International Convention)
SPF Sun protection factor
SPOC Search and rescue point of contact
SRR Search and rescue region
SSA Surface supplied air
STOP Stay/stop, think, observe, plan
TFL Task force leader (US&R)
TIS Technical information specialist (US&R)
TLL Track line length
Topo Topographical map
UAS Unmanned aircraft systems
US&R Urban search and rescue (do not confuse with USAR, below)
USAID U.S. Agency for International Development
USAR U.S. Army Reserves (do not confuse with US&R, above)
USCG U.S. Coast Guard (U.S. Department of Homeland Security)
USGS U.S. Geological Survey
UTC Universal time coordinate
UTM Universal Transverse Mercator
UV Ultraviolet
VIPS Volunteers in police service
VPA Volunteer Protection Act
WAAS Wide area augmentation system
WEA Wireless emergency alert
WRS Water rescue specialist (US&R)

Appendix E:

Correlation to NFPA 1006

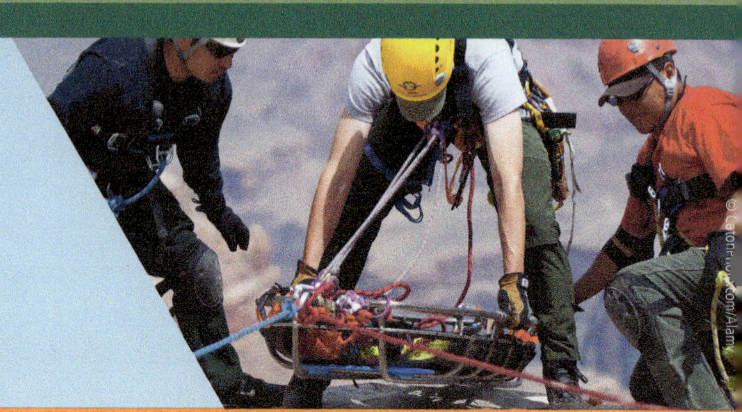

NFPA 1006, *Standard for Technical Rescue Personnel Professional Qualifications, 2017 Edition* and the Corresponding Chapter(s)

Section	Chapter(s)
10.1	2
10.1.1	8, 12
10.1.1(A)	8, 12
10.1.1(B)	8, 12
10.1.2	3, 15
10.1.2(A)	3, 8, 15
10.1.2(B)	3, 8, 15
10.1.3	15
10.1.3(A)	15
10.1.3(B)	15
10.1.4	3, 15
10.1.4(A)	3, 15
10.1.4(B)	3, 15
10.1.5	2–3, 11, 14–15
10.1.5(A)	2–3, 14
10.1.5(B)	14–15
10.2	2
10.2.1	8
10.2.1(A)	8
10.2.1(B)	8
10.2.2	2
10.2.2(A)	2
10.2.2(B)	2
10.2.3	3, 11
10.2.3(A)	3
10.2.3(B)	3, 11
10.2.4	15
10.2.4(A)	14–15
10.2.4(B)	15
10.2.5	13
10.2.5(A)	13
10.2.5(B)	13
10.2.6	6, 8–9, 12
10.2.6(A)	5–6, 8–9, 12
10.2.6(B)	6, 8–9, 14
10.2.7	10
10.2.7(A)	10
10.2.7(B)	10
10.2.8	3, 11
10.2.8(A)	3, 11
10.2.8(B)	3, 11
10.2.9	8
10.2.9(A)	8
10.2.9(B)	8
10.2.10	16
10.2.10(A)	16
10.2.10(B)	16
10.2.11	3, 15
10.2.11(A)	3, 9, 15
10.2.11(B)	3, 9, 15
10.2.12	12
10.2.12(A)	12
10.2.12(B)	12
10.3	2
10.3.1	8
10.3.1(A)	8
10.3.1(B)	8
10.3.2	6, 8, 10
10.3.2(A)	8, 10
10.3.2(A)(1)	8
10.3.2(A)(2)	8
10.3.2(A)(3)	8
10.3.2(A)(4)	8
10.3.2(A)(5)	8
10.3.2(A)(6)	8
10.3.2(A)(7)	8
10.3.2(A)(8)	8
10.3.2(A)(9)	8
10.3.2(A)(10)	8
10.3.2(A)(11)	10
10.3.2(A)(12)	8
10.3.2(B)	8, 10
10.3.3	—
10.3.3(A)	—
10.3.3(B)	—
10.3.4	6
10.3.4.1	6
10.3.4.2	6
10.3.5	3, 15
10.3.5(A)	2–3
10.3.5(B)	2–3
10.3.6	—
10.3.6(A)	—
10.3.6(B)	—
10.3.7	10, 13–14
10.3.7(A)	10, 14
10.3.7(B)	10
10.3.8	3
10.3.8(A)	3
10.3.8(B)	3
10.3.9	15
10.3.9(A)	13, 15
10.3.9(B)	13, 15
10.3.10	6
10.3.10(A)	—
10.3.10(B)	6
10.3.11	12
10.3.11(A)	12
10.3.11(B)	12

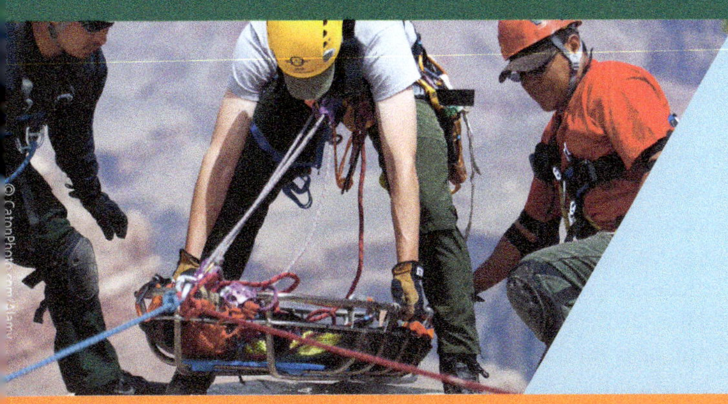

Glossary

24-hour pack Also called a *ready pack*, the suggested minimum equipment and pack that SAR personnel should carry at all times during a mission. It allows the person carrying it to be self-reliant and comfortable should a bivouac become necessary while waiting for help or rescue.

A

Abandonment The unilateral termination of care without assuring continuation of care at the same level or higher.

Acute mountain sickness (AMS) A collection of symptoms that commonly occur to people who travel to over 8,000 feet in altitude without acclimating (taking time to reach that altitude).

Aerobic exercise Exercise that combines food (often fat) with oxygen to produce energy for the body and that leads to cardiorespiratory endurance.

Agency A division of government with a specific function, or a nongovernmental organization (e.g., private contractor, business) that offers a particular kind of assistance. In ICS, agencies are defined as jurisdictional (having statutory responsibility for incident mitigation) or assisting and/or cooperating (providing resources and/or assistance).

Agency administrator A chief executive officer (or designee) of an agency or jurisdiction that has responsibility for the incident.

Agency representative An individual assigned to an incident from an assisting or cooperating agency that has been delegated authority to make decisions on matters affecting that agency's participation at the incident. Agency representatives report to the incident liaison officer.

All-risk Any incident or event, natural or human-caused, that warrants action to protect life, property, environment, public health or safety, and minimizes disruption of government, social, or economic activities.

Anterior A medical term used to refer to something toward the front of the body or toward the head.

Arch The bottom, medial part of the foot, just forward of the ankle, that curves above the ground. It stretches from the calcaneus to the three medial metatarsals and is sometimes referred to as the medial longitudinal arch.

Area effectively swept Also called *search effort*, a measure of the area that can be (or was) effectively searched by searchers within the limits of search speed, endurance, and effective sweep width. This area (Z) is computed as the product of the effective sweep width (W) times search speed (V) times hours spent in the search area (T). That is, $Z = W \times V \times T$ for one searcher or one resource (such as a ground searcher, dog team, boat, or aircraft and its crew) "Search effort is computed as the product of search speed (V), search endurance (T), and sweep width (W), or $Z = V \times T \times W$" (NSARC, 2011, p. xxiii).

Area search When a bounded segment of the search area is searched in an organized manner by a specific resource.

Assault Unlawfully placing a person in fear of immediate bodily harm without the person's consent.

Assigned resources Resources checked in and assigned work tasks on an incident.

Assistants Subordinates of command staff positions. The title indicates a level of technical capability, qualifications, and responsibility subordinate to the primary positions. Assistants may also be assigned to unit leaders.

Assisting agency An agency or organization providing personnel, services, or other resources to the agency with direct responsibility for incident management.

Available resources Resources assigned to an incident, checked in, and available for a mission assignment, normally located in a staging area.

Avalanche path A terrain feature where an avalanche occurs. Composed of a starting zone, track, and runout zone.

Avalanche starting zones The portions of an avalanche path where an avalanche releases.

Avalanche track The portion of an avalanche path between the starting zone and the runout zone.

Azimuth See *bearing*.

B

Back azimuth 180 degrees opposite from one's azimuth, bearing, or heading.

Back stop The linear feature bounding the far side of the segment that defines the endpoint of one search pass and serves as the baseline of the return search lanes.

Basal metabolic rate The amount of energy required to sustain the body's functions at rest.

Baseline A line, perpendicular to the direction of travel, on which searchers line up to begin their search.

Battery Unlawfully touching a person.

Bearing The direction of an object measured in degrees from north. Azimuth, bearing, and heading are often used interchangeably.

Bend A knot used to join two pieces, or ends, of a rope.

Bivouac Temporary camp without a tent or cover.

Bloodborne pathogens Microorganisms—such as viruses, bacteria, and similar microbes—that are present in human blood and can cause disease in humans.

Bracketing An occasionally acceptable method of interpolation that uses a predetermined stride to skip one step in sequence to find the next, and then use it to find the one skipped.

Branches The organizational level having functional or geographic responsibility for major parts of the operations or logistics functions. The branch level is organizationally between section and division/group in the operations section and between section and units in the logistics section. Branches are identified by Roman numerals or by functional name (e.g., medical, security). A branch is led by a branch director who reports to the operations chief.

Breaking strength The point at which a rope fails under a load.

Briefing Exchange of information, usually at the onset of a situation, that conveys important knowledge from the upper levels of a hierarchy to the lower, for example information from the Incident Commander conveyed to a field team before they begin their assignment. A summary of the situation, past and present, conveyed by those who know to those who need to know and that provides information that will help orient personnel to all facets of the problem.

Buoyancy The tendency of a body to float or sink in water or any other fluid.

C

Calorie The amount of heat required to raise the temperature of 1 gram of water 1 degree Celsius.

Camps Geographical sites, within the general incident area, separate from the incident base, equipped and staffed to provide sleeping, food, water, and sanitary services to incident personnel.

Candle ice Ice that resembles many candles bundled together; commonly found in late winter or early spring.

Carabiner A load-bearing connector with a self-closing gate used to join other elements of a rescue system.

Cardinal directions The four principal points of the compass: north, south, east, and west.

Catastrophic incident Any natural or manmade incident, including terrorism, that results in extraordinary levels of mass casualties, damage, or disruption severely affecting the population, infrastructure, environment, economy, national morale, or government functions.

Chain of command The orderly line of authority within the ranks of the incident management organization.

Check-in The process whereby resources first report to an incident. All responders, regardless of agency affiliation, must report in to receive an assignment in accordance with the procedures established by the incident commander. Check-in locations include: incident command post (resources unit), incident base, camps, staging areas, helibases, helispots, and division supervisors (for direct line assignments).

Chilblains Itchy, reddish and purple, swollen lesions that occur primarily on the extremities due to longer exposure to temperatures just above freezing or sudden rewarming after exposure to cold.

Clarification For water, the act of removing or filtering sediment and debris from water to make it clearer.

Clear ice New ice formed by a long, hard freeze; considered to be the strongest ice.

Clear text The use of plain English in radio communications transmissions. No ten codes or agency-specific codes are used when utilizing clear text.

Clue conscious Aware that clues exist.

Comfort zone Any area of human existence, based on a state of physical ease and freedom from pain or constraints, with which people become accustomed (habit) and from which people do not wish to deviate.

Command staff The staff who report directly to the incident commander, including the public information officer, safety officer, liaison officer, and other positions as required. They may have an assistant or assistants, as needed.

Command The act of directing and/or controlling resources by virtue of explicit legal, agency, or delegated authority. May also refer to the incident commander.

Common terminology Normally used words and phrases—avoiding the use of different words/phrases for the same concepts—to ensure consistency and to allow diverse incident management and support organizations to work together across a wide variety of incident management functions and hazard scenarios.

Communications unit Functional unit in the logistics section responsible for providing communication services at an incident. A communications unit may also be a facility (e.g., a trailer or mobile van) used to provide the major part of an incident communications center.

Compensation/claims unit Functional unit within the finance/administration section responsible for financial concerns resulting from property damage, injuries, or fatalities at the incident.

Complete print The entire impression is visible.

Conclusively human sign Evidence (sign) that, on its own, can be said to have been definitely caused by a person and not an animal.

Condition yellow A relaxed, heightened situational awareness where no threat exists but the individual is alert, observant, aware of his or her surroundings, and ready to respond to a problem or threat.

Confinement see *Containment*.

Containment Steps taken to ensure that the subject does not leave the search area; also called *confinement*.

Continuous limited search (CLS) An indirect, last resort search technique in which the use of any direct tactics in the search area are suspended, but the incident management team may opt to continue the investigation and/or use the area for regular training purposes.

Contour lines On a map, contour lines represent relative elevation and connect all points at the same elevation above sea level. On a USGS topographical map, it is brown and may be either darker brown and include elevation numbers (called an index contour line) or a lighter brown that is not numbered and falls between the index contour lines (called an intermediate contour line).

Contrast The difference in luminance (intensity of light) or color that makes an object visually distinguishable.

Cooperating agency An agency supplying assistance other than direct operational or support functions or resources to the incident management effort.

Coordinates A set of values represented by the letters x, y, and optionally z or m (measure) that define a position within a spatial reference. Coordinates are used to represent locations in space relative to other locations.

Coordinate system A reference system consisting of a set of points, lines, and surfaces, and a set of rules, used to define the positions of points in space in either two or three dimensions.

Coordination centers Facilities that are used for the coordination of agency or jurisdictional resources in support of one or more incidents.

Corroborant sign Disturbance that is not decisively human and could have been caused by an animal. It cannot be determined to have been definitely caused by a person, but it may confirm or substantiate other evidence with which it may be found.

Cost unit Functional unit within the finance/administration section responsible for tracking costs, analyzing cost data, making cost estimates, and recommending cost-saving measures.

Course Plan of travel using a compass, map, or both.

Coverage (coverage factor) "The ratio of the search effort (Z) to the area searched (A); C = Z/A. For parallel sweep searches, it may be computed as the ratio of sweep width (W) to track spacing (S). C = W/S". Coverage may be thought of as a measure of "thoroughness." The probability of detection (POD) of a search is a function of coverage.

Coverage factor (C) The ratio of the search effort (Z) to the area searched (A); C = Z/A. For parallel sweep searches, it may be computed as the ratio of sweep width (W) to track spacing (S), or C = W/S. Coverage may be thought of as a measure of thoroughness. The probability of detection (POD) of a search is a function of coverage.

Crampons A lightweight frame of steel spikes that can be attached to one's boots; for walking or climbing on ice.

Credentialing The authentication and verification of the certification and identity of designated incident managers and emergency responders.

Crew See *single resource*.

Cuttable area A reasonably good area for cutting sign.

D

Datum The reference specifications of a measurement system, usually a system of coordinate positions on a surface (a horizontal datum) or heights above or below a surface (a vertical datum).

Debriefing Exchange of information, usually at the close of a situation, that conveys important knowledge and experience from the lower levels of a hierarchy to the upper; that is, information conveyed to the incident commander from a field team after completing an assignment.

Decision points Locations, usually on linear features such as trails, paths, and roads, where the subject had to decide which path or road to take.

Declination The horizontal angle between geographic north and magnetic north from the point of observation.

DEET Abbreviation for chemical name, N,N-diethyl-meta-toluamide, a potent insect repellant.

Delegation of authority A statement provided to the incident commander by the agency executive delegating authority and assigning responsibility. The delegation of authority can include objectives, priorities, expectations, constraints, and other considerations or guidelines as needed. Many agencies require written delegation of authority to be given to incident commanders prior to their assuming command on larger incidents. Also known as *letter of expectation*.

Demobilization The orderly, safe, and efficient return of an incident resource to its original location and status.

Demobilization unit Functional unit within the planning section, responsible for assuring orderly, safe, and efficient demobilization of incident resources.

Deputy A fully qualified individual who, in the absence of a superior, could be delegated the authority to manage a functional operation or perform a specific task. In some cases, a deputy could act as relief for a superior and, therefore, must be fully qualified in the position. Deputies can be assigned to the incident commander, general staff, and branch directors.

Design factor The ratio of the strength of a rope to the intended load.

Direction-of-travel arrow The arrow or line on the base plate of an orienteering compass that points in the direction of travel when the compass is oriented.

Direction The relative location of one terrain feature to another; similar to bearing, azimuth, and heading but usually described in terms of points of the compass rather than degrees.

Director The ICS title for individuals responsible for supervision of a branch and who answer to the operations chief.

Direct tactics Tactics that include all organized methods used to move through the search area to detect a lost subject or clues.

Disinfection For water, the removal or destruction of harmful microorganisms in drinking water.

Divisions The organizational level having responsibility for operations within a defined geographic area. A division is located within the ICS organization between the branch and the task force/strike team. (See *group*.) Divisions are identified by alphabetic characters for horizontal applications and, often, by floor numbers when used in buildings. A division is led by a division supervisor.

Documentation unit Functional unit within the planning section responsible for collecting, recording, and safeguarding all documents relevant to the incident.

Dry suits Neoprene suits that trap air against the skin to provide both warmth and buoyancy while in the water.

Duty of care A requirement that a person act toward others with the watchfulness, attention, caution, and prudence that a reasonable person in the circumstances would use.

Duty to act An individual's responsibility to provide care or services. This responsibility may come from law or be secondary to the function being performed.

E

Easting A figure or a line representing eastward distance on a map (expressed by convention as the first part of a grid reference, before northing).

Emergency locator transmitters (ELTs) An emergency radio beacon that usually operates on both 121.5 MHz and 406 MHz; used by most aircraft.

Emergency position indicating radio beacons (EPIRBs) A distress radio beacon for use in maritime applications; used to alert search and rescue services in the event of an emergency. It does this by transmitting a coded message on the 406-MHz distress frequency via satellite and Earth stations to the nearest rescue coordination center. Some EPIRBs also have built-in GPS, which enables the rescue services to more accurately locate the device.

Engendered reliance The assumption by SAR service users that a SAR provider will provide a certain level of service.

Ephemeris A table giving the coordinates of GPS satellites at several specific times during a given period.

Event A planned, nonemergency activity. ICS can be used as the management system for a wide range of events, for example, parades, concerts, or sporting events.

Evidence Something legally acceptable before a court, such as an object or a witness, that bears on or establishes an issue. In tracking, evidence is divided into physical and incorporeal.

Expressed consent Consent granted when a person expressly authorizes another—usually verbally—to provide care or transportation.

F

Facilities unit Functional unit within the support branch of the logistics section that provides fixed facilities for the incident. These facilities may include the incident base, feeding areas, sleeping areas, sanitary facilities, etc.

Fall factor The ratio computed by dividing the fall distance of a climber attached to an anchored rope by the length of the rope between the load and the anchor or belay. For example, a 9-foot (3-meter) fall on a 9-foot (3-meter) rope would be a fall factor of 1.

Feature (1) an object in a landscape or on a map, or (2) a shape in a spatial data layer, such as a point, line, or polygon, that represents a geographic object.

Finance/administration section The incident command system section responsible for all administrative and financial considerations surrounding an incident. Includes the time unit, procurement unit, compensation/claims unit, and cost unit.

First notice The initial notification of responders to a search and rescue incident.

Flankers Members of a three-person tracking team standing on either side of the point person who help discover sign, usually from a standing position.

Food unit Functional unit within the service branch of the logistics section responsible for providing meals for incident personnel.

Forefoot The larger part of the foot, forward of the ankle.

Frazil ice The first type of ice to form; a thin, opaque film that floats to the surface.

Frazil slush Soft collections of frazil crystals that form in moving water where a current prevents a solid freeze.

Frostbite Partial or complete freezing of the skin and deeper tissues caused by exposure to the school.

Frost nip Early frostbite, characterized by numbness and pallor without significant tissue damage.

Functions The five major activities in the incident command system: command, operations, planning, logistics, and finance/administration. A sixth function, intelligence/investigations, may be established, if required, to meet incident management needs. The term *function* is also used when describing the activity involved (e.g., the planning function).

G

Gaiters Garments worn over the shoe and/or lower leg that protect the wearer from abrasion, dirt, debris, snow, moisture, insects, snakes, and other foreign objects.

Gait The pattern of how a person walks.

General staff A group of incident management personnel organized according to function and reporting to the incident commander. The general staff normally consists of the operations section chief, planning section chief, logistics section chief, and finance/administration section chief. An intelligence/investigations chief may be established, if required, to meet incident management needs.

Geographic coordinate system Navigating using a system of reference lines called parallels of latitude and meridians of longitude.

Georeferencing Defining and establishing the location of an object in physical space.

Global positioning system (GPS) A space-based radio navigation system consisting of a constellation of satellites and a network of ground stations used for monitoring and control.

Good Samaritan laws Laws that limit liability when one person provides reasonable help to another in good faith.

Granular convection A phenomenon where granular material subjected to vibration or shaking causes separation of the various sizes of the granules with larger ones rising to the surface.

Graticule A network of longitude and latitude lines on a map or chart that relates points on a map to their true locations on the Earth.

Grid north The north established by the vertical UTM grid lines on the map. In the declination diagram of a USGS topographical map, grid north is usually indicated by the letters "GN," and the grid north line has no arrow on it.

Grid search Search method in which human, visual search crews systematically line search a bounded, well-defined, usually relatively small segment.

Gross negligence A form of negligence in which one's failure to exercise reasonable care constitutes an extreme departure from the ordinary standard.

Ground searchers Searchers used to conduct confinement, attraction, rapid (hasty), and area searches.

Ground support unit Functional unit within the support branch of the logistics section responsible for the fueling, maintaining, and repairing of vehicles, and the transportation of personnel and supplies.

Groups Organizational subdivisions established to divide the incident management structure into functional areas of operation. Groups are composed of resources assembled to perform a special function not necessarily within a single geographic division. (See *Division*.) Groups are located between branches (when activated) and resources in the operations section. A group is led by a group supervisor.

Guide line A linear feature, parallel to the search track, to which a searcher refers for guidance regarding the general direction of the search track; also called *control line*.

Guide person The searcher on the search line who provides guidance regarding the general direction of the search track. On guide right situations, this person is on the right of the search line and guides on a feature to his or her right. On guide left situations, this person is on the left of the search line and guides on a feature to his or her left. On guide center situations, this person is in or near the middle of the search line.

H

Hardware In rescue, any rescue equipment not considered software.

Hazard controls Procedures adopted to minimize injury, reduce adverse health effects, and control damage to property.

Hazard mitigation Any sustained action taken to reduce or eliminate the long-term risk to people and property from hazards and their effects.

Hazard Something that has the potential for harm.

Heading See *bearing*.

Heat cramps Muscle spasms that usually occur after vigorous exercise in hot weather and are generally relieved by rest and drinking water.

Heat exhaustion A form of shock that occurs when the body loses too much water and too many electrolytes through very heavy sweating after exposure to heat.

Heatstroke A condition of rapidly rising internal body temperature that occurs when the body's mechanisms for the release of heat are overwhelmed. Untreated, it can lead to death.

Heat transfer The movement of heat between the body and the environment through radiation, conduction, convection, or evaporation.

Heel The back part of the foot below the ankle.

Helibase The main location for parking, fueling, maintenance, and loading of helicopters operating in support of an incident. It is usually located at or near the incident base.

Helispots Any designated locations where a helicopter can safely take off and land. Some helispots may be used for loading of supplies, equipment, or personnel.

Hierarchy of hazard controls A system used to minimize or eliminate exposure to hazards.

High-altitude cerebral edema (HACE) An altitude illness in which there is a change in mental status and/or ataxia in a person with acute mountain sickness or the presence of mental status changes and ataxia in a person without acute mountain sickness.

High-altitude pulmonary edema (HAPE) An altitude illness characterized by at least two of the following: dyspnea at rest, cough, weakness or decreased exercise performance, or chest tightness or congestion. Also at least two of the following signs: central cyanosis, audible rales or wheezing in at least one lung field, tachypnea, or tachycardia.

High-coverage search A systematic area search, accomplished by searchers usually lining up on a baseline at relatively small between-searcher track spacing, with the goal of spending enough time and resources in a segment to achieve a relatively high coverage. The coverage achieved is often equal to or greater than 0.5.

Hitch A knot used to attach a rope to a fixed object or fixed rope.

Hydraulic In river rescue, a backwash that traps and recirculates anything that floats.

Hydrophilic Refers to fabric that absorbs water.

Hydrophobic Refers to fabric that repels and does not absorb water.

Hyperthermia Condition or illness caused by the body's core temperature being significantly higher than normal (normal is 98.5°F/37°C).

Hypothermia A lowering of body temperature, which can endanger survival.

Hypothermia Condition or illness caused by the body's core temperature being significantly lower than normal (normal is 98.5°F/37°C).

I

Identifiable A complete or partial print that has at least one characteristic that differentiates it from others similar to it.

Implied consent Consent granted when a person is injured and unable to provide expressed consent, and the law assumes the person would grant permission for treatment and transportation.

Incident action plans (IAPs) Oral or written plans containing general objectives reflecting the overall strategy for managing an incident. It may include the identification of operational resources and assignments. It may also include attachments that provide direction and important information for management of the incident during one or more operational periods.

Incident base Location at the incident where the primary logistics functions are coordinated and administered. (Incident name or other designator will be added to the term *base*.) The incident command post may be co-located with the base. There is only one base per incident.

Incident commander (IC) The individual responsible for all incident activities, including the development of strategies and tactics and the ordering and the release of resources. The IC has overall authority and responsibility for conducting incident operations and is responsible for the management of all incident operations at the incident site.

Incident command post (ICP) The field location at which the primary tactical-level, on-scene incident command functions are performed. The ICP may be co-located with the incident base or other incident facilities and is normally identified by a green rotating or flashing light.

Incident command system (ICS) A standardized on-scene emergency management construct specifically designed to provide for the adoption of an integrated organizational structure that reflects the complexity and demands of single or multiple incidents, without being hindered by jurisdictional boundaries. ICS is the combination of facilities, equipment, personnel, procedures, and communications operating within a common organizational structure, designed to aid in the management of resources during incidents. It is used for all kinds of emergencies and is applicable to small as well as large and complex incidents. ICS is used by various jurisdictions and functional agencies, both public and private, to organize field-level incident management operations.

Incident management team (IMT) An incident commander and the appropriate command and general staff personnel assigned to an incident. The level of training and experience of the IMT members, coupled with the identified formal response requirements and responsibilities of the IMT, are factors in determining "type," or level, of IMT.

Incident management The broad spectrum of activities and organizations providing effective and efficient operations, coordination, and support applied at all levels of government, utilizing both governmental and nongovernmental resources to plan for, respond to, and recover from an incident regardless of cause, size, or complexity.

Incident objectives Statements of guidance and direction necessary for the selection of appropriate strategies and the tactical direction of resources. Incident objectives are based on realistic expectations of what can be accomplished when all allocated resources have been effectively deployed. Incident objectives must be achievable and measurable, yet flexible enough to allow for strategic and tactical alternatives.

Incidents Occurrences or events, natural or human-caused, that require an emergency response to protect life or property. Incidents can, for example, include major disasters, emergencies, terrorist attacks, terrorist threats, wildland and urban fires, floods, hazardous materials spills, nuclear accidents, aircraft accidents, earthquakes, hurricanes, tornadoes, tropical storms, war-related disasters, public health and medical emergencies, and other occurrences requiring an emergency response.

Incident types Incidents are categorized by five types based on complexity. Type 5 incidents are the least complex, and Type 1 incidents are the most complex.

Incorporeal evidence Nonphysical information or knowledge; intangible evidence that cannot be touched or held. Examples include the subject's age, a whistle blowing, a flashing light, or a report from a witness.

Indirect tactics Tactics that do not involve physically moving through the search area to detect lost subjects or clues. Examples include fact finding (investigation), attraction, containment, and continuous limited search.

Individual resources One person; in contrast to a "single resource," which describes a piece of equipment and its personnel complement. Individual resources are often called responders or specialists.

Inflatable Dependent on flexible air chambers that can be filled with air or other gas (usually carbon dioxide) for flotation.

Information Data, knowledge, and facts about someone or something gained from somewhere.

Intelligence Information that has been verified, analyzed, collated, evaluated, and prepared for use in making decisions.

Intelligence officer The intelligence officer is responsible for managing internal information, intelligence, and operational security requirements supporting incident management activities. These may include information security and operational security activities, as well as the complex task of ensuring that sensitive information of all types (e.g., classified information, law enforcement sensitive information, proprietary information, or export-controlled information) is handled in a way that not only safeguards the information but also ensures that it gets to those who need access to it to perform their missions effectively and safely.

Intercardinal directions The four points of the compass between the four cardinal points: northeast, southeast, northwest, and southwest.

International conventions Written agreements between countries, used to establish rules between them.

Intoeing See *pigeon toed.*

J

Jam holds Climbing holds that involve jamming any part of the body or extremity into a crack. This is done by putting the hand into the crack and clenching it into a fist, or by placing the arm into the crack and twisting the elbow against one side and the hand against the other side.

Jump tracking An unskilled form of tracking that involves finding an obvious footprint, then proceeding along the presumed direction of travel until another obvious track is found.

Jurisdiction A range or sphere of authority. Public agencies have jurisdiction at an incident related to their legal responsibilities and authority. Jurisdictional authority at an incident can be political or geographical (e.g., city, county, tribal, state, or federal boundary lines) or functional (e.g., law enforcement, public health).

K

Kernmantle rope Rope construction with two parts: a tightly woven outer sheath that serves to support a load and protects the inner core, and an inner core consisting of strands of fibers that are bundled together to provide most of the rope's strength.

Kilocalorie One thousand calories, or the amount of heat required to raise the temperature of 1 kilogram of water 1 degree Celsius.

Kindling The initial fuel stage of a fire; used to ignite sustaining fuel.

Kinds of resources Describe what the resource is (e.g., medic, fire fighter, planning section chief, helicopters, ambulances, combustible gas indicators, bulldozers).

L

Landing zones (LZs) See *helispots.*

Landmark A feature in the landscape that can be readily recognized—anything from a prominent tree or rock to a building or lake.

Last known position (LKP) (1) The last substantiated position based on clues or evidence belonging to the missing subject and indicating that the missing subject was known to be at that location. (2) Last witnessed, reported, or computed position of a distressed person or craft.

Lateral A medical term used to describe something situated away from the middle or to the side of the body; usually to the left or the right.

Latitude The angular distance along a meridian north or south of the equator, usually measured in degrees. Lines of latitude are called *parallels.*

Layered ice Ice formed from many layers of frozen and refrozen snow.

Leader The incident command system title for an individual responsible for a task force, strike team, or functional unit.

Lensatic compass A (formerly) typical military, field, magnetic compass having a magnifying lens for reading the compass scale.

Liaison A form of communication for establishing and maintaining mutual understanding and cooperation.

Liaison officer A member of the command staff responsible for coordinating with representatives from cooperating and assisting agencies or organizations. The liaison officer may have assistants.

Litter Body-length transfer device used to support and protect an injured subject during movement; also called a *stretcher.*

Logistics section The section responsible for providing facilities, services, and materials for the incident.

Logistics The process and procedure for providing resources and other services to support incident management.

Longitude The angular distance, expressed in degrees, minutes, and seconds, of a point of the Earth's surface east or west of a prime meridian (usually the Greenwich meridian). All lines of longitude are great circles that intersect the equator and pass through the north and south poles. Lines of longitude are called *meridians.*

Low-coverage search A systematic area search, accomplished by searchers usually lining up on a baseline at relatively wide between-searcher track spacing, with the goal of covering larger geographic segments with fewer resources in a relatively short period of time. The coverage achieved is often less than 0.5.

Low head dam A man-made structure, typically built to back up water in a reservoir.

Luminance The intensity of light emitted from a surface per unit of area in a given direction.

M

Magnetic declination (or just declination) See *declination.*

Magnetic north The direction to which the compass points. In the declination diagram of a USGS topographical map, magnetic north is usually indicated by the letters "MN," and the magnetic north line has an arrow on it.

Major disaster As defined under the Robert T. Stafford Disaster Relief and Emergency Assistance Act, "any natural catastrophe (including any hurricane, tornado, storm, high water, wind-driven water, tidal wave, tsunami, earthquake, volcanic eruption, landslide, mudslide, snowstorm, or drought), or, regardless of cause, any fire, flood, or explosion, in any part of the United States, which in the determination of the President causes damage of sufficient severity and magnitude to warrant major disaster assistance under this Act to supplement the efforts and available resources of States, tribes, local governments, and disaster relief organizations in alleviating the damage, loss, hardship, or suffering caused thereby" (Robert T. Stafford Disaster Relief and Emergency Assistance Act, 2013).

Management by objectives A management approach that involves a five-step process for achieving the incident goal. The management by objectives approach includes the following: establishing overarching incident objectives; developing strategies based on overarching incident objectives; developing and issuing assignments, plans, procedures, and protocols; establishing specific, measurable tactics or tasks for various incident management functional activities and directing efforts to attain them, in support of defined strategies; and documenting results to measure performance and facilitate corrective action.

Managers Individuals within an incident command system organizational unit who are assigned specific managerial responsibilities (e.g., staging area manager or camp manager).

Map scale The ratio or relation between distance or area on a map and the corresponding distance or area on the ground.

Medial A medical term that describes something that is situated toward the middle or midline of the body.

Medical unit Functional unit within the service branch of the logistics section responsible for the development of the medical emergency plan and for providing emergency medical treatment of incident personnel.

Meridians Lines of longitude.

Micropores Pores with a diameter less than 2 nanometers.

Mobilization center Off-incident location at which emergency service personnel and equipment are temporarily located pending assignment, release, or reassignment.

Modular organization An organization that can be expanded or contracted as the incident warrants by adding (activating) or removing (demobilizing) organizational elements such as functional sections and units, as needed.

Moisture regain The amount of water a completely dry fiber absorbs from the air at a standard condition of 70° F and a relative humidity of 65%, expressed as a percentage of the dry fiber weight.

Multiagency coordination (MAC) entities or groups Administrators or executives, or their appointed representatives, working together, who are typically authorized to commit agency resources and funds. A MAC group can provide coordinated decision-making and resource allocation among cooperating agencies and may establish the priorities among incidents, harmonize agency policies, and provide strategic guidance and direction to support incident management activities. MAC groups may also be known as multiagency committees, emergency management committees, or as otherwise defined by the multiagency coordination system.

Multiagency coordination systems (MACS) Systems that provide the architecture to support coordination for incident prioritization, critical resource allocation, communications systems integration, and information coordination. MACS assist agencies and organizations responding to an incident. The elements of a MACS include facilities, equipment, personnel, procedures, and communications. Two of the most commonly used elements are emergency operations centers and MAC groups.

N

National Incident Management System (NIMS) A set of principles that provides a systematic, proactive approach guiding government agencies at all levels, nongovernmental organizations, and the private sector to work seamlessly to prevent, protect against, respond to, recover from, and mitigate the effects of incidents, regardless of cause, size, location, or complexity, in order to reduce the loss of life or property and harm to the environment.

National Integration Center The U.S. Department of Homeland Security's facility responsible for managing the implementation and administration of the National Incident Management System (NIMS).

National Preparedness Goal U.S. national goal established secondary to Presidential Policy Directive 8 (2011) that identifies the core capabilities necessary for preparedness and a national preparedness system to guide activities that will provide systematic preparation for national threats including acts of terrorism, cyberattacks, pandemics, and catastrophic natural disasters. The goal itself is "A secure and resilient nation with the capabilities required across the whole community to prevent, protect against, mitigate, respond to, and recover from the threats and hazards that pose the greatest risk" (DHS, 2015, p. 1).

National Response Framework (NRF) "A guide to how the United States responds to all types of disasters and emergencies. It is built on scalable, flexible, and adaptable concepts identified in the National Incident Management System (NIMS) to align key roles and responsibilities across the Nation. The NRF describes specific authorities and best practices for managing incidents that range from the serious but purely local to large-scale terrorist attacks or catastrophic natural disasters." This framework is always in effect, and elements can be implemented at any time.

Negligence Deviation from the accepted standard of care resulting in further injury to the patient. Components include a duty to act, breach of that duty, injury/damages inflicted (physical or psychological), and that the actions of the individual rendering care caused the injury/damage.

Normalcy bias The tendency of an individual to underestimate the possibility of something bad happening.

Northing A figure or line representing northward distance on a map (expressed by convention as the second part of a grid reference, after easting).

O

Officer The incident command system title for the personnel responsible for the command staff positions of safety, liaison, and public information.

Operational period The time scheduled for executing a given set of operation actions, as specified in the incident action plan. Operational periods can be of various lengths, although usually they last 12 to 24 hours.

Operations section The incident command system section responsible for all tactical incident operations and implementation of the incident action plan. In ICS, the operations section is led by the operations section chief and normally includes subordinate branches, divisions, and/or groups, task forces, strike teams, single resources, and staging areas.

Orientation The process of determining one's location in the field with the help of landscape features, map, or compass, or with all three combined.

Orienteering compass A compass especially designed to simplify the process of finding one's way with map and compass. It usually has a compass housing mounted on a rectangular base plate in such a way that it can be turned easily.

Orthotic An artificial support, brace, or splint used to support, align, or correct the function of movable parts of the body. Shoe inserts are orthotics that are intended to correct an abnormal or irregular walking pattern by altering slightly the angles at which the foot strikes a walking or running surface.

Out-of-service resources Resources assigned to an incident but unable to respond for mechanical, rest, or personnel reasons.

P

Parallels Lines of latitude.

Partial Only part of the impression is visible.

Pasteurization For water, applying enough heat to water (< boiling point) to reduce the number of surviving microorganisms in the water to such a low level that they are unlikely to cause illness or disease.

Perimeter cutting Sign cutting around the boundary or outer edge of an area.

Personal flotation device (PFD) A device designed to maintain the wearer's head above water.

Personal locator beacons (PLBs) Portable units that operate much the same as EPIRBs or ELTs. They are designed to be carried by an individual person instead of on a boat or aircraft.

Personnel accountability reports (PAR) Periodic reports verifying the status of responders assigned to an incident.

Phalanges The bones of the toes (and fingers).

Physical fitness The ability to perform daily tasks vigorously and alertly, with energy left over for enjoying leisure-time activities and meeting emergency demands.

Pigeon toed When one walks with the toes pointed medially. This is sometimes called *intoeing*, and the medical terms *metatarsus varus* or *metatarsus adductus* may also be used.

Planning meeting A meeting held as needed throughout the duration of an incident, to select specific strategies and tactics for incident control operations, and for service and support planning. On larger incidents, the planning meeting is a major element in the development of the incident action plan.

Planning section The incident command system section responsible for the collection, evaluation, and dissemination of operational information related to the incident, and for the preparation and documentation of the incident action plan. This section also maintains information on the current and forecasted situation and on the status of resources assigned to the incident. This section includes the situation, resources, documentation, and demobilization units, as well as technical specialists.

Point last seen (PLS) The point where the search object was last seen by a witness or captured on video at a specific time and location.

Point person Member of a three-person tracking team that leads the act of sign discovery, usually from a position just ahead of, and between, the flankers.

Positive control "The separation of all air traffic within designated airspace by air traffic control" (USDOT FAA, 2015a).

Possibility area (1) The smallest area containing all possible survivor or search object locations. (2) For a scenario, the smallest area containing all possible survivor or search object locations that are consistent with the facts and assumptions used to form the scenario.

Posterior A medical term used to describe something toward the back of the body.

Print Impression left from the passage of a person that can be positively identified as being human.

Probability density (Pden) Probability of containment per unit area; often POC or POA/mi^2. Pden is constant throughout any given region.

Probability of area (POA) The probability that the search object (or subject) is contained within the boundaries of an area, subarea, or grid cell; also called *probability of containment (POC)*.

Probability of detection (POD) The probability of the search object being detected, assuming it was in the areas that were searched. POD is a function of coverage factor, sensor, search conditions, and the accuracy with which the search unit navigates its assigned search pattern. Measures sensor effectiveness under the prevailing search conditions.

Probability of success (POS) The probability of finding the search object with a particular search. For each subarea searched, POS = POA × POD. Measures overall search effectiveness. The accumulated probability of finding the search object with all the search effort expended over all searches to date is called *cumulative POS (POScum)*.

Probability theory A branch of mathematics used to systematically deal with uncertain events.

Procurement unit Functional unit within the finance/administration section responsible for financial matters involving vendor contracts.

Pronation Rotation of the medial bones in the midtarsal region of the foot inward and downward so that in walking the foot tends to come down on its inner margin.

Protractor Instrument for measuring angles, usually in degrees.

Public information officer A member of the command staff responsible for interfacing with the public and media or with other agencies with incident-related information requirements.

Purification For water, the removal of pathogenic (disease causing) microorganisms in the water such as bacteria, viruses, and parasites.

Q

Qualified A person meeting a recognized level of training, experience, and certification for the assigned position.

Quarry Anything being pursued.

R

Range of detection (Rd) The linear distance at which a search object is first detected when moving toward it from multiple angles.

Rapid (hasty) search Quickly looking for the search object along likely routes of travel, along linear geographical features, or in high probability locations; also called *initial reflex search.*

Rapid (hasty) search teams Small (usually three members), well-trained, highly mobile, rapidly deployable, self-sufficient, clue-conscious search teams.

Region "A delineated portion or subset of the search area within which there is a nearly uniform distribution of likelihood for containing the search subject or object." (NSARC, 2011, p. xxii).

Reporting location Location or facility where incoming resources can check in at the incident. (See *check-in.*)

Rescue An operation to retrieve persons in distress, provide for their initial medical or other needs, and deliver them to a place of safety.

Rescue coordination center (RCC) A unit, recognized by a cognizant international body, responsible for promoting efficient organization of SAR services and for coordinating the conduct of SAR operations within a Search and Rescue Region (SRR).

Resource management A system for identifying available resources at all jurisdictional levels to enable timely, efficient, and unimpeded access to resources needed to prepare for, respond to, or recover from an incident. Resource management under the National Incident Management System includes mutual aid agreements and assistance agreements; the use of special federal, state, tribal, and local teams; and resource mobilization protocols.

Resources Personnel and major items of equipment, supplies, and facilities available or potentially available for assignment to incident operations and for which status is maintained. Resources are described by kind and type and may be used in operational support or supervisory capacities at an incident or at an emergency operations center.

Resources unit Functional unit within the planning section responsible for recording the status of resources committed to the incident. The unit also evaluates resources currently committed to the incident, the impact that additional responding resources will have on the incident, and anticipated resource needs. The resources unit is led by the resources unit leader, who reports to the planning section chief.

Resource tracking A standardized, integrated process conducted prior to, during, and after an incident by all emergency management/response personnel and their associated organizations.

Risk An estimate of the probability of a hazard-related incident or exposure occurring.

Risk assessment A process to identify potential hazards and analyze what could happen if a hazard occurs.

Rotten ice Old ice that is honeycombed with pockets of air bubbles; may crumble under the slightest pressure.

Runout zone The portion of an avalanche path where the debris typically comes to rest.

S

Safety culture The attitude, beliefs, perceptions and values that people, usually in one industry or in one organization, share in relationship to safety.

Safety Freedom from unreasonable risk.

Safety officer A member of the command staff responsible for monitoring incident operations and advising the incident commander on all matters relating to operational safety, including the health and safety of emergency responder personnel. The safety officer may have assistants.

Scenario A consistent set of known facts and assumptions describing what may have happened to the survivor(s) (search subject).

Scope of practice In health care, the procedures, actions, and processes that a healthcare practitioner is permitted to undertake in keeping with the terms of his or her professional license. In the context of SAR, the services a SAR organization is able to provide.

Scree slopes Areas consisting of small rocks and gravel that have collected below rock ridges and cliffs.

Search and rescue coordinator "One or more persons or agencies within an Administration with overall responsibility for establishing and providing SAR services, and ensuring that planning for those services is properly coordinated" (NSARC, 2016, p. 2).

Search and rescue region (SRR) "An area of defined dimensions, associated with a rescue coordination center (RCC), within which SAR services are provided".

Search An operation using available personnel and facilities to locate persons in distress.

Search area The area, determined by the search planner, that is to be searched. This area may be subdivided into search subareas for the purpose of assigning specific responsibilities to the available search facilities. It includes the smallest area, consistent with all available information, which contains all possible search object locations and, therefore, includes all regions and segments that are consistent with a particular scenario. This area may be divided into regions based on the probable scenarios and into segments for assigning specific tasks to the available search resources.

Search lane The area an individual searcher is assigned to scan during a search.

Search line A series of searchers forming a line to conduct an area search.

Search object A ship, aircraft, or other craft missing or in distress, or survivors or related search objects or evidence for which a search is being conducted. A generic term used to indicate the lost subject or evidence (clues) related to a lost subject. A live human search object is often referred to as a search subject.

Search speed The average rate of travel (speed over the ground) of searchers while engaged in search operations within a segment.

Search subarea A designated area to be searched by a specific assigned search facility, or possibly two facilities working together in close coordination.

Search subject The person being searched for, commonly referred to as the "subject." Searches focusing primarily on the discovery of objects as opposed to persons (e.g., aircraft or vessels) commonly use the term *search object.*

Search track The general line of travel a searcher or search line takes through the search area during a search.

Section chief The incident command system title for individuals responsible for management of functional sections: operations, planning, logistics, finance/administration, and intelligence/investigations (if established as a separate section). A section chief answers to the incident commander.

Section The organizational level having responsibility for a major functional area of incident management, for example, operations, planning, logistics, finance/administration, and intelligence (if established). The section is organizationally situated between the branch and the incident command and is led by a section chief.

Segment A delineated portion or subset of the search area bounded and sized to be searchable by assigned facilities. Segments and their boundaries are based on factors that affect the searchers, and the search planner determines the size of a segment. The boundaries of a segment are identifiable both in the field and on a map and are based on suitability for assigning search resources, not probability of the search object's location.

Sensor Human senses (sight, hearing, touch, etc.), those of specially trained animals (such as dogs), or electronic devices used to detect the object of a search. A human, multisensor platform is often referred to as a *searcher.*

Service branch A branch within the logistics section responsible for service activities at the incident. Includes the communication, medical, and food units. A branch is led by a branch director who reports to the operations chief.

Shank In a boot or a shoe, a part of the supportive structure between the insole and the outsole traditionally made of steel but often made from polymer materials.

Sign Any evidence of change from the natural state that is inflicted on an environment by a person's or an animal's passage.

Sign-cutting stick A walking stick-type device used by trackers to measure stride. Furthermore, it assists in focusing attention where the tracker should be looking for sign and not everywhere else. Also called a *tracking stick.*

Sign cutting The process of looking for the first piece of evidence from which to track. Also called *cutting sign.*

Sign Discoverable evidence located in an area where a subject would likely have passed.

Single resource A piece of equipment and its personnel complement, or a crew or team of individuals with an identified work supervisor that can be used on an incident.

Situational awareness The ability to identify, process, and comprehend the critical elements of information about what is happening to the team with regards to the mission. In short, having situational awareness is knowing what is going on around you.

Situation unit Functional unit within the planning section responsible for the collection, organization, and analysis of incident status information, and for analysis of the situation as it progresses. The situation unit is led by the situation unit leader, who reports to the planning section chief.

Snow blindness Essentially a sunburn of the eyes. Symptoms may not occur for many hours after the injury but include the sensation of a foreign body or sand in the eyes. Sensitivity to light (photophobia) is also common. Also called *photokeratitis.*

Snow ice Opaque or milky-colored ice that is formed from the freezing of water-soaked snow; considered to be very weak.

Software In rescue, any soft, pliable material that can be tied into knots. Examples are rope, webbing, and cordage.

Sound sweep An effective search technique that combines a sound attraction tactic with the direct tactic of wide-spaced grid searching. The use of sound, typically whistle blasts, is closely choreographed with simultaneous blasts followed by a uniform listening period for subject response. The use of this technique presumes a responsive subject and, thus, is most effectively utilized in the early stages of a search.

Span of control The number of resources for which a supervisor is responsible, usually expressed as the ratio of supervisors to individuals. (Under NIMS, an appropriate span of control is between 1:3 and 1:7, with optimal being 1:5, or between 1:8 and 1:10 for many large-scale law enforcement operations.)

Spatial Of or relating to space.

Splayed feet When the toes point outward (laterally) when walking; the opposite of intoeing. Sometimes referred to as *toe out.*

Staging areas Temporary locations for available resources. A staging area can be any location in which personnel, supplies, and equipment can be temporarily housed or parked while awaiting operational assignment. The operations section manages staging areas.

Standard of care How a reasonably prudent person with similar training and experience would act under similar circumstances, with similar equipment, and in the same place.

Standard precautions Precautions applied to the care of patients in all healthcare settings, regardless of the suspected or confirmed presence of an infectious agent, for the purpose of preventing the transmission of infectious agents. Standard precautions include the use of personal protective equipment such as gloves, face masks, eye protection (goggles), and gowns (clothing covers). Formerly called *body substance isolation.*

Step-by-step tracking A disciplined tracking methodology and teaching system where a tracker sees each step in sequence and proceeds no further than the last visible track, using the stride to determine where next to look for sign.

Steppage gait When one walks with a footdrop where the foot hangs with the toes pointing down, causing the toes to scrape the ground while walking and requiring the walker to lift the leg higher than normal when walking.

Sterilization For water, raising the temperature of water high enough, and for long enough, to completely remove or destroy all living microorganisms.

Straddle The lateral distance between footfalls, perpendicular to the direction of travel.

Strainer In swift water, an obstacle that moving water can flow through, but that a swimmer or boat cannot. Some examples include trees, human-made obstacles, and debris. In swift water, strainers are life-threatening obstacles that should be avoided whenever possible.

Strategy The general direction selected to accomplish incident objectives set by the incident commander.

Stride Measured distance from the heel of the rear print to the heel of the next front print.

Strike teams Specified combinations of the same kind and type of resources with common communications and a leader.

Sunburn A first-degree burn (superficial, thermal burn) that causes reddening and pain of the skin after being exposed to sunlight. Swelling might accompany the reddening, and more prolonged exposure to sunlight might cause severe pain and blistering.

Sun protection factor (SPF) A measure of how well a sunscreen protects skin from UVB rays, which is radiation that causes sunburn, damages skin, and can contribute to skin cancer.

Supervisor The ICS title for individuals responsible for a division or group.

Supination A movement of the foot and the leg in which the foot rolls outward with an elevated arch so that in walking the foot tends to come down on its outer edge.

Supply unit Functional unit within the support branch of the logistics section responsible for ordering equipment and supplies required for incident operations.

Support branch A branch within the logistics section responsible for providing personnel, equipment, and supplies to support incident operations. Includes the supply, facilities, and ground support units. A branch is led by a branch director, who reports to the operations chief.

Supporting agency An agency that provides support and/or resource assistance to another agency. See *assisting agency.*

Sustaining fuel Anything that burns for an extended period of time.

Sweep width A measure of the effectiveness with which a particular sensor can detect a particular object under specific environmental conditions; a measure of detectability. Sweep width depends on the characteristics of the search object, the sensor, and the environmental conditions prevailing at the time and place of the search. Also called *effective sweep width.*

Swiftwater Water moving at greater than 1 nautical mile per hour (1.15 [statute] mile per hour).

Switchback A zigzag pattern used to traverse steep slopes.

System safety factor The ratio between the weakest link in a rescue system and the load to be supported.

T

Tactics The deployment and directing of resources on an incident to accomplish the objectives designated by strategy.

Talus The term sometimes used by climbers to describe something similar to scree, except the rock pieces are larger, and the rocks do not slide as much. Geologists use the term to describe the slope on which scree is found.

Target heart rate The heart rate you should maintain during exercise.

Tarsals The big bones of the foot below and including the ankle and the calcaneus.

Task forces Combination of single resources assembled for a particular tactical need with common communications and a leader.

Technical specialists Personnel with special skills that can be used anywhere within the ICS organization and who are activated only when needed.

Tendinitis An inflammation of the sheath of the Achilles tendon, or soreness above the heel, caused by continuous pressure over long periods of time.

Time unit Functional unit within the finance/administration section responsible for recording time for incident personnel and hired equipment.

Tinder Anything that ignites at a very low temperature, with a spark, small flame, or other heat source.

Toe out See *splayed feet.*

Topographical (topo) maps Type of map that portrays the shape and the elevation of the terrain with lines, while showing a graphic representation of selected man-made and natural features on a part of the Earth's surface plotted to a definite scale.

Topography The shape or configuration of the land, represented on a map by contour lines, hypsometric tints, and/or relief shading.

Track An impression left from the passage of a person or an animal.

Track aware Conscious that sign, tracks, and prints exist and may be useful.

Tracking Following someone or something by stringing together a continuous chain of their sign. Following a chronology of sign.

Tracking stick See *sign-cutting stick.*

Tracking team A three-person group, comprising a point and two flankers, and organized specifically to track.

Track line length (TLL) Total distance traveled by a sensor (i.e., searcher, boat, or aircraft) while searching in the assigned segment; also called *effort.* It is the sum of all track lines lengths used on a search.Track spacing The distance between the centers of each adjacent search lane.

Track trap An area particularly good for detecting sign (e.g., sand, mud, snow). May be human-made by clearing off an area so that sign would be more easily detected if a subject subsequently passed through.

Trail mix A type of snack mix, specifically a combination of granola, dried fruit, nuts, and sometimes chocolate, developed as a food to be taken along on hikes; also called *gorp.*

Trail tape, ribbon, or string line The use of markers to install a guide line where no visible guide line exists. Toilet paper, surveyor's tape, survey markers, evidence markers, string, and other similar material can be tied, placed, or anchored to indicate a line or boundary of a search lane.

Trench foot A process similar to frostbite but caused by prolonged exposure to cool, wet conditions.

Trespassing The act of passing beyond a boundary onto one's property without the owner's permission.

True north A line from any position on the Earth's surface to the North Pole. All lines of longitude are true north lines. In the declination diagram of a USGS topographical map, true north is usually indicated by a star.

Type An incident command system resource classification that refers to capability. Type 1 is generally considered to be more capable than Types 2, 3, or 4, respectively, because of size, power, capacity, or (in the case of incident management teams) experience and qualifications.

U

Unified command (UC) An incident command system application used when more than one agency has incident jurisdiction or when incidents cross political jurisdictions. Agencies work together through the designated members of the UC, often the senior persons from agencies and/or disciplines participating in the UC, to establish a common set of objectives and strategies and a single incident action plan.

United States National Grid (USNG) An unambiguous, nationally consistent, alpha-numeric georeferencing system that can be easily implemented using both printed maps and USNG-enabled GPS devices.

Unit leaders The individuals in charge of managing units within an incident command system (ICS) functional section. The unit can be staffed by many support personnel providing a wide range of services. Some of the support positions are preestablished within ICS (e.g., base/camp manager), but many others will be assigned as technical specialists.

Units The organizational element having functional responsibility for a specific incident planning, logistics, or finance/administration activity.

Unity of command An incident command system principle stating that each individual involved in incident operations will be assigned to only one supervisor.

Universal Transverse Mercator (UTM) Navigation grid system used worldwide.

V

Visual cues Visible indications that something does not belong and may be part of a track (sign). There are five common visual cues: outline, shape, contrast, color, and texture.

W

Waddling gait A duck-like walk where the lateral distance between footfalls can be larger than a normal gait.

Waterproof and breathable Material that is nearly impermeable to water droplets (waterproof) and yet allows water vapor to pass (breathable).

Waterproof Material that is impermeable to water, even water under pressure.

Water-repellent Sheds water that is not under pressure; however, falling or wind-blown rain may penetrate the fabric.

Water-resistant The material temporarily resists water under pressure.

Waypoint Set of coordinates that identifies a point in physical space.

Wilderness An uninhabited region devoid of any synthetic amenities.

Index

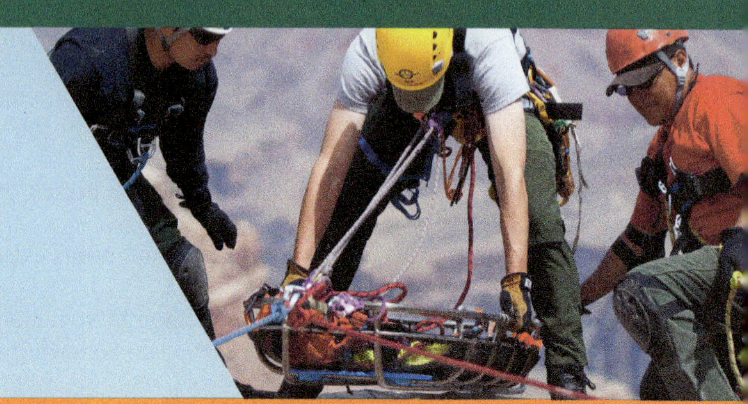

Note: Page numbers followed by *f*, or *t* indicate material in figures, or tables, respectively.

D

E

F

G

J

K

L

Q

R

V

W

Z